MEDICAL
ETHICS

MEDICAL ETHICS

Applying Theories

and

Principles

to the

Patient Encounter

edited by

Matt Weinberg, M.B.

with a foreword by
Arthur Caplan, Ph.D.

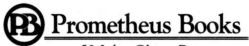

Prometheus Books

59 John Glenn Drive
Amherst, New York 14228-2197

Published 2001 by Prometheus Books

Medical Ethics: Applying Theories and Principles to the Patient Encounter. Copyright © 2001 by Matt Weinberg. All rights reserved. No part of this publication may be reproduced, stored in a retrieval system, or transmitted in any form or by any means, digital, electronic, mechanical, photocopying, recording, or otherwise, or conveyed via the Internet or a Web site without prior written permission of the publisher, except in the case of brief quotations embodied in critical articles and reviews.

Inquiries should be addressed to
Prometheus Books
59 John Glenn Drive
Amherst, New York 14228–2197
VOICE: 716–691–0133, ext. 207
FAX: 716–564–2711
WWW.PROMETHEUSBOOKS.COM

04 03 02 01 00   5 4 3 2 1

Library of Congress Cataloging-in-Publication Data

Medical ethics : applying theories and principles to the patient encounter / edited by Matt Weinberg ; foreword by Arthur Caplan.
    p. cm.
  Includes bibliographical references.
  ISBN 1–57392–652–3 (pbk. : alk. paper)
  1. Medical ethics–Study and teaching–United States. 2. Medical ethics–United States–Examinations, questions, etc. 3. Correspondence schools and courses–United States. I. Weinberg, Matt.

R724 .M2935 2000
174'.2–dc21   00–040658

Printed in the United States of America on acid-free paper

For my dad, from a loving and grateful son.
Jeffrey Jay Weinberg
January 10, 1942–February 22, 1997

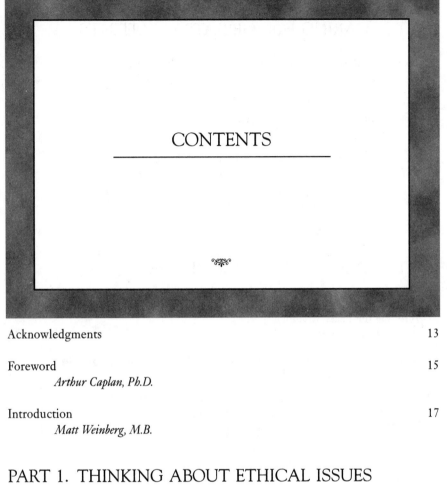

CONTENTS

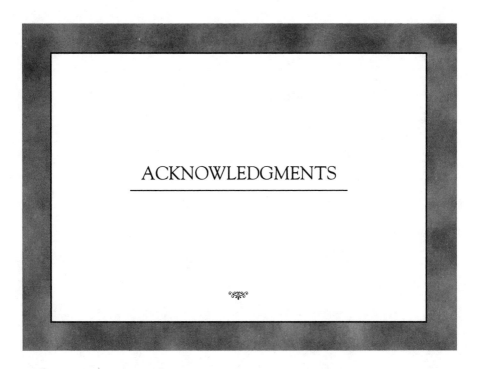

ACKNOWLEDGMENTS

A s this book is an edited anthology both my colleagues and friends were spared the burden of reviewing draft upon draft; however, I still owe many debts. To my teachers, who provided me with the intellectual foundation that allowed me to conceive of this book: Arthur Caplan, Glenn McGee, David Magnus, Paul Wolpe, Arnold Rosoff, Nancy Dubler, and Cliff Anderson. To my friends and family for their unending encouragement: Marlene Weinberg, Ameen Nassiri, Constantine Marinakos, Tim Kirk, Sefi Knoble, and Fr. W. D. Peckenpaugh. And to my best friend and wife, Michelle Weinberg, who is everything.

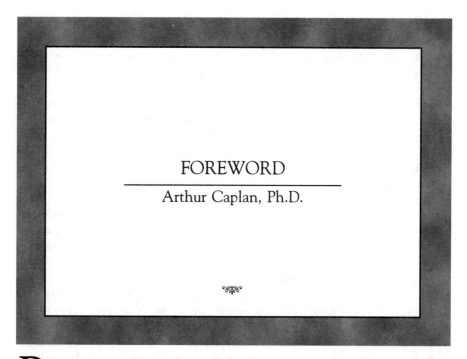

FOREWORD

Arthur Caplan, Ph.D.

Physicians, nurses, social workers, and the other health-care providers who work in hospitals, hospices, and nursing homes struggle almost daily with deeply personal ethical issues. On some occasions it is obvious that the issue at hand is an ethical one—whether to enroll a child dying of cancer in a trial studying the toxic effects of a drug when the child cannot consent, or wrestling with the question of what to do when an elderly, demented patient has no family or friends to guide crucial medical decisions. More often, however, the ethical issue is subtle. Sometimes it is classified simply as a problem of "staffing" or "resources"; say, when assigning fewer ICU nurses to the night shift. At other times what is clearly ethical—what to do with a patient who is noncompliant—is treated as a psychological or legal matter. The identification and classification of ethical issues is the single most important step in analyzing moral quandaries in health care.

What makes the obvious issues harder to address, and the subtler issues harder to recognize, is that those who must struggle with them are rarely afforded the opportunity to gain formal instruction in medical ethics. It is this educational void that gave rise to this anthology. Matt Weinberg has thoughtfully edited this book with the goal of helping health-care providers and ethics committee members recognize and address many of the everyday ethical issues and concerns they confront. He has provided those facing both the tough and the not-so-tough moral challenges of medicine a most useful tool—whatever side of the bed they may find themselves on.

Ironically, while we have become sophisticated enough to put a human liver on a plane for two hours and then reimplant it, and to correct deformities in a fetus through in utero surgery, it is not the issues these technologies raise that cause the most problems. It is the relationships among health-care providers themselves and the relationships between health-care providers, patients, and families that without fail brings about the most fodder for those concerned with medical ethics. Weinberg appreciates this irony and has chosen numerous readings that address it head on. Included are articles on the health-care provider–proxy relationship, the nurse's role in a parent's decision-making process for her critically sick newborn, and how to help the family of an Alzheimer's patient adjust to the "loss" of their loved one.

To give readers a language for talking about these and other issues, the anthology's first section looks at the various ethical theories that are widely invoked in the medical ethics literature. This section begins with a discussion of what it means for a choice, or a person, to be right or wrong, good or bad. From this the reader will develop an understanding of what it means for a health-care provider to have a duty or obligation, as well as what it means to allocate a scarce resource fairly. The next reading explores the central concept of patient autonomy in an unusual but effective way. This selection makes us ask the rarely asked question of how cultural beliefs shape a patient's expression of his or her autonomy. Weinberg concludes his first section with an article that considers how health-care providers can respond to patients whose culturally based values fundamentally conflict with their own.

From there the book goes on to address geriatric issues, end-of-life care, consent, pain management and palliative care, the art of medicine, health law, AIDS, pediatric issues, organ transplantation, managed care, allocation of resources, organizational ethics, genetic testing, clinical integrity, and professionalism. The reader will find recent empirical studies, court decisions, and federal regulations to help ground the more philosophical analysis.

Overall, the ideas and issues raised in this anthology will greatly benefit health-care providers who want to gain a more sophisticated understanding of the issues they face in order to be better prepared to address them. Agreement may not always be possible in ethics as to what answer is best, but this anthology goes a long way toward making it possible for the reader to agree on why ethical problems at the bedside are so vexing.

Arthur Caplan, Ph.D.
Center for Bioethics
University of Pennsylvania

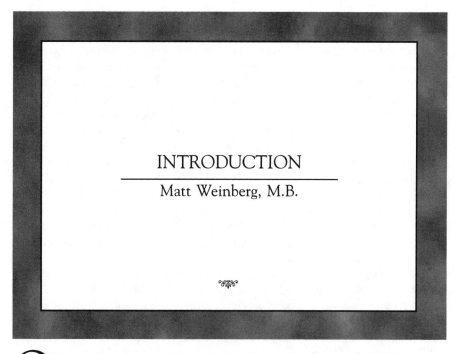

INTRODUCTION

Matt Weinberg, M.B.

Over the past few years it has become a common occurrence for the nightly news to excitedly report on yet another cutting-edge medical breakthrough. I think most of us would be hard pressed to recall a week when the media did not report on a discovery or development that was going to revolutionize how a certain disease would be tested or treated. Gene therapy, bioengineering, human cloning, and stem cell research are all examples of the "breaking news" attitude that seems to characterize modern health care.

Following such media announcements are the exclusive interviews, Op-Ed pieces, and scholarly articles, along with the occasional congressional hearing, presidential moratorium, and report by the National Bioethics Advisory Commission. Yet for all the hoopla these and other "breakthroughs" muster, the issues they raise and consequences they entail are, for most health-care providers and ethics committee members, neither relevant nor informative. It is ironically the mundane issues that the media tend to eschew, such as how health-care providers and patients can form trusting relationships, that health-care providers and ethics committee members *need* to see addressed. While ethical issues of this sort are not discussed on *Larry King Live* or *60 Minutes*, they are fortunately starting to be discussed where they should be—at the patient's bedside, at the nurse's station, in the back of paramedic units, at morning rounds, and in ethics committee meetings. It is these discussions for which this anthology was borne, as health-care providers and ethics committee members struggle daily with deeply personal ethical issues—with little help from lofty commissions or high-minded journal articles.

To be of any use to health-care providers and ethics committee members, an introductory anthology on medical ethics must appreciate the world in which they work. My graduate school advisor, Glenn McGee, made this point abundantly clear several years ago at a conference on managed care. While participating on a panel discussion he was asked to prove his claim that patients have actually been harmed by capitation. He responded: "I am a philosopher, I don't need no stinking data." Glenn's point was not lost on anyone. Without an understanding of the actual context in which ethical issues arise, principles, theories, and maxims have little to offer in the way of addressing or resolving ethical issues in health care. To that end, the following readings were chosen because they provide theoretical, empirical, and practical foundations for thinking about everyday ethical issues faced by health-care providers and ethics committee members, for example, withdrawing life-sustaining treatment, restraining patients with dementia, helping surrogates make difficult decisions, pain management issues, and the like.

The readings that fall under the guise of *theoretical* provide the intellectual tools needed to consider, discuss, and apply our values and beliefs to health care. Those readings considered *empirical* use surveys and interviews to take account of, for example, how a patient's culture can influence how she expresses her autonomy. And those readings conceived of as *practical* use a case study approach in order to draw out the issues and provide the reader with suggestions as to how ethical concerns can be addressed and resolved. With these three approaches in mind, this anthology consists of forty-one readings divided into sixteen sections. Of these readings, six are recent empirical studies, two are full-text court decisions, and two are federal regulations.

As this anthology originally began as a training manual for hospital ethics committees, it was developed with the notion that time is by far a health-care provider's and ethics committee member's most scarce resource. To account for this, each section can stand on its own, so long as the opening section on ethical theory is attended to first. Therefore, when confronted with a concern or conflict, the reader can turn to the relevant section in order to gain insight into the issue at hand. Ideally, the readings will provide clarity and understanding to what may be an extremely complex, confusing, and emotionally charged situation.

By working through this anthology, health-care providers and ethics committee members will gain a solid foundation for thinking about the everyday ethical issues they face. This anthology, however, is only a starting point; learning how to apply theories and principles to the patient encounter is a lifelong endeavor.

Part 1
THINKING ABOUT ETHICAL ISSUES IN HEALTH CARE

I t seems reasonable to begin this anthology with a section on the dominant theories and principles of medical ethics. As there are thousands of articles on this topic, I decided to narrow the field by using two requirements. First, the articles would have to provide a basic framework for thinking and talking about ethical issues in health care. Second, they could not be boring; I have never seen health-care providers or ethics committee members become more uninterested than when the words "ethical" and "theory" are put together. Finding readings that met both of these requirements took a good deal of searching. The articles that I ultimately selected not only meet these requirements, but they do so in such a way as to help us gain some insight into why people make the health-care decisions they do.

When reading the first piece, "A Pluralistic Approach to Moral Issues," by Lawrence Hinman, it is important to appreciate that he is only trying to give the reader a brief sketch. As such, I strongly encourage additional reading in order to gain a broader understanding of the theories he presents.

An example of ethical theory's relevance to our daily lives can be found in the daily newspaper, quite literally. A group of people recently volunteered to be subjects in a research trial that was testing an experimental Lyme disease vaccine. Many of those who volunteered did so because they lived in a wooded area. Importantly, even though they enrolled hoping to help themselves, enrolling was still a sacrifice as the vaccine was unproven and the side effects unknown. With knowledge of this risk, they enrolled with the hope that the burdens they endured would ultimately benefit many people, including themselves. In this way, the volunteers were trying to increase happiness (by being protected from Lyme disease) for the greatest number of people, by risking unhappiness to a small number of people (themselves). Without realizing it, volunteers in such circumstances are apllying John Stuart Mill's philosophy of utilitarianism.

Another example of how we use ethical theory every day is when we talk about the health-care providers who have cared for us. We usually use such terms as compassionate, caring, understanding, and kind. Unfortunately we sometimes also use terms such as mean, uncaring, and arrogant. When we use these terms—and we all have—we are talking about virtue. Virtue ethics is a very old ethical theory and one that we use throughout our lives. Without thinking about what it means to be a good person, how would we decide who we are going to be friends with or who we are going to marry?

The next two articles will help us to see how the theoretical framework Hinman provided us with plays out in the real world of patients, families, and health-care providers.

"Ethnicity and Attitudes Toward Patient Autonomy," a study by Leslie Blackhall and colleagues, looks at two hundred adults, aged sixty-five and older, who fall into one of four ethnic categories: (1) Korean American, (2) Mexican American, (3) European American, or (4) African American. Blackhall and her colleagues try to understand how different groups of patients might go about making a medical decision. More specifically, they want to see what role ethnicity plays in the decision-making process, particularly when those decisions concern care at the end of life.

They found that European and African Americans tend to hold a patient-centered decision-making process, whereas Mexican and Korean Americans tend to prefer a family-centered decision-making process. These results draw out two very important points. First, as Hinman discussed, we ought to respect a patient's right to decide not only what treatments he does or does not want, but how he wants to go about making his decision. Second, health-care providers need to ask their patients how they want to express their autonomy.

This study provides a wonderful, nonthreatening opening for such a discussion, as physicians can say to their patients: "I just read a study that looked at how some people prefer to make their health-care decisions. Some wanted their families to make their decisions for them, and others wanted to make their own decisions. I have also had patients who have made their decisions with the help of their families. How do you want to make important health-care decisions? Do you prefer one of these methods, or is there some other way you would prefer to make decisions?"

The final article in this section is titled "Ethical Relativism in a Multicultural Society." Ruth Macklin takes the issues Blackhall raises and discusses the various decision-making preferences and how they can, at times, fundamentally conflict with a health-care provider's sense of professional ethics.

Macklin appreciates the position health-care providers are in when a patient, or a patient's parent, chooses a course of action that is grounded in what the provider sees as an irrational belief that may actually harm the patient if carried out. Examples of requests that have caused conflict include female genital mutilation, the withholding of a cancer diagnosis from patient, and the use of mercury in healing rituals. There are countless other examples of culturally derived treatments that are harmful and can exacerbate a patient's illness by delaying appropriate medical care. An example that I have seen numerous times is "coining." Coining is a technique that is used to cure illness, usually in children, by continually rubbing a coin up and down a child's back until large welts appear. Sometimes the welts bleed and/or become severely infected. Another example I encountered was a request for a treatment that the patient knew would not work, but which he wanted anyway because the treatment would cause him to suffer. Suffering, he and his wife believed, would bring him closer to God and salvation.

It is important to remember that even though some requests may seem strange or even silly, that does not in and of itself make such requests harmful or inappropriate. And I cannot emphasize this enough: If a practice does actually harm a patient, as with the children who were "coined," it does not necessarily mean the parents are guilty of child abuse or of being bad parents. My goals for including this piece were threefold: first, to help health-care providers and ethics committees understand why patients and families make such requests; second, to help health-care providers think about how they might respond to such requests; and finally, to give flesh to the ideas that Hinman raises, such as moral relativism and moral pluralism.

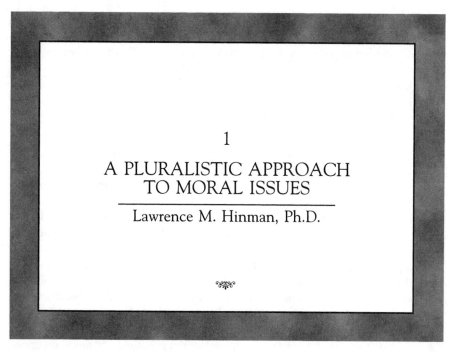

1

A PLURALISTIC APPROACH
TO MORAL ISSUES

Lawrence M. Hinman, Ph.D.

MORAL DISAGREEMENT

The Apparent Prevalence of Moral Disagreement

As we move through the chapters of tills book, we will see one area of moral disagreement after another. Abortion, surrogacy, euthanasia, the death penalty, racism, sexism, homosexuality, welfare, world hunger, animal rights, and environmental issues—all are areas characterized by fundamental disagreements that are often intense, sometimes bitter and acrimonious.

This situation is made even more perplexing by the fact that in all of these debates, each side has good arguments in support of its position. In other words, these are not debates in which one side is so obviously wrong that only moral blindness or ill will could account for its position. Thus we cannot easily dismiss such disagreements by just saying that one side is wrong in some irrational or malevolent way. Ultimately, these are disagreements among intelligent people of good will. And *it is precisely this fact that makes them so disturbing.* Certainly part of moral disagreement can be attributed to ignorance or ill will, but the troubling part is the moral disagreement among informed and benevolent people.

Contemporary Moral Issues: Diversity and Consensus 2/E by Hinman, Lawrence M., ©1995. Reprinted by permission of Prentice-Hall, Inc., Upper Saddle River, NJ.

What kind of sense can we make of such disagreement? Three possible responses deserve particular attention.

Moral Absolutism

The first, and perhaps most common, response to such disagreements is to claim that there is a single, ultimate answer to the questions being posed. This is the answer of the moral absolutists, those who believe there is a single Truth with a capital *T*. Usually, absolutists claim to know what that truth is—and it usually corresponds, not surprisingly, to their own position.

Moral absolutists are not confined to a I single position. on. Indeed, absolutism is best understood as much as a way of *holding* certain beliefs as it is an item of such belief. Religious fundamentalists—whether Christian, Muslim, or some other denomination—are usually absolutists. Some absolutists believe in others believe just as absolutely in free-market economics. Some moral philosophers are absolutists, believing that their moral viewpoint is the only legitimate one. But what characterizes all absolutists is the conviction that their truth is *the* truth.

Moral absolutists may be right, but there are good reasons to be skeptical about their claim. If they are right, how do they explain the persistence of moral disagreement? Certainly there are disagreements and disputes in other areas (including the natural sciences), but in ethics there seems to be a persistence to these disputes that we usually do not find in other areas. It is hard to explain this from an absolutist standpoint without saying such is due to ignorance or ill will.

Certainly this is part of the story, but can it account for all moral disagreement? Absolutists are unable to make sense out of the fact that sometimes we have genuine moral disagreements among well-informed and good-intentioned people who an honestly and openly seeking the truth.

Moral Relativism

The other common response to such disagreement effectively denies that there is a truth in this area, even with a lowercase *t*. *Moral relativists* maintain that moral disagreements stein from the fact that what is right for one is not necessarily right for another. Morality is like beauty, they claim, purely relative to the beholder. There is no ultimate standard in terms of which perspectives can be judged. No one is wrong; everyone is right within his or her own sphere.

Notice that these relativists do more than simply acknowledge the existence of moral disagreement. just to admit that moral disagreement exists is called *descriptive relativism*, and this is a comparatively uncontroversial claim. There is plenty of disagreement in the moral realm, just as there is in most other areas of life. However, *normative relativists* go further. They not only maintain that such disagreement exists; they also say that each is right relative to his or her own culture. Incidentally, it is also worth noting that relativists disagree about precisely what morality is relative *to*. At the one end of the spectrum are those (*cultural moral relativists*) who say that morality is relative to culture; at the other end of the spectrum are those (*moral subjectivists*) who argue that morality is relative to each individual. When we refer to moral relativists here, we will be talking about normative relativists, including both cultural moral relativists and moral subjectivists.

Although moral relativism often appears appealing at first glance, it proves to be singularly unhelpful in the long run. It provides an explanation of moral disagreement, but it fails to provide a convincing account of how moral *agreement* could be forged. In the face of disagreement, what practical advice can relativists offer us? All they can say, it would seem, is that we ought to follow the customs of our society, our culture, our age, or our individual experience. Thus cultural moral relativists tell us, in effect, "When in Rome, do as the Romans do." Moral subjectivists tell us that we should be true not to our culture, but to our individual selves. But relativists fall to offer us help in how to resolve disputes when they arise. To say that each is right unto itself is of no help, for the issue is what happens when they come together.

While this might have been helpful advice in an age of moral isolationism when each society (or individual) was an island unto itself, it is of little help today. In our contemporary world, the pressing moral question is how we can live together, not how we can live apart. Economies are mutually interdependent; corporations are often multinational; products such as cars are seldom made in a single country. Communications increasingly cut across national borders. Satellite-based telecommunication systems allow international television (MTV is worldwide, and news networks are sure to follow) and international telephone communications. Millions of individuals around the world dial into the Internet, establishing a virtual community. In such a world, relativism fails to provide guidance for resolving disagreements. All it can tell us is that everyone is right in their own world. But the question for the future is how to determine what is right when those worlds overlap.

Moral Pluralism

Let's return to our problem: In some moral disputes, there seem to be well-informed and good-intentioned people on opposing sides. Absolutism falls to offer a convincing account of how opposing people could be both well-informed and good-intentioned. It says there is only one answer, and those who do not see it are either ignorant or ill-willed. Relativism fails to offer a convincing account of how people can agree. It says no one is wrong, that each culture (or individual) is right unto itself. However, it offers no help about how to resolve these moral disputes.

There is a third possible response here, which I will call *moral pluralism*. Moral pluralists maintain that then am moral truths, but they do not form a body of coherent and consistent truths in the way that one finds in the sciences or mathematics. Moral truths are real, but partial. Moreover, they am inescapably *plural*. There are many moral truths, not just one—and they may conflict with one another.

Let me borrow an analogy from government. Moral absolutists are analogous to old fashioned monarchists: There is one leader, and he or she has the absolute truth. Moral relativists are closer to anarchists: Each person or group has its own truth. The U.S. government is an interesting example of a tripartite pluralist government. We don't think that the president, the Congress, or the judiciary alone has an exclusive claim to truth. Each has a partial claim, and each provides a check on the other two. We don't—at least not always—view conflict among the three branches as a bad thing. Indeed, such a system of overlapping and at times conflicting responsibilities is a way of hedging our bets. If we put all of our hope in only one of the branches of government, we would be putting ourselves at greater risk. If that one branch is wrong, then everything is wrong. However, if there are three (at least partially conflicting) branches of government then the effect of one branch's being wrong are far less catastrophic. Moreover, the chance that mistakes will be uncovered earlier is certainly increased when each branch is being scrutinized by the others.

We have an analogous situation in the moral domain. As we shall see, there are conflicting theories about goodness and rightness. Such conflict is a good thing. Each theory contains important truths about the moral life, and none of them contains the whole truth. Each keeps the others honest, as it were, curbing the excesses of any particular moral absolutism. Yet each claims to have the truth, and refuses the relativist's injunction to avoid making judgments about others. Judgment—both making judgments and being judged—is crucial to the moral life, just as it is to the political life. We have differing moral perspectives, but we must often inhabit a common world.

It is precisely this tension between individual viewpoints and living in a common world that lies at the heart of this book. The diversity of viewpoints is not intended to create a written version of those television news shows where people constantly shout at one another. Rather, these selections indicate the range of important and legitimate insights with which we approach the issue in question. The challenge, then, is for us—as individuals, and as a society-to forge a common ground that acknowledges the legitimacy of the conflicting insights but also establishes a minimal area of agreement so that we can live together with our differences. The model this book strives to emulate is not the one-sided monarch who claims to have the absolute truth, nor is it the anarchistic society that contains no basis for consensus. Rather, it is the model of a healthy democracy in which diversity, disagreement, compromise, and consensus are signs of vitality.

A Pluralistic Approach to Moral Theories

Just as in the political realm there are political parties and movements that delineate the contours of the political debate so also in philosophy there are moral theories that provide characteristic ways of understanding and resolving particular moral issues. In the readings throughout this book, we will see a number of examples of these theories in action. Before we examine these theories, it is helpful to look at some of the main characteristics of each of these theories. just as Republicans and Democrats, liberals and conservatives, and libertarians and socialists all have important, and often conflicting, insights about the political life, so, too, does each of these theories have valuable insights into the moral life. Yet none of them has the whole story. Let's look briefly at each of

MORALITY AS CONSEQUENCES

What makes an action morally good? For many of us, what counts are consequences. The right action is the one that produces good consequences. If I give money to Oxfam to help starving people, and if Oxfam saves the lives of starving people and helps them develop a self-sustaining economy, then I have done something good. It is good because it produced good consequences. For this reason, it is the right thing to do. Those who subscribe to this position are called *consequentialists*. All consequentialists share a common belief that it is consequences that make an action good, but they differ among themselves about precisely which consequences.

Ethical Egoism

Some consequentialists, called *ethical egoists* maintain that each of us should look only at the consequences that affect us. In their eyes, each person ought to perform those actions that contribute most to his or her own self-interest. Each person is the best judge of his or her own self-interest, and each person is responsible for maximizing his or her own self-interest. The political expression of ethical egoism occurs most clearly in libertarianism, and the best-known advocate of this position was probably Ayn Rand.

Ethical egoism has been criticized on a number of counts, most notably that it simply draws the circle of morality much too closely around the isolated individual. Critics maintain that self-interest is precisely what morality has to overcome, not what it should espouse. Egoism preaches selfishness, but morality should encourage altruism, compassion, love, and a sense of community—all, according to critics, beyond the reach of the egoist.

Utilitarianism

Once we begin to enlarge the circle of those affected by the consequences of our actions, we move toward a utilitarian position. At its core, *utilitarianism* represents the belief that one ought to do what produces the greatest overall good for *everyone*, not just for oneself. One determines what to do by examining the various courses of action open to us, calculating the consequences associated with each, and then deciding on the one that produces the consequences that provide the greatest overall good for everyone. Utilitarianism is consequentialist and computational. It holds out the promise that moral disputes can be resolved objectively by computing consequences. Part of the attraction of utilitarianism is precisely this claim to objectivity based on a moral calculus.

This is a very demanding moral doctrine for two reasons. First, it asks people to set aside their own individual interests for the good of the whole. Often this can result in great individual sacrifice, if taken seriously. For example, the presence of hunger and starvation in our society (as well as outside of it) places great demands on the utilitarian, for often more good would be accomplished by giving food to the hungry than by eating it oneself. Second, utilitarianism asks us to do whatever produces the *most* good. Far from being a doctrine of the moral minimum, utilitarianism always asks us to do the maximum.

Utilitarians disagree among themselves about what the proper standard is for judging consequences. What are "good" consequences? Are they the ones that produce the most *pleasure*? The most *happiness*? The most truth, beauty, and the like? Or, simply the consequences that satisfy the most people? Each of these standards of utility has its strengths and weaknesses. Jeremy Bentham originally proposed pleasure as the standard of utility. *Pleasure* is comparatively easy to measure, but in many people's eyes it seems to be a rather base standard. Can't we increase pleasure just by putting electrodes in the proper location in a person's brain? Presumably we want something more, and better, than that. John Stuart Mill criticized Bentham's standard of pleasure and argued that happiness should be the standard of utility. *Happiness* seems a more plausible candidate, but the difficulty with happiness is that it is both elusive to define and extremely difficult to measure. This is particularly a problem for utilitarianism, since its initial appeal rests in part on its claim to objectivity. *Ideals* such as truth and beauty are even more difficult to measure. *Preference satisfaction* is more measurable, but it provides no foundation for distinguishing between morally acceptable preferences and morally objectionable preferences such as racism.

The other principal disagreement that has plagued utilitarianism centers around the question of whether we look at the consequences of each individual act—this is called *act utilitarianism*—or the consequences that would result from everyone following a particular rule—this is called *rule utilitarianism*. The danger of act utilitarianism is that it may justify some particular acts that most of us would want to condemn, particularly those that sacrifice individual life and liberty for the sake of the whole. This classic problem occurs in regard to punishment. We could imagine a situation in which punishing an innocent person—while concealing his innocence, of course—would have consequences that imparted the greatest overall good. If doing so would result in the greatest overall amount of pleasure or happiness, then it would not only be permitted by act utilitarianism, it would be morally required. Similar difficulties arise in regard to an issue such as euthanasia. It is conceivable that overall utility might justify active euthanasia of the elderly and infirm, even involuntary euthanasia, especially of those who leave no one behind to mourn their passing. Yet are there things we cannot do to people, even if utility seems to require it? Many of us would answer such a question affirmatively.

In response to such difficulties, utilitarian theorists pointed out that, while consequences may justify a particular act of punishing the innocent, they could never justify living by a *rule* that said it was permissible to punish the innocent when doing so would produce the greatest utility. Rule utilitarians agree that we should look only at consequences, but maintain that we should look at the consequences of adopting a particular rule for everyone, not the consequences of each individual action. This type of utilitarianism is less likely to generate the injustices associated with act utilitarianism, but many feel that it turns into rule worship. Why, critics ask, should we follow the rule in those instances where it does not produce the greatest utility?

Feminist Consequentialism

During the last twenty years, much interesting and valuable work has been done in the area of feminist ethics. It would be misleading to think of feminist approaches to ethics as falling into a single camp, but certainly some feminist moral philosophers have sketched out accounts of the moral life in at least two different ways.

First, some feminists have argued that morality is a matter of consequences but that consequences are not best understood or evaluated in the traditional model offered by utilitarianism. Instead, they focus primarily on the ways in which particular actions have consequences for relationships and feelings. Negative consequences are those that destroy relationships and that hurt others, especially those that hurt others emotionally. Within this tradition, the morally good course of action is that one that preserves the greatest degree of connectedness among all those affected by it. Carol Gilligan has described this moral voice in her book *In a Different Voice.*

Second, other feminists have accepted a roughly utilitarian account of consequences but have paid particular attention to—and often given special weight to—the consequences that affect women. Such consequences, they argue, have often been overlooked by traditional utilitarian calculators, supposedly impartial but often insensitive to harms to women. Unlike the work of Gilligan and others mentioned In the previous paragraph, feminists in this tradition do not question the dominant utilitarian paradigm, but rather question whether it has in fact been applied impartially.

Conclusion

Despite these disagreements about the precise formulation of utilitarianism, most people would admit that utilitarianism contains important insights. into the moral life. Part of the justification for morality, and one of the reasons people accept the" burdens of morality, is that it promises to produce a better world than we would have without it. This is undoubtedly part of the picture. But is it the whole picture?

MORALITY AS ACT AND INTENTION

Critics of utilitarianism point out that, for utilitarianism, no actions are good or bad in themselves. All actions in themselves are morally neutral, and, for pure consequentialists, no action is intrinsically evil. Yet this seems to contradict the moral intuition of many people—people who believe that some actions are just morally wrong, even if they have good results. Killing innocent human beings, torturing people, raping them—these are but a few of the actions that many would want to condemn as wrong in themselves, even if in unusual circumstances they may produce good consequences.

How can we tell if some actions are morally good or bad in themselves? Clearly, we must have some standard against which they can be judged. Various standards have been proposed, and most of these again capture important truths about the moral life.

Conforming to God's Commands

In a number of religious traditions, including some branches of Judaism, Christianity, and Islam, what makes an act right is that it is commanded by God and what makes an act wrong is that it is forbidden by God. In these traditions, certain kinds of acts are wrong just because God forbids them. Usually such prohibitions are contained in sacred texts such as the Bible or the Koran.

There are two principal difficulties with this approach, one external, one internal. The external problem is that, while this may provide a good reason for believers to act in particular ways, it hardly gives a persuasive case to nonbelievers. The internal difficulty is that it is often difficult, even with the best of intentions, to discern what God's commands actually are. Sacred texts, for example, contain numerous injunctions, but it is rare that any religious tradition takes *all* of them seriously. (The Bible tells believers to pick up venomous vipers, but only a handful of Christians engage in this practice.) How do we decide which injunctions to take seriously and which to ignore or interpret metaphorically?

Natural Law

There is a long tradition, beginning with Aristotle and gaining great popularity in the Middle Ages, that maintains that acts which are "unnatural" are always evil. The underlying premise of this view is that the natural is good, and, therefore, what contradicts it is bad. Often, especially in the Middle Ages, this was part of a larger Christian worldview that saw nature as created by God, who then was the ultimate source of its goodness. Yet it has certainly survived in twentieth-century moral and legal philosophy quite apart from its theological underpinnings. This appeal to natural law occurs at a number of junctures in our readings, but especially in the discussions of reproductive technologies and those of homosexuality. Natural law arguments lead quite easily into considerations of human nature, again with the implicit claim that human nature is good.

Natural law arguments tend to be slippery for two closely interrelated reasons. First, for natural law arguments to work, one has to provide convincing support for the claim that the natural is (the only) good-or at least for its contrapositive, the claim that the "unnatural" is bad. Second, such arguments presuppose that we can clearly differentiate between the natural and the unnatural. Are floods and earthquakes natural? Is disease natural? Either the natural is not always good, or else we have to adopt a very selective notion of the "natural."

Proper Intention

A second way in which acts can be said to be good or bad is that they are done for the proper motivation, with the correct intention. Indeed, intentions are often built into our vocabulary for describing actions. The difference between stabbing a person and performing surgery on that person may well reside primarily in the intention of the agent.

Acting for the sake of duty

Again, there is no shortage of candidates for morally acceptable intentions. A sense of duty, universalizability, a respect for other persons, sincerity or authenticity, care compassion—these are but a few of the acceptable moral motivations. Consider, first of all, the motive of duty. Immanuel Kant argued that what gives an action moral worth is that it is done for the sake of duty. In his eyes, the morally admirable person is the one who, despite inclinations to the contrary, does the right thing solely because it is the right thing to do. The person who contributes to charities out of a sense of duty is morally far superior to the person who does the samething in order to look good in the eyes of others, despite the fact that the consequences may be the same in both cases.

Universalizability

Yet how do we know what our duty is? Kant wanted to avoid saying duty was simply a matter of "following orders." Instead he saw duty as emanating from the nature of reason itself. And because reason is universal, duty is also universal. Kant suggested an important test whether our understanding of duty was rational in any particular instance. We always act, he maintained, with a subjective rule or maxim that guides our decision. Is this maxim one that we can will that everyone accept, or is it one that falls this test of universalizability?

Consider cheating. If you cheat on an exam, it's like lying: You are saying something is your work when it is not. Imagine you cheat on all the exams in a course and finish with an average of 98 percent. The professor then gives you a grade of *D*. You storm into the professor's office, demanding an explanation. The professor calmly says, "Oh, I lied on the grade sheet." Your natural reply would be: "But you can't lie about my grade!" Kant's point is that, by cheating, you've denied the validity of your own claim. You've implicitly said that it is morally all right for people to lie. But of course you don't believe it's permissible for your professor to lie—only for you yourself to do so. This, Kant says, fails the test of universalizability.

Notice that Kant's argument isn't a consequentialist one. He's not asking what would happen to society if everyone lied. Rather, he's saying that certain maxims are inconsistent and thus irrational. You cannot approve of your own lying without approving of everyone else's, and yet the advantage you get depends precisely on other people's honesty. It is the irrationality of making an exception of my own lying in this way that Kant feels violates the moral law. Indeed, we should all examine our own past actions to see where we may have made an exception for ourselves that we know (at least in retrospect) isn't morally justified.

Kant has captured something valuable about the moral life: the insight that what's fair for one is fair for all. Yet Kant's critics were quick to point out that this can hardly be the entire story. Consequences count, and intentions are notoriously slippery. A given act can be described with many different intentions—to cheat on a test, to try to excel, to try to meet your parents' expectations, to be the first in the class—and not all of them necessarily fall the test of universalizability.

Respect for other persons

Kant offered another formulation of his basic moral insight, one that touches a responsive chord in many of us. We should never treat people merely as things, Kant argued. Rather, we should always respect them as autonomous (i.e., self-directing) moral agents. Both capitalism and technology pressure us to treat people merely as things, and many have found Kant's refusal to do this to be of crucial moral importance.

It is easy to find examples at both ends of this spectrum. We use people merely as things when we do not let them make their own decisions and when we harm them for our own benefit without respect for their rights. Consider the now infamous Tuskegee experiment, in which medical researchers tracked the development of syphilis in a group of African American men for over thirty years, never telling them the precise nature of their malady and never treating them—something that would have been both inexpensive and effective. Instead, the researchers let the disease proceed through its ultimately fatal course in order to observe more closely the details of its progress. These men were used merely as means to the researchers' ends

Similarly, we have all—I hope—experienced being treated as ends in ourselves. If I am ill, and my physician gives me the details of my medical condition, outlines the available options for treatment (including nontreatment), and is supportive of whatever choice I finally make in this matter, then I feel as though I have been treated with respect.

The difficulty with this criterion is that there is a large middle ground where it is unclear if acting in a particular way is really using other people merely as things. Indeed, insofar as our economic system is based on the exchange of currency for commodities, we can be assured that this will be a common phenomenon in our society. To what extent is respect for persons attainable in a capitalist and technological society?

Compassion and caring

Some philosophers—particularly, but not exclusively, feminist—have urged the moral importance of acting out of motives of care and compassion. Many of these philosophers have argued that caring about other persons is the heart of the moral life, and that a morality of care leads to a refreshingly new picture of morality as centering on relationships, feelings, and connectedness rather than on impartiality, justice, and fairness. In a moral dispute, the justice-oriented person will determine the fair thing to do, and then proceed to follow that course of action, no matter what effect that has on others. The care-oriented individual, on the other hand, will try to find the course of action that best preserves the interests of all involved and does the least amount of damage to the relationships involved.

Many in this tradition have seen the justice orientation as characteristically male and the care orientation as typically female. (Notice that this is not the same as claiming that these orientations are exclusively male or female.) Critics have argued that such correlations are simplistic and misleading. Both orientations may be present to some degree in almost everyone, and particular types of situations may be responsible for bringing one or the other to the fore.

Respect for Rights

Kant, as we have just seen, told us that we ought to respect other persons. Yet what specific aspects of other persons ought we to respect? One answer, which has played a major political as well as philosophical role during the past two centuries, has been framed in terms of human rights. The Bill of Rights was the first set of amendments to the U.S. Constitution. At approximately the same time, the French were drafting the *Declaration of the Rights of Man and Citizen*. Concern for human rights has continued well into the twentieth century, and the last forty years in the United States have been marked by an intense concern with rights—the civil rights movement for racial equality, the equal rights movement for women, the animal rights movement, the gay rights movement, and the movement for equal rights for Americans with disabilities. Throughout the selections in this book, we will see continual appeals to rights, debates about the extent and even the existence of rights, and attempts to adjudicate conflicts of rights.

Rights provide the final criterion to be considered here for evaluating acts. Those acts that violate basic human rights are morally wrong, this tradition suggests. Torture, imprisoning, and executing the innocent, denial of the right to vote, denial of process—these are all instances of actions that violate human rights. (The fact that an act does not violate basic human rights does not mean that it is morally unobjectionable; there may be other criteria for evaluating it as well as rights.) Human rights, defenders of this tradition maintain, are not subject to nationality, race, religion, class, or any other such limitation. They cannot be set aside for reasons of utility, convenience, or political or financial gain. We possess them simply by virtue of being human beings, and they thus exhibit a universality that provides the foundation for a global human community.

Criticisms of the rights tradition abound. First, how do we determine *which* rights we have? Rights theorists often respond that we have a right to those things—

such as life, freedom, and property—which are necessary to human existence itself. Yet many claim that such necessities are contextual, not universal. Moreover, they maintain that there is something logically suspicious about proceeding from the claim that "I need something" to the claim that "I have a right to it." Needs, these critics argue, do not entail rights. Second, critics have asked whether these rights are *negative rights* (i.e., freedoms from certain kinds of interference) or *positive rights* (i.e., entitlements). This is one of the issues at the core of the welfare debate currently raging in the United States. Do the poor have any positive rights to welfare, or do they only have rights not to be discriminated against in various ways? Finally, some critics have argued that the current focus on rights has obscured other, morally relevant aspects of our lives. Rights establish a a moral minimum for the ways in which we interact with others, especially strangers we do not care about. But when we we dealing with those we know and care about, more may be demanded of us morally than just respecting their rights.

MORALITY AS CHARACTER

It is rare that a philosophy anthology reaches the best-seller lists, and it is even more unusual when that book is a relatively traditional work about character. William Bennett's *The Book of Virtues*, however, has done just that. Staying on the best-seller list for week after week, Bennett's book indicates a resurgence of interest in a long-neglected tradition of ethic: Aristotelian virtue theory.

The Contrast between Act-Oriented Ethics and Character-Oriented Ethics

This Aristotelian approach to ethic, sometimes called *character ethics* or *virtue ethics*, is distinctive. In contrast to the preceding act-oriented approaches, it does not focus on what makes acts right or wrong. Rather, it focuses on people and their moral character. Instead of asking, "What should I do?" those in this tradition ask, "What kind of person should I strive to be?" This gives a very different focus to the moral life.

An analogy with public life may again be helpful. Consider the American judiciary system. We develop an elaborate set of rules through legislation, and these rules are often articulated in excruciating detail. However, when someone is brought to trial, we do not depend solely on the rules to guarantee justice. Ultimately, we place the fate of accused criminals in the hands of people—a judge and jury. As a country, we bet on both rules and people.

A similar situation exists in ethics. We need good rules-and the preceding sections have described some attempts to articulate those rulesbut we also need good people to have the wisdom and good will to interpret and apply those rules. Far from being in conflict with each other, act-oriented and character-oriented approaches to ethics complement one another.

Human Flourishing

The principal questions that character-oriented approaches to ethics pose are the following: What strengths of character (i.e., virtues) promote human flourishing? And, correlatively, what weaknesses of character (i.e., vices) impede human flourishing? *Virtues* are thus those strengths of character that contribute to human flourishing, while *vices* are those weaknesses that get in the way of flourishing.

In order to develop an answer to these questions, the first thing that those in this tradition must do is to articulate a clear notion of human flourishing. Here they depend as much on moral psychology as moral philosophy. Aristotle had a vision of human flourishing, but it was one that was clearly limited to his time—one that excluded women and slaves. In contemporary psychology, we have seen much interesting work describing flourishing in psychological terms—Carl Rogers and Abraham Maslow have made but two of the better-known attempts at describing human flourishing in psychological terms. The articulation of a well-founded and convincing vision of human flourishing remains one of the principal challenges of virtue ethics today.

The Virtue of Courage

We can better understand this approach to ethics if we look at a sample virtue and its corresponding vices. Consider courage. Aristotle analyzes it primarily in military terms, but we now see that it is a virtue necessary to a wide range of human activities—and those who lack courage will rarely flourish. Courage is the strength of character to face and overcome that which we fear. Fears differ from one person to the next, but we all have them. Some may fear physical danger; some may fear intimacy and the psychological vulnerability that comes with it; some may fear commitment; some may fear taking risks to gain what they desire. We all have things we fear, and we must overcome those fears if we are to achieve our goals, to attain what we value in life.

Imagine people who lack the courage to take chances in their careers. They desire a more challenging position, but they are unwilling to give up the old one in order to make the move. Imagine those who fear the vulnerability that comes with genuinely intimate relationships. They long for intimacy, but are unable or unwilling to take the risk necessary to attain it. Those who lack courage will be unable to take the necessary risks, and this is the sense in which cowardice is a vice: It prevents us from flourishing.

Yet Aristotle also suggests that virtues are usually a mean between two extremes. One of the extremes here is clear: cowardice. But what would it mean to have too much courage? It is easy to imagine examples. First, one could be willing to risk too quickly. Rashness is one way of having too much courage. Or one could risk much for too little. To run into a burning building to save a trapped child is courageous; to run into the same building to save an old pair of shoes is foolhardy. Foolhardiness is another way of having too much courage. Of course, the phrase "too much courage" here can be misleading. In the end, too much courage isn't really courage, it's something else.

Compassion

Aristotle talked a lot about virtues such as proper pride, courage, fortitude, and the like. Compassion was not among them. Yet many today would argue that compassion is a virtue—and this becomes a pivotal issue in a number of our readings in this book. What would an Aristotelian analysis of compassion look like?

First, let's define compassion and bracket it between its two extremes, the vices that correspond to a deficiency or an excess of compassion. *Compassion* itself is a feeling for our fellow moral beings (human beings and perhaps animals). It is literally a "feeling with . . . ," an ability to identify with the feelings of another being, especially feelings of suffering. Moreover, it is usually oriented toward action. The compassionate person is moved to help those who are suffering, and we would doubt the genuineness of the compassion if it never led to action. Those with too little compassion are cold-hearted, indifferent to the suffering of others. Unfortunately, there is no shortage of examples here. Yet what is "too much" compassion? Presumably, it is being overly concerned with the suffering of others. There are several ways in which this could occur. First, we might be so concerned with the suffering of others that we neglect ourselves and those to whom we have direct duties. Second, we might be so concerned with the suffering of others that we neglect the nonsuffering parts of their personalities, turning them into pure victims when they are not. Third, we may be appropriately concerned with the suffering of others, but we may manifest this in inappropriate ways. If compassion for a child crying in pain during a medical procedure leads us to kidnap the child to save it from suffering, we have expressed our compassion in an inappropriate way.

Compassion has an emotional element to it, but it is not just a blind feeling. Rather, it is also a way of perceiving the world—the world looks different through the eyes of the compassionate person than through the eyes of the sociopath. Moreover, it is also a way of thinking about the world, a way of understanding it. Compassion has to make judgments about the nature and causes of suffering, and also about the possible remedies for suffering. Compassion, finally, is also a way of acting, a way of responding to the suffering of the world. Compassion can be both deeply passionate and smart at the same time. As we shall see in our discussion of issues about poverty and starvation, it is not enough to feel compassion. We also have to know how to respond to suffering in effective ways that not only relieve the immediate suffering but also help the sufferers to free themselves from future suffering. Compassion needs to be wise, not just strongly felt.

Virtue Ethics As the Foundation of Other Approaches to Ethics

We can conclude this section by reflecting once again on the relationship between virtue ethics and action-oriented approaches to ethics. One of the principal problems faced by moral philosophers has been how to understand the continuing disagreement among the various ethical traditions sketched out above. It seems implausible to say that one is right and all the rest are wrong, but it also seems impossible to say that they are all right, for they seem to contradict each other. If we adopt a pluralistic approach, we may say that each contains partial truths about the moral life, but none contains the whole truth. But then the question is: How do we know which position should be given precedence in a particular instance?

There is, I suspect, no *theoretical* answer to this question, no metatheory that integrates all these differing and at times conflicting theories. However, I think there is a *practical* answer to this question: We ultimately have to put our trust in the wise person to know when to give priority to one type of moral consideration over another. Indeed, it is precisely this that constitutes moral wisdom.

ANALYZING MORAL PROBLEMS

As we turn to consider the various moral problems discussed in this book, each of these theories will help us to understand aspects of the problem that we might not originally have noticed, to see connections among apparently unconnected factors, and to formulate responses that we might not previously have envisioned. Ultimately, our search is a personal one, a search for wisdom.

But it is also a social approach, one that seeks to discern how to live a good life with other people, how to live well together in community. As we consider the series of moral issues that follows in this book, we will be attempting to fulfill both the individual and the communal goals. We will be seeking to find the course of action that is morally right for us as individuals, and we will be developing our own account of how society as a whole ought to respond to these moral challenges.

2

ETHNICITY AND ATTIDUES TOWARD PATIENT AUTONOMY

Leslie J. Blackhall, M.D., M.T.S.,
Sheila T. Murphy, Ph.D., Gelya Frank, Ph.D.,
Vicki Michel, M.A., J.D., and Stanley Azen, Ph.D.

❦

For the past 25 years, ethical and legal analysis of medical decision making in the United States has revolved around the idea of patient autonomy. The principle of patient autonomy asserts the rights of individuals to make informed decisions about their medical care. Thus, patients should be told the truth regarding their diagnosis and prognosis, as well as the risks and benefits of proposed treatments, and should be allowed to make choices based on this information. Although this ethical ideal is imperfectly realized in actual practice, the standard of care in this country is to tell patients the truth about even fatal illnesses,[1,2] to obtain their informed consent for major procedures,[3,4] and to involve them in decisions about withholding resuscitation.[5,6] The ideal of patient autonomy is so powerful that attempts have been made to extend patient control over medical decision making even to those circumstances in which the patient has lost the capacity to make decisions through advance care directives, such as the durable power of attorney for health care.[7–11] A federal statute, the Patient Self-Determination Act, has been enacted to enhance and preserve patient autonomy. Recently, however, it has been suggested that this focus on patient autonomy has become overly narrow and that other values, such as family integrity[12-14] and physician responsibility,[15,16] have been ignored. In particular, some have argued that this preoccupation with individual rights to the exclusion of other values may

Blackhall LJ, Murphy ST, Frank G, Michel V, Azen S. "Ethnicity and Attitudes toward Patient Autonomy." *Journal of the American Medical Association.* 1995;274(10):820–825. © American Medical Association. Reprinted by permission.

reflect a cultural bias on the part of the Western medical and bioethics communities.[13,14,17] To determine the attitudes of individuals of varying ethnic backgrounds, toward patient autonomy in medical decision making, we surveyed 800 Korean American, Mexican American, African American, and white (European American) subjects as part of a larger study examining the attitudes of older Americans of varying ethnicities toward health care and medical decision making.

MATERIALS, SUBJECTS, AND METHODS

Materials

The Ethnicity and Attitudes Toward Advance Care Directives Questionnaire is an hour-long instrument whose content and format was developed after an extensive review of the relevant anthropologic and medical literature, as well as consultation with clinicians, anthropologists, and experts in health beliefs. The instrument includes both previously validated scales and scales designed specifically to measure issues relevant to this study.

New sections were tested for internal (construct and content) and external validity, including extensive pilot testing. Once finalized, the instrument was translated into Korean and Spanish and back-translated into English by an independent agency with experience in translation of medical and technical documents.

In this article, we focus on the relationship between attitudes toward patient autonomy and demographic factors, including ethnicity, age, religion, level of education, and income. We also evaluate functional status (as measured by the Duke Activity Status Index[18] and the Katz Index of Activities of Daily Living[19]), acculturation (as measured by the Marin Short Acculturation Scale[20]), access to health care,[21] and the subject's experience with illness and with withholding and withdrawing care (as measured by subscales developed specifically for this project). The Marin Short Acculturation Scale, originally developed for use with a Latino population, consists of items that measure language use, use of Englishlanguage media (television and radio), and ethnic social relations. For use with the Korean population, the word "Korean" was substituted for "Spanish" or "Latino." Access to health care was based on four items from the Edgecombe hypertension study[21] relating to structural barriers (such as difficulty obtaining physician appointments and in obtaining transportation to appointments) and financial barriers (including insurance status) to care. Experience with health care was measured by asking subjects if they had ever been admitted to a hospital or an intensive care unit, or had received mechanical ventilation. Subjects were also asked whether close friends or family members had undergone these experiences. If so, subjects were asked if they visited the family members while they were hospitalized, in the intensive care unit, or receiving mechanical ventilation.

The dependent variable—attitudes toward patient autonomy—was measured as responses to a series of questions regarding attitudes toward truth telling (diagnosis and prognosis) and toward decision making with respect to the use of life support (see Table 2–1).

Subjects

Interviews were conducted with 200 individuals aged 65 years and older who identified themselves as belonging to one of the following four ethnic groups: African American, European American, Korean American, and Mexican American (N=800). Care was taken to include an equal number of men and women within each group and to maintain a similar age distribution across all four groups. Because a simple random sample of individuals older than 65 years would have yielded a sample that was heavily skewed in terms of sex and age, a stratified quota sampling technique was used. Attempts were made to minimize selection bias by sampling from a wide range of sites. Participation was strictly voluntary, and respondents were given twenty dollars in exchange for their time. This study was approved by the University of Southern California Institutional Review Board.

Procedure

All interviewers were trained by one of us (S.T.M.) during a half-day seminar. The interviewers' ethnic backgrounds matched those of the four groups of interest. Korean American and Mexican American interviewers were bilingual. Interviews were conducted in a one-on-one private setting. A list of senior citizen centers in Los Angeles County was obtained from the Los Angeles County Agency on Aging. To ensure that ethnicity and not income would be the primary variable differentiating our respondents, we further reduced our sampling frame to thirty-one sites located in areas with comparable socioeconomic distributions. Directors in each site were contacted for permission to recruit at the center. Recruitment procedures included flyers, handouts, direct approach, and announcements at times of congregate activities, such as meals. Once an individual expressed interest, either in response to a direct solicitation or by calling a telephone number listed on a flyer, an interviewer proceeded to determine eligibility. If the individual met the eligibility criteria of minimum age of 65 years and self-identification as a member of one of the four ethnic groups of interest, he was given a consent form and an appointment was made with an interviewer of the same ethnic background. Respondents were interviewed at the time of enrollment or an appointment for a more convenient time was made. Although Mexican American and Korean American respondents were given a choice of being interviewed in English or their native language, all subjects chose their native language.

Statistical Analyses

Differences in the independent and dependent variables across the four ethnic groups were assessed with the use of analysis of variance or χ^2 procedures. For the analyses of variance, pairwise comparisons between ethnic groups used Scheffé's multiple comparison procedure with a significance level of $P<.001$.

Table 2–1. Measures of Patient Autonomy

Diagnosis: A physician diagnoses a person as having cancer that has spread to several parts of their body.
   (a) The physician believes that the cancer cannot be cured. Should he or she tell the patient that they have cancer? <u>Yes or No</u>
   (b) Should the physician tell the patient's family about the cancer? <u>Yes or No</u>

Prognosis: The physician believes that the patient will probably die of the cancer.
   (a) Should the physician tell the patient that he or she will probably die? <u>Yes or No</u>
   (b) Should the physician tell the patient's family that the patient will probably die of the cancer? <u>Yes or No</u>

Decision regarding life-prolonging technology: The patient becomes very ill and a decision must be made about whether to put the patient on life-prolonging machines. The machines will prolong the patient's lite for a little while but will not cure the illness and may be uncomfortable. Who should make the decision about whether to put the patient on the machine?
   (a) It should be mainly the physician's decision.
   (b) It should be mainly the family's decision.
   (c) It should be mainly the patient's decision.

Estimates of the odds ratio (OR) were calculated for each independent variable with the use of univariate logistic regression analysis. The OR is the extent to which being a member of a specific category increases or decreases the probability of an individual agreeing with the patient autonomy model of truth telling and patient decision making. Indicator variables were used for independent variables that were categorical. Odds ratios greater than 1 represent how much more likely it was for subjects in a specified category to believe that a patient should have autonomy with regard to knowing her diagnosis and prognosis and making a decision regarding life-prolonging machines. The significance level was also set at $P<.001$.

In addition, stepwise multiple regression analyses were performed for each dependent variable to assess which of the independent variables "best" predicted attitudes toward truth telling and medical decision making. Finally, within-group χ^2 analyses were performed to identify factors significantly related to measures of autonomy after controlling for ethnicity. For these multivariate and within-group analyses, the significance level was set at $P<.05$.

RESULTS

Ethnic Differences in Attitudes Toward Patient Autonomy

Table 2–2 describes the characteristics of the survey sample, and the figure displays the effect of ethnicity on measures of attitudes toward patient autonomy. Korean Americans (47%±4% [SE]) were less likely than African Americans (89%±2%) and European Americans (87%±2%) to believe that a patient with metastatic cancer should be told the truth about that diagnosis (*P*<.001). Similarly, Korean Americans (35%±3%) were less likely than African Americans (63%±3%) and European Americans (69%±3%) to believe that the patient should be informed of a terminal prognosis and were also less likely to believe that the patient should make the decision about the use of life-supporting technology (28%±3% vs. 60%±3% and 65%±3%, all *P*<.001). Instead, most Korean Americans (57% ± 3%) believed that the family should make decisions about the use of life support.

Mexican Americans tended to fall between African Americans and Korean Americans, with 65%±3% supporting truth telling in diagnosis (statistically different from European Americans and African Americans at the *P*<.001 level). Forty-eight percent (±3%) of Mexican Americans believed that the patient should be told the truth about the prognosis, and only 41% (±3%) chose the patient as primary decision maker. Forty-five percent (±3%) of Mexican Americans believed that the family should make such decisions. Although the groups differed in their opinions about whether the patient should be told the truth, 90% or more of the subjects in all ethnic groups believed that the family should be told the truth about the patient's diagnosis and prognosis. The difference was that the Korean American and Mexican American subjects were more likely to believe that only the family, and not the patient, should be told the truth.

To determine whether acculturation (as measured by the Marin Short Acculturation Scale) affected the attitudes of Mexican Americans toward truth telling and decision making, subjects were categorized as "high" (score ≥3) versus "low" (score <3) acculturation. The majority (79%) of the Mexican-American subjects had low Marin Short Acculturation Scale scores. Acculturated Mexican Americans (i.e., those who spoke and read more English and associated more with "Anglos") were more likely to believe that the patient should be told the truth about the diagnosis (83% vs. 60%, *P*=.005) and prognosis (62% vs. 44%, *P*<.05). Choice of patient as primary decision maker was not affected by acculturation (36% vs. 42%, *P*=.42). Analyses could not be performed for Korean Americans because 100% of this group had scores below 3 on the Korean version of the Marin Short Acculturation Scale.

To better understand the relationship between acculturation and socioeconomic status in the Mexican American population, we analyzed the correlation between the Marin Short Acculturation Scale score, personal income, and education. Mexican American subjects with annual incomes above $10,000 (*P*<.0l) or more than six years of education (*P*<.001) were more likely to have a high Marin Short Acculturation

Table 2–2. Demographic Characteristics of Ethnic Groups (n=200/Group; N=800)*

Characteristic	African American	European American	Korean American	Mexican American	P
Age, y					
64–70	57 (29)	57 (28)	57 (29)	64 (32)	
71–75	56 (28)	49 (25)	54 (27)	57 (29)	.96
76–80	49 (25)	57 (28)	53 (27)	46 (23)	
≥ 81	38 (19)	37 (19)	37 (18)	33 (17)	
Religion					
Protestant/Christian	188 (94)	81 (40)	39 (19)	5 (2)	
Catholic	4 (2)	58 (29)	10 (5)	195 (98)	
Jewish	0	48 (24)	0	0	<.001
Buddhist	0	0	92 (46)	0	
Other	8 (4)	13 (7)	59 (30)	0	
Schooling, y					
1–6	23 (11)	6 (3)	53 (29)	116 (61)	
7–12	132 (66)	103 (51)	89 (49)	57 (30)	<.001
>12	45 (23)	91 (46)	39 (22)	16 (8)	
Personal annual income					
<$10000	106 (55)	87 (45)	192 (96)	153 (84)	
$10000–$25000	81 (42)	80 (42)	8 (4)	25 (14)	<.001
>$25000	5 (3)	25 (13)	0	5 (3)	
Functional status					
Katz Index	11.9 (0.4)[a]	11.4 (1.0)[b]	11.8 (0.6)[a]	11.3 (1.2)[b]	<.001
Duke Index	22.0 (10.6)[b]	23.5 (10.9)[a,b]	20.6 (8.6)[b]	27.4 (9.9)[a]	
Personal experience with illness					
0=none	22 (11)[a]	9 (5)[a]	88 (44)[b]	45 (23)[a]	<.001
≥1 =some	178 (89)	191 (95)	112 (56)	155 (77)	
Personal experience with withholding care					
0=none	166 (83)[b,c]	89 (45)[a]	181 (91)[c]	136 (68)[b]	<.001
≥1=some	34 (17)	111 (55)	19 (9)	64 (32)	
Access to care					
Structural	4.3 (2.1)[a]	3.6 (2.2)[a]	3.4 (1.8)[a]	6.3 (2.9)[b]	<.001
Financial	0.3 (0.3)[b]	0.1 (0.2)[a]	0.5 (0.0)[c]	0.4 (0.2)[d]	

*Means with the same letter (a, b, or c) are not significantly different at the $P<.001$ level with use of the Scheffé multiple comparison procedure.

Scale score. Acculturation does not appear to be a simple function of years lived in the United States. The majority (66%) of Korean Americans had lived in the country for more than 10 years. Likewise, more than 90% of the Mexican American sample had lived in the United States at least 10 years; of those, 78% had a low Marin Short Acculturation Scale score.

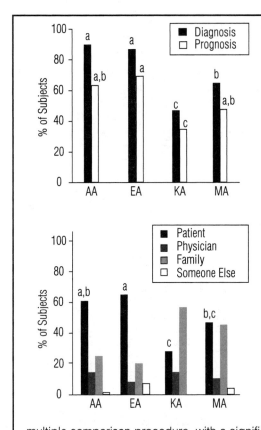

Top: The percentages of African American (AA), European American (EA), Korean American (KA), and Mexican American (MA) subjects who believe that the physician should inform the patient that they have cancer (diagnosis) and that the physician should inform the patient that they will probably die (prognosis). **Bottom**: The percentages of subjects who believe that the decision about whether to put the patient on a life-support machine should be made by the patient, physician, family, or someone else. Differences in percentages of subjects who believed in patient autonomy with regard to diagnosis, prognosis, and the use of a life-support machine were assessed with use of one-way analysis of variance. Pairwise comparisons across ethnic groups used Scheffé's multiple comparison procedure, with a significance level set at *P*<.001. For each measure of patient autonomy, ethnic groups that were not significantly different are indicated in the figure with the same letter (a, b, or c).

Univariate Logistic Regression Analyses of Factors Related to Patient Autonomy

Differences in attitudes toward patient autonomy among the ethnic groups are borne out in the logistic regression analyses presented in Table 2–3. Relative to European Americans, Korean Americans and Mexican Americans were less likely to favor telling the truth about diagnosis and prognosis and less likely to choose the patient as primary decision maker (ORs <1, *P*<.001). Religion and socioeconomic status were also related to our measures of patient autonomy. Because these variables were strongly associated with ethnicity, multivariate and within-group analyses were performed and are reported below. With respect to age, the oldest subjects (aged 81 years and older) were less likely to believe that the patient should be told the truth about a terminal prognosis than were the youngest subjects (ORs <1, $P<.001$). Subjects with personal experience with illness and withholding and withdrawing care were more likely to favor truth telling (ORs >1, $P<.001$). No relationships were found for sex, functional status, and access to care.

Stepwise Multiple Logistic Regression Analyses of Factors Related to Patient Autonomy

To further examine the relative contribution of each of the factors related to our measures of autonomy, we performed a stepwise logistic regression (see Table 2–4). Because no associations were found for sex, functional status (Katz Index of Activities of Daily Living and Duke Activity Status Index), and access to care indexes in the univariate analysis (see Table 2–3), these variables were not included in the model. Years of schooling and income were analyzed as continuous (rather than categorical) variables.

For all three measures of attitudes toward patient autonomy, the primary factor related to attitude was ethnicity. Relative to European Americans (the reference group), Korean Americans and Mexican Americans were least likely to favor truth telling about the diagnosis and prognosis and least likely to believe that the patient should make the decision about the use of life support. After controlling for ethnic differences, the second most important factor associated with attitudes toward truth telling was years of education. Patients with more education were more likely to favor telling the truth about the diagnosis and prognosis. In contrast, years of education did not predict who would be selected to make the decision about the use of life-sustaining technology. Finally, patients with some personal experience with illness were more likely to favor truth telling with respect to diagnosis.

Within-Group Analyses of Factors Related to Patients Autonomy

To further explicate the relationship between socioeconomic status, ethnicity, and attitudes, we performed within-group χ^2 analyses to examine the relationship between these and our measures of patient autonomy within each ethnic group. Socioeconomic status (as measured by income and years of schooling) was not related to attitudes in the European American and African American groups. In the Korean American and Mexican American groups, however, some relationships emerged. Mexican Americans with more years of education (≥ 7 years) were more likely to believe that the patient should be told the diagnosis (79% vs. 57%, $P<.05$), and those with higher annual incomes (≥ $10,000) were more likely to favor truth telling about the diagnosis (93% vs. 61%, $P<.001$) and prognosis (70% vs. 45%, $P<.01$). Korean Americans with higher levels of education were more likely to believe that the patient should make the decision about the use of life support (32% vs. 19%, $P<.05$). Similarly, within-group analyses of age revealed that although age was not related to attitudes in the European American and African American subjects, it was a predictor in the Korean American and Mexican

Table 2–3. Odds Ratios (95% Confidence Intervals) of Measures of Autonomy			
	Tell diagnosis	Tell Prognosis	Decision maker about life support
Ethnic group			
European American	1.0	1.0	1.0
African American	1.2 (0.7–2.3)	0.8 (0.5–1.1)	0.8 (0.6–1.2)
Mexican American	0.3* (0.2–0.5)	0.4* (0.3–0.6)	0.4* (0.3–0.6)
Korean American	0.1* (0.1–0.2)	0.2* (0.1–0.4)	0.2* (0.1–0.3)
Sex			
Male	1.0	1.0	1.0
Female	1.1 (0.8–1.4)	0.8 (0.6–1.1)	1.2 (0.9–1.5)
Age, y			
64–70	1.0	1.0	1.0
71–75	1.1 (0.7–1.7)	0.8 (0.6–1.2)	0.9 (0.7–1.4)
76–80	1.0 (0.7–1.6)	0.9 (0.6–1.4)	0.8 (0.6–1.2)
≥ 81	0.7 (0.4–1.0)	0.6* (0.4–0.9)	0.7 (0.5–1.1)
Religion			
Protestant/Christian	1.0	1.0	1.0
Catholic	0.6* (0.4–0.8)	0.7 (0.5–1.0)	0.6* (0.5–0.9)
Jewish	1.0 (0.5–2.2)	0.7 (0.4–1.3	1.3 (0.7–2.4)
Buddhist	0.2* (0.1–0.3)	0.2* (0.1–0.4)	0.4* (0.2–0.6)
Schooling, y			
1–6	1.0	1.0	1.0
7–12	2.1* (1.4–3.0)	1.3 (0.9–1.8)	1.8 (1.2–2.5)
>12	3.3* (2.1–5.4)	2.0* (1.4–3.1)	2.5* (1.7–3.8)
Personal annual income			
<$10,000	1.0	1.0	1.0
$10,000–$25,000	4.3* (2.7–7.0)	2.4* (1.7–3.4)	2.4* (1.7–3.3)
>$25,000	3.1 (1.2–8.0)	2.3 (1.1–4.8)	2.0 (1.0–4.1)
Functional status			
Katz Index	0.9 (0.8–1.1)	1.0 (0.8–1.1)	1.1 (0.9–1.3)
Duke Index	1.0 (1.0–1.0)	1.0 (1.0–1.0)	1.0 (1.0–1.0)
Experience with			
Illness	3.0* (2.1–4.3)	2.1* (1.5–3.0)	1.3 (0.9–1.9)
Withholding care	2.1* (1.3–3.0)	1.8* (1.3–2.6)	1.5 (1.0–2.1)
Access to care			
Structural	1.0 (0.9–1.0)	1.0 (0.9–1.0)	1.0 (1.0–1.0)
Financial	1.1 (1.1-1.1)	1.1 (1.0–1.1)	1.0 (0.9–1.1)

*Odds ratio significantly different from 1, $P < .001$.

American groups. Older Korean Americans and Mexican Americans (81 years or older) were less likely than younger subjects of the same ethnicity to favor telling the patient the diagnosis (25% vs. 52%, $P < .01$, for Korean Americans; 45% vs. 69%, $P < .01$, for Mexican Americans).

In the European American and Korean American groups, religion was related to differences in attitudes toward some of the autonomy indexes. In the European American group, Protestants were more likely than non-Protestants to believe that

Table 2–4. Stepwise Multiple Logistic Regression Analysis of Factors Predictive of Measures of Autonomy

Step	Variable	Odds Ratio (95% Confidence Interval)	P	Model P
		Diagnosis		
1	Ethnic group			
	European American	1.0	. . .	
	African American	1.4 (0.7–2.7)	.31	
	Mexican American	0.5 (0.2–0.9)	<.02	
	Korean American	0.2 (0.1–0.3)	<.001	<.001
2	Years of schooling	1.1 (1.0–1.1)	<.01	
3	Personal experience: illness	1.7 (1.0–2.5)	<.03	
		Prognosis		
1	Ethnic group			
	European American	1.0	. . .	
	African American	0.8 (0.5–1.3)	.39	
	Mexican American	0.6 (0.3–0.9)	<.03	<.001
	Korean American	0.3 (0.2–0.4)	<.001	
2	Years of schooling	1.0 (1.0–1.1)	<.05	
		Patient as Decision Maker		
1	Ethnic group			
	European American	1.0	. . .	
	African American	0.8 (0.5–1.2)	.27	
	Mexican American	0.3 (0.2–0.6)	<.001	<.001
	Korean American	0.2 (0.1–0.3)	<.001	

the patient should be told about a terminal prognosis (81% vs. 61%, $P<.01$) and were more likely to believe that the patient should be the primary decision maker (73% vs. 59%, $P<.05$). Jewish subjects were less likely than non-Jewish subjects to believe in telling the truth about the prognosis (52% vs. 75%, $P<.01$). In the Korean American group, Buddhists were less likely to believe that the patient should be told the prognosis (27% vs. 41%, $P<.05$). The African American and Mexican American groups had very little religious diversity, with 98% of the Mexican American group being Catholic and 94% of the African American group being Protestant; thus, further analyses of religious differences within these groups could not be conducted.

COMMENT

Korean American and Mexican American subjects were less likely than European American and African American subjects to believe that the patient should be told the truth about the diagnosis and prognosis of a serious illness and were less likely to believe that the patient should make decisions about the use of life support. Within the Korean American and Mexican American groups, older subjects and those with lower socioeconomic status tended to be opposed to truth telling and patient decision making even more strongly than their younger, wealthier, and more highly educated counterparts.

Our study suggests that the attitudinal differences among these ethnic groups are related to cultural rather than demographic variables, such as socioeconomic status, which tend to vary with ethnicity. In the Mexican American group, in which the subjects had variable levels of acculturation, more acculturated subjects were more likely to share the patient autonomy model with the European American and African American subjects. As they begin to speak, think, and read more in English, and associate more with Anglos, they tend to take on the attitudes that are expressed by the English-speaking groups in our study. Socioeconomic status does not predict attitudes in the European American and African American groups. Instead, socioeconomic status may be acting as a marker for acculturation. Wealthier, more educated Mexican Americans are more likely to speak English and be in contact with values promoted in the English-speaking sectors of American society and more likely to adopt those values with respect to medical decision making.

There are several limitations to the generalizability of our data. Subjects aged 65 years and older are more likely to be faced with serious health-care decisions for themselves or their loved ones; younger subjects may hold different views. Moreover, to prevent skewing our population toward younger, female subjects, we used a quota sampling technique rather than a true random sample of the entire elderly population of these four ethnic groups. Although we attempted to minimize selection bias by sampling from a wide variety of sites, our subjects may not represent all portions of those groups. Finally, our sample was from urban southern California; the attitudes of the elderly may differ by geographic location.

The decision-making style exhibited by most of the Mexican American and Korean American subjects in our study might best be described as family centered. Although the patient autonomy model does not exclude family involvement, in this family-centered model, it is the sole responsibility of the family to hear bad news about the patient's diagnosis and prognosis and to make the difficult decisions about life support. Several prior studies of the issue of telling the diagnosis of cancer with different ethnic groups have yielded similar results. In one recent report, an Italian oncologist described the approach toward decision making in Italy as one in which the patient is frequently "protected" from bad news by the family and physicians.[22] Autonomy is not viewed as empowering. Rather, it is seen as isolating and burdensome to patients who are too sick and too ignorant about their condition to be able to make meaningful choices. In a survey from Greece, only a third of those questioned believed that patients should be told the truth about a terminal illness.[23] As in our study, older subjects with less education were more likely to be opposed to truth telling. Anecdotal reports also note the tendency of Chinese and Ethiopian families to oppose truth telling on the grounds that it harms patients by causing them to lose hope.[24,25] Other studies have shown that Latinos are more likely than Anglos to believe that cancer is a death sentence.[26] Finally, studies of physicians' attitudes and practice show that those in

Spain, France, Japan, and Eastern Europe rarely tell patients with cancer their diagnosis or prognosis, usually informing the family instead.[27-29]

Thus, belief in the ideal of patient autonomy is far from universal. In this country, as recently as 1961, Oken[30] documented that 90% of physicians did not inform their patients of the diagnosis of cancer. By 1979, when this survey was repeated, this attitude had completely reversed. By 1979, 97% of physicians made it their policy to inform patients with cancer of their diagnosis.[1] Most of the literature that discusses this change views it as simple progress from an uninformed paternalism to a more enlightened and respectful attitude toward patients. Indeed, there have been many benefits to more open discussion and increased patient involvement in medical decision making. It is probably impossible to completely deceive seriously ill patients when, despite all reassurance, they continue to deteriorate physically and to require hospitalization and medical care. Acknowledgment of the truth lets patients express their feelings and receive the emotional and spiritual comfort appropriate to the crisis they are experiencing. Allowing patients to choose from the range of treatment options available ensures that the treatment will conform to their preferences. However, the high value placed on open expression of emotion and on the rights of individuals to control their destiny are not necessarily shared by all segments of American society. For those who hold the family-centered model, a higher value may be placed on the harmonious functioning of the family than on the autonomy of its individual members. Although the patient autonomy model is founded on the idea of respect for persons, people live, get sick, and die while embedded in the context of family and culture and inevitably exist not simply as individuals but in a web of relationships. Insisting on the patient autonomy model of medical decision making when that model runs counter to the deepest values of the patient may ironically be another form of the paternalistic idea that "doctor knows best."

Many questions remain to be answered about how this family-centered model functions in actual practice. Do patients who are not told the diagnosis usually know it anyway? Is this information later communicated by verbal or nonverbal means? Is the interaction between patient and family different when the patient is the head of the household? What is the perceived harm when the medical community violates cultural conventions and insists on telling the truth to the patient? What disruptions occur in the coping mechanisms of the individual and the family? In what ways does acculturation change the beliefs of patients of various ethnicities, i.e., how are the cultures of immigrants transformed and combined with the culture of their adopted country? We plan to explore these and other issues through in-depth ethnographic interviews with 10% of the study sample.

The purpose of our study was not to convince ethicists that there should be one set of moral rules for Korean Americans and another for European Americans, and we do not expect that the information we have obtained will allow physicians to predict with certainty the attitude of any given person from a particular ethnic group. As our study demonstrates, much diversity of opinion about these issues occurs not only between ethnic groups but also within each ethnic group. Rather, we believe that it is vital to uncover the usually unspoken beliefs and assumptions that are common among patients of particular ethnicities to raise the sensitivity of physicians and others who work with these groups. Understanding that such attitudes exist will allow physicians to recognize and avoid potential difficulties in communication and to elicit and negotiate differences when they occur. In particular, we suggest that physicians ask patients if they wish to be informed about their illness and be involved in making decisions about their care or if they prefer that their family handles such matters.[31] In either case, the patient's wishes should be respected. Allowing patients to choose a family-centered decision-making style does not mean abandoning our commitment to individual autonomy or its legal expression in the doctrine of informed consent. Rather, it means broadening our view of autonomy so that respect for persons includes respect for the cultural values they bring with them to the decision-making process.

This project was supported by grant 1 R01 HS07001 01A1 from the Agency for Health Care Policy and Research, Washington, DC.

We thank Alex Capron, LL.B.; David Goldstein, M.D., Barbara Malcolm, M.A.; and Elena Taylor-Muhoz, M.A., for their help and support.

REFERENCES

1. Novack DH, Plumer R, Smith PL, Ochitill H, Morrow GR, Bennett JM. Changes in physicians' attitudes toward telling the cancer patient. *JAMA.* 1979;241:897–900.

2. President's Commission for the Study of Ethical Problems in Medicine and Biomedical and Behavioral Research. *The Ethical and Legal Implications of Informed Consent in the Patient-Practitioner Relationship.* Washington, DC: US Government Printing Office; 1982;1:74–76.

3. *Cobbs* v *Grant*, 8 C. 3d 229, 242–3 (1972).

4. Beauchamp TL, Faden RR. *A History and Theory of Informed Consent.* Oxford, England: Oxford University Press; 1986:88–98.

5. American Thoracic Society. Withholding and withdrawing life-sustaining therapy. *Annals of Internal Medicine.* 1991;115:478–484.

6. Council on Ethical and Judicial Affairs, American Medical Association. Guidelines for the appropriate use of do-not-resuscitate orders. *JAMA.* 1991; 265:1868–1871.

7. Steinbrook R, Lo B. Decision making for incompetent patients by designated proxy. *New England Journal of Medicine.* 1984;310:1598–1601.

8. Schneiderman LJ, Arras JD. Counseling patients to counsel physicians on future care in the event of patient incompetence. *Annals of Internal Medicine.* 1985;102: 693–698.

9. Annas GJ. The health care proxy and the living will. *New England Journal of Medicine.* 1991;324:1210–1213.

10. Emanuel L. Does the DNR order need lifesustaining intervention? time for comprehensive advance directives. *American Journal of Medicine.* 1989;86:87–90.

11. Emanuel E, Emanuel L. Living wills: past, present and future. *Journal of Clinical Ethics.* 1990;1:9–18.

12. Sehgal A, Galbraith A, Chesney M, Schoenfeld P, Charles G, Lo B. How strictly do dialysis patients want their advance directives followed? *JAMA.* 1992;277:59–63.

13. Nelson JL. Taking families seriously. *Hastings Center Report.* 1992;22:6–12.

14. Orona CJ, Koenig BA, Davis AJ. Cultural aspects of nondisclosure. *Cambridge Quarterly of Healthcare Ethics.* 1994;3:338–346.

15. Blackhall LJ. Must we always use CPR? *New England Journal of Medicine.* 1987;317:1281–1284.

16. Schneiderman LJ, Jecker NS, Jonsen AR. Medical futility: its meaning and ethical implications. *Annals of Internal Medicine.* 1990;112:949–954.

17. Levine RJ. Informed consent: some challenges to the universal validity of the Western model. *Law, Medicine & Health Care.* 1991;19:207–213.

18. Hlatsky M, Boireu RE, Higgenbotham MB, et al. A brief self-administered questionnaire to determine functional capacity (the Duke Activity Status Index). *American Journal of Cardiology.* 1989;64:651–654.

19. Katz S, Ford AB, Moskowitz RW, Jackson BA, Jaffe MW. Studies of illness in the aged: the index of ADL, a standardized measure of biological and psychosocial function. *JAMA.* 1963;185:914–919.

20. Marin G, Sabogal F, Marin BV, Otero-Sabogal R, Perez-Stable E. Development of a short acculturation scale for Hispanics. *Hispanic Journal of Behavioral Science.* 1987;9:183–205.

21. James SA, Wagner EH, Strogatz DS, et al. The Edgecombe high blood pressure control program, II: barriers to the use of medical care among hypertensives. *American Journal of Public Health.* 1984;74:468–472.

22. Surbone A. Truth telling to the patient. *JAMA.* 1992;268:1661–1662.

23. Dalla-Vorgia P, Katsouyanni K, Garanis TN, Toulourni G, Drogari P, Koutselinis A. Attitudes of a Mediterranean population to the truth-telling issue. *Journal of Medical Ethics.* 1992;18:67–74.

24. Muller JH, Desmond B. Ethical dilemmas in a cross-cultural context: a Chinese example. *Western Journal of Medicine.* 1992;157:323–327.

25. Beyene Y. Medical disclosure and refugees: telling bad news to Ethiopian patients. *Western Journal of Medicine.* 1992;157:328–332.

26. Pérez-Stable EJ, Sabogal F, Otero-Sabogal R, Hiatt RA, McPhee SJ. Misconceptions about cancer among Latinos and Anglos. *JAMA.* 1992;268:3219–3223.

27. Holland JC, Geary N, Marchini A, Tross S. An international survey of physician attitudes and practice in regard to revealing the diagnosis of cancer. *Cancer Investigation.* 1987;5:151–154.

28. Estapé E, Palombo H, Herruindez, et al. Cancer diagnosis disclosure in a Spanish hospital. *Annals of Oncology.* 1992;3:451–454.

29. Thomsen O, Wulff H, Martin A, Singer P. What do gastroenterologists in Europe tell cancer patients? *Lancet.* 1993;341:473–476.

30. Oken D. What to tell cancer patients. *JAMA.* 1961;175:86–94.

31. Freedman B. Offering truth: one ethical approach to the uninformed cancer patient. *Archives of Internal Medicine.* 1993;153:572–576.

3

ETHICAL RELATIVISM IN A MULTICULTURAL SOCIETY

Ruth Macklin, Ph.D.

Cultural pluralism poses a challenge to physicians and patients alike in the multicultural United States, where immigrants from many nations and diverse religious groups visit the same hospitals and doctors. Multiculturalism is defined as "a social-intellectual movement that promotes the value of diversity as a core principle and insists that all cultural groups be treated with respect and as equals."[1(p609)] This sounds like a value that few enlightened people could fault, but it produces dilemmas and leads to results that are, at the least, problematic if not counterintuitive.

Critics of mainstream bioethics within the United States and abroad have complained about the narrow focus on autonomy and individual rights. Such critics argue that much—if not most—of the world embraces a value system that places the family, the community, or the society as a whole above that of the individual person. The prominent American sociologist Renée Fox is a prime example of such critics: "From the outset, the conceptual framework of bioethics has accorded paramount status to the value-complex of individualism, underscoring the principles of individual rights, autonomy, self-determination, and their legal expression in the jurisprudential notion of privacy."[2(p206)]

The emphasis on autonomy, at least in the early days of bioethics in the United States, was never intended to cut patients off from their families by

R. Macklin. "Ethical Relativism in a Multicultural Society." *Kennedy Institute of Ethics Journal.* 1998;8(1):1–22. ©The Johns Hopkins University Press.

focusing monistically on the patient. Instead, the intent was to counteract the predominant and long-standing paternalism on the part of the medical profession. In fact, there was little discussion of where the family entered in and no presumption that a family-centered approach to sick patients was somehow a violation of the patient's autonomy. Most patients want and need the support of their families, regardless of whether they seek to be autonomous agents regarding their own care. Respect for autonomy is perfectly consistent with recognition of the important role that families play when a loved one is ill. Autonomy has fallen into such disfavor among some bioethicists that the pendulum has begun to swing in the direction of families, with urgings to "take families seriously"[3] and even to consider the interests of family members equal to those of the competent patient.[4]

The predominant norm in the United States of disclosing a diagnosis of serious illness to the patient is not universally accepted even among long-standing citizens comprising ethnic or religious subcultures. Moreover, "respect for autonomy" as an ethical principle continues to be misunderstood and perhaps even deliberately misrepresented. The following episode is illustrative.

An orthodox rabbi was invited to deliver a lecture on Jewish medical ethics at a medical school. The rabbi outlined some of the leading precepts of Jewish medical ethics and sought to compare them with their counterparts in contemporary secular bioethics. Understandably, given his commitment to Orthodox Judaism, he undertook to defend the precepts of Jewish medical ethics in those instances where they conflict with the secular version. The rabbi told the story of a man with an abiding fear of cancer who visited his doctor because he was worried about a small growth on his upper lip. The pair had a long-standing physician-patient relationship, and the doctor was aware of the patient's deep fear of cancer. When the patient paid a return visit following a delay in which the biopsy was examined, he said to the doctor: "It isn't cancer, is it?" The physician, after a brief hesitation, reassured the patient that he did not have cancer.

The rabbi commended the physician's action, saying that secular bioethics would insist on patient autonomy and require that the doctor tell the truth, thereby instilling great anxiety in the patient. The rabbi went on to say that Jewish medical ethics does not place autonomy above all other values, noting that respect for autonomy has little place in Jewish medical ethics. Instead, the physician, as the person with medical expertise, has the obligation to do whatever is best for the patient, based on that expertise, and the patient—a layperson—does not have "a right to know" everything the doctor may discover. The impression the rabbi sought to convey was that secular bioethics mandates truth telling to patients even when it means inflicting unwanted information. In contrast, the more benevolent Jewish medical ethics allows for withholding diagnostic information and can support telling "white lies" in order to avoid harming the patient.

I am not concerned here to debate the general merits of the contemporary practice of disclosing a diagnosis of cancer. Nor do I intend to argue that a value placed on truth telling should prevail universally, inside medical practice as well as in the world at large. But I did object, when I listened to the rabbi's lecture, to his omission of a few critical pieces of information. He had taken the story of the patient fearful of cancer from an article in a medical journal written by the physician who also was a protagonist in the story. In the published article, the physician explained his action and sought to justify it, not by defending the tradition of medical paternalism but with a different rationale.

The physician believed he had an obligation to be truthful to his patients. He normally does disclose a diagnosis of cancer. However, reflecting in this case on the patient's extreme and irrational fear, the physician reasoned as follows. Although the patient did, indeed, have a form of cancer, it was a tiny growth confined to a small region of the skin, of a type that does not spread and could not have metastasized. The growth could be completely removed and there would be no further consequences. What this patient thought of as cancer—what he feared so deeply—was not the condition he actually had. So, the doctor reasoned, he could be conveying as much of an untruth by telling this man he had cancer, given the patient's conception of that disease. Telling the patient he did not have cancer was the doctor's way of saying that the man did not have what he most feared—a fatal illness. And that was being truthful.

One might quibble with the semantics of this little story: Did the doctor lie, or not? Wasn't it literally a lie? Or was the "larger" truth the physician intended to convey the "real" truth? Is it correct to say that the doctor was being truthful, even though he did not literally "tell the truth"? However those philosophical questions may be answered, the lessons that flow from the tale are several. The first lesson highlights the difference between an absolutist ethics and a universalist ethics. An absolutist ethics contains exceptionless rules: "Never lie. Never break promises. Always tell the truth." Few people anywhere (rigid Kantians excepted) defend this form of absolutism. Every ethical rule has some exceptions, which can be justified in the usual manner by appealing to higher principles that would be violated if one adhered to the rule.

A universalist ethics, on the other hand, holds that fundamental ethical principles exist and can be used to justify specific rules. This brings us to the second lesson of the story: the fundamental principle that underlay the physician's response to the patient was the "respect for persons" principle. The rabbi who recounted the story sought to demonstrate the superiority of Jewish medical ethics because the beneficence of the physician's white lie was ethically defensible. And so it was.

Where the rabbi erred, however, was in his contention that secular medical ethics, with its reigning principle of "respect for autonomy," would require inflicting on the patient the unwanted information that he had cancer. The principle of "respect for persons" is broader than the principle of "autonomy," although the latter concept is often the relevant interpretation of what follows from "respect for persons." In this episode, the concept of autonomy played a different role from what usually follows from "respect for persons." This was a matter of the physician revealing to the patient the nature of his ailment, and describing it to him in a way that the patient would properly understand. In recognizing and being sensitive to the patient's fear of cancer, the physician showed respect for the patient's beliefs and values. The physician reasoned that this patient would misunderstand a diagnosis of cancer. Neither respect for persons nor beneficence mandates providing information that a patient would not fully comprehend.

The third lesson from this story is a reminder that the much-maligned principles of bioethics are often misused or abused by people conducting an ethical analysis. I neither know nor care whether the rabbi was intentionally distorting the application of the principle of "respect for autonomy" in order to demonstrate the beneficent nature of Jewish medical ethics. But it was simply a mistake to say that the principle of autonomy as employed in secular bioethics requires that doctors always "tell the truth" to patients, even when it may cause terrible harm.

PERSPECTIVES OF HEALTH-CARE WORKERS AND PATIENTS

A circumstance that arises frequently in multicultural urban settings is one that medical students bring to ethics teaching conferences. The patient and family are recent immigrants from a culture in which physicians normally inform the family rather than the patient of a diagnosis of cancer. The medical students wonder whether they are obligated to follow the family's wish, thereby respecting their cultural custom, or whether to abide by the ethical requirement at least to explore with patients their desire to receive information and to be a participant in their medical care. When medical students presented such a case in one of the conferences I codirect with a physician, the dilemma was heightened by the demographic picture of the medical students themselves. Among the fourteen students, eleven different countries of origin were represented. Those students either had come to the United States themselves to study or their parents had immigrated from countries in Asia, Latin America, Europe, and the Middle East.

The students began their comments with remarks like, "Where I come from, doctors never tell the patient a diagnosis of cancer" or, "In my country, the doctor always asks the patient's family and abides by their wishes." The discussion centered on the question of whether the physician's obligation is to act in accordance with what contemporary medical ethics dictates in the United States or to respect the cultural differences of their patients and act according to the family's wishes. Not surprisingly, the medical students were divided on the answer to this question.

Medical students and residents are understandably confused about their obligation to disclose information to a patient when the patient comes from a culture in which telling a patient she has cancer is rare or unheard of. They ask: "Should I adhere to the American custom of disclosure or the Argentine custom of withholding the diagnosis?" That question is miscast, since there are some South Americans who want to know if they have cancer and some North Americans who do not. It is not, therefore, the cultural tradition that should determine whether disclosure to a patient is ethically appropriate, but rather the patient's wish to communicate directly with the physician, to leave communications to the family, or something in between. It would be a simplistic, if not unethical, response on the part of doctors to reason that "this is the United States, we adhere to the tradition of patient autonomy, therefore I must disclose to this immigrant from the Dominican Republic that he has cancer."

Most patients in the United States do want to know their diagnosis and prognosis, and it has been amply demonstrated that they can emotionally and psychologically handle a diagnosis of cancer. The same may not be true, however, for recent immigrants from other countries, and it may be manifestly untrue in certain cultures. Although this, too, may change in time, several studies point to a cross-cultural difference in beliefs and practice regarding disclosure of diagnosis and informed consent to treatment.

One survey examined differences in the attitudes of elderly subjects from different ethnic groups toward disclosure of the diagnosis and prognosis of a terminal illness and regarding decision making at the end of life.[5] This study found marked differences in attitudes between Korean Americans and Mexican Americans, on the one hand, and African Americans and Americans of European descent, on the other. The Korean Americans and Mexican Americans were less likely than the other two groups to believe that patients should be told of a prognosis of terminal illness and also less likely to believe that the patient should make decisions about the use of life-support technology. The Korean Americans and Mexican Americans surveyed were also more likely than the other groups to have a family-centered attitude toward these matters; they believed that the family and not the patient should be told the truth about the patient's diagnosis and prognosis. The authors of the study cite data from other countries that bear out a similar gap between the predominant "autonomy model" in the United States and the family-centered model prevalent in European countries as well as in Asia and Africa.

The study cited was conducted at thirty-one senior citizen centers in Los Angeles. In no ethnic group did 100 percent of its members favor disclosure or nondisclosure to the patient. Forty-seven percent of Korean Americans believed that a patient with metastatic cancer should be told the truth about the diagnosis, 65 percent of Mexican Americans held that belief, 87 percent of European Americans believed patients should be told the truth, and 89 percent of African Americans held that belief.

It is worth noting that the people surveyed were all sixty-five years old or older. Not surprisingly, the Korean American and Mexican American senior citizens had values closer to the cultures of their origin than did the African Americans and European Americans who were born in the United States. Another finding was that among the Korean American and Mexican American groups, older subjects and those with lower socioeconomic status tended to be opposed to truth telling and patient decision making more strongly than the younger, wealthier, and more highly educated members of these same groups. The authors of the study draw the conclusion that physicians should ask patients if they want to receive information and make decisions regarding treatment or whether they prefer that their families handle such matters.

Far from being at odds with the "autonomy model," this conclusion supports it. To ask patients how much they wish to be involved in decision making does show respect for their autonomy: Patients can then make the autonomous choice about who should be the recipient of information or the decision maker about their illness. What would fail to show respect for autonomy is for physicians to make these decisions without consulting the patient at all. If doctors spoke only to the families but not to the elderly Korean American or Mexican American patients without first approaching the patients to ascertain their wishes, they would be acting in the paternalistic manner of the past in America, and in accordance with the way many physicians continue to act in other parts of the world today. Furthermore, if physicians automatically withheld the diagnosis from Korean Americans because the majority of people in that ethnic group did not want to be told, they would be making an assumption that would result in a mistake almost 50 percent of the time.

INTOLERANCE AND OVERTOLERANCE

A medical resident in a New York hospital questioned a patient's ability to understand the medical treatment he had proposed and doubted whether the patient could grant truly informed consent. The patient, an immigrant from the Caribbean islands, believed in voodoo and sought to employ voodoo rituals in addition to the medical treatment she was receiving. "How can anyone who believes in that stuff be competent to consent to the treatment we offer?" the resident mused. The medical resident was an observant Jew who did not work, drive a car, or handle money on the sabbath and adhered to Kosher dietary laws. Both the Caribbean patient and the Orthodox Jew were devout believers in their respective faiths and practiced the accepted rituals of their religions.

The patient's voodoo rituals were not harmful to herself or to others. If the resident had tried to bypass or override the patient's decision regarding treatment, the case would have posed an ethical problem requiring resolution. Intolerance of another's religious or traditional practices that pose no threat of harm is, at least, discourteous and, at worst, a prejudicial attitude. And it does fail to show respect for persons and their diverse religious and cultural practices. But it does not (yet) involve a failure to respect persons at a more fundamental level, which would occur if the doctor were to deny the patient her right to exercise her autonomy in the consent procedures.

At times, however, it is the family that interferes with the patient's autonomous decisions. Two brothers of a Haitian immigrant were conducting a conventional Catholic prayer vigil for their dying brother at his hospital bedside. The patient, suffering from terminal cancer and in extreme pain, had initially been given the pain medication he requested. Some time later a nurse came in and found the patient alert, awake, and in excruciating pain from being undermedicated. When questioned, another nurse who had been responsible for the patient's care said that she had not continued to administer the pain medication because the patient's brothers had forbidden her to do so. Under the influence of the heavy dose of pain medication, the patient had become delirious and mumbled incoherently. The brothers took this as an indication that evil spirits had entered the patient's body and, according to the voodoo religion of their native culture, unless the spirit was exorcised it would stay with the family forever, and the entire family would suffer bad consequences. The patient manifested the signs of delirium only when he was on the medication, so the brothers asked the nurse to withhold the pain medication, which they believed was responsible for the entry of the evil spirit. The nurse sincerely believed that respect for the family's religion required her to comply with the patient's brothers' request, even if it contradicted the patient's own expressed wish. The person in charge of pain management called an ethics consultation, and the clinical ethicist said that the brothers' request, even if based on their traditional religious beliefs, could not override the patient's own request for pain medication that would relieve his suffering.

There are rarely good grounds for failing to respect the wishes of people based on their traditional religious or cultural beliefs. But when beliefs issue in actions that cause harm to others, attempts to prevent those harmful consequences are justifiable. An example that raises public health concerns is a ritual practiced among adherents of the religion known as Santería, practiced by people from Puerto Rico and other groups of Caribbean origin. The ritual involves scattering mercury around the household to ward off bad spirits. Mercury is a highly toxic substance that can harm adults and causes grave harm to children. Shops called "botánicas" sell mercury as well as herbs and other potions to Caribbean immigrants who use them in their healing rituals.

The public health rationale that justifies placing limitations on people's behavior in order to protect others from harm can justify prohibition of the sale of mercury and penalties for its domestic use for ritual purposes. Yet the Caribbean immigrants could object: "You are interfering with our religious practices, based on your form of scientific medicine. This is our form of religious healing and you have no right to interfere with our beliefs and practices." It would not convince this group if a doctor or public health official were to reply: "But ours is a well-confirmed, scientific practice while yours is but an ignorant, unscientific ritual." It may very well appear to the Caribbean group as an act of cultural imperialism: "These American doctors with their Anglo brand of medicine are trying to impose it on us." This raises the difficult question of how to implement public health measures when the rationale is sufficiently compelling to prohibit religious or cultural rituals. Efforts to eradicate mercury sprinkling should enlist members of the community who agree with the public health position but who are also respected members of the cultural or religious group.

BELIEF SYSTEM OF A SUBCULTURE

Some widely held ethical practices have been transformed into law, such as disclosure of risks during an informed-consent discussion and offering to patients the opportunity to make advance directives in the form of a living will or appointing a health-care agent. Yet these can pose problems for adherents of traditional cultural beliefs. In the traditional culture of Navajo Native Americans, a deeply rooted cultural belief underlies a wish not to convey or receive negative information. A study conducted on a Navajo reservation in Arizona demonstrated how Western biomedical and bioethical concepts and principles can come into conflict with traditional Navajo values and ways of thinking.[6] In March 1992, the Indian Health Service adopted the requirements of the Patient Self-Determination Act, but the Indian Health Service policy also contains the following proviso: "Tribal customs and traditional beliefs that relate to death and dying will be respected to the extent possible when providing information to patients on these issues."[6(p828)]

The relevant Navajo belief in this context is the notion that thought and language have the power to shape reality and to control events. The central concern posed by discussions about future contingencies is that traditional beliefs require people to "think and speak in a positive way." When doctors disclose risks of a treatment in an informed-consent discussion, they speak "in a negative way," thereby violating the Navajo prohibition. The traditional Navajo belief is that health is maintained and restored through positive ritual language. This presumably militates against disclosing risks of treatment as well as avoiding mention of future illness or incapacitation in a discussion about advance care planning. Western-trained doctors working with the traditional Navajo population are thus caught in a dilemma. Should they adhere to the ethical and legal standards pertaining to informed consent now in force in the rest of the United States and risk harming their patients by "talking in a negative way"? Or should they adhere to the Navajo belief system with the aim of avoiding harm to the patients but at the same time violating the ethical requirement of disclosure to patients of potential risks and future contingencies?

The authors of the published study draw several conclusions. One is that hospital policies complying with the Patient Self-Determination Act are ethically troublesome for the traditional Navajo patients. Since physicians who work with that population must decide how to act, this problem requires a solution. A second conclusion is that "the concepts and principles of Western bioethics are not universally held."[6(p829)] This comes as no surprise. It is a straightforward statement of the thesis of descriptive ethical relativism, the evident truth that a wide variety of cultural beliefs about morality exist in the world. The question for normative ethics endures: What follows from these particular facts of cultural relativity? A third conclusion the authors draw, in light of their findings, is that health-care providers and institutions caring for Navajo patients should reevaluate their policies and procedures regarding advance care planning.

This situation is not difficult to resolve, ethically or practically. The Patient Self-Determination Act does not mandate patients to actually make an advance directive; it requires only that health-care institutions provide information to patients and give them the opportunity to make a living will or appoint a health-care agent. A physician or nurse working for the Indian Health Service could easily fulfill this requirement by asking Navajo patients if they wish to discuss their future care or options, without introducing any of the negative thinking. This approach resolves one of the limitations of the published study. As the authors acknowledge, the findings reflect a more traditional perspective and the full range of Navajo views is not represented. So it is possible that some patients who use the Indian Health Service may be willing or even eager to have frank discussions about risks of treatment and future possibilities, even negative ones, if offered the opportunity.

It is more difficult, however, to justify withholding from patients the risks of proposed treatment in an informed-consent discussion. The article about the Navajo beliefs recounts an episode told by a Navajo woman who is also a nurse. Her father was a candidate for bypass surgery. When the surgeon informed the patient of the risks of surgery, including the possibility that he might not wake up, the elderly Navajo man refused the surgery altogether. If the patient did indeed require the surgery and refused because he believed that telling him of the risk of not waking up would bring about that result, then it would be justifiable to withhold that risk of surgery. Should not that possibility be routinely withheld from all patients, then, since the prospect of not waking up could lead other people—Navajos and non-Navajos alike—to refuse the surgery? The answer is no, but it requires further analysis.

Respect for autonomy grants patients who have been properly informed the right to refuse a proposed medical treatment. An honest and appropriate disclosure of the purpose, procedures, risks, benefits, and available alternatives, provided in terms the patient can understand, puts the ultimate decision in the hands of the patient. This is the ethical standard according to Western bioethics. A clear exception exists in the case of patients who lack decisional capacity altogether, and debate continues regarding the ethics of paternalistically overriding the refusal of marginally competent patients. This picture relies on a key feature that is lacking in the Navajo case: a certain metaphysical account of the way the world works. Western doctors and their patients generally do not believe that talking about risks of harm will produce those harms (although there have been accounts that document the "dark side" of the placebo effect). It is not really the Navajo values that create the crosscultural problem but rather, their metaphysical belief system holding that thought and language have the power to shape reality and control events. In fact, the Navajo values are quite the same as the standard Western ones: fear of death and avoidance of harmful side effects. To understand the relationship between cultural variation and ethical relativism, it is essential to distinguish between cultural relativity that stems from a difference in values and that which can be traced to an underlying metaphysics or epistemology.

Against this background, only two choices are apparent: insist on disclosing to Navajo patients the risks of treatment and thereby inflict unwanted negative thoughts on them, or withhold information about the risks and state only the anticipated benefits of the proposed treatment. Between those two choices, there is no contest. The second is clearly ethically preferable. It is true that withholding information about the risks of treatment or potential adverse events in the future radically changes what is required by the doctrine of informed consent. It essentially removes the 'informed" aspect, while leaving in place the notion that the patient should decide. The physician will still provide some information to the Navajo patient, but only the type of information that is acceptable to the Navajos who adhere to this particular belief system. True, withholding certain information that would typically be disclosed to patients departs from the ethical ideal of informed consent, but it does so in order to achieve the ethically appropriate goal of beneficence in the care of patients.

The principle of beneficence supports the withholding of information about risks of treatment from Navajos who hold the traditional belief system. But so, too, does the principle of respect for autonomy. Navajos holding traditional beliefs can act autonomously only when they are not thinking in a negative way. If doctors tells them about bad contingencies, that will lead to negative thinking, which in their view will fail to maintain and restore health. The value of both doctor and patient is to maintain and restore health. A change in the procedures regarding the informed-consent discussion is justifiable based on a distinctive background condition: the Navajo belief system about the causal efficacy of thinking and talking in a certain way. The less-than-ideal version of informed consent does constitute a "lower" standard than that which is usually appropriate in today's medical practice. But the use of a "lower" standard is justified by the background assumption that that is what the Navajo patient prefers.

What is relative and what is nonrelative in this situation? There is a clear divergence between the Navajo belief system and that of Western science. That divergence leads to a difference in what sort of discussion is appropriate for traditional Navajos in the medical setting and that which is standard in Western medical practice. According to one description, "always disclose the risks as well as the benefits of treatment to patients," the conclusion points to ethical relativism. But a more general description, one that heeds today's call for cultural awareness and sensitivity, would be: "Carry out an informed-consent discussion in a manner appropriate to the patient's beliefs and understanding." That obligation is framed in a nonrelative way. A heart surgeon would describe the procedures, risks, and benefits of bypass surgery in one way to a patient who is another physician, in a different way to a mathematician ignorant of medical science, in yet another way to a skilled craftsman with an eighth-grade education, and still differently to a traditional Navajo. The ethical principle is the same; the procedures differ.

OBLIGATIONS OF PHYSICIANS

The problem for physicians is how to respond when an immigrant to the United States acts according to the cultural values of her native country, values that differ widely from accepted practices in American medicine. Suppose an African immigrant asks an obstetrician to perform genital surgery on her baby girl. Or imagine that a Laotian immigrant from the Iu Mien culture brings her four-month-old baby to the pediatrician for a routine visit and the doctor discovers burns on the baby's stomach. The African mother seeks to comply with the tradition in her native country, Somalia, where the vast majority of women have had clitoridectomies. The Iu Mien woman admits that she has used a traditional folk remedy to treat what she suspected was her infant's case of a rare folk illness.

What is the obligation of physicians in the United States when they encounter patients in such situations? At one extreme is the reply that in the United States, physicians are obligated to follow the ethical and cultural practices accepted here and have no obligation to comply with patients' requests that embody entirely different cultural values. At the other extreme is the view that cultural sensitivity requires physicians to adhere to the traditional beliefs and practices of patients who have emigrated from other cultures.

A growing concern on the part of doctors and public health officials is the increasing number of requests for genital cutting and defense of the practice by immigrants to the United States and European countries. A Somalian immigrant living in Houston said he believed his Muslim faith required him to have his daughters undergo the procedure; he also stated his belief that it would preserve their virginity. He was quoted as saying, "It's my responsibility. If I don't do it, I will have failed my children."[7(p1)] Another African immigrant living in Houston sought a milder form of the cutting she had undergone for her daughter. The woman said she believed it was necessary so her daughter would not run off with boys and have babies before marriage. She was disappointed that Medicaid would not cover the procedure, and planned to go to Africa to have the procedure done there. A New York City physician was asked by a father for a referral to a doctor who would do the procedure on his three-year-old daughter. When the physician told him this was not done in America, the man accused the doctor of not understanding what he wanted.[7(pp1,9)]

However, others in our multicultural society consider it a requirement of "cultural sensitivity" to accommodate in some way to such requests of African immigrants. Harborview Medical Center in Seattle sought just such a solution. A group of doctors agreed to consider making a ritual nick in the fold of skin that covers the clitoris, but without removing any tissue. However, the hospital later abandoned the plan after being flooded with letters, postcards, and telephone calls in protest.[7]

A physician who conducted research with East African women living in Seattle held the same view as the doctors who sought a culturally sensitive solution. In a talk she gave to my medical school department, she argued that Western physicians must curb their tendency to judge cultural practices different from their own as "rational" or "irrational." Ritual genital cutting is an "inalienable" part of some cultures, and it does a disservice to people from those cultures to view it as a human rights violation. She pointed out that in the countries where female genital mutilation (FGM) is practiced, circumcised women are "normal." Like some anthropologists who argue for a "softer" linguistic approach,[8] this researcher preferred the terminology of "circumcision" to that of "female genital mutilation."

One can understand and even have some sympathy for the women who believe they must adhere to a cultural ritual even when they no longer live in the society where it is widely practiced. But it does not follow that the ritual is an "inalienable" part of that culture, since every culture undergoes changes over time. Furthermore, to contend that in the countries where FGM is practiced, circumcised women are "normal" is like saying that malaria or malnutrition is "normal" in parts of Africa. That a human condition is statistically normal implies nothing whatever about whether an obligation exists to seek to alter the statistical norm for the betterment of those who are affected.

Some Africans living in the United States have said they are offended that Congress passed a law prohibiting female genital mutilation that appears to be directed specifically at Africans. France has also passed legislation, but its law relies on general statutes that prohibit violence against children.[7] In a recent landmark case, a French court sent a Gambian woman to jail for having had the genitals of her two baby daughters mutilated by a midwife. French doctors report an increasing number of cases of infants who are brought to clinics hemorrhaging or with severe infections.

Views on what constitutes the appropriate response to requests from parents to health professionals for advice or referrals regarding the genital mutilation of their daughters vary considerably. Three commentators gave their opinions on a case vignette in which several African families living in a U.S. city planned to have the ritual performed on their daughters. If the procedure could not be done in the U.S., the families planned to have it done in Africa. One of the parents sought advice from health professionals.

One commentator, a child psychiatrist, commented that professional ethical practice requires her to respect and try to understand the cultural and religious practices of the group making the request.[9] She then cited another ethical requirement of clinical practice: her need to promote the physical and psychological well-being of the child and refusal to condone parenting practices that constitute child abuse according to the social values and laws of her city and country. Most of what this child psychiatrist would do with the mother who comes to her involves discussion, mutual understanding, education, and the warning that in this location performing the genital cutting ritual would probably be considered child abuse.

The psychiatrist would remain available for a continuing dialogue with the woman and others in her community, but would stop short of making a child-abuse report since the woman was apparently only considering carrying out the ritual. However, the psychiatrist would make the report if she had knowledge that the mother was actually planning to carry out the ritual or if it had already been performed. She would make the child-abuse report reluctantly, however, and only if she believed the child to be at risk and if there were no other option. She concluded by observing that the mother is attempting to act in the best interest of her child and does not intend to harm her. The psychiatrist's analysis demonstrates the possible ambiguities of the concept of child abuse. Is abuse determined solely by the intention of the adult? Should child abuse be judged by the harmful consequences to the child, regardless of the adult's intention? Of course, if a law defines the performance of female genital mutilation as child abuse, then it is child abuse, from a legal point of view, and physicians are obligated to report any case for which there is a reasonable suspicion. Legal definitions aside, intentions are relevant for judging the moral worth of people, but not for the actions they perform. This means that the good intentions of parents could exonerate them from blame if their actions cause harm to their children, but the harmful actions nevertheless remain morally wrong.

The second commentator, a clinical psychologist and licensed sex therapist, would do many of the same things as the child psychiatrist, but would go a bit further in finding others from the woman's community and possibly another support network.[10] Like most other commentators on female genital mutilation, this discussant remarked that "agents of change must come from within a culture."[10(p289)]

The third commentator on this case vignette was the most reluctant to be critical. A British historian and barrister, he began with the observation that "a people's culture demands the highest respect."[11] On the one hand, he noted that custom, tradition, and religion are not easily uprooted. But on the other hand, he pointed out that no human practice is beyond questioning. He contended that the debate over the nature and impact of female circumcision is a "genuine debate," and the ritual probably had practical utility when it was introduced into the societies that still engage in it. Of the three commentators, he voiced the strongest opposition to invoking the child abuse laws because it "would be an unwarranted criminalization of parents grappling in good faith with a practice that is legal and customary in their home country."[11(p291)] In the end, this discussant would approach the parents "much as a lawyer would address a jury," leaving the parents (like a jury) to deliberate and come to an informed decision. He would also involve the girls in this process, since they are adolescents, and should have input into the deliberations.

It is tempting to wonder whether the involvement of adolescent girls in deliberations of their parents would, in traditional Gambian culture, be even remotely considered, much less accepted. The "lawyer-jury-adolescent involvement" solution looks to be very Western. If these families living in the United States still wish to adhere to their cultural tradition of genital mutilation, is it likely that they will appreciate the reasoned, deliberative approach this last commentator proposed?

Exactly where to draw the line in such cases is a difficult matter. Presumably, one could go further than any of these commentators and inform the African families that since U.S. law prohibits female genital mutilation, which has been likened to child abuse, a health professional would be obligated to inform relevant authorities of an intention to commit child abuse. Conceivably, U.S. authorities could prevent immigrants from returning to this country if they have gone to Africa to have a procedure performed that would be illegal if done within the United States. But this is a matter of law, not ethics, and would involve a gross invasion of privacy since to enforce the ruling it would be necessary to examine the genitals of the adolescent girls when these families sought reentry into the United States. That would be going too far and probably deserves condemnation as "ethical imperialism." Since the cutting would already have been done, punitive action toward the family could not succeed in preventing the harm.

Another case vignette describes a Laotian woman from the Mien culture who immigrated to the United States and married a Mien man. When she visited her child's pediatrician for a routine four-month immunization, the doctor was horrified to see five red and blistered quarter-inch round markings on the child's abdomen.[12] The mother explained that she used a traditional Mien "cure" for pain, since she thought the infant was experiencing a rare folk illness among Mien babies characterized by incessant crying and loss of appetite, in addition to other symptoms. The "cure" involves dipping a reed in pork fat, lighting the reed, and passing the burning substance over the skin, raising a blister that "pops like popcorn." The popping indicates that the illness is not related to spiritual causes; if no blisters appear, then a shaman may have to be summoned to conduct a spiritual ritual for a cure. As many as eleven burns might be needed before the end of the "treatment." The burns are then covered with a mentholated cream.

The Mien woman told the pediatrician that infection is rare and the burns heal in a week or so. Scars sometimes remain but are not considered disfiguring. She also told the doctor that the procedure must be done by someone skilled in burning, since if a burn is placed too near the line between the baby's mouth and navel, the baby could become mute or even retarded. The mother considered the cure to have been successful in the case of her baby, since the child had stopped crying and regained her appetite. Strangely enough, the pediatrician did not say anything to the mother about her practice of burning the baby, no doubt from the need to show "cultural sensitivity." She did, however, wonder later whether she should have said something since she thought the practice was dangerous and also cruel to babies.

One commentator who wrote about this case proposed using "an ethnographic approach" to ethics in the crosscultural setting.[13] This approach need not result in a strict ethical relativism, however, since one can be respectful of cultural differences and at the same time acknowledge that there are limits. What is critical is the perceived degree of harm; some cultural practices may constitute atrocities and violations of fundamental human rights. The commentator argued that the pediatrician must first seek to understand the Mien woman in the context of her world before trying to educate her in the ways of Western medicine. The commentator stopped short of providing a solution, but noted that many possible resolutions can be found for crosscultural ethical conflicts. Be that as it may, we still need to determine which of the pediatrician's obligations should take precedence: to seek to protect her infant patient (and possibly also the Mien woman's other children) from harmful rituals or to exhibit cultural sensitivity and refrain from attempts at reeducation or critical admonitions.

A second pair of commentators assumed a nonjudgmental stance. These commentators urged respect for cultural diversity and defended the Mien woman's belief system as entirely rational: "It is well grounded in her culture; it is practiced widely; the reasons for it are widely understood among the Iu Mien; the procedure, from a Mien point of view, works."[14(p17)] This is a culturally relative view of rationality. The same argument could just as well be used to justify female genital mutilation. Nevertheless, the commentators rejected what they said was the worst choice: simply to tolerate the practice as a primitive cultural artifact and do nothing more. They also rejected the opposite extreme: a referral of child abuse to the appropriate authorities. The mother's actions did not constitute intentional abuse, since she actually believed she was helping the child by providing a traditional remedy. Here I think the commentators are correct in rejecting a referral to the child-abuse authorities, since a charge of child abuse can have serious consequences that may ultimately run counter to the best interests of the child.

What did these commentators recommend? Not to try to prohibit the practice directly, which could alienate the parent. Instead, the pediatrician could discuss the risk of infection and suggest safer pain remedies. The doctor should also learn more about the rationale for and technique of the traditional burning "cure." The most she should do, according to these commentators, is consider sharing her concerns with the local Mien community, but not with the mother alone.

There is in these commentaries a great reluctance to criticize, scold, or take legal action against parents from other cultures who employ painful and potentially harmful rituals that have no scientific basis. This attitude of tolerance is appropriate against the background knowledge that the parents do not intend to harm the child and are simply using a folk remedy widely accepted in their own culture. But tolerance of these circumstances must be distinguished from a judgment that the actions harmful to children should be permitted to continue. What puzzles me is the notion that "cultural sensitivity" must extend so far as to refrain from providing a solid education to these parents about the potential harms and the infliction of gratuitous pain. In a variety of other contexts, we accept the role of physicians as educator of patients. Doctors are supposed to tell their patients not to smoke, to lose weight, and to have appropriate preventive medical checkups such as pap smears, mammograms, and proctoscopic examinations.

Pediatricians are thought to have an even more significant obligation to educate the parents of their vulnerable patients: inform them of steps that minimize the risks of sudden infant death syndrome, tell them what is appropriate for an infant's or child's diet, and give them a wide array of other social and psychological information designed to keep a child healthy and flourishing. Are these educational obligations of pediatricians only appropriate for patients whose background culture is that of the United States or Western Europe? Should a pediatrician not attempt to educate parents who, in their practice of the Santería religion, sprinkle mercury around the house? The obligation of pediatricians to educate and even to urge parents to adopt practices likely to contribute to the good health and well-being of their children, and to avoid practices that will definitely or probably cause harm and suffering, should know no cultural boundaries.

My position is consistent with the realization that Western medicine does not have all the answers. This position also recognizes that some traditional healing practices are not only not harmful but may be as beneficial as those of Western medicine. The injunction to "respect cultural diversity" could rest on the premise that Western medicine sometimes causes harm without compensating benefits (which is true) or on the equally true premise that traditional practices such as acupuncture and herbal remedies, once scorned by mainstream Western medicine, have come to be accepted side by side with the precepts of scientific medicine. Typically, however, respect for multicultural diversity goes well beyond these reasonable views and requires toleration of manifestly painful or harmful procedures such as the burning remedy employed in the Mien culture. We ought to be able to respect cultural diversity without having to accept every single feature embedded in traditional beliefs and rituals.

The reluctance to impose modern medicine on immigrants from a fear that it constitutes yet another instance of "cultural imperialism" is misplaced. Is it not possible to accept non-Western cultural practices side by side with Western ones, yet condemn those that are manifestly harmful and have no compensating benefit except for the cultural belief that they are beneficial? The commentators who urged respect for the Mien woman's burning treatment on the grounds that it is practiced widely; the reasons for it are widely understood among the Mien; and the procedure works, from a Mien point of view, seemed to be placing that practice on a par with practices that "work" from the point of view of Western medicine. Recall that if the skin does not blister, the Mien belief holds that the illness may be related to spiritual causes and a shaman might have to be called. Should the pediatrician stand by and do nothing if the child has a fever of 104° and the parent calls a shaman because the skin did not blister? Recall also that the Mien woman told the pediatrician that if the burns are not done in the right place, the baby could become mute or even retarded. Must we reject the beliefs of Western medicine regarding causality and grant equal status to the Mien beliefs? To refrain from seeking to educate such parents and to not exhort them to alter their traditional practices is unjust, as it exposes the immigrant children to health risks that are not borne by children from the majority culture.

It is heresy in today's postmodern climate of respect for the belief systems of all cultures to entertain the notion that some beliefs are demonstrably false and others, whether true or false, lead to manifestly harmful actions. We are not supposed to talk about the evolution of scientific ideas or about progress in the Western world, since that is a colonialist way of thinking. If it is simply "the white man's burden, medicalized"[15] to urge African families living in the United States not to genitally mutilate their daughters, or to attempt to educate Mien mothers about the harms of burning their babies, then we are doomed to permit ethical relativism to overwhelm common sense.

Multiculturalism, as defined at the beginning of this paper, appears to embrace ethical relativism and yet is logically inconsistent with relativism. The second half of the definition states that multiculturalism "insists that all cultural groups be treated with respect and as equals." What does this imply with regard to cultural groups that oppress or fail to respect other cultural groups? Must the cultural groups that violate the mandate to treat all cultural groups with respect and as equals be respected themselves? It is impossible to insist that all such groups be treated with respect and as equals, and at the same time accept any particular group's attitude toward and treatment of another group as inferior. Every cultural group contains subgroups within the culture: old and young, women and men, people with and people without disabilities. Are the cultural groups that discriminate against women or people with disabilities to be respected equally with those that do not?

What multiculturalism does not say is whether all of the beliefs and practices of all cultural groups must be equally respected. It is one thing to require that cultural, religious, and ethnic groups be treated as equals; that conforms to the principle of justice as equality. It is quite another thing to say that any cultural practice whatever of any group is to be tolerated and respected equally. This latter view is a statement of extreme ethical relativism. If multiculturalists endorse the principle of justice as equality, however, they must recognize that normative ethical relativism entails the illogical consequence of toleration and acceptance of numerous forms of injustice in those cultures that oppress women and religious and ethnic minorities.

This article is adopted from a chapter in the author's Against Relativism: Cultural Diversity and the Search for Ethical Universals in Medicine. *New York, NY: Oxford Univesity Press; 1999.*

REFERENCES

1. Fowers BJ, Richardson FC. Why is multiculturalism good? American Psychologist. 1996;51:609–621.

2. Fox RC. The evolution of American bioethics: a sociological perspective. In: Weisz G.

Social Science Perspectives on Medical Ethics. Philadelphia, PA: University of Pennsylvania Press; 1990.

3. Nelson KL. Taking families seriously. *Hastings Center Report.* 1992;22(4):6–12.

4. Hardwig J. What about the family? *Hastings Center Report.* 1990;20(2):5–10.

5. Blackhall L, Murphy ST, Frank G, Michel V, Azen S. Ethnicity and attitudes toward patient autonomy. *JAMA.* 1995;274:820–825.

6. Carrese J, Rhodes L. Western bioethics on the Navajo reservation: benefit or harm? *JAMA.* 1995;274:826–829.

7. Dugger CW. Tug of taboos: African genital rite vs. U.S. law. *New York Times.* December 28, 1996: 1, 9.

8. Lane SD, Rubinstein RA. Judging the other: responding to traditional female genital surgeries. *Hastings Center Report.* 1996;26(5):31–40.

9. Brant R. Child abuse or acceptable cultural norms: child psychiatrist's response. *Ethics & Behavior.* 1995;5:284–287.

10. Wyatt GE. Ethical issues in culturally relevant intervention. *Ethics & Behavior.* 1995;5:288–290.

11. Martin T. Cultural contexts. *Ethics & Behavior.* 1995;5:290–292.

12. Case study: culture, healing, and professional obligations. *Hastings Center Report.* 1993;23(4):15.

13. Carrese J. Culture, healing, and professional obligations: commentary. *Hastings Center Report.* 1993;23(4):16.

14. Brown K, Jameton A. Cutlure, healing, and professional obligations: commentary. *Hastings Center Report.* 1993;23(4):17.

15. Morsy SA. Safeguarding women's bodies: the white man's burden medicalized. *Medical Anthropology Quarterly.* 1991;5(1):19–23.

Part 2

CARING FOR GERIATRIC PATIENTS

❦

Older Americans face a number of problems and concerns with regard to health care. Deciding which ethical issues to address in this section made evident just how stacked the deck is against them. Those not on the higher end of our socioeconomic scale have to spend a large portion of their fixed monthly income on medications. Others have to use all of their financial reserves and then go on Medicaid in order to afford nursing home care. To make maters worse, our health-care system is in large part an acute-care system; leaving chronic and long-term care by the wayside, as evidenced by the morally repugnant conditions that are present in many nursing homes. In the end, the three issues addressed in this section, which are pervasive throughout our health-care system, are issues that individual health-care providers can do something about. These issues are (1) the use of restraints, (2) caring for patients with Alzheimer's, and (3) the lack of appropriate pain management.

The first article, by Susan Dodds, is titled "Exercising Restraint: Autonomy, Welfare, and Elderly Patients." Dodds clearly and succinctly discusses the harm that is done when a geriatric patient is restrained, whether physically or chemically. Harm can be seen in terms of the patient's freedom, dignity, sense of worth, and health. Another effect brought about by the use of restraints, although Dodds does not explicitly discuss it, is damage to the patient–health-care provider relationship. One patient described being restrained as feeling "like I was a dog and [I] cried all night. It hurt me to have to be tied up. I felt like I was nobody, that I was dirt."[1] After this experience, how could that patient—or any of us—feel safe and protected? More to the point, without trust there is no health-care provider–patient relationship. And forming a trusting relationship with the health-care providers who used restraint, would, to say the least, be problematic. Although Dodds discusses restraints primarily within the nursing home context, these issues are just as relevant to hospital patients.

Importantly, there are certainly situations when the use of restraints is appropriate. In such situations, health-care providers know that there are two ways a patient can be restrained. The first respects the patient as someone who needs to be restrained because she is ill, and may hurt herself or, inadvertently, someone else. This way promotes a patient's dignity as best as possible under the circumstances. The second way views the patient as someone who deserves to be restrained because she is "bad," or, to use the more common euphemism, she is combative. This way is demeaning, painful, and often abusive. Those who are subjected to the latter may be patients with dementia who grab or scratch, or patients who have overdosed and are uncooperative. Ultimately, restraints can either further the interests of the patient by protecting her from harm, or they can be used as a means of punishment.

The next article, "The Fear of Forgetfulness: A Grassroots Approach to an Ethics of Alzheimer's Disease," by Stephen Post, is a nice segue from Dodds, as many Alzheimer's patients are restrained and/or confined to a hospital or nursing home "lock-down unit." Although the use of restraints with this patient population is decreasing, it is still by no means uncommon.

Post goes on to point out that this disease is not a disease just of the patient, but of all his informal caregivers, typically friends and family. This disease brings about circumstances in which the patient loses his understanding of who he is, as well as of the world around him. Caregivers must help him to do those things he used to enjoy—even though he is no longer the "person" who once enjoyed them. Interestingly, by helping the patient participate in once-loved activities, the caregiver is often in some sense trying to get back the person she loved by doing those activities that made the patient who he was, for those activities now only have meaning for the informal caregiver.

It is issues such as this that health-care providers need to consider when treating patients with Alzheimer's. When a health-care provider asks an informal caregiver how a patient is doing—"Does she still remember you? Your children?"—he is talking to someone whose sense of connectedness to the patient has been crushed. Therefore, on many levels the health-care provider has to *care* for both the patient and patient's informal caregiver(s). This is the underlying theme of Post's article.

Post does a wonderful job discussing what autonomy means to someone who no longer has a sense self. He raises other important issues, such as whether patients should be told of their diagnosis, genetic testing, the use of feeding tubes, and how the use of antidementia medications can actually bring about harm.

This section ends with a study that first appeared in the June 1998 issue of the *Journal of the American Medical Association*. In "Management of Pain in Elderly Patients with Cancer," Roberto Bernabei and colleagues look at the adequacy of pain management in nursing homes. The authors found that 26 percent of those who had chronic cancer-related pain received nothing for it; additionally, they "found a strong inverse correlation between the presence of pain and increasing age and an equally strong relationship between pain and belonging to minority groups." As with Dodds, this study discusses this issue from within the nursing home context; this issue, however, is endemic to our entire health-care system. From physician offices in rural America to the most sophisticated academic medical centers, patients are not receiving appropriate care for their pain—nursing home residents, our most vulnerable population, just have it the worst. These results evoke a great number of ethical issues that health-care providers must begin to address, primarily justice and dignity.

There are many ways to conceive of justice, but for our purpose we can take it mean that each patient ought to be treated equally and fairly. For example, a patient being treated for cancer deserves appropriate therapies (e.g., medications, chemotherapy, radiation, etc.) that are necessary to either cure or ameliorate his illness. Patients are owed these benefits because health-care providers have a duty to provide them. So when such benefits are withheld based on advanced age or minority status, these patients are being treated unfairly and unequally in light of what health-care providers owe them; in short, they are being treated unjustly.

Dignity is another key issue this study raises. True pain is all-consuming. By true pain, I mean pain caused by ailments such as cancer, severe peripheral neuropathy, severe burns, and spinal injuries. It is these kinds of pain that force a patient to reformulate her goals, activities, and sense of hope. She may no longer be able to play her favorite sport, hold her child, take a romantic walk with her spouse, or even continue doing the job she loves. It is these cherished activities that give our lives meaning.

Those who have spent years training and working toward the goal of being a professional athlete, firefighter, nurse, or teacher may no longer be able to perform their duties. As a result of no longer being able participate in those activities that many of a patient's relationships were based on, these relationships may be compromised or lost.

Hope is also forced to accommodate the burdens of pain. Initially, a patient hopes his diagnosis is wrong. When it is not, he hopes that the treatments will cure him. When they do not, he hopes that the pain will not be too bad. When it is, he hopes that his pain will be treated. When it is not, he just hopes that each day will not be as bad as the one before. With these consequences of untreated (or undertreated) severe pain in mind, imagine the anger and the feelings of abandonment that patients experience, knowing that their health-care providers could easily treat their pain, but do not.

To have dignity is to be able to take care of oneself, to be able to fulfill one's own basic needs. When any of us can no longer do this, we see ourselves as belittled and humiliated. These are burdens that individual health-care providers can help to prevent or relieve.

REFERENCE

1. Dodds S. Exercising restraint: autonomy, welfare, and elderly patients. In this volume: 55.

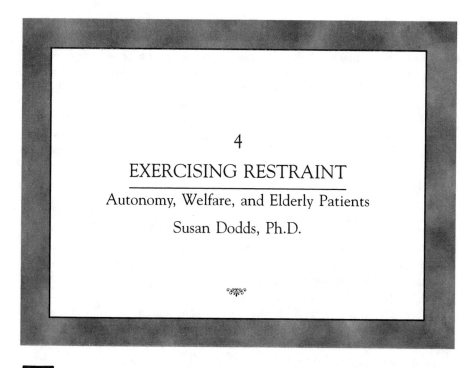

4

EXERCISING RESTRAINT

Autonomy, Welfare, and Elderly Patients

Susan Dodds, Ph.D.

The use of mechanical restraints to limit the freedom of individuals poses a great threat to personal dignity. People whose freedom is reduced through the use of restraints often become agitated, angry, and, eventually, resigned to their loss of freedom.[1-3] Testimony of patients who have been so restrained reveals the sense of loss of personal integrity and dignity that accompanies this loss of freedom. Evans and Strumpf quote two patients' experiences of restraint in hospital. A seventy-two-year-old man said: "I felt like I was a dog and cried all night. It hurt me to have to be tied up. I felt like I was nobody, that I was dirt. It makes me cry to talk about it.... The hospital is worse than a jail."[2] An eighty-four-year-old woman recalled her experience this way: "I don't remember misbehaving, but I may have been deranged from all the pills they gave me. Normally, I am spirited, but I am also good and obedient. Nevertheless, the nurse tied me down, like Jesus on the cross, by bandaging both wrists and ankles.... It felt awful, I hurt and I worried, 'What if I get leg cramps; what will I do then if I can't move?' It was miserable ... and an awful shock.... Because I am a cooperative person, I felt so resentful. Callers, including men friends, saw me like that and I lost something; I lost a little personal prestige. I was embarrassed, like a child placed in a corner for being bad.... I haven't forgotten the pain and indignity of being tied."[2]

S. Dodd. "Exercising Restraint: Autonomy, Welfare and Elderly Patients." *Journal of Medical Ethics.* 1996;22:160–163. Reprinted by permission of the BMJ Publishing Group.

It is not surprising that health professionals considering whether to use mechanical restraints to limit the actions of elderly patients are often deeply distressed by the prospect. Those who have to make such decisions may feel themselves confronted by two conflicting moral obligations: the duty to protect those in their care from harm and the duty to respect the autonomy of other persons. This paper argues that justifications for the use of restraints based on the duty to protect elderly patients from harm are much weaker than many who rely on them may hope, in light of empirical evidence and a careful articulation of "harm." Moreover, it argues that the duty to respect an individual's remaining autonomy persists, even after the individual ceases to be legally competent. The imposition of physical restraints on paternalistic grounds, thus, has very limited justification. Further, the imposition of restraints in order to protect third parties, such as health-care staff or other patients, is rarely justified. Finally, while in the United States restraints are frequently applied to protect nursing homes from litigation in the event of a fall or accident,[4-6] those medico-legal issues are not addressed here, in part because litigation should be informed by ethics, rather than ethics responding to litigation.

To clarify what I mean by restraints: Restraints are any intentionally placed impediment to another's freedom of action. For older patients in nursing homes these impediments may include mechanical restraints, for example vest, pelvic, or waist restraints that are attached to standard chairs, wheelchairs, or to geriatric recliner chairs, and raised side rails on hospital beds (with or without ankle and wrist bandages tied to them); and the use of locked doors and barred windows to restrict the movement of patients. Chemical restraints—the use of psychotropic drugs where there is no recorded diagnosis of mental disorder—are also used to reduce patients' desire to move about.[7] As the use of chemical restraints raises issues that fall outside the scope of this paper, this discussion is restricted to the use of mechanical restraints in nursing homes.

Restraints may be placed on a person with her or his consent. For example, a woman who has cerebral palsy and is unable to hold herself in an upright sitting position may choose to have her freedom of movement restrained so that she may engage in various activities that she would otherwise be unable to do. Alternatively, a man can be bound by a waist restraint to his chair without his consent and against his will. My concern here is whether a policy of routine use of mechanical restraints in geriatric care without consent is morally justified.

None of us would think it morally justifiable to have others bind us to our chairs, to imprison us against our will, without very good reasons. Given that use of restraints limits personal freedom in a way which we would usually think reprehensible, the onus must be on those who advocate use of restraints to establish the justifiability of their use. Many sincere health professionals working in nursing homes would defend limited use of mechanical restraints on the grounds that the restraints are required to protect their patients from harm. Their argument might be of the following form. A special relationship exists between residents of nursing homes and those who have responsibility for their care. This special relationship gives rise to a moral duty on the part of the caregivers to protect those in their care from harm. Frail, elderly patients may sometimes lose their balance or become confused and disoriented and, as a result, risk harming themselves or others unless their movements are restricted. Thus, in certain circumstances, health professionals are morally obliged to place mechanical restraints on patients to protect them from harm.

This argument needs to be filled out to be at all useful in practice. We would need to know what harm is supposedly protected against by use of restraints and how serious or probable that harm needs to be before application of restraints is justified. Further, we would need to know how strong the moral duty to protect those in one's care from harm is and how it compares with other duties (such as the duty to respect autonomy) that health-care workers may have. When we examine some of the assumptions implicit in this defense of the use of restraints we find that this argument would only justify very limited use of restraints.

What harm is being prevented by use of restraints? Harm that restraint use is intended to avoid includes: physical injury such as stumbling and breaking a hip (with the attendant grave effects on older patients); falling out of bed or a chair; risks of physical harm associated with wandering; and harms associated with failing to receive adequate treatment.[8] Sometimes restraints are used in the hopes they will reduce psychological harm such as agitation, anxiety about falling out of bed, confusion that may result from wandering, and so on. Some of these can be serious, even fatal, and restraints may serve to reduce them, but we must also consider whether restraints are effective at protecting against these harms, whether there are equivalent harms associated with use of restraints, and whether effective alternatives to restraints are available.

Empirical research has indicated there is little evidence to suggest that restraints are effective;[6] various authors cite as evidence that restrained residents in a nursing home setting exhibited the same, or more agitated, behaviors than unrestrained residents;[3] that the use of bed rails is not effective at preventing falling out of bed in acute hospital settings;[3] "that the risk of injury from falls out of bed actually increases when restraints are applied and that restraints do not remove risk of injury";[2,5] and that previously restrained nursing home residents experience no greater incidence of serious falls once their restraints are removed and, while they experience more nonserious falls than when they were restrained, they experience no greater incidence of nonserious falls than those residents who have never been restrained.[9] Further, two nursing homes that have never used restraints in their many years of service record, "no more injuries from falls than do facilities that use restraints."[1] The evidence suggests that risk of some of the harm that use of restraints is intended to protect against may be increased by their use. Indeed, accidental death has been reported after patients have attempted to escape from beds or chairs while restrained.[2,3]

Further, there is a body of evidence to suggest that restrained older patients suffer other ill effects from being restrained. Restrained patients "often suffer from chronic constipation; incontinence; pressure sores; loss of bone mass, muscle tone, and the ability to walk independently."[1,3] Other harm associated with restraint use includes: skin abrasions; abnormal changes in body chemistry, basal metabolic rate, and blood volume; lower extremity edema; contractures; cardiac stress; and reduced functional capacity.[2] The psychological harm associated with restraint is also significant: mechanical restraint may contribute to sensory deprivation, disorganized behavior, loss of self-image, and dependency; restraint may "increase confusion or precipitate regressive behavior and withdrawal";[1,2] agitation is often increased,[8] as is anger and demoralization of residents.[3] It appears that regular use of one's limbs and intellectual capacities of the sort that occurs when a person moves about freely assists in the preservation of these abilities and of health more generally.[10] All in all, while restraints are intended to protect against harm, they may actually contribute to reduced health. At the very least this empirical evidence gives us reason to question the efficacy of restraints and indicates that alternatives to restraints should be sought to avoid the health risks posed by their use.

Evans has conducted crosscultural research that indicates that refraining from use of restraints can be consistent with good health practice.[4,11] This study points out the differences between American and Scottish nursing home staff in their attitudes towards the use of restraints. In Scotland, restraints are rarely used and it is accepted that while there are certain risks associated with unrestrained patients moving about, taking these risks is justified by respect for patients' autonomy and awareness of the benefits of continued mobility.[4,11]

Blakeslee's account of her nursing experience[1] describes some alternative ways of protecting older patients from harm that she has developed in nursing home settings. She has been involved with two nursing homes in which restraints have never been used. Rearrangement of ward design, physical and behavioral therapy, and cooperation among all staff made it possible to protect patients from harm without depriving them of their freedom.[1]

A policy of justified restraint use must involve an assessment of the risk of harm posed by the absence of restraint as compared with the risk of harm posed by the imposition of restraints. This assessment must attend to both the seriousness of the harm and the probability of the harm occurring. A very low probability of a serious injury occurring if no restraints are imposed may well be outweighed by a very high probability of less serious injury occurring if restraints are used. The degree to which alternatives to restraint reduce the probability of harm occurring must also be assessed.

The availability of alternatives will frequently depend on resources, attitudes, and policies of health professionals, institutions, and governments. Nonetheless, whoever claims that restraints are required to protect those in nursing home care from harm should be prepared to examine the empirical evidence concerning the use or avoidance of mechanical restraints, in order to make a genuine assessment of the risk of harm to those who would be restrained.

Although harm to health is the most frequently cited (and most easily tabulated) in the literature, the relative harm to physical and emotional health risked by restraint use or abeyance is not the only kind of harm at stake. To be deprived of freedom and to have one's capacity for self-determination limited without consent are, in themselves, great harms—or simply wrongs—to individuals, even if done from a worthy motive. As the testimonials above imply, use of restraints threatens our sense of ourselves as persons, and may lead to a loss of self-respect. To feel like "a dog," "a nobody," "dirt," or to suffer loss of personal dignity are surely indications that the debate concerning use of restraints is not simply about protecting patients from harm to their health, but also about treating patients of all ages as persons worthy of respect. Imposing restraints on a person without consent may very well indicate a lack of respect for the patient as a person, a moral agent who has an interest in his or her own welfare and freedom.

The past twenty years have seen a shift in emphasis in health care from a strongly paternalistic approach to greater concern and respect for the personal autonomy of patients. No longer can health-care workers assume that the sole issue at stake in health care is the health of the patient. The language of patients' rights and self-determination has permeated medical schools, nursing faculties, and health-care institutions. When one is assessing the merits of restraints, one must count all harm to a person's interests. Some of those interests are in health and physical well-being, but others are interests in freedom, personal dignity, autonomy, and respect by others.

Patients in nursing homes are very often people who were active in pursuing various interests for most of their lives. They have made autonomous choices about their careers, their families, their values, their health, and the course of their lives. These choices would often have involved taking risks. For example, in deciding to marry, a person risks hurting her or himself deeply if the marriage fails; rock climbing risks serious physical harm, perhaps even death; and investing all one's savings in one particular venture may lead to financial ruin. The choices made and the risks taken by these people throughout their lives reflect the interests and the values that are part of their identities as autonomous individuals. There is no reason to believe that when people become older and less able to live fully independently, they lose all interests beyond protection of their health. On the contrary, many people, despite sometimes experiencing lapses of memory or periods of confusion, have a clear view that life and health are just two values among many and a firm idea of how they want to live out the rest of their lives.[12,13]

Nursing homes are designed to look after the health interests of those in their care and health-care professionals in such homes have special responsibilities to protect the health of those in their care. Such professionals also have immense control over the lives of patients, who are often entirely dependent on nursing home staff in order to pursue any of their interests. From this disproportionate power also arises the special responsibility of nursing home staff to respect the autonomy of patients. They may have to look beyond conventional practices to ensure that their policies do respect the dignity, freedom, and autonomy of their patients.

That a person is frail and unsteady on her or his feet does not render her or him incapable of making autonomous choices, even if the frailty and unsteadiness increases the risk that she or he will be harmed. Further, the loss of some mental functioning may be good reason for limiting a person's responsibilities concerning her or his affairs (for example, the appointment of a guardian responsible for managing the person's financial affairs). But to say that a person lacks sufficient capacity to exercise autonomy in these areas is not to say that she or he lacks autonomy outright. Thus, a person may lack legal competence and yet still be a person whose autonomy ought to be respected. The ability to understand or retain sufficient information to make complex choices about treatment (that is competence to consent to that treatment), may be lost without loss of all competence to make choices or to express preferences. Autonomy develops by degrees; so, too, can it diminish over time. In some cases respect for autonomy requires that health professionals act on the previously articulated preferences and attitudes of a person who is no longer able to express her or his autonomy. In such cases a guardian may be able to articulate the autonomous interests of a patient.

Neither nursing home residents nor those outside nursing homes have a moral obligation to preserve their own health above all else. Residents are owed the respect due to persons: They are entitled to have their interests respected even if pursuit of their interests means that they might hurt themselves. To deprive a person of freedom of action without consent is, prima facie, a violation of the duty to respect persons. If use of restraints is proposed, then consent from either the patient or from the patient's proxy (who is charged to act in the interests of the patient), must be sought and granted. Such consent should only be given where adequate information is offered about the nature and duration of the restraint, the reason for its use, and the risks associated with the use of restraint as opposed to absence of restraint (or other alternatives).

Where it is genuinely the best available course of care, use of constraints may be justified without the patient's consent if the patient lacks sufficient autonomy to make any kind of choice, or to recognize in very basic terms the nature of her or his choice. However, her or his guardian or proxy must consent to the use of restraints in light of the guardian's knowledge of the patient and the evidence given to support restraint use.

Some may argue that use of restraints on a patient, without consent, can be justified to protect other patients and staff from harm. One question to be asked is whether this kind of restraint is proposed as protection or as punishment.[8] It is generally accepted that the only authority that can legitimately deprive adults of their liberty, as punishment, is the state (through the court system) and, thus, that it would be illegitimate for nursing home staff to deprive individuals of their liberty as a form of punishment. If restraints are to be used as protection for others, one must ask on what grounds the other patients or staff are believed to be at risk. Surely the test for use of restraints in these cases must take into account the risk of harm posed by restraint to the person to be restrained as compared to the risk of harm posed to the staff or other patients. If nursing home staff have no business using restraints as punishment (as it would be a form of illegal and unjustified imprisonment), then the harm that is to be avoided must be at least as great as the harm that is risked through use of restraints, in order to justify this limitation of freedom.

Two weaknesses in the standard defense of the use of mechanical restraints on elderly nursing home patients have been uncovered: firstly, empirical evidence suggests that restraints may cause the kinds of harm they are intended to protect against; secondly, restraints frequently involve an unjustified limitation of the autonomy of patients. This is not to claim that all possible arguments for restraint use have been defeated. Rather, the onus is placed firmly on those who wish to restrain elderly patients to provide adequate justification for their decision. Thorough assessment of the harm that use of restraints may avoid or cause in a particular case, and the requirement of consent to use of restraints, should serve to reduce risk of harm while protecting the freedom and autonomy of elderly patients. A challenge is made, then, to nursing home administrators and staff to attempt to avoid the need for restraints by taking on the task of assessing why a particular patient wanders, or sleeps poorly, or poses a risk to others. Further effort should go into developing alternatives to the use of mechanical restraints. Care for residents can be improved if the possibilities for safe, restraint-free nursing homes that protect personal freedom are thoroughly examined.

REFERENCES

1. Blakeslee JA. Speaking out: untie the elderly. *American Journal of Nursing.* 1988;88:833–834.

2. Evans LK, Strumpf NE. Myths about elder restraint. *Image. Journal of Nursing Scholarship.* 1990;22:124–128.

3. Moss RJ, La Puma J. The ethics of mechanical restraints. *Hastings Center Report.* 1991;21:22–25.

4. Anonymous [editorial]. Cotsides—protecting whom against what? *Lancet.* 1984;2:383–384.

5. Collopy B, Boyle P, Jennings B. New direction in nursing home ethics. *Hastings Center Report* (special supp.). 1991;21:3–15.

6. Evans LK, Strumpf NE. Tying down the elderly. *Journal of the American Geriatrics Society.* 1989;37:65–74.

7. Jencks SF, Clauser SB. Managing behavior problems in nursing homes. *JAMA.* 1991;265(4):502–503.

8. Tinetti M, Liu W, Marottoli R, Ginter S. Mechanical restraint use among residents of skilled nursing facilities. *JAMA.* 1991;265:468–471.

9. Ejaz FK, Jones JA, Rose MS. Falls among nursing home residents. *Journal of the American Geriatrics Society.* 1994;42:960–64.

10. Hogue CC. Falls and mobility late in life. *Journal of the American Geriatrics Society.* 1984;32:82–85.

11. Evans L. Restraint use with the elderly patient. *Nursing Research and Clinical Management of Alzheimer's Disease Proceedings.* Minneapolis, MN: University of Minnesota; 1989:41–57.

12. Schaffer A. Restraints and the elderly. *Canadian Medical Association Journal.* 1985;132:1257–1260.

13. Agich GJ. Reassessing autonomy in long term care. *Hastings Center Report.* 1990;20:12–17.

5

THE FEAR OF FORGETFULNESS

A Grassroots Approach to an Ethics of Alzheimer's Disease

Stephen G. Post, Ph.D.

❧

The perils of forgetfulness are especially evident in our culture of independence and economic productivity, which so values intellect, memory, and self-control. Alzheimer's disease (AD)[1] is a quantifiable neurological atrophy that objectively assaults normal human functioning;[2] alternatively, as medical anthropologists highlight, AD is also viewed within the context of socially constructed images of the human self and its fulfillment.[3] A longitudinal study carried out in urban China, for example, reported that dementia does not seem to evoke the same level of dread there as it does among Americans.[4] Thus, the stigma associated with the mental incapacitation of dementia varies according to culture.[5]

This article focuses on issues that emerged from dialogues with AD caregivers and mildly affected individuals across the United States during an estimated forty ethics workshops, panels, and focus groups at annual meetings of chapters of the Alzheimer's Disease and Related Disorders Association, Inc. (ADRDA), between 1996 and 1997 (with support from the Ethical, Legal, and Social Implications Program of the National Human Genome Research Institute of the National Institutes of Health and the ADRDA). Through participating in these meetings, I am able to introduce the

S. Post. "The Fear of Forgetfulness: A Grassroots Approach to an Ethics of Alzheimer's Disease." *Journal of Clinical Ethics.* 1998;9(1). Copyright 1998 by *The Journal of Clinical Ethics.* All rights reserved. Reprinted from *The Journal of Clinical Ethics.*

latest developments in socially and clinically relevant topics that affect people with AD, their caregivers, and health-care professionals.

I will not discuss some issues because they are gradually being resolved. For instance, the use of physical restraints is diminishing. Studies have reported that the use of restraints accelerates deconditioning and dependence, increases the use of major and minor tranquilizers (administered in response to the agitation caused by the fear and humiliation felt by those restrained), and increases cognitive deterioration.[6] This and other issues, including restriction of driving, have been discussed previously, based on community dialogues within the Cleveland Area Chapter of the ADRDA.[7] In this article, I will focus on overarching themes, in particular, that in the world of AD there is no hegemonic place for the principle of respect for autonomy; that as the disease progresses the ethics of care comes to the forefront; and that the "being with" of care in the culture of dementia holds moral hope, despite the pressure to flee from the deeply forgetful.

THEORIES OF PERSONHOOD, EXCLUSION, AND STIGMA

In response to the voices of caregivers across the country, I have grown increasingly critical of personhood theories of ethics, for they bestow a higher moral status on human beings who are envisioned as self-legislating moral agents than on people with cognitive impairment. Those philosophers who emphasize the superior moral status of the cognitively intact have excluded the person with severe dementia from moral standing. However, in fairness, H. Tristram Engelhardt Jr., a relatively inclusive proponent of personhood theory, has argued that while people with severe AD are objectively nonpersons (defined strictly as moral agents), they may still be persons in a "social sense" within a particular community, and thus would be protected.[8(p150)] But David H. Smith writes that even such a "conferred" or "social" sense of persons means that "at some point someone entering into a dementia begins to count less than, or have a different status than, the rest of us."[9(p47)] He describes caring for his AD-affected mother-in-law and contends that personhood theories can diminish our sensitivity to the well-being of those with AD: "Used as an engine of exclusion, the personhood theory easily leads to insensitivity, if not to great wickedness."[9(p47)]

In *The Moral Challenge of Alzheimer Disease*, I warn against the tendencies of a "hypercognitive culture" to exclude the deeply forgetful by reducing their moral status or by neglecting the emotional, relational, aesthetic, and spiritual aspects of well-being that are open to them, even in the advanced stage of the disease.[10] I reject categorizing people with dementia as nonpersons, because this fails to affirm the capacities that remain.

In stark contrast to personhood theorists, I believe that persons who lack certain empowering cognitive capacities are not nonpersons; rather, they have become the weakest among us and are worthy of care. The hypercognitivist value system that shapes personhood theories of ethics is merely an example of how our culture's criteria of rationality and productivity blind us to other ways of thinking about the meaning of our humanity and the nature of humane care. I am impressed with anthropologist Charlotte Ikels's work; she points out that in Chinese culture, "the cognitive domain is not taken to be the total sum of the person," nor is the self conceptualized as essentially independent and autonomous.[4] Thus in the eyes of the Chinese family, the person with dementia is still "there." Fortunately, not everyone in the world bows before the exclusionary phrase of the error-prone Descartes, "I think, therefore, I am." In Japanese culture, there are some who find in the image of dementia a release from the fetters of everyday cares and occupations.[11]

People with AD and their caregivers have convinced me that the arrogant hyper-cognitive ideology of human worth is of little help; however, they do require more people who are ready to lend a hand in the world of the forgetful. For nine years, I have devoted most of my professional life to people with AD through service, community dialogue, and work with national associations. I work in the context of the Judeo-Christian tradition of ethics, which chiefly asserts the moral principle of protecting the most vulnerable and "least" among us.[12(pp508–512)] A basic moral problem in AD care is that many people want to separate themselves from the presence of those with dementia. Love (synonymous with "care," "*chesed*," or "*agape*"), a basic solicitude, can overcome the tendency to exclude the forgetful.[13] This care is often best expressed in "being with" the forgetful, rather than by the "doing to" of invasive medical technologies.

For care to succeed, we must struggle to overcome the problem of stigma. Across the United States, people with mild AD described this problem. One of the finest autobiographical accounts of living with the diagnosis and initial decline of AD is Rev. Robert Davis's *My Journey into Alzheimer's Disease*.[14] As Davis "mourned the loss of old abilities," he nevertheless could draw on his faith: "I choose to take things moment by moment, thankful for everything that I have, instead of raging wildly at the things that I have lost."[14(p57)] Even as he struggled to find a degree of peace through his religious faith, he was also keenly aware of people who "simply cannot handle being around someone who is mentally and emotionally impaired."[14(p115)]

We must not separate "them" from "us." Instead, we must support the remaining capacities and enhance the relational well-being of persons with AD using data that indicate which interventions are most helpful.[15]

DIAGNOSTIC DISCLOSURE AND A SIGNIFICANT ROLE FOR AUTONOMY

Telling a patient the truth about a diagnosis of "probable AD" should be less controversial than it is. Doing it sensitively and in a way that does not cause unnecessary despair requires more focused attention than it has currently received. Disclosure should include mention of AD as a disease of the brain, expectations for the future, and the fact that while the condition cannot be cured, its effects can be treated. As

Joseph M. Foley, M.D., observes, all experienced health-care professionals have participated in the agonizing of the family about whether to tell the patient about AD, only to have the patient say, "That's what I've thought all along."[16] The discovery of inheritance patterns, emerging treatments, and the general public awareness of AD all contribute to a noticeable swing toward diagnostic truth telling. By informing the person of the AD diagnosis, we enable him or her to: (a) plan for optimal life experiences in remaining years of intact capacities; (b) prepare a durable power of attorney for health-care decisions—some may prepare a living will also—to be implemented upon eventual incompetence; (c) consider possible enrollment in AD research programs based on comprehended choice (I prefer "comprehended choice" to "informed consent," because the latter seems to imply that consent is normative);[17] (d) participate actively in AD support groups; (e) make the highly personal decision about taking available antidementia compounds.[18]

Regrettably, some clinicians still hide the diagnosis from the affected individual.[19] In my panel work, I have found that these clinicians reference the one case they encountered (or heard about) in which the diagnosis was given in an unsupportive way and had some adverse consequence. The ADRDA recently issued national guidelines strongly recommending diagnostic disclosure of AD to patients.[20] Nevertheless, a large (but diminishing) minority of clinicians remain extremely reluctant to disclose a diagnosis of AD to the patient. This may be bound up with the problem of stigma.

In the face of this reluctance to impart diagnostic information, it seems ironic that most older people with serious memory problems suspect that they have AD. In one instance, an older man named Murray C. knew his memory was weak, and asked his wife to take him to a speech on AD that he saw advertised in the local newspaper. Afterward, he insisted on a formal diagnostic workup. He received the diagnosis, and went door-to-door in his neighborhood informing old friends that he was not a "schmuck" because he forgets their names and what they have experienced together; he just has a disease called Alzheimer's. For Murray, the diagnosis was quite liberating.[10]

Diagnostic truth telling is the necessary beginning point for an AD ethics of autonomy. There are several ethicists who extol the value of autonomy in the context of AD, as do McCullough and Ronald Dworkin.[21] Although I, too, appreciate the value of respect for precedent autonomy in AD for those who wish to exercise it and are still able,[22] I firmly adhere to diagnostic disclosure to patients, and I reject any diminution of the status of human choice in the face of the erosions of dementia. On the other hand, some ethicists have rightly underscored the value of a current best-interest approach to the care of persons with AD, suggesting that a person's autonomy prior to his or her decline is limited by the fact that the still-intact self has never experienced dementia, and therefore knows nothing of how she or he might adjust to it. Further, the caring impulses of caregivers are undermined by decisions to allow the person with moderate dementia to die.[23]

Practically speaking, proponents of an ethics of autonomy do face an uphill struggle: Many AD patients suffer incapacitating cognitive decline long before having a diagnostic workup; those who are diagnosed early enough to exercise their autonomy can become quickly incapacitated; some ethnic traditions (for example, Korean Americans and Mexican Americans) entrust choices to family members and do not accept the principle of respect for autonomy;[24] and, short of assisted suicide, entrusting one's self to the hands of a loved one or other proxy is necessary and inevitable.

The best mechanism for empowering autonomy through self-control is the implementation of durable power of attorney for health care, which is, paradoxically, the act of relinquishing self-control by placing one's self in the loving hands of another. It thus seems to combine precedent autonomy with an ethics of care. The ADRDA's guidelines on issues in death and dying strongly urge the use of a durable power of attorney.[20] The guidelines indicate the right to forego life-sustaining treatment (specifying "use of artificial feeding, mechanical ventilators, cardiopulmonary resuscitation, antibiotics, dialysis, and other invasive technologies").

ANTIDEMENTIA DRUGS

The absence of clear outcomes data necessitates the use of caution when addressing the ethical implications of new antidementia compounds. Some major ethical quandaries are, however, already identifiable.[25]

The recent introduction of the acetylcholinesterase inhibitor donepezil for treatment of mild to moderate AD is, on the one hand, promising. Some patients may briefly regain their sense of self-identity or experience liberation from the isolation of speech limitations. There is anecdotal evidence of this effectiveness: a mildly demented woman insisted that, with the help of donepezil, she can now find her words; a woman who was too forgetful to cook any more regained sufficient memory to begin cooking again in relative safety. Donepezil can be effective, and it represents a point of hope.[26]

This hopefulness does not eliminate ethical problems. Temporary partial "awakenings" in the context of an irreversible progressive dementing condition create enormously difficult ethical issues. Patients and caregivers who have already navigated certain crises of cognitive decline may have to repeat the process. The individual who has lost insight into his or her losses may regain insight, along with renewed anxiety. Under the influence of the drug, aggressive behavioral problems that had been successfully treated may resurface. Thus, for AD patients who have already navigated significant decline, the sudden intrusion of a temporary awakening may not necessarily enhance quality of life; for caregivers, some of the most taxing phases of care may need to be repeated, resulting in renewed stress.

Some case examples about Aricept (the brand name for donepezil) will clarify this scenario.

Case 1: Aricept Family Story

"Katie S. (wife) shared with Dorothy how much Aricept has changed the situation with her husband. He is once again obsessing about finances, whereas, before Aricept, he had finally gotten to the point where he wasn't aware anymore—which was a relief for the family. He was very frustrated and suspicious about the financial situation earlier in the disease. Also, Katie shared that the children can no longer come over and talk openly about their problems and issues at home and with their own families, because he is now aware enough to be concerned and start worrying again. You might want to follow up with her and get the whole story, and hear the good aspects too."[27]

Case 2: A Mute Man Speaks

Mr. K. is mute, largely sedentary, and expressionless. With the help of behavioral medications and strenuous caregiving, he has moved past a period of violence and aggression. He can eat with some assistance. He lives at home, and his wife remains convinced that there is more of her husband left than the observer might think.

Mr. K.'s neurologist recommended Aricept. Neither Mrs. K. nor the neurologist doubted that prescribing an antidementia compound might enhance Mr. and Mrs. K.'s well-being. Mrs. K. described the results as nearly miraculous, "like a ray of light." Mr. K. regained his ability to speak a few words ("he was suddenly able to speak, even if not coherently"), he was able to smile, and he began to wander again. In addition, he again became "quite agitated and somewhat aggressive," as well as sleepless as night. Mrs. K. and her neurologist decided to lower the dosage of Aricept in the hope that his behavioral problems would cease while allowing his symptomatic gains to continue.

Case 3: Jenny Was Content!

Mrs. W. described the case of her mother-in-law, Jenny, who was previously well adjusted to the routine in her nursing home. She was in a relatively benign emotional state and seemed to be enjoying the art and music programs in which she actively participated. She was described as your "ideal dementia patient, seemingly happy, content." After beginning Aricept, Jenny regained insight into her situation. For example, she remembered that she did not want to be in a nursing home, and she insisted that she be allowed to leave. She also refused to participate in any support programs because the participants "are too slow for me."

Recommendations

New antidementia compounds are very promising, but should not be prescribed without attention to individual cases. Each patient's response must be carefully monitored with regard to his or her quality of life. Every caregiver should know that the use of a compound such as Aricept is a deeply personal and value-laden decision that requires the careful exercise of compassion and good judgment. Caregivers should know that there is nothing wrong with withdrawing an antidementia treatment that does not seem to have a positive result. Modest improvement or temporary stabilization of cognitive decline will be viewed by some caregivers as gratifying—but certainly not by all.

These concerns *do not* arise for the patient who receives an antidementia compound early in the disease, preferably on initial diagnosis. In such cases, some patients will retain insights and capacities throughout the mild and perhaps the early-moderate phases of AD. In these cases, the mitigation of symptoms enhances quality of life. Because these compounds do not affect the underlying process of neurological deterioration, however, there will eventually be losses in capacity; but the losses will come more slowly and the patient will need to adjust to these losses only once.

How long into the progression of AD should clinically important functional deterioration be delayed? While donepezil does not slow the underlying loss of neurons, it may ameliorate symptoms of cognitive decline. At some threshold of cognitive decline, however, the level of fragmentation reaches a point where an antidementia compound can offer no benefit. One concerned group of British observers stated: "No scientific data exist on the effects of stopping treatment with a cholinesterase inhibitor. Patients who took part in the clinical trials continued to take the active drugs with no defined end point."[28]

WHEN THE PERSON CAN
NO LONGER SWALLOW

In general terms, no caregiver should feel that the ability of technology to extend the morbidity of severe AD is necessary or beneficent. The patient's inability to swallow is one clear marker of AD's severe stage. Artificial nutrition and hydration are generally not a solution, because patients almost invariably perceive such intrusions as unwelcome. Physical discomfort and iatrogenic complications are equally serious considerations. No wonder the person with AD repeatedly pulls out feeding tubes. The ADRDA guidelines for the treatment of patients with severe dementia are clear:

> Severely and irreversibly demented patients need only care given to make them comfortable. If such a patient is unable to receive food and water by mouth, it is ethically permissible to choose to withhold nutrition and hydration artificially administered by vein or gastric tube. Spoon feeding should be continued if needed for comfort.[29]

In case consultations, caregivers who have already rejected the use of a feeding tube ask how aggressively they should encourage eating and drinking by mouth in patients who are losing these capacities. As long as a person retains capacity, food and water should be offered and encouraged by spoon feeding, When the person no longer is able to swallow, it is of no benefit to fill the mouth with food and water.

After the patient loses the capacity for natural eating and drinking, caregivers should understand that a decision against artificial nutrition must also be a decision against artificial hydration (administration of fluids intravenously). Clinicians should inform families that their loved one will likely die within two weeks, and that dehydration has sedating effects that ensure a more peaceful dying. Continuing artificial hydration makes the person less comfortable, often leading to uremia and bloating; in addition, the process of dying will be extended several more weeks. In some cases, a room humidifier can be used to avoid dryness of the skin.

The clinician should proactively clarify for caregivers the burdens of invasive treatments in order to spare them the sense of guilt associated with not doing everything to prolong life. Chaplains should advise caregivers that their love is better expressed through compassion, commitment, and humble entry into the culture of dementia to facilitate whatever "resurrection" is possible.[30]

THE LIMITS OF GENETIC TESTING

Every caregiving family at some point asks the question: Will I be next? Genetic testing, however, has important and often negative social implications. A nationally recognized insurance medical director, Robert J. Pokorski, recently published an article in the leading genetics journal entitled "Insurance Underwriting in the Genetic Era."[31] In it, he argues, "It will be virtually impossible for insurers to avoid using this information; genetic parameters are becoming an integral part of medical practice." Pokorski uses AD genetics and long-term care insurance as a primary example. In response to suggestions put forward by the ADRDA for anonymous genetic testing, he reports that his professional peers "view these pronouncements with mounting frustration." He points out the expense of long-term care, and asserts that limitations on access to AD-related genetic information represent "a frontal assault on a fundamental business practice." A consensus statement on AD and genetics and ethics published in *JAMA* takes up the urgent possibility of discrimination, and sharply rejects the use of AD-related genetic information for the purposes of actuarial discrimination.[32]

AD is the object of intense genetic analysis. It is a genetically heterogeneous disorder—that is, to date, it is associated with three determinative or causal (disease) genes and one susceptibility (risk) gene. The three determinative AD genes (located on chromosomes 21, 14, and 1) were discovered in the last decade. These autosomal-dominant genes pertain to early-onset forms of Alzheimer's (in which onset is usually manifested in one's early forties to midfifties), which, according to one estimate, account for possibly less than 1 percent of all cases. These families are usually well aware of their unique histories. Only in these very few tragic families is genetic prediction possible.

There is no clearly predictive test for ordinary late-onset AD. In 1993, investigators discovered that an apolipoprotein E ∈4 allele on chromosome 19 [apoE - protein; apoE - gene] was associated with susceptibility to late-onset AD (after age 60). A single ∈4 gene (found in about one-third of the general population) is not predictive of AD in asymptomatic individuals—that is, it does not approach being able to be used to foretell disease. Among those 2 percent of people with two of the ∈4 genes, AD may not manifest. All the major consensus groups recommend against susceptibility testing in asymptomatic individuals because the data are not useful.[33] If other susceptibility genes are found, this prevailing view may change. At the moment, however, the real debate concerns the use of APOE genotyping as an adjunct diagnostic test for those patients already presenting with the symptoms of dementia.

Robert N. Butler, editor of *Geriatrics*, urged clinicians to be cautious.[34] He emphasized that the APOE testing was not yet established as a diagnostic or predictive marker, that people should avoid the emotional toll of thinking that the APOE genotype means they are doomed after forgetting the car keys, and that discrimination in employment and insurance was likely. At a time when there is increasing public concern about genetic privacy and discrimination, a new magnitude of genetic knowledge has emerged. The growing long-term care insurance industry will make actuarial use of genetic information, which will become more precise as other susceptibility genes are discovered.

On the one hand, the ADRDA strongly endorses the research plan of coupling enhanced susceptibility analysis with treatments to delay or prevent disease. Genetically defined at-risk populations could engage in prophylactic efforts—for example, estrogen replacement and ibuprofen (risking potential adverse side effects such as increased risk for breast cancer or liver failure). At the very moment when delay of onset may be possible in at-risk populations, the possibilities for discrimination are, paradoxically, very real.[35]

QUALITY OF LIFE AS CARE'S CREATION

Emotional, relational, aesthetic, and spiritual forms of well-being are possible to varying degrees in people with progressive dementia.

Emotional and Relational Well-Being

Tom Kitwood and Kathleen Bredin developed a description of the "culture of dementia" that is useful in appreciating emotional and relational aspects of quality of life. They provide indicators of well-being in people with severe dementia: the assertion of will or desire, usually in the form of dissent despite various coaxings; the ability to express a range of emotions; the initiation of social contact (for instance, a person with dementia has a small toy dog that he treasures and places it before another person with dementia in order to attract attention); affectional warmth (for instance, a woman wanders back and forth in the facility without much socializing, but when people say hello to her she gives them a kiss on the check and continues her wandering).[36]

There is no need to add to the above description, except to state the obvious: if a man mistakes his wife for a hat, fine, no need for correction. Many a person with dementia has been badgered by those who wish to impose reality on him or her long past the point when it was a serious possibility. In the mild stage of AD, there is much to be said for trying to orient a person to reality; at some point in moderate AD, however, it becomes oppressive to impose reality upon him or her.

Aesthetic and Spiritual Well-Being

The aesthetic well-being available to people with AD is obvious to anyone who has watched art or music therapy sessions. In some cases, a person with advanced AD may still draw the same valued symbol, as though through art a sense of self is retained.[37,38] The abstract expressionist Willem de Kooning painted his way through much of his struggle with AD. Various art critics commented that his work, while not what it had been, was nevertheless impressive. As Kay Larson, former art critic for *New York* magazine wrote:

> It would be cruel to suggest that de Kooning needed his disease to free himself. Nonetheless, the erosions of Alzheimer's could not eliminate the effects of a life-time of discipline and love of craft. When infirmity struck, the artist was prepared. If he didn't know what he was doing, maybe it didn't matter—to him. He knew what he loved best, and it sustained him.[39]

A review of de Kooning's late art indicates, on the one hand, a loss of the sweeping power and command of brush typical of his work in the 1950s; but there is also a quality to the late work that should not be diminished.

Spiritual Well-Being

David McCurdy has addressed spiritual well-being. Chaplains can engage people with AD and their caregivers in a clinically relevant minstry. As Chaplain Debbie Everett of Edmonton, Alberta, Canada, said at a national meeting of the U.S. Alzheimer's Association:

> If a deeper experience of life could be realized by myself through a greater aware-ness of touch, music, human presence, love, smell, color, play, laughter, nature, and so on, what could this mean in the lives of those with Alzheimer's disease? In dis-covering how better to meet the spiritual needs of these people, in essence I found what spirituality means in a wider context beyond intellect, in the realm of our bodies and emotions.[40]

Everett adds that if part of spirituality in Eastern and Western religions includes an awareness of the present moment, there may even be something to learn from people with AD. She writes, "The paradigm shift that I advocate in the care of those affected by AD is to discover and appreciate a wider range of communication possibilities."

Spirituality may also play an important role in the experience of some care-givers. A recent study of the variables related to the rewards that caregivers perceive from their caregiving reports that "indicators of religiosity" (that is, "prayer, comfort from religion, self-rated religiosity, attendance at religious services") are especially significant as coping resources in female caregivers who are African American.[41] Because it clearly deters stress, spirituality also affects the rate of depression, which is extraordinarily high in AD caregivers. These authors suggest, "If religiosity indicators are shown to enhance a caregiver's perceived rewards, health-care professionals could encourage caregivers to use their religiosity to reduce the negative consequences and increase the rewards of caregiving."[41(p89)] (It should be added that this path makes sense only if caregivers have some interest in using spirituality and religion to cope with stress.)

CONCLUSIONS

AD has only received serious attention from bioethicists over the last several years. There appears to be a certain tension between advocates/ethicists such as myself, who are steeped in the voices of the marginalized forgetful, and foundationalist philosophers who struggle to apply ethical theories and personhood models to the very complex world of dementia.

The image of denying moral consideration to people with dementia that is equal to that of the nondemented is nicely illustrated in the 1982 film *Blade Runner* in which human beings have created artificial "replicants" to take on hazardous work "off-world." Rachel, a young female replicant, has been given implanted childhood memories (as a means of improving on previous replicants). It is the presence of these memories that moves Deckard (the hero, whose job it is to "terminate" unruly replicants) to see that Rachel is not a thing to be terminated. In future decades, as more people lose their memories, will we find ourselves so burdened by economic and caregiving pressures that nonvoluntary euthanasia of the most deeply forgetful becomes commonplace?

In an aging society, dementia is, as Lewis Thomas has often proclaimed it, "the disease of the century." The most urgent bioethical problem of our time may not be death, but dementia and the hypercognitive idea that the forgetful are already in the house of the dead. Such ideas have consequences for the forgetful that are hardly salutary.

REFERENCES

1. Gilman S. Alzheimer's disease. *Perspectives in Biology and Medicine.* 1997;40(2):230–243.

2. Fox NC, Freeborough PA, Rossor MN. Visualisation and quantification of rates of atrophy in Alzheimer's disease. *Lancet.* 1996;348(9020):94–97.

3. Herskovitz E. Struggling over subjectivity: debates about the "self" and Alzheimer's disease. *Medical Anthropology Quarterly.* 1995;9(2):146–164.

4. Ikels C. The experience of dementia in China. *Culture, Medicine and Psychiatry.* 1998; 22(3):257–283.

5. Yeo G, Gallagher-Thompson D (ed.). *Ethnicity & the Dementias.* Bristol, PA: Taylor & Francis; 1996.

6. Miles SH, Meyers R. Untying the elderly. *Clinics in Geriatric Medicine.* 1994;10(3):513–523.

7. Post SG, Whitehouse PJ. Fairhill Guidelines on ethics of the care of people with

Alzheimer's disease: a clinical summary. *Journal of the American Geriatrics Society.* 1995;43:1423–1429.

8. Engelhardt HT. *The Foundations of Bioethics.* 2d ed. New York, NY: Oxford University Press; 1996.

9. Smith DH. Seeing and knowing dementia. In: Binstock RH, Post SG, Whitehouse PJ (eds.). *Dementia and Aging: Ethics, Values, and Policy.* Baltimore, MD: Johns Hopkins University Press; 1992:44–54.

10. Post SG. *The Moral Challenge of Alzheimer Disease.* Baltimore, MD: Johns Hopkins University Press; 1995.

11. Ariyoshi S. *The Twilight Years.* New York, NY: Kodansha International; 1984.

12. Harrelson W. Prophetic ethics. In: Childress JF, Macquarries J (eds.). *The Westminster Dictionary of Christian Ethics.* Philadelphia, PA: Westminster Press; 1986.

13. Martin RJ, Post SG. Human dignity, dementia, and the moral basis of caregiving. In: Binstock RH, Post SG, Whitehouse PJ. *Dementia and Aging: Ethics, Values, and Policy.* Baltimore, MD: Johns Hopkins University Press; 1992:55–68.

14. Davis R, Davis B. *My Journey into Alzheimer's Disease: Helpful Insights for Family and Friends.* Wheaton, IL: Tyndale House; 1989.

15. Sabat SR. Recognizing and working with remaining abilities: toward improving the care of Alzheimer's disease sufferers. *American Journal of Alzheimer's Care and Related Disorders & Research.* 1994;9(3):8–16.

16. Foley JM, Post SG. Ethical issues in dementia. In: Morris JC (ed.). *Handbook of Dementing Illnesses.* New York, NY: Marcel Dekker; 1994:3–22.

17. Keyerslingk EW et al. Proposed guidelines for the participation of persons with dementia as research subjects. *Perspectives in Biology and Medicine.* 1995;38(2):319–362.

18. Post SG. Slowing the progression of Alzheimer disease: ethical issues. *Alzheimer Disease and Associated Disorders.* 1997;11(supp. 5):34–39.

19. Drickamer MA, Lachs MS. Should patients with Alzheimer's disease be told their diagnosis? *New England Journal of Medicine.* 1992;326(14):947–951.

20. *Ethical Considerations: Issues in Diagnostic Disclosure.* Chicago, IL: ADRDA; 1997.

21. Dworkin R. *Life's Dominion: An Argument about Abortion, Euthanasia, and Individual Freedom.* New York, NY: Vintage; 1993.

22. Post SG. Alzheimer disease and the "then" self. *Kennedy Institute of Ethics Journal.* 1995;5(4):307–321.

23. Dresser R. Missing persons: legal perceptions of incompetent patients. *Rutgers Law Review.* 1994;46(2):609–619.

24. Blackhall LJ et al. Ethnicity and attitudes toward patient autonomy. *JAMA.* 1995;274:820–825.

25. Mohr E, Feldman H, Gauthier S. Canadian guidelines for the development of anti-dementia therapies: a conceptual summary. *Canadian Journal of Neurosciences.* 1995;22(1):62–71.

26. Rogers SL, Friedhoff LT, the Donepezil Study Group. The efficacy and safety of Donepezil in patients with Alzheimer's disease: results of a U.S. multicenter, randomized, double-blind, placebo-controlled trial. *Dementia.* 1996;7:293–303.

27. E-mail from the Cleveland, OH, area chapter of ADRDA.

28. Kelly CA, Harvey RJ, Cayton H. Drug treatments for Alzheimer's disease raise clinical and ethical problems. *British Medical Journal.* 1997;314:693–694.

29. *Guidelines for the Treatment of Patients with Advanced Dementia.* Chicago, IL: ADRDA; 1994.

30. Weaver GD. Senile dementia and a resurrection theology. *Theology Today.* 1986;43(4): 444–456.

31. Pokorski RJ. Insurance underwriting in the genetic era. *American Journal of Human Genetics.* 1997;60:205–216.

32. Post SG et al. The clinical introduction of genetic testing for Alzheimer disease: an ethical perspective. *JAMA.* 1997;277:832–836.

33. Mayeux R et al. Utility of the A polipoproten E genotype in the diagnosis of Alzheimer's disease. *New England Journal of Medicine.* 1998;338:506–511.

34. Butler R. ApoE: new risk factor for Alzheimer's. *Geriatrics.* 1994;49:10–11.

35. Post SG, Whitehouse PJ (eds.). *Genetics, Ethics, and Alzheimer Disease.* Baltimore, MD: Johns Hopkins University Press; 1998.

36. Kitwood T, Bredin K. Towards a theory of dementia care: personhood and well-being. *Ageing and Society.* 1992;12:269–297.

37. Firlik AD, Margo's logo. *JAMA.* 1991;265:201.

38. Clair AA. *Therapeutic Uses of Music with Older Adults.* Baltimore, MD: Health Professions Press; 1996.

39. Larson K. Willem de Kooning and Alzheimer's. *World & I.* 1997;12(7):297–299.

40. Everett D. Forget me not: the spiritual care of people with Alzheimer's. *Proceedings of the Sixth National Alzheimer's Disease Education Conference.* Chicago, IL: ADRDA; 1997:A4.

41. Picot SJ et al. Religiosity and perceived rewards of black and white caregivers. *Gerontologist.* 1997;37(1):89–101.

6

MANAGEMENT OF PAIN IN ELDERLY PATIENTS WITH CANCER

Roberto Bernabei, M.D., Giovanni Gambassi, M.D.,
Kate Lapane, Ph.D., Francesco Landi, M.D.,
Constantine Gatsonis, Ph.D., Robert Dunlop, M.D.,
Lewis Lipsitz, M.D., Knight Steel, M.D.,
and Vincent Mor, Ph.D., for the SAGE Study Group

T he prevalence of cancer increases with age,[1] and pain is one of cancer's most frequent and disturbing symptoms.[2] Despite the widespread dissemination of the World Health Organization's (WHO) three-level ladder,[3] and the demonstration that its appropriate use can relieve pain in more than 90% of cases,[4-5] pain management remains poor. A high prevalence of unrelieved cancer pain has been documented in a variety of clinical settings, including general medical and surgical units,[6] oncology wards,[7] emergency departments,[8] and pediatric wards.[9] Even in oncology outpatient clinics, the management of pain falls well below accepted standards.[10,11] Although there is no physiologic basis for a decrease in pain with increasing age, pain is believed to be less prevalent among the aged and is historically underreported and undertreated. While the WHO ladder approach is applicable to older patients with cancer,[12] limited attention has been devoted to the management of pain in this age group.

With hospital length of stay declining and the elderly segment of the population increasing, the role of nursing homes is expanding to provide both postacute care and rehabilitation.[13] These trends are forcing more complex clinical care problems onto facilities that are still tainted by an image as the poorest-quality providers in the U.S. health care system.[14] Indeed, a new study reports that the prevalence of pain among

Bernabei R, Gambassi G, Lapane K, et al. "Management of Pain in Elderly Patients with Cancer." *Journal of the American Medical Association.* 1998;279(23):1877–1882. © American Medical Association. Reprinted by permission.

nursing home patients has increased in recent years.[15] Yet, data on the management of cancer pain in this population are lacking.

This study characterizes the treatment of pain among nearly 15,000 elderly cancer patients admitted to U.S. nursing homes, and specifically examines independent predictors of pain and prescribed analgesics in elderly and minority patients.

METHODS

The Systematic Assessment of Geriatric Drug Use via Epidemiology Database

Data were from the Systematic Assessment of Geriatric Drug Use via Epidemiology (SAGE) database described in detail elsewhere.[16-18] Briefly, SAGE is a population-based, multilinked database that includes computerized data collected as part of the Health Care Financing Administration's Multistate, Nursing Home Case-Mix and Quality Demonstration Project. Since 1992, nursing home staff in all Medicare and Medicaid facilities of five states have evaluated patients using the Resident Assessment Instrument, which includes a more than 350-item Minimum Data Set (MDS), a comprehensive instrument.[19] Over 350,000 patients had an MDS completed on admission to one of 1492 facilities in Kansas, Maine, Mississippi, New York, and South Dakota, during the 1992 to 1995 period.

The MDS includes sociodemographic information, numerous clinical items ranging from the degree of functional dependence to cognitive functioning, and all clinical diagnoses.[20,21] The MDS also includes an extensive array of signs, symptoms, syndromes, and treatments being provided.[20,21] A variety of different, multi-item summary scales are embedded in the MDS measuring, among others, physical function (activities of daily living)[22] and cognitive status (cognitive performance scale).[23]

In addition to MDS data, nursing staff recorded up to eighteen different medications received by each resident in the prior seven days. Drug information included brand and/or generic name, dosage, route, and frequency of administration.[16-18] Drugs were coded according to the national drug codes, and we used the Master Drug Data Base (MediSpan Inc, Indianapolis, Ind.) to translate them into therapeutic classes and subclasses.[17]

Study Sample

Of a total population of 363,354 persons, we identified 30,039 patients (8.3%) with a diagnosis of cancer. We subsequently excluded (1) patients younger than 65 years (n = 2105), (2) patients not admitted from a hospital (n = 4292), (3) persons who were residents when the use of MDS was initiated (n = 9120), (4) comatose patients (n = 60), and (5) patients admitted after October 1, 1995, in New York State, because facilities no longer uniformly collected drug information (n = 837). As a result, the final study sample comprised the 13,625 remaining individuals.

Pain Measurement

A multidisciplinary team of various professionals evaluated signs and symptoms of pain, but as the experience of pain is subjective, assessors were instructed to rely on self-report, when possible.[20] The team started the assessment within hours of admission to the facility, but subsequently allowed for a period of observation (at least seven days) to repeatedly interact with the patient and to integrate the observations of family and staff who regularly provided direct care. Daily pain was defined as any type of physical pain or discomfort in any part of the body that was manifested daily. Specifically, staff making the ratings were instructed to ask simple, direct questions about whether the patient had experienced pain. Because some residents did not complain verbally, or were unable to speak, the assessors were instructed to observe such persons for indicators of pain, including moaning, crying, wincing, frowning, or other facial expressions or posturing such as guarding or protecting an area of the body. If the assessor had difficulty determining the frequency, pain was coded as daily. Independent, dual assessment of pain items in a diverse sample of residents during testing and revision of the MDS showed an average weighted κ exceeding 0.7.[15]

Drug Information

We classified analgesics into three groups according to the WHO ladder[3-5]; level 1: salicylates, acetaminophen, and nonsteroidal anti-inflammatory drugs; level 2: codeine phosphate or codeine sulfate, oxycodone hydrochloride, hydrocodone bitartrate, propoxyphene hydrochloride or propoxyphene napsylate, meperidine hydrochloride, pentazocine hydrochloride or pentazocine lactate, buprenorphine hydrochloride, nalbuphine hydrochloride, butorphanol tartrate and any combination of these compounds with WHO level 1 drugs (mostly with acetaminophen and aspirin); and level 3: morphine sulfate, hydromorphone hydrochloride, oxymorphone hydrochloride, methadone hydrochloride, levorphanol tartrate, and fentanyl citrate. Corticosteroids, antidepressants, benzodiazepines, and anesthetics as well as antineoplastic hormones were considered to be adjuvant medications.[5]

Analytical Approach

We evaluated age trends of sociodemographic variables and indicators of disease severity using Mantel-Haenszel χ^2 tests for categorical variables. For continuous variables with skewed distributions, we used a nonparametric method (i.e., Wilcoxon tests) to evaluate age differences. To identify predictors of unresolved daily pain, we constructed a multiple logistic regression model. Independent variables considered for the model included sociodemographic variables and indicators of severity of ill-ness (e.g., explicit terminal prognosis, low body weight defined as body mass index of 19 kg/m^2 or less, presence of feeding tubes, immediate history of radiation or chemotherapy). Using a forward model-building approach (not computer driven), we first evaluated crude associations between each independent variable of interest and daily pain. At each stage in the modeling process, we selected the strongest predictor for inclusion in the model, then considered the remaining variables in the presence of those selected for the model. We evaluated and ruled out the presence of collinearity in the model by examining changes in the estimates and their SEs. From the final model, we derived odds ratios (ORs) and corresponding 95% confidence intervals (CIs). Also, we identified predictors of no analgesic use among patients who had daily pain using a similar modeling approach. Statistical analyses were performed using SAS statistical package.[24]

RESULTS

Patients were predominantly female (57%) and white (89%), and had a mean (SD) age of 81 (8) years (65–74 years: n = 2949, 21%; 75–84 years: n = 6004, 44%; >85 years: n = 4672, 35%) (see Table 6-1). The prevalence of moderate-to-severe cogni-tive impairment increased progressively with age, while the opposite was true for depressive symptoms. An explicit terminal prognosis was indicated in 18% of patients aged 65 to 74 years compared with 12% and 9% among patients aged 75 to 84 and 85 years and older, respectively ($P<.001$ for age trend; see Table 6-1). The mean number of active medical conditions increased with age ($P<.001$), but patients aged 85 years and older received fewer drugs than their younger counterparts (6.2 ± 3.9 vs 7.3 ± 4.2 in the 65-year to 74-year group; $P<.001$ for age trend). Daily pain was recorded (after an observation period that lasted, on average, seven days) in 38% of patients aged 65 to 74 years, 29% in those aged 75 to 84 years, and 24% in those aged 85 years and older. Localized pain—joint, chest, or mouth—did not differ among age groups. In contrast, clinical conditions potentially associated with pain were more prevalent with increasing age. A diagnosis of arthritis was made in 11%, 17%, and 25% of patients in the 65-year to 74-year, 75-year to 84-year, and 85-year and older age groups, respectively; the prevalence was 4%,7%, and 9% for osteoporosis, and 10%, 14%, and 18% for recent fractures. There were no differences for decubiti, sur-gical lesions, or amputations.

Table 6-2 presents the predictors of daily pain. Age was inversely associated with daily pain. Patients from racial or ethnic minority groups were less likely to have pain recorded relative to whites, although the 95% CI included unity for all groups except African Americans. Independent of age, patients with low cognitive perfor-mance were less likely to have documented daily pain. Marital status, terminal prog-nosis, compromised physical function, depressed mood, the presence of an indwelling catheter, and the use of restraints were associated with daily pain.

Table 6-1. Characteristics of Patients with Cancer*

Variable	Patient Age Group		
	65–74 y (n = 2949)	75–84 y (n = 6004)	>85 y (n = 4672)
Female	1626 (55)	3335 (56)	2799 (60)
Race			
White	2452 (83)	5320 (89)	4266 (91)
African American	355 (12)	436 (7)	250 (5)
Hispanic	52 (2)	66 (1)	45 (1)
Asian	25 (1)	50 (1)	32 (1)
American Indian	65 (2)	132 (2)	79 (2)
Marital status, widowed	1087 (37)	3103 (52)	3137 (67)
Degree activities of daily living compromised†			
Moderately	1427 (49)	3021 (51)	2392 (51)
Severely	1117 (38)	2311 (39)	1894 (41)
Degree of impaired cognitive performance‡			
Moderately	938 (32)	2305 (39)	1995 (43)
Severely	244 (8)	594 (10)	490 (11)
Depressed mood§	619 (21)	1170 (20)	808 (17)
Bedridden	462 (16)	665 (11)	358 (8)
Explicit terminal prognosis‖	517 (18)	742 (12)	433 (9)
No. of diagnoses, mean ± SD (range)	3.9 ± 2.0 (1–14)	4.2 ± 2.0 (1–24)	4.4 ± 1.9 (1–13)
No. of drugs, mean ± SD (range)	7.3 ± 4.2 (1–18)	6.7 ± 3.9 (1–18)	6.2 ± 3.9 (1–18)
Daily pain¶	1119 (38)	1756 (29)	1128 (24)

*Data are given as number (percent) unless otherwise indicated.

†Based an a 6–level scale.[22] Activities of daily living scare is 2 to 3 for moderately compromised and 4 to 5 for severely compromised.

‡Based on a 7–level scale.[23] Cognitive performance scale score is 2 to 4 for moderately impaired and 5 to 6 for severely impaired.

§Based on criteria derived from the American Psychiatric Association's *Diagnostic and Statistical Manual of Mental Disorders, Third Edition Revised.* Washington, DC: American Psychiatric Association; 1987.

‖Indicated conditions with less than six months of expected survival.

¶Resident complains or shows evidence of pain daily (as assessed by the nursing home staff over a seven-day period).

Table 6-3 presents the pattern of analgesic drug use among patients stratified by the presence of daily pain. Twenty-six percent of the individuals who reported having daily pain received no analgesics. Nonnarcotic analgesics (WHO level 1) were used by 16% of patients in pain. Weak opiates (WHO level 2) and strong opiates (WHO level 3) were administered in only 32% and 26% of the residents in pain, respectively. Acetaminophen was the most common drug prescribed, accounting for more than 55% of WHO level 1 drugs, (27% aspirin, 18% anti-inflammatory drugs).

Table 6-2. Predictors of Daily Pain*

Variable	Daily Pain (n = 4003)	No Pain (n = 9610)	Univariate Odds Ratio (95% Confidence Interval)		Adjusted Model† Odds Ratio (95% Confidence Interval)	
Age, y						
65–74	1119	1826	1.0	(Referent)	1.0	(Referent)
75–84	1756	4244	0.68	(0.62–0.74)	0.71	(0.64–0.78)
≥85	1128	3540	0.52	(0.47–0.58)	0.56	(0.50–0.63)
Gender						
Male	1528	4320	1.0	(Referent)	1.0	(Referent)
Female	2472	5283	1.32	(1.23–1.43)	1.32	(1.21–1.44)
Race						
White	3697	8332	1.0	(Referent)	1.0	(Referent)
African American	188	852	0.50	(0.42–0.58)	0.55	(0.46–0.66)
Hispanic	23	140	0.37	(0.24–0.58)	0.70	(0.43–1.14)
Asian	21	86	0.55	(0.34–0.89)	0.80	(0.45–1.40)
American Indian	74	200	0.83	(0.64–1.09)	0.88	(0.65–1.17)
Marital status						
Not	1836	4455	1.0	(Referent)	1.0	(Referent)
Widowed	2167	5155	1.18	(1.12–1.31)	1.24	(1.10–1.39)
Religious faith	2061	4423	1.25	(1.16–1.35)	1.16	(1.07–1.26)
Compromised activities of daily living function‡	2875	6513	1.24	(1.14–1.35)	1.19	(1.08–1.31)
Impaired cognitive performance§	1608	4955	0.63	(0.58–0.68)	0.72	(0.64–0.80)
Depressed mood	1026	1568	1.77	(1.62–1.94)	1.56	(1.41–1.72)
No feeding tube	3816	8920	1.0	(Referent)	1.0	(Referent)
Feeding tubes	183	684	0.63	(0.53–0.74)	0.57	(0.47–0.68)
No catheter	3120	8058	1.0	(Referent)	1.0	(Referent)
Indwelling catheter	827	1502	1.42	(1.29–1.56)	1.16	(1.04–1.30)
No restraints	934	2836	1.0	(Referent)	1.0	(Referent)
Use of restraints‖	3069	6774	1.38	(1.26–1.50)	1.21	(1.10–1.33)
Ambulatory	3213	8900	1.0	(Referent)	1.0	(Referent)
Bedridden	787	697	3.13	(2.80–3.49)	2.60	(2.29–2.97)
Prognosis not terminal	3109	8814	1.0	(Referent)	1.0	(Referent)
Explicit terminal prognosis	894	796	3.18	(2.87–3.53)	2.53	(2.25–2.83)

*Twelve patients have missing pain data.
†Adjusted simultaneously for all the variables listed in Table 6-1 and variables describing participation in the assessment (family, spouse, resident) and communication skills.
‡Activities of daily living scores are at least 2.
§Cognitive performance scale scores equal 2 or more.
‖Includes trunk and limb restraints as well as chairs to prevent raising.

Propoxyphene and codeine (53% and 25% of prescriptions, respectively) among WHO level 2 drugs and morphine and fentanyl (65% and 18% of prescriptions, respectively) among WHO level 3 drugs were the agents used most often. In nearly all cases, a WHO level 1 (93%) and WHO level 2 (97%) drug was administered

Table 6-3. Use of Analgesics by Patients With Cancer*

Analgesic Use	Patient Pain Group, No. (%)	
	Daily (n = 4003)	None (n = 9610)
None	1019 (26)	6053 (63)
Any	2984 (74)	3557 (37)
Nonnarcotic†	659 (16)	2297 (24)
Weak opiates‡	1293 (32)	870 (9)
Morphine or like substances§	1029 (26)	390 (4)

*Twelve patients have missing pain data.
†Classified by the WHO as a level 1 drug.
‡Classified by WHO as level 2.
§Classified by WHO as level 3.

orally, whereas WHO level 3 drugs were commonly given as skin patches (17%) or by injection (subcutaneous 5%, intramuscular 7%, intravenous 6%).

The figure reveals the relationship between age and analgesic use. As age increased, a greater proportion of patients in pain received no analgesic drugs (21%, 26%, and 30% of patients in the 65-year to 74-year, 75-year to 84-year, and 85-year and older age groups, respectively; $P<.001$ for age trend). Patients aged 85 years and older received morphine or other strong opiates one-third less frequently than patients aged 65 to 74 years (13% vs. 38%, respectively; $P<.001$).

The use of adjuvant drugs was relatively uncommon. An adjuvant was given to 27% of patients in pain who were already receiving a WHO analgesic drug, with no age-related differences. Use of corticosteroids (10%), antineoplastic hormones (9%), and anesthetics (2%) was not correlated with a complaint of pain or analgesic use. Antidepressants were used in 12% of those taking an analgesic agent as compared with 9% of those who were not. Similarly, benzodiazepines were taken by 9% of patients taking analgesics and 4% of others.

The age-related differences in the use of narcotic analgesics could not be accounted for by potential contraindications. As age increased. a decrease in the prevalence of seizures (8% in patients aged 65–74 years versus 3% in those aged >85 years), dyspnea (17% vs. 11%), vomiting (7% vs. 5%), and hallucinations (3% vs. 2%) was observed. Constipation (26%), dizziness (3%), and syncope (1%) did not differ by age.

Table 6-4 shows predictors of analgesia use among persons with cancer in daily pain. Patients older than 75 years were more likely to have no analgesia relative to patients aged 65 to 74 years (OR, 1.27; 95% CI, 1.06–1.52; and OR, 1.54; 95% CI, 1.27–1.86, for patients aged 75–84 and >85 years, respectively). This association remained significant in a multivariable model adjusting for several variables, including gender, cognitive status, communication skills, and indicators of disease severity, such as explicit terminal prognosis, being bedridden, number of diagnoses,

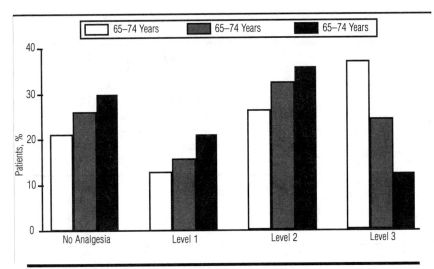

Pharmacological treatment of cancer patients with pain according to the World Health Organization's (WHO's) 3-level ladder. The WHO's level 1 is nonnarcotic analgesics; level 2, weak opiates; and level 3, morphine or like substances.

and the use of other medications. Minority patients were more likely to receive no analgesia. In the adjusted model, African Americans appeared to have a 63% increased probability of being untreated relative to whites (OR, 1.63; 95% CI, 1.18-2.26). Similar results were observed for patients belonging to other race minority groups, although the CIs were wide because of small numbers.

COMMENT

This study reveals that between 25% and 40% of elderly patients with cancer experience daily pain. We found a strong inverse correlation between the presence of pain and increasing age and an equally strong relationship between pain and belonging to minority groups.

While data describing the extent of cancer pain in the elderly are sparse, two studies that included the elderly estimated that more than half the patients had pain.[10,25] No physiologic changes in pain perception in the elderly have been demonstrated.[26] In fact, the elderly may experience more pain than younger people,[27,28] although they may be less likely to complain of it.[29] However, the assessment of pain in elderly individuals with cancer may pose significant and specific challenges.[30] Residents may be reluctant to report pain, often viewing it to be an expected concomitant of aging. The presence of multiple concurrent medical problems, the increased likelihood of cognitive[31] and sensory impairment,[32] and the presence of depression[33] may all contribute to underreporting of pain. Our study

Table 6-4. Predictors of Receiving No Analgesia Among Patients with Cancer with Daily Pain

Variable	No Analgesia (n = 1022)	Analgesia (n = 2981)	Univariate Odds Ratio (95% Confidence Interval)	Adjusted Model* Odds Ratio (95% Confidence Interval)
Age, y				
65–74	239	880	1.0 (Referent)	1.0 (Referent)
75–84	451	1305	1.27 (1.06–1.52)	1.19 (1.00–1.45)
≥85	332	796	1.54 (1.27–1.86)	1.40 (1.13–1.73)
Gender				
Male	417	1111	1.0 (Referent)	1.0 (Referent)
Female	603	1869	0.86 (0.74–0.99)	0.91 (0.78–1.07)
Race				
White	927	2770	1.0 (Referent)	1.0 (Referent)
African American	64	124	1.54 (1.13–2.10)	1.63 (1.18–2.26)
Hispanic	8	15	1.59 (0.67–3.76)	1.35 (0.53–3.43)
Asian	7	14	1.49 (0.60–3.70)	1.40 (0.54–3.65)
American Indian	16	58	0.82 (0.47–1.44)	0.84 (0.46–1.54)
No. of medications				
1–5	551	1198	1.0 (Referent)	1.0 (Referent)
6–10	372	1331	0.84 (0.72–0.99)	0.85 (0.72–1.00)
>11	99	452	0.66 (0.52–0.84)	0.65 (0.50–0.84)
Compromised activities of daily living function†	748	2127	1.08 (0.92–1.27)	1.10 (0.91–1.31)
Impaired cognitive performance‡	458	1150	1.29 (1.12–1.49)	1.23 (1.05–1.44)
No restraints	241	693	1.0 (Referent)	1.0 (Referent)
Use of restraints	781	2288	1.09 (0.87–1.38)	1.09 (0.87–1.38)
Ambulatory	852	2361	1.0 (Referent)	1.0 (Referent)
Bedridden	170	617	0.76 (0.63–0.92)	0.80 (0.65–0.99)
Prognosis not terminal	827	2282	1.0 (Referent)	1.0 (Referent)
Explicit terminal prognosis	195	699	0.77 (0.65–0.92)	0.74 (0.60–0.90)

*Adjusted simultaneously for all the variables listed in Table 6-1 and variables describing participation in the assessment (family, spouse, resident) and communication skills.
†Activities of daily living scores are at least 2.
‡Cognitive performance scale scores equal 2 or more.

revealed that impaired cognitive function was independently associated with a decreased notation of pain, as reported by others.[31,32] However, several authors have suggested that there appears to be no valid difference of pain complaints among cognitively intact and markedly impaired individuals,[34,35] yet the issue remains controversial.[36,37] The relationship between depression and pain may suggest that elderly patients with depression are more sensitive to pain caused by the coexisting physical condition, as others have concluded.[33-38]

Women were more likely than men to have pain recorded. Recent experimental data would support the notion of a biologically different susceptibility,[39] but an increased interaction with staff might have favored the recording of pain in men.[40] Yet, women with cancer appear to have more knowledge than men about pain and its management.[41]

Minority patients were also less likely than whites to have pain recorded even after adjustment for language differences. Statistical significance was reached only for African Americans, but a similar trend was noted for Hispanics, Asians, and American Indians. These results are concordant with recent findings by Cleeland et al,[42] who speculated that language barriers accounted for some or all of these differences. Indeed, cultural and linguistic backgrounds affect ratings of pain's interference with physical function, mood, and sleep.[43] Furthermore, there is evidence that Hispanics are more reluctant to report pain and, like African Americans, less willing to complete advanced directives.[44] We found that of those in daily pain, about one-fourth of patients did not receive any analgesic medications. Older individuals were less likely to receive any analgesia, especially morphine or another WHO level 3 drug.

Overall, these findings are in agreement with the notion that there are age and racial or ethnic differences in the management of patients with cancer.[45-47] More specifically, our data concur with those of Cleeland et al,[10] who reported that outpatients aged 70 years or older with cancer were less likely to receive adequate analgesic treatment than a younger population.[10] In the same study, members of ethnic groups, when in pain, also were less likely to receive analgesic treatment when compared with whites. In a more recent report, the same authors confirmed and extended these results, noting that 65% of minority patients who had pain received inadequate analgesia compared with 50% of nonminority patients.[42]

Elderly and minority cancer patients may receive inadequate analgesia in part due to an underestimation or underreporting of pain. In the study by Cleeland et al.[42] Hispanics reported more frequently concerns about receiving too many analgesics and were more worried about side effects. Some authors have suggested that older patients also may have less knowledge about pain management and a disproportionate fear of addiction.[41] Of interest, elderly patients and especially those aged 85 years and older in our study appeared to have fewer possible contraindications to the use of opiates than younger persons. With regard to racial or ethnic minority patients, no data are available to determine whether cultural, social, or economic factors could explain our findings, or whether more disturbing hypotheses should be formulated.

Several limitations of our study need to be recognized. Although the MDS is a standardized, comprehensive assessment instrument, and each of its components is a prerequisite to effective pain management,[30] the recording of pain was not a special focus. Pain was assessed based on observational evaluation of the nursing home staff, and the potential for underestimation remains a concern, especially so among older patients or those with difficulty communicating. However, in 86% of cases, regardless of age, patients were the primary source of information, although the participation of family members in completing the MDS assessment increased progressively with the age of patients. This was true although communication skills (e.g., the ability to understand others or to make oneself understood) were only slightly worse in those aged 85 years and older. Consistent with previous reports, family members of Hispanic and

Asian patients were more frequently involved in the collection of information. Interestingly, this would likely result in a bias toward overreporting of pain.[48,49]

The proportion of patients in pain in all groups was lower than that found in some other studies because we included only daily pain. Despite being a more restricted observation, this symptom unquestionably deserves attention. We were not able to identify the site of pain with certainty and were unable to attribute the pain to cancer definitively. However, other studies on the relationship of pain to a given cancer site also did not reveal a consistent relationship.[10,50,51]

The use of analgesics refers to the first seven to fifteen days in the facility only, and therefore no statements can be made about pain management in those residents who lived longer in the facility. No data about analgesic dose or frequency of administration are presented. Although these issues warrant further study, it has been noted that as age increases, both the dose and frequency of administration of analgesic drugs decrease progressively.[52] No specific intervention was made for patients as a result of this study because it was observational. However, ongoing research should help better define high-risk groups to target for improved pain control.

The results of our study are not generalizable to all elderly cancer patients. This study focused on patients admitted to nursing homes following discharge from a hospital. This is the group for which we could verify conclusively the diagnosis of cancer and identify the specific nature of the neoplasm. Usually when persons are sent from a hospital to a nursing home, staff receive considerable medical information including the need for pain medication. Financial issues were unlikely to play a role in whether pain medications were provided since all the patients, regardless of their own insurance status, had Medicare coverage extended to include medication costs. Geographical, market, and facility variations could have existed, although we repeated the entire set of analyses varying the inclusion criteria of the study sample and the results were consistent across all samples studied.

In conclusion, a practical solution to the management of persons with cancer pain in long-term care facilities is required, as recently attempted in acute care hospitals.[53] Any approach must take into account barriers to appropriate pain management such as the unwillingness of many nursing homes to stock opiates, inadequate staff to provide and monitor frequent analgesia administration, and the inadequate knowledge and failure of many physicians to use analgesic agents aggressively.[54] Experts agree about the need to educate individual clinicians and patients to influence their routine behaviors.[54] Disappointingly, in a recent multicenter trial, enhancing opportunities for more patient-physician communication did not change established practices.[55] Other projects have suggested that other strategies may be more effective.[56,57] Failure to prevent and/or treat pain effectively at virtually all times is no longer acceptable and should be considered a first-line indicator of poor quality of medical care.

This study was supported in part by grant 17C90428 from the U.S. Department of Health and Human Services, Health Care Financing Administration, to the University of Michigan with a contract to Brown University. Dr. Steel is supported in part by a grant from the John A. Hartford Foundation and by the Hunterdon Health Fund.

REFERENCES

1. Parker SL, Tong T, Bolden S, Wingo PA. Cancer statistics, 1996. *CA: A Cancer Journal for Clinicians.* 1996;46:5–27.

2. Daut RL, Cleeland CS. The prevalence and severity of pain in cancer. *Cancer.* 1982;50:1913–1918.

3. Stjernsward J. WHO cancer pain relief programme. *Cancer Surv.* 1988;7:195–208.

4. Zech DFJ, Grond S, Lynch J, Hertel D, Lehmann K. Validation of World Health Organization guidelines for cancer pain relief: a 10-year prospective study. *Pain.* 1995;63:65–76.

5. Levy MH. Pharmacologic treatment of cancer pain. *New England Journal of Medicine.* 1996;335:1124–1132.

6. Donovan M, Dillon P, McGuire L. Incidence and characteristics of pain in a sample of medical-surgical inpatients. *Pain.* 1987;30:69–87.

7. Foley KM. Pain relief into practice: rhetoric without reform. *Journal of Clinical Oncology.* 1995;13:2149–2151.

8. Todd K, Sarnaroo N, Hoffmann JR. Ethnicity as a risk factor for inadequate emergency department anesthesia. *JAMA.* 1993;269:1537–1539.

9. Schechter NL. The undertreatment of pain in children: an overview. *Pediatric Clinics in North America.* 1989;36:631–646.

10. Cleeland CS, Gonin R, Hatfield AK, et al. Pain and its treatment in outpatients with metastatic cancer. *New England Journal of Medicine.* 1994;330:592–596.

11. Portenoy RK, Kornbhth AB, Wong G, et al. Pain in ovarian cancer patients: prevalence, characteristics, and associated symptoms. *Cancer.* 1994;74:907–915.

12. Portenoy RK. Pain management in the older cancer patient. *Oncology.* 1992;6:86–98.

13. Kahn KL, Keeler EB, Sherwood MJ, et al. Comparing outcomes of care before and after implementation of DRG-based prospective payment system. *JAMA.* 1990;264:1984–1988.

14. Shaughnessy PW, Kramer AM. The increased needs of patients in nursing homes and patients receiving home health care. *New England Journal of Medicine.* 1990;322:2127.

15. Fries BE, Hawes C, Morris JN, Phillips CD, Mor V, Park PS. Effect of the national Resident Assessment Instrument on selected health conditions and problems. *Journal of the American Geriatric Society.* 1997;45:994–1001.

16. Bernabei R, Gambassi G, Mor V. The SAGE database: introducing functional outcomes in geriatric pharmaco-epidemiology. *Journal of the American Geriatric Society.* 1998;46:250–252.

17. Gambassi G, Landi F, Peng L, et al. Validity of diagnostic and drug data on standardized nursing home resident assessments: potential for geriatric pharmaco-epidemioiogy. *Medical Care.* 1998;36:167–169.

18. Bernabei R, Gambassi G, Lapane K, et al. Characteristics of the SAGE database, a new resource for research on outcomes in long-term care. *Journals of Gerontology. Series A, Biological Sciences and Medical Sciences.* 1999;54(1):M25–33.

19. Schroll M. Effect of systematic geriatric assessment. *Lancet.* 1997;350:604–605.

20. *Minimum Data Set Plus Training Manual.* Natick, MA: Eliot Press; 1991.

21. Morris JN, Hawes C, Fries BE, et al. Designing the national resident assessment instrument for nursing homes. *Gerontologist.* 1990;30:293–297.

22. Phillips C, Morris JN, Hawes C, et al. Association of the Resident Assessment Instrument (RAI) with changes in function, cognition, and psychosocial status. *Journal of the American Geriatric Society.* 1997;45:986–993.

23. Morris JN, Fries BE, Mehr DR, et al. MDS Cognitive Performance Scale. *Journals of Gerontology. Series A, Biological Sciences and Medical Sciences.* 1994;49:MI74–MI82.

24. SAS Institute. *SAS Users Guide. Statistics.* 5th ed. Cary, NC: SAS Institute; 1985.

25. Stein WM, Miech RP. Cancer pain in the elderly hospice patient. *Journal of Pain and Symptom Management.* 1993;8: 474–482.

26. Kwentus JA, Harkins SW, Lignon N, et al. Current concept of geriatric pain and its treatment. *Geriatrics.* 1985;40:48–57.

27. Corran TM, Gibson SJ, Farrell MJ, Helme RD. Comparison of chronic pain experience between young and elderly patients. In: Gebhart GF, Hammond DL, Jensen TS, eds. *Proceedings of the 7th World Congress on Pain, Vol 2: Progress in Pain Research and Management.* Seattle, WA: IASP Press; 1994:895–906.

28. Institute of Medicine. *Approaching Death: Improving Care at the End of Life.* Washington, DC: National Academy Press; 1997:51–86.

29. Melding PS. Is there such a thing as geriatric pain? *Pain.* 1991;46:119–121.

30. Vallerand AH. Measurement issues in the comprehensive assessment of cancer pain. *Seminars in Oncology Nursing.* 1997;13:16–24.

31. Sengstaken EA, King SA. The problem of pain and its detection among geriatric nursing home residents. *Journal of the American Geriatric Society.* 1993;41:541–544.

32. Ferrell BA, Ferrell BR, Rivera L. Pain in cognitively impaired nursing home patients. *Journal of Pain and Symptom Management.* 1995;10:591–598.

33. Cohen-Mansfield J, Marx MS. Pain and depression in the nursing home: corroborating results. *Journal of Gerontology. Series B, Psychological Sciences and Social Sciences.* 1993;48:P96–P97.

34. Parmalee PA, Smith BD, Katz IR. Pain complaints and cognitive status among elderly institution residents. *Journal of the American Geriatric Society.* 1993;41:517–522.

35. Porter FL, Malhotra KM, Wolf CM, Morris JC, Miller JP, Smith MC. Dementia and response to pain in the elderly. *Pain.* 1996;68:413–421.

36. Fisher-Morris M, Gellalty A. The experience and expression of pain in Alzheimer patients. *Age and Ageing.* 1997;26:497–500.

37. Scherder EJ, Bouma A. Is decreased use of analgesics in Alzheimer disease due to a change in the affective component of pain? *Alzheimer Disease and Associated Disorders.* 1997;11:171–174.

38. Parmalee PA, Katz IR, Lawton MP. Depression among institutionalized aged: assessment and prevalence estimation. *Journals of Gerontology. Series A, Biological Sciences and Medical Sciences.* 1989;41:M22–M29.

39. Mogil JS, Richards SP, O'Toole LA, Helms ML, Mitchell SR, Belknap JK. Genetic sensitivity to hotplate nociception in DBA/2J and C57BL/6J inbred mouse strains: a possible sex-specific mediation by delta2-opioid receptors. *Pain.* 1997;70:267–277.

40. Lindesay J, Skea D. Gender and interactions between care staff and elderly nursing home residents with dementia. *International Journal of Geriatric Psychiatry.* 1997; 12:344–348.

41. Yeager KA, Miaskowski C, Dibble S, Wallhagan M. Differences in pain knowledge in cancer patients with and without pain. *Cancer Pract.* 1997;5:39–45.

42. Cleeland CS, Gonin R, Baez L, Loehrer P, Pandya KJ. Pain and treatment of pain in minority patients with cancer. *Annals of Internal Medicine.* 1997;127:813–816.

43. Cleeland CS, Nakamura Y. Mendoza TR, Edwards KR, Douglas J, Serlin R C. Dimensions of the impact of cancer pain in a four country sample: new information from multidimensional scaling. *Pain.* 1996;67:267–273.

44. Caralis PV, Davis B, Wright K. Marcial E. The influence of ethnicity and race on attitudes toward advance directives, life-prolonging treatments, and euthanasia. *Journal of Clinical Ethics.* 1993:4:155–165.

45. McDonald DD. Gender and ethnic stereotyping and narcotic analgesic administration. *Research in Nursing and Health.* 1994;17:45–49.

46. Ball JK, Elixhauser A. Treatment differences between blacks and whites with colorectal cancer. *Medical Care.* 1996;34:970–984.

47. Repetto L, Venturino A, Vercelli M, et al. Performance status and comorbidity in elderly cancer patients compared with young patients with neoplasia and elderly without neoplastic conditions. *Cancer.* 1998;82:760–765.

48. Higginson I, Priest P, McCarthy M. Are bereaved family members a valid proxy for a patient's assessment of dying? *Social Science and Medicine.* 1994;38: 553–554.

49. Sneeuw KCA, Aaronson NK. Osoba D, et al. The use of significant others as proxy raters of the quality of life of patients with brain cancer. *Medical Care.* 1997;35:490–506.

50. Greenwald HP, Bonica JJ, Bergber M. The prevalence of pain in four cancers. *Cancer.* 1987;60:2563–2569.

51. Portenoy RK. Cancer pain: epidemiology and syndromes. *Cancer.* 1989;63:2298–2307.

52. Goldberg RJ, Mor V, Wiemann M, Greer DS, Hiris J. Analgesic use in terminal cancer patients: report from the National Hospice Study. *Journal of Chronic Disease.* 1986;39:37–45.

53. Rischer JB, Childress SB. Cancer pain management: pilot implementation of the AHCPR guideline in Utah. *Joint Commission Journal on Quality Improvement.* 1996;22:683–700.

54. American Pain Society Quality of Care Committee. Quality improvement guidelines for the treatment of acute pain and cancer pain. *JAMA.* 1995;274:1874–1880.

55. The SUPPORT Principal Investigators. A controlled trial to improve care for seriously ill hospitalized patients. *JAMA.* 1995;274:1591–1598.

56. Elliott TE, Murray DM, Oken MM, et al. Improving cancer pain management in communities: main results from a randomized controlled trial. *Journal of Pain and Symptom Management.* 1997;13:191–203.

57. Bookbinder M, Coyle N, Kiss M. et al. Implementational standards for cancer pain management: program model and evaluation. *Journal of Pain and Symptom Management.* 1996;12:334–347.

Part 3

CARE AT THE END OF LIFE

❧

T alking about end-of-life issues is never easy. This is because, more than any other topic in medical ethics, this issue is something everyone has experienced in some deeply personal way. These personal experiences come in many forms: a parent who dies suddenly, at home, with no history of disease; a spouse who suffers a stroke and lingers on a ventilator for six months prior to dying; a child who dies at home on hospice, pain-free and surrounded by family. Such experiences can play a large part in how end-of-life issues are addressed by health-care providers and ethics committee members.

This seems obvious enough, yet often physicians, nurses, paramedics, and ethics committee members respond to end-of-life dilemmas in such a way that it is obvious they are "mapping" their own experiences onto the current dilemma. When this happens, the questions they ask and the recommendations they make may not be entirely for the situation at hand. Although this can be problematic at times, it is understandable; it is such experiences that allow health-care providers to be truly empathetic to patients and families that come before them. An experience that creates a powerful connection with a patient can certainly bring about better end-of-life care, but only if providers realize that they are, in fact, "mapping." It is this realization that will be the focus of this section.

The goal for this section is twofold: first, that you think about these issues as they relate to your experiences and obligations as a health-care provider or ethics committee member; and second, that you acknowledge what these issues mean within the context of your experiences, familial and professional.

This section begins with "The Persistent Vegetative State: The Medical Reality," by Ronald Cranford. This article is a response to an important and obvious realization: Discussing end-of-life issues is of little value unless we "collect the facts and . . . understand the medical reality."[1] To that end, Cranford guides us through the commonly confused syndromes of coma, brain death, persistent vegetative state, dementia, neocortical death, and locked-in syndrome. By clearly defining these conditions and providing actual cases in which they were misconstrued, he makes explicit the harm that can be done to patients and their families when health-care providers are not careful with the terms they use.

The next four articles raise some of the most troubling end-of-life issues. Phyllis Schmitz begins with "The Process of Dying With and Without Feeding and Fluids by Tube." She takes on what it actually means to die without food or fluids, and she shows us the reality of our fears. Many patients, families, and health-care providers cast withholding and withdrawing nutrition and hydration as an act of cruelty. Not only do some see this as causing severe pain, but many families consider this a deprivation of their ability (and right) to nurture and comfort their dying loved one. When a dying patient no longer wants to eat, or when the health-care team suggests to the family that they should no longer feed the patient, the loving bond that arises from feeding and nurturing our loved ones is denied.

Schmitz helps us to understand that, in spite of all of our basic instincts, sometimes the kindest act to a dying patient is to not make him feel that he must eat. And sometimes the kindest thing a health-care provider can do for a family that has decided to forgo nutrition and hydration is to help them understand, and continually reinforce, that their decision will not cause pain or discomfort.

The next reading, a study originally published in the *American Journal of Respiratory and Critical Care Medicine,* is titled "Decisions to Limit or Continue Life-sustaining Treatment by Critical Care Physicians in the United States: Conflicts Between Physicians' Practices and Patients' Wishes." Drs. David Asch, John Hansen-Flaschen, and Paul Lanken surveyed 879 intensive care physicians regarding whether they had ever continued or withdrawn life sustaining treatment without the consent of, or over the objections of, patients and families.

The patients' rights movement has helped patients and families become, ideally, equal partners with their physicians in the medical decision-making process. Unfortunately, this movement has also set the stage for conflict, as the topic of this survey makes clear: patients struggling for personal autonomy versus physicians struggling for professional autonomy. We call this struggle "futility."

Futility comes from the Latin word *futilis,* meaning leaky. The term originated from the story of Danaus's daughters, who were condemned in Hades to draw water for eternity using leaky containers. Likewise, there are some goals in medicine that could *possibly* be achieved, but which experience has time and again shown this to be highly unlikely. One such example can be an emergency room team trying high-dose epinephrine on a fifty-year-old man in cardiac arrest, after they have spent forty-five minutes trying everything else they can think of, to no avail. They are almost certain this will not work, but there is that faint, far-off hope that maybe, just maybe, this will be the patient it works for.

It is important to realize that it can mean two very different things when health-care providers, patients, and families claim something ought not to be done because it is "futile." One version of futility is referred to as *physiologic futility*. When a health-care provider invokes this sense she is saying that no matter what we try or how hard we try it, nothing will work. This is the fifty-year-old man scenario; he could have been given every drug in the hospital and nothing would have changed. The other sense of futility is referred to by some as *medical futility*. This version brings forth the idea that some drug might have resuscitated the fifty-year-old, but he would have gained no significant benefit or improvement as a result. Yes, he would have a heartbeat, but he would also be on a ventilator in a coma from which he would, most likely, not wake.

With the concept of futility in hand, consider how the medical-industrial complex has bombarded the public with the notion that health-care providers can save just about anyone from just about anything. We have TV shows, such as *ER*, in which even the most catastrophically injured or devastatingly ill patients can be saved. There is the $3-billion Human Genome Project that will result in a cure for all diseases with a few puffs from an inhaler containing modified genes. So are patients and their families truly being unreasonable when they insist that "everything" be done? At the same time, are health-care providers truly being unreasonable when they refuse a request that they know will not work, or will not achieve the ends the patient and/or their family are hoping for?

This article should foster an appreciation as to why health-care providers, patients, and families insist on particular courses of action. Too easily are patients and families seen as being unreasonable by requesting "futile" care. Health-care providers, on the other hand, are frequently portrayed in these situations as denying care in order to save money, or when they refuse to withdraw care they are seen as cruel and only protecting themselves from a lawsuit. Once these dice are cast, communication is no longer possible. To prevent this, patients, families and health-care providers must consider together the patient's prognosis, current condition, preferences, goals, the benefits and burdens of possible interventions (including doing nothing), and the expected quality of life associated with each possible intervention. It is this kind of dialogue that will promote patient and professional autonomy, as well as good end-of-life care.

The final two readings are the yearly reports from the Oregon Heath Division's (OHD) Center for Disease Prevention and Epidemiology. As required by Oregon's Death with Dignity Act, the OHD developed a reporting system to monitor and collect information on physician-assisted suicide. The reports included here are "Oregon's Death with Dignity Act: The First Year's Experience (1998)" and "Oregon's Death with Dignity Act: The Second Year's Experience (1999)."

The Death with Dignity Act was passed in 1994 by popular referendum with a 2 percent margin. Not surprisingly, immediately after its passage an injunction preventing its implementation was imposed. After three years of legal battles, all hurdles were finally cleared—or so everyone thought. Oregon's legislators placed on the November 1997 ballot a measure calling for the repeal of the act. The measure was voted down by a 20 percent margin. The act allows adult residents of Oregon who are capable of making health-care decisions and who are terminally ill to request from their physician a prescription for a lethal medication.

Prior to the act, those on both sides of the debate made claims as to what would happen if society allowed physicians to write a prescription for a lethal dose of medicine. There were concerns that thousands of people would flock to Oregon to die; that unscrupulous physicians would set up "death clinics;" and most of all that the uninsured, the handicapped, and the unwanted would be coerced into asking for such a prescription. The American Medical Association also believed that allowing physicians to do this would destroy the public's trust in the medical profession and severely harm its integrity. On the other side, there were claims that this would bring about better overall end-of-life care as physicians would do whatever it took to make sure their patients were comfortable and cared for so that they would not ask for such prescriptions. Many also believed this would make physicians in other states better at caring for the dying so that their states would not pass such a law.

These reports seem to show that both fears and hopes were misplaced. No one flocked anywhere; no death clinics were established; the disabled, the poor and the unwanted were not done away with; and the integrity of the medical profession still seems to be intact. Improved end-of-care in the state of Oregon and beyond has also not come to fruition, as Bernabei and colleagues make clear. Ironically, last September, in one of the first cases of its kind, a physician was sanctioned by a state medical board for underprescribing pain medication. That state was Oregon.

By taking account of what actually has happened nationally and in Oregon since this option was made available, our discussions about how to improve end-of-life care will be guided more by facts and less by uniformed rhetoric. The OHD reports will go a long way in this pursuit.

REFERENCE

1. Cranford R. The persistent vegetative state: the medical reality. In this volume: 111.

7

THE PERSISTENT VEGETATIVE STATE

The Medical Reality (Getting the Facts Straight)

Ronald E. Cranford, M.D.

T he first step in any bioethical dilemma is to collect the facts and to understand the medical reality of the situation. Nowhere is this more necessary than in treatment decisions concerning patients with serious neurologic impairments. Modern medicine's halfway technologies have produced new neurologic creatures and require new terminology to describe syndromes both more complex and more common than anticipated a few decades ago.

Unfortunately, enormous conceptual and scientific confusion persists concerning the characteristics of these new syndromes, which include brain death (whole brain death), persistent vegetative state (PVS), permanent unconsciousness, coma, dementia, irreversible coma, chronic and irreversible coma, neocortical death, and locked-in syndrome.

For example, many over the last ten years mistakenly believed that Karen Quinlan was brain dead. Others, including neurological specialists, continue to consider the persistent vegetative state a form of coma. Many, including physicians, still believe that permanently unconscious patients, such as those in a persistent vegetative state, can experience pain and suffering.

In addition, there is little consensus about the appropriate terminology to describe such syndromes. In its 1986 statement on fluids and nutrition, the American

R. Cranford. "The Persistent Vegetative State: The Medical Reality." *Hastings Center Report.* 1988; February/March. Reproduced by permission. © The Hastings Center.

Medical Association's Council on Ethical and Judicial Affairs used the misleading term "irreversible coma." British physicians continue to apply broadly the phrase "brain stem death," a medical syndrome that simply does not exist except in extremely rare situations. Many physicians, especially in Europe, use imprecise and antiquated language such as "coma vigile," "akinetic mutism," and "apallic state" to describe some syndromes. The term "chronically and irreversibly comatose" as used in the Child Abuse Amendments of 1984 will be an endless source of confusion.

If the medical profession persists in failing to understand these syndromes and continues using inconsistent and incorrect terminology, how can the rest of society begin to unravel the complexities of neurology and lay the foundation for a moral and legal analysis of the issues emanating from these neurologic conditions? A full understanding of the medical facts about persistent vegetative state, including an examination of the significant similarities and differences between it and several other syndromes, is essential before we can begin to apply appropriate moral and legal principles to individual cases and to develop meaningful social policies.

THE MEDICAL REALITY

It is first important to differentiate *brain death* (whole brain death) from the *persistent vegetative state*.[1] The brain stem, the lower center of the brain, basically controls vegetative functions, such as respiration, and primitive stereotyped reflexes, such as the pupillary response to light. Additionally, it contains the activating or arousal system for the entire brain called the *ascending reticular activating system*. The cerebral hemispheres, in turn, contain the function of consciousness or awareness (which is more precisely located in the outer layers of the cerebral hemispheres, the cerebral cortex), as well as other important voluntary and involuntary actions, such as control of movements.

When brain death occurs, these higher cerebral functions cease; in addition, all brain stem functions are lost—eye movements; pupillary response to light; the most primitive protective reflexes such as the cough, gag, and swallowing; and spontaneous respiration. Heart beat, as well as other vegetative functions related to internal homeostasis, can continue, since these functions are semiautonomous, that is, they are not completely dependent on the integrity of the brain stem.

By contrast, in cases of patients in a persistent vegetative state, the brain stem, including the ascending reticular activating system, is relatively intact. The brunt of neurological destruction is located in the cerebral hemispheres. This state often results when a patient suffers a cardiac or respiratory arrest with lack of blood flow (*ischemia*) or oxygen (*hypoxia*) to the brain for a matter of minutes. The cerebral cortex is the part of the brain most vulnerable to this deprivation because of its high metabolic rate, requiring a constant supply of oxygen, glucose, and blood. The brain stem, however, is fairly resistant to ischemia or hypoxia. It is commonly accepted in medicine that approximately four to six minutes of complete loss of blood flow or oxygen to the brain can result in extensive destruction of the cerebral cortex while relatively sparing the brain stem.

After experiencing ischemia or hypoxia, the patient often will be in a coma that may persist for a few days or from two to four weeks. This transient coma results from a temporary dysfunction of the brain stem, which is not totally immune to the effects of hypoxicischernic injury. After this period, the patient will awaken and evolve into a condition of eyes-open unconsciousness, that is, the vegetative state.

Patients in a fully developed persistent vegetative state do manifest a variety of normal brain stem functions. The patient's eyes are open at times, and periods of wakefulness and sleep are present. The eyes wander, but without sustained visual pursuit (that is, following people or objects in the room in a consistent, meaningful, purposeful fashion). The pupils respond normally to light. Such a patient commonly requires a respirator initially, but this technology is usually unnecessary within a few days or weeks. The protective gag and cough reflexes are usually normal, which partially accounts for the long-term survival of these patients.

The patient is also completely unconscious, that is, unaware of him- or herself or the surrounding environment.[2] Voluntary reactions or behavioral responses reflecting consciousness, volition, or emotion at the cerebral cortical level are absent. PVS patients, then, are awake but unaware.

These characteristics allow a distinction to be made between comatose patients and patients in a persistent vegetative state. A coma is a state of sleeplike (eyes-closed) unarousability due to extensive damage to the reticular activating system of the brain stem. Patients in this condition often have impaired cough, gag, and swallowing reflexes with a resultant inability (involuntary) to clear the passages of the throat and lungs. This impairment leads to frequent, often fatal, respiratory infections—a common cause of death in comatose patients, and one of the major reasons why truly comatose patients typically do not experience the long-term survival period associated with the vegetative state. Thus, in one sense it is reasonable to describe comatose patients as "terminally ill," with death anticipated in six months to a year, unless extremely vigorous therapeutic efforts are made to sustain life.

If PVS patients are unconscious, but not comatose, as many mistakenly believe, what is their medical status? *Permanent unconsciousness*, as used by the President's Commission for the Study of Ethical Problems in Medicine and Biomedical and Behavioral Research and others, is the best term to apply to the broad category of patients with complete and permanent loss of consciousness or awareness.[3(pp171-192)] Permanently unconscious patients fall into two major categories: eyes-closed unconsciousness (coma) and eyes-open unconsciousness (persistent vegetative state and anencephaly). In these patients there are no cerebral cortical functions on clinical examination indicative of consciousness or behavioral interaction with the environment.

The persistent vegetative state should also be distinguished from the medical syndrome of dementia. Neurological impairment of cerebral cortical functions causes abnormalities of content of consciousness. Progressive loss of cerebral cortical functions is termed dementia, which in the case of Alzheimer's disease occurs over a period of years. By contrast, the catastrophic injury that results in the persistent vegetative state produces complete loss of cerebral cortical functions over a period of minutes. Patients in a persistent vegetative state are not simply demented, but amented (a complete loss of mental functions).

The term *irreversible coma* is frequently used with clinically and morally confusing consequences. In retrospect, those who drafted the Harvard Committee criteria for brain death erred in using the term "irreversible coma" as synonymous with brain death.[4] In a superficial sense, the terminology is correct; brain death is the ultimate irreversible coma—there is total destruction of the brain with the deepest possible coma and no possibility of reversibility. Beginning in the 1970s, however, neurological specialists began using the same term to apply to patients in the persistent vegetative state, such as Karen Quinlan. Thus, some physicians would use irreversible coma to mean brain death while others used it to mean the persistent vegetative state. Even today, physicians use the term irreversible coma in at least three different ways: whole brain death, persistent vegetative state, or as a general term for all types of permanently unconscious patients.

The term *chronically and irreversibly comatose* is even more misleading and should be rejected. The life span of a truly comatose patient is limited to weeks or months, rarely years, hardly the duration appropriately characterized as "chronic." When applied to the persistent vegetative state, such language is medically wrong. Nevertheless, this medical oxymoron now will be emblazoned forever in the annals of medical ethics by its inclusion in the Amendments to the Child Abuse Prevention and Treatment Act of 1984 and the implementing Health and Human Services regulations of 1985.[5] I doubt that the various parties responsible for the language of the amendments had a clear idea of what they intended to mean and which specific neurologic conditions fell under the designation "chronically and irreversibly comatose."

The case of Lance Steinhaus in Minnesota graphically illustrates the confusion that ensues when unclear or medically inaccurate language is relied on in legal decisions.[6] Lance was a normally developing five-week old child who was assaulted by his father on April 23 and 24, 1986, sustaining multiple abdominal and chest injuries and severe brain damage. Subsequent to the father's conviction on assault charges, Lance's mother requested that life-sustaining treatment be discontinued. When local authorities were alerted to the possibility that the case could fall under the jurisdiction of the Child Abuse Amendments and a corresponding state statute, a preliminary hearing was held to assess the mother's request. Prior to the hearing, briefs were submitted that claimed the vegetative state was not a form of coma. In testimony before the court, a pediatric intensivist asserted that Lance was in a persistent vegetative state. Based on this testimony, and interpreting the law in its most literal sense, the judge ruled that treatment could not be discontinued because the child was not "chronically and irreversibly comatose."

Subsequently, a pediatric neurologist, who was familiar with both the new neurologic syndromes and the precise terminology, was asked to see the child as an independent medical expert. After carefully examining Lance on several occasions, and reviewing the results of the the magnetic resonance imaging scan (MRI), the physician testified at a second hearing that Lance was in a coma from which he would not recover. The neurologist noted that Lance exhibited no sleep-wake cycles and only extremely infrequent and brief episodes of eye opening; there was significant impairment of brain stem functions on clinical examination; and the MRI scan showed extensive damage to the cerebral hemispheres and brain stem.

On the basis of this evaluation, the judge concluded that Lance was in a chronic and irreversibly comatose state and thus fell within that exception to the Child Abuse Amendments treatment requirements. With respect to the mother's decision, he ruled that some forms of treatment could be withheld (e.g., no cardiopulmonary resuscitation and no reintubation), but that other forms should be continued (appropriate nutrition, hydration, and medication).

The child, following a course typical of one who is truly comatose and has impaired brain stem functions, died of recurrent infections three months after this second ruling. Yet it would have been a far more tragic situation had the child been in a vegetative state, for the Child Abuse Amendments would have supported the initial decision to continue maximal treatment indefinitely. Lance could have then survived for months or perhaps years in this hopeless condition. Applied literally, which is surely the intent of some, the amendments permit nontreatment of a newborn who is unconscious (comatose) and who will die soon, but do not permit nontreatment of an equally unconscious (but amented) child who could live in this condition for years.

DIAGNOSTIC AND PROGNOSTIC COMPLEXITIES

The Steinhaus case also indicates some of the difficulties involved in clinical diagnosis of the persistent vegetative state. Indeed, in the minds of many, the reliability of a diagnosis of persistent vegetative state is a controversial issue that has yet to be adequately resolved.

A diagnosis of the persistent vegetative state usually can be made with a reasonably high degree of reliability within weeks or months after the original injury by a physician skilled in neurological diagnoses. However, for several reasons, the degree of certainty about diagnosis of this syndrome is less absolute than a diagnosis of brain death.

In the majority of cases, the diagnosis of brain death is not extremely difficult for a neurological specialist (neurologist, neurosurgeon, or pediatric neurologist) or physician knowledgeable and experienced in neurological diagnosis. If the accepted criteria are properly applied, the diagnosis reaches absolute certainty. The current national standards for the diagnosis of brain death are presented in the report of the Consultants to the President's Commission for the Study of Ethical Problems in Medicine and Biomedical and Behavioral Research.[7] In addition to the clinical criteria, these standards recommend specific confirmatory studies, for example, no blood flow to the brain as measured by various blood flow studies, or a flat electroencephalogram (electrocerebral silence).

With the persistent vegetative state, however, there is no broadly accepted, published set of specific medical criteria with as much clinical detail and certainty as the brain death criteria. Furthermore, even the generally accepted criteria, when properly applied, are not infallible. There have been a few unexpected, but unequivocal and well-documented, recoveries of cognitive functions in situations where it was believed that the criteria were correctly applied by several neurologists experienced in the diagnosis of this condition. In cases in New Mexico and Minnesota, the patients recovered full cognitive functioning, although they were left with a severe and permanent paralysis of all extremities and some paralysis of facial and head movements, that is, a locked-in syndrome.[3(pp179–180)] The locked-in syndrome is a medical condition in which, though both level and content of consciousness may be fairly normal, the patient is so severely paralyzed it may appear on superficial examination that he or she has diminished consciousness.

Presently, there are no specific laboratory studies to confirm the clinical diagnosis of the persistent vegetative state. After a variable period of time (weeks to months), some studies such as MRI and computerized axial tomography (CAT) scanning will show extensive structural damage to the cerebral hemispheres consistent with the clinical diagnosis, but these studies are not quantifiable. The most promising test on the horizon that will be of value in confirming a clinical diagnosis of the persistent vegetative state is the positron emission tomography (PET) scan.[8] This test measures in a quantitative fashion the metabolic rates of glucose and oxygen in various parts of the brain, including the cerebral cortex, an important index since consciousness cannot be sustained below certain quantifiable levels of metabolism. This method was used in the Nancy Jobes case in New Jersey to support the clinical diagnosis of the persistent vegetative state. However, PET scanning is new and extremely expensive; only a few centers in the country currently have the equipment necessary to carry out PET scanning. Furthermore, there is not yet sufficient data to document unequivocally the value of this test in the diagnosis of the persistent vegetative state.

The electroencephalogram (EEG) also does not provide absolute certainty because the degree of abnormality of the EEG will vary widely in individual cases. Some appear remarkably normal considering the extent of damage to the cerebral hemispheres. In a small percentage (probably less than 5 percent) of persistent vegetative cases, the EEG will display no electrical activity whatsoever, that is, electrocerebral silence, as in brain death. Thus it is possible for a patient whose eyes are open and who manifests sleep/wake cycles to have a completely flat EEG. Some neurologists refer to this specific neurologic syndrome as *neocortical death*. It is important to note that neocortical death is now being used in two different ways. Physicians may use this term in a very specific way: to denote persistent vegetative state patients with no electrical activity on the EEG. Others, such as philosophers and lawyers, use this term in a much more general sense—for patients permanently unconscious (whether persistently vegetative or permanently comatose) who have lost all neocortical functions.

Prognostic assessments of patients in a persistent vegetative state are not free of controversy. A major problem is attributable to the multiple causes and pathophysiologic changes associated with the syndrome. In brain death, the underlying cause of the brain injury is not so important once the basic sequence of pathophysiologic events begins and leads inexorably to its conclusion (severe primary injury–brain swelling–marked increase in intracranial pressure–increased intracranial pressure exceeding blood pressure, causing secondary loss of blood flow to the entire brain–infarction of cerebral hemispheres and the brain stem). In the persistent vegetative state, however, there are multiple causes for the syndrome, and no single pathophysiologic sequence of events. Therefore, the prognosis about recovery of neurologic function, when the prognosis can be made, and its degree of certainty will vary considerably according to the underlying cause of the brain damage and the specific pathophysiology.

For example, hypoxic-ischemic injuries to the brain, such as those experienced by Karen Quinlan and Nancy Jobes, result primarily in the death of neurons of the cerebral cortex.[9] Other injuries may cause the persistent vegetative state by different mechanisms, and the primary damage may not even be to the cerebral cortex itself. In head trauma the damage may be due to shearing injuries (mechanical distortion) of the subcortical white matter, the fiber tracts deep in the cerebral hemispheres. In Paul Brophy's case, the primary damage was to the upper brain stem and deep cerebral hemispheres.[10] This resulted from the rupture of a saccular, berry aneurysm (a ballooning of a blood vessel secondary to weakening of the arterial wall), which caused a vasospasm (constriction of the arteries) that resulted in infarction of the brain tissue. This brain destruction disrupted the connections between the cerebral cortex and the rest of the brain.

LONG-TERM SURVIVAL

It is abundantly clear that with the combination of cardiopulmonary resuscitation, more effective means of intubation, intensive care units, and other emergency resuscitative measures, there will continue to be an increase in the disparity between the effectiveness of cardiac and pulmonary resuscitation and the relative ineffectiveness thus far of cerebral (brain) resuscitation. The most commonly cited estimate of the number of PVS patients in the United States is 5,000 to 10,000, and this number can be anticipated to significantly increase in the future, especially when coupled with their increased longevity.[11]

It is not uncommon for patients to survive in this condition for five, ten, and twenty years. The longest reported, well documented, survival (without recovery) was thirty-seven years, 111 days.[12] In a recent medical/legal case involving an adolescent in a persistent vegetative state for several years, I testified that it was more likely than not that he would not be alive in ten years, and much more likely than not that he would not be alive in twenty years. I was not willing to be more specific than that. These were the limits of my certainty.

The duration is contingent upon several major factors: (1) age (elderly patients develop more medical complications secondary to prolonged immobility and unresponsiveness than younger patients); (2) economic, family, and institutional factors (in general, wealthier patients receive better care and more attention than indigent patients); (3) natural resistance of the body to infections and the effectiveness of cough and gag reflexes; and (4) changing moral and social views on the appropriateness of stopping treatment, especially medical means of providing nutrition and hydration. The variable survival periods of patients in persistent vegetative state makes it important to examine what forms of care can be provided to such patients and the costs of this care.

Because PVS patients often have an intact involuntary swallowing reflex in addition to intact gag and cough reflexes, it is theoretically, and in rare cases practically, possible to feed these patients by hand. However, this usually requires an enormous amount of time and effort by health-care professionals and families. If the patient is positioned properly, and food is carefully placed in the back of the throat, the patient's involuntary swallowing reflex will be activated. However, the overwhelming majority of patients are given fluids and nutrition by nasogastric tubing, gastrostomy, or other medical means.

Withholding of all fluids and nutrition will normally result in death within one to thirty days. If given adequate nursing care during this withdrawal, including good oral hygiene, PVS patients will not manifest the horrible signs ascribed to this process by some (e.g., mouth dried out and caked or coated with thick material; lips parched and cracked or fissured; tongue swollen and cracked; eyes sunk back into their orbits; cheeks hollow; lining of the nose cracked; nose bleeding; skin dry, scaly, and hanging loosely from the body; lining of stomach dried out causing dry heaves and vomiting; hyperthermia; brain cells dried out causing convulsions) nor will they experience consciously any symptoms (burning of urine, hunger, thirst).

Of related concern is the question of whether such patients experience any pain and suffering. While this has been much debated, it is not difficult to answer. The neurologic substratum for genuine human thinking and emotions and experiencing pain and suffering at a conscious level is the cerebral cortex. The American Academy of Neurology, in its amicus curiae brief filed in the *Brophy* case, took an unequivocal position on this issue: patients in a persistent vegetative state cannot experience pain and suffering.

> No conscious experience of pain and suffering is possible without the integrated functioning of the brainstem and cerebral cortex. Pain and suffering are attributes of consciousness, and PVS patients like Brophy do not experience them. Noxious stimuli may activate peripherally located nerves, but only a brain with the capacity for consciousness can translate that neural activity into an experience. That part of Brophy's brain is forever lost.[13]

There may be, and often are, facial movements and other signs indicating an apparent manifestation of conscious human suffering, but these actions result from subcortical (structures deep in the cerebral hemispheres that may be relatively undamaged) and brain stem actions of a primitive stereotyped, reflexive nature. In other words, PVS patients may "react" to painful and other noxious stimuli, but they do not "feel" (experience) pain in the sense of conscious discomfort of the kind that physicians would be obligated to treat and of the type that would seriously disturb the family. Families are often quite distressed by these subcortical and brainstem reflex responses, which they mistakenly interpret as a conscious interaction with the environment and an indication that the patient is experiencing distress. The family needs constant reassurance on this matter and, of course, the physician must be extremely confident of the diagnosis.

The cost of maintaining these patients varies substantially by state, type of institution, and support systems. In some states, like Minnesota, daily costs are usually $50 to $70 per day, about $1,500 to $2,000 a month, or approximately $18,000 to $25,000 a year. In Massachusetts, the charges in Paul Brophy's case were approximately $10,000 per month. Extrapolating from a monthly low of $2,000 to a high of $10,000, and assuming there are five thousand to ten thousand patients in a vegetative state in the United States, the annual national health bill for these patients is from $120 million to $1.2 billion. This does not include the extremely high costs of the first year of care after the original injury when the patient may have spent extensive time in an intensive care unit. In cases with which I am personally familiar, costs during the first year (especially in young people) were $200,000 to $250,000. The precise cost will vary depending on how much time is spent in an intensive care unit and at what point the patient is transferred from an acute care hospital to a chronic care facility.

THE NEED FOR CLARITY, CONSISTENCY, AND CONSENSUS

The vast majority of termination of treatment cases before the courts in recent years have involved neurologically impaired patients. One major lesson we have learned from these landmark legal cases, and from the thousands of cases occurring regularly in American hospitals today, is the critical need for better understanding of the medical facts and for clarity and consistency in medical terminology.

Physicians should stop using confusing and in many cases inaccurate language. For example, it makes no sense to talk about "comfort measures" or "pain and suffering" in patients in a persistent vegetative state. Physicians should bring to the attention of Congress the fact that the class of patients called "chronically and irreversibly comatose" simply does not exist in any meaningful sense. The term "irreversible coma" should be completely abandoned. Physicians should educate the public that the withdrawal of artificial feeding from patients in persistent vegetative state does not lead to the horrible signs and symptoms attributed to this process by special interest groups; this is misleading rhetoric, not medical reality.

The medical, ethical, and legal issues in the near future will be far more complex and common than those faced thus far. It is time that medical professionals, especially the national medical and neurological specialty societies, undertake a much more active leadership role by developing position papers on the medical aspects of these neurological syndromes, forging a consensus through increased interdisciplinary dialogue, and developing broader guidelines on the appropriate care and management of these patients.

Families, physicians, the public, and the courts can only make informed, humane, and fitting decisions after understanding the relevant and correct medical facts. Once the medical reality of these syndromes is appreciated, I believe that certain logical, moral, and legal conclusions will naturally follow.[14]

REFERENCES

1. Cranford RE, Smith HL. Some critical distinctions between brain death and the persistent vegetative state. *Ethics in Science and Medicine*. 1979;6:199–209.

2. Jennett B, Plum F. Persistent vegetative state after brain damage. *Lancet*. 1972;1:734–737.

3. President's Commission for the Study of Ethical Problems in Medicine and Biomedical and Behavioral Research. *Deciding to Forego Life-Sustaining Treatment*. Washington, DC: US Government Printing Office; 1983.

4. Report of the Ad Hoc Committee of the Harvard Medical School to Examine the Definition of Brain Death. A definition of irreversible coma. *JAMA*. 1968;205(6):85–88.

5. Child Abuse and Neglect Prevention and Treatment, 45 C.F.R. Secs. 1340.1–1340.20. 1986.

6. New "Baby Doe" ethics tested. *American Medical News*. October 10, 1986: 1, 45.

7. Consultants to the President's Commission for the Study of Ethical Problems in Medicine and Biomedical and Behavioral Research. Guidelines for the determination of death. *JAMA*. 1981;246(19):2184–2186.

8. Levy D, Sidtis J, Rottenberg D, et al. Positron emission tomography in the diagnosis of the vegetative state. Forthcoming.

9. In re Quinlan, 70 N.J. 10, 355 A.2d 647, *cert denied* 429 U.S. 922 (1976); In re Jobes, 108 N.J. 394, 529 A.2d 434 (1987).

10. *Brophy* v. *New England Sinai Hospital, Inc.* 398 Mass. 417, 497 N.E.2d 626 (1986).

11. This estimate is based on epidemiological studies from Japan showing approximately 2,000 to 3,000 patients in this condition in that country, and an extrapolation of that data to the United States, taking into account both a doubling in population and our more advanced (and more indiscriminately applied) life-support systems.

12. Cranford RE. Termination of treatment in the persistent vegetative state. *Seminars in Neurology*. 1984;4(1):36–44.

13. *Brophy* v. *New England Sinai Hospital, Inc.* Amicus Curiae Brief, American Academy of Neurology, Minneapolis, MN. 1986.

14. Cranford RE. Consciousness as the critical moral (constitutional) threshold for life. Presented at the annual General Meeting of the American Society of Law and Medicine, *Justice Blackmun, the Supreme Court, and the Limits of Medical Privacy*. October 23–24, 1987, Boston, MA.

8

THE PROCESS OF DYING WITH AND WITHOUT FEEDING AND FLUIDS BY TUBE

Phyllis Schmitz, R.N.

The process of dying, ultimately, is an experience that will be common to us all. Considering the current trends in health care, I would guess that most of us give more than a passing thought to how that final phase of life will be played out on a personal level. Undoubtedly, that image is shaped by our attitudes and experiences. In addition, each of us recognizes that we have had or are likely to have an impact on the dying in our role as family or friend, health-care provider, or interpreter of the legal or ethical issues. As a member of a hospice team, I have personally cared for hundreds of terminally ill patients, and based on these experiences, I present the following observations regarding the process of dying, with and without feeding and fluid by tube.

J. R. was a successful business executive until AIDS intervened; within an eight-month period, he was forced to give up both his position and independence because of severe peripheral neuropathy which left him minimally functional and in constant pain. He came to us embittered and depressed. Our initial goals were to treat his mental and physical anguish. Once these were managed, his angry outbursts settled into gentler protests. We planned his care using criteria similar to those by which he conducted his office affairs: All aspects of his care were given a relative value and prioritized. Compromises were carefully negotiated and eventually a routine was estab-

P. Schmitz. "The Process of Dying, With and Without Feeding and Fluids by Tube." *Law, Medicine & Health Care*. 1991;19(1–2):23–27. ©1991. Reprinted with the permission of the American Society of Law, Medicine & Ethics. All rights reserved.

lished. He was comforted by gentle massage, a cigarette, conversation that included anything from politics to the merits of classic Coke, and a promise that we would not torture him with tubes. His appetite, always poor, seemed to diminish daily, but he consistently refused medical intervention. For days, his intake consisted of sips of water, juice, or Coke and an occasional spoonful of ice cream. He became progressively weaker and dyspneic because of profound anemia.

One morning, about a month after his admission to our unit, he awoke and asked for a cigarette. His oxygen was discontinued, he took two short puffs, frowned, and motioned for me to extinguish it. He then asked for a favorite psalm to be read and quietly closed his eyes. No further words were necessary; we both knew the end would come soon.

Two doors down the hall, Anna sat and stared at the calendar on the wall next to her bed. Each day, she crossed off the date with her red marker. In a week, she would have a new grandchild. Children had always been important to her. She had been a teacher's aide for many years and had raised her two children as a single parent. A malignant tumor had invaded her pharynx two years earlier, and she had consented to the radical surgery and subsequent radiation therapy. She had become quite competent and proud of her ability to care for her tracheostomy and feeding tubes. She communicated by writing and took delight in simple pleasures: sitting outdoors, chewing on some favorite foods just for the taste of it. But she was getting weaker, the tumor was growing rapidly, now erupting to the surface of her neck. We often found her looking at the tumor and then glancing at the calendar. We knew that time was a critical issue. She kept a rigid feeding schedule, and at times overfed herself, which resulted in episodes of vomiting or diarrhea. We continued to work with her, changing both formulas and schedules several times. Her granddaughter arrived and Anna had the opportunity to hold her several times, to the delight of us all. Soon afterward, Anna began to retreat: less communication, refusal of feedings, and general apathy. She seemed to like company, though, and would frequently reach over and pat our hands when we sat with her. But we all agreed that it appeared that on some level, she had already left us.

I present these two cases in order to point out the link between life and death, as no mere presentation of clinical data could do. The threads of dying are in fact woven into the fabric of living and I would like the reader to hold that image as I continue.

Giving food and drink is basic to human relationships and has been so across time and culture. We have heard so often that the ministering of food and water to the vulnerable is a powerful symbol that expresses care and compassion and so communicates significant societal values. These are wonderful ideals that are important to establishing the appropriate moral climate. But what of the ordinary experiences of eating? Think of your favorite food. Can you taste it, smell it? Can you remember eating just to console yourself over a disappointment, or perhaps to avoid dealing with a difficult issue? The bottom line is that some people live to eat and others eat to live and this should be an important consideration as well when food and water are offered. Those who care for the dying have found that individual values play an important part in accepting or rejecting symbols. I think it is essential to balance the tension between the symbolic meaning of food and water and the patient's wishes.

In general, providing appropriate nutritional intake for the dying frequently improves the sense of well-being and quality of life, at least for a while. Patients seem to do best when there is a minimum of restrictions in food selection and a relaxation of rigid schedules. Even those who are fed through tubes benefit from individualizing their therapy. For family and caregivers, continued intake means continued life, and when the dying patient is unable to tolerate feeding, the stress level of concerned others escalates sharply. It is at this time that family and caregivers are likely to attempt force feeding, indicating their inability to deal with their impending loss. While pointing out the burdens of such an approach, it is helpful to offer suggestions that are more appropriate for the dying patient but also respect the sensitivity of family and/or friends.

Weakness and diminished intake, either abrupt or gradual, are common manifestations of the dying trajectory. These changes seem to occur as part of an overall disengagement process in which the patient withdraws on a physical, emotional, and social level. At this time, less communication takes place, but an awareness continues and, in fact, hearing becomes more acute. There is often a focus on important objects in the person's life: a person, a pet, a particular food. Overall, there is a tendency to lethargy, somnolence, and a quiet resignation. These behavioral changes occur in all dying patients, with and without feeding tubes.

At about the same time, those who have foregone artificial nutrition and hydration will begin to exhibit signs of fluid deficit: reduced peripheral circulation with accompanying skin changes, decreased urinary output, restlessness, muscular irritability, cardiac arrhythmias, mental status changes, and dry skin and and mucus membranes, all indicative of electrolyte imbalance. Those who receive food and fluids by tube may not experience this in the same manner; however, continued feeding and hydration, especially utilizing normal parameters, frequently creates other hardships which I will describe shortly. It is important to remember that these signs and symptoms will vary greatly, depending on the underlying pathology and rate of system failure.

Patients who remain alert do not seem greatly disturbed by these changes. They will note their increased weakness but very few appear concerned. Frequently, they are experiencing less discomfort at this time. The symptoms of electrolyte imbalance can be treated with mild sedatives. However, this is often a period of heightened anxiety as patients sense something is happening and consequently are fearful of being left alone. It is frequently a time of conversation that is focused on the topic, "What will it be like?"

The issue of dehydration continues to be controversial, and many continue to believe that dying from a lack of fluids is exceedingly painful, something our society should not permit. The subject is debated in our courts and in our healthcare institutions.

Before the advent of feeding tubes, intravenous feeding, and total parenteral nutrition, little could be done for those patients who were unable to ingest sufficient food or fluid. Caregivers provided intake as long as was possible and patients eventually succumbed to their illnesses, often in a state of malnutrition or dehydration. Available literature does not indicate that the lack of food or fluid had a deleterious effect on the nature of the death.

Since the advent of the medical technologies that efficiently deliver food and fluids through an array of conduits, efforts are made to utilize one of the many options to treat the medically malnourished. Aggressive nutritional support has well-documented benefits for the critically ill, but there is little evidence that the dying benefit from measures to correct malnutrition and dehydration. In fact, use of such techniques can harm the patient, or at the very least worsen the quality of life.

For the dying patient, the experience of dehydration is the result of decreased water or fluids over time, related to pathology and a gradual biological deterioration. A few recent articles appear to describe symptoms that would occur in an otherwise healthy person who experienced acute water deprivation. Terminal dehydration is generally an isotonic dehydration, with mixed disorders of salt and water depiction. Hospice workers consistently state that patients report dry mouth and occasional thirst, but rarely encounter nausea, vomiting, or cramps. When these do occur, they are usually the result of other pathology, such as obstruction or renal failure. Dying patients who are subjectively dehydrated are often more comfortable in their last days. Decreased gastrointestinal fluid results in fewer bouts of vomiting; reduced pulmonary secretions bring relief from congestion, coughing, and fear of choking; decreased urinary output means less struggling with the bedpan or fewer linen changes for the incontinent. The discomfort of peripheral and pulmonary edema is relieved as this fluid is gradually resorbed during the last days of life. One of the more significant findings is that patients dying of terminal dehydration rarely need oral-pharyngeal suctioning. Hospice workers have long felt that the disinterest in food and fluid exhibited in the last days of life is part of an adaptive process that allows the patient to die with less suffering. In the end, the patient becomes obtunded and death generally occurs peacefully.

Patients receiving food and fluids through tubes often experience the distress of fluid overload and depending on the preexisting disease process, an increase in distressing symptoms, such as vomiting, diarrhea, and pulmonary congestion. If the patient has edema, excess body fluid can aggravate discomfort. The patient may be awake and therefore painfully aware of the suffering.

How, then, should we meet the nutritional needs of dying patients, with and without feeding and fluids by tube? On a basic level, it begins with health-care providers who are willing to walk with patients in the dying process rather than focus efforts on rescuing them from their disease. A health-care institution is served well by having in place a philosophy that defines the framework for making decisions with regard to nutrition and hydration, and describes the available options and under what conditions they are used. It is essential that all involved care providers are made aware of this document and communicate its content to patients and families.

A general assessment is crucial to providing optimal supportive care and, in the context of history taking and a physical exam, the capabilities of the patient to receive nutrition can be evaluated. In addition, a values history contributes important information that can help the health-care team determine the patient's priorities and goals.

The needs of the dying patient are best met when the goals are focused on promoting optimum comfort, advancing the priorities of the patient, and making available those experiences that allow the patient to live as fully as possible.

Decreasing the distressing symptoms of advanced disease that interfere with nutritional intake is essential. When pain is eliminated, depression, anxiety, and fatigue usually decrease in intensity. Vomiting, diarrhea, and constipation often improve with the appropriate drug therapy, and the discomfort associated with dry mouth and dysphagia are easily remedied with local measures.

Once the patient has achieved a satisfactory level of comfort, a creative combination of options should be made available. Frequent small meals are best, the amount and type of food dependent on appetite and preferences. Dietary restrictions can be comfortably eliminated if the rescue mentality is abandoned. Attention in providing favorite foods is generally appreciated, and cultural and ethnic dishes provided by family and friends also encourage oral intake.

For those patients receiving food and fluids by tube, efforts can be made to closely approximate normal feeding. Adapting the feeding schedule for patient comfort and providing occasional treats, such as coffee, homemade soup, or a beer, are expressions of caring and sensitivity to individual needs that provide priceless experiences for the dying. Patients should be offered small amounts of food orally if they are capable of swallowing, and if not they may still be open to enjoying the taste.

If we agree that death is the extinguishing of a life, then those who provide the care for a dying patient must do so with the utmost respect for the patient as a person. Decisions relevant to food and fluids, as well as other aspects of care, should take into consideration the patient's wishes. For some, eating and drinking are of vital importance; for others, they are of minimal interest. But our commitment to care for the dying implies that food and water should always be offered. In the final analysis, medical care of the dying ought to be shaped by patient's values and priorities and not the other way around.

J. R. awoke one afternoon and asked that his sisters, friend, and minister be summoned. He continued to accept sips of water but refused all other care. He was rallying his energy for something quite different. After sleeping much of the day, he began to call each person into his room to give a final message. As his primary nurse, I, too, was summoned. His words were brief: "Thank you for the care and for letting me be me."

Anna died a week after the birth of her granddaughter. She generally continued to refuse feedings but did allow us to give her water and juice. She became incontinent and after each episode she wept, sometimes inconsolably. Her tumor began to bleed, heightening her anxiety, but she always seemed to derive comfort from a staff presence. Her death was peaceful, following a brief loss of consciousness. Though their family members and friends grieved, they recognized and appreciated that death had occurred in an acceptable fashion, reflecting the lives that preceeded it. J. R.'s sister commented that he had orchestrated his dying much as he did his living.

In conclusion, I would like to leave the reader with some food for thought. My experiences over the last nine years have taught me how truly impoverished our language can be. Caring for the dying has challenged me to look beyond our limited definition of nurture. Besides to nourish, does it not include the obligation to cherish, to support self-respect and self-determination as long as possible, to sustain the dying in their weakness? Expanding our perspective can lead to a whole new repertoire of behaviors toward the dying. I believe dialogue about end-of-life decisions ought to be an integral part of any physiciant/patient relationship. I see this as an expression of nurturing at the highest level.

Suffering is the state of anguish of one who bears pain, injury, or loss. As such it is a subjective experience. However, when health-care providers focus on "pathology," they are less likely to understand the patient's experience. Elizabeth O'Connor, in her book, *Our Many Selves*, states, "The sick [dying] in their suffering are closer to what is real. They see things that really matter and are in possession of different values." A little later, she adds, "As it is, we often have learned very little and so are destined to suffer in the same ways again."

Dying patients frequently report that health-care providers are unable to relieve their suffering. When the emphasis is on "medical things," caregivers have done little to enter into the patient's experience where multiple losses and injury are usually at the heart of the pain.

J. R. and Anna taught us well. They provided guideposts in their dying that helped us to care for them, to nurture them and to relieve their suffering.

As we continue to struggle to learn how to make good medical decisions, let us not forget that death is not a separate phenomenon, but a part of life, and each passing is a loss as we share in the solidarity of our mortality. We must look to the patients for answers in this struggle. Their experiences can enrich us and help us to better understand and serve those in the process of dying, with and without feeding and fluid by tube.

BIBLIOGRAPHY

Andrews MR, Levine AM. Dehydration in the terminal patient: perception of hospice nurses. *American Journal of Hospice Care.* January/February 1989: 31–34.

Annas GJ. Do feeding tubes have more rights than patients? *Hastings Center Report.* February 1986: 26–28.

Arnold C. Nutrition intervention in the terminally ill cancer patient. *Journal of the American Dietetic Association.* 1986;86:522–523.

Billings JA. Comfort measures for the terminally ill—is dehydration painful? *Journal of the American Geriatric Society.* 1985;33:808–810.

Cox SS. Is dehydration painful? *Ethics & Medics.* 1987;12:1–2.

Guidelines on the Termination of Life-Sustaining Treatment and the Care of the Dying. New York, NY: Hastings Center; 1987.

Lo B, McLeod GA, Saika G. Patient attitudes to discussing life-sustaining treatment. *Archives of Internal Medicine.* 1986;146:1613–1615.

Lynn J, Childress JF. Must patients always be given food and water? *Hastings Center Report.* 1983;10:17–21.

Lynn J (ed.). *By No Extraordinary Means.* Bloomington, IN: Indiana University Press; 1989.

Miles SH. The terminally ill elderly: dealing with the ethics of feeding. *Geriatrics.* 1985;40:112–120.

Miller RJ, Albright PG. What is the role of nutritional support and hydration in terminal cancer patients? *American Journal of Hospice Care.* November/December 1989: 33–38.

O'Connor E. *Our Many Selves.* New York, NY: Harper & Row; 1971.

Paris JJ. When burdens of feeding outweigh benefits. *Hastings Center Report.* February 1986: 30-32.

President's Commission for the Study of Ethical Problems in Medicine and Biomedical Research. *Deciding to Forego Life-Sustaining Treatment: A Report on the Ethical, Medical, and Legal Issues in Treatment Decisions.* Washington, DC: US Government Printing Office; 1983.

Ramsay P. *The Patient As Person.* New Haven, CT: Yale University Press; 1970.

Steinbrook R, Lo B. Artificial feeding—solid ground, not a slippery slope. *New England Journal of Medicine.* 1988;318:286–290.

Watts DT, Cassel CK. Extraordinary nutritional support: a case study and ethical analysis. *Journal of the American Geriatric Society.* 1984;32:237–242.

Zerwekh JV. The dehydration question. *Nursing.* 1983;1:47–51.

9

DECISIONS TO LIMIT OR CONTINUE LIFE-SUSTAINING TREATMENT BY CRITICAL CARE PHYSICIANS IN THE UNITED STATES

Conflicts Between Physicians' Practices and Patients' Wishes

David A. Asch, M.D., John Hansen-Flaschen, M.D., and Paul N. Lanken, M.D.

꽃

Decisions to forgo life-sustaining treatment are among the most challenging that physicians and patients face. In response to this challenge, many institutions and authorities have proposed guidelines for withholding and withdrawing life-sustaining treatment.[1-5] These efforts have converged toward a series of ethical principles. Perhaps the most central principle is that patients have the right to forgo life-sustaining treatment based on their preferences and goals. This ethical principle of self-determination has gained legal support from the 1990 *Cruzan* decision by the Supreme Court [6] and the 1990 Patient Self-Determination Act.[7,8] If this consensus has helped guide clinicians in practices that previously were much more controversial, we would expect to find widespread physician acceptance of decisions to forgo life support.

In fact, studies of physicians' attitudes toward the withholding and withdrawing of life-sustaining treatment suggest that physicians generally accept decisions to limit life-sustaining treatments—at least in the abstract—as a legitimate part of clinical practice.[9-17] At the same time, some investigators have demonstrated significant variation in physicians' attitudes in this area, and have identified factors that may explain this variation, including differences in physicians' rank or experience,[9,12] specialty,[16]

D. Asch, J. Hansen-Flaschen, P. Lanken. "Decisions to Limit or Continue Life-Sustaining Treatment by U.S. Critical Care Physicians: Conflicts between Physicians' Practices and Patients' Wishes." *American Journal of Respiratory and Critical Care Medicine.* 1999;151(2):288–292. Reprinted by permission of the American Thoracic Society.

preferences for risk,[15] social attributes,[14] and specific biases in the way they make their decisions.[13]

Fewer investigators have extended this research beyond physician attitudes to physician practice. Some studies suggest that the withholding or withdrawing of life-sustaining treatment accounts for a large proportion of hospital deaths,[18,19] but studies rarely address practices at the level of the individual physician. Surveys of physicians in Rhode Island[11] and Pennsylvania,[13] and physician and nonphysician critical care practitioners more nationally,[17] suggest that in these populations the practice of forgoing life support is widespread.

However, we are unaware of attempts to gauge practices in more controversial areas. As the practice of forgoing life-sustaining treatment in response to patients' wishes becomes less controversial, physicians have begun to question whether they must always comply with requests to continue or limit such treatment, even when they disagree with the rationale or intent of those requests. This question may result from a greater understanding among physicians of the limits of medical technology; from physicians' increasing acceptance of their role as stewards of societal resources; or perhaps as a reaction to rising patient consumerism and a perceived decline in physician authority. Whatever the explanation, ethicists have responded by reexamining the line between patient autonomy and physician authority, and by trying to define the concept of medical futility and its meaning in clinical practice. Although futility is not a new concept in medicine, defining its practical implications represents a new social and clinical frontier.

Most published work on medical futility consists of ethical analyses of alternative definitions of futility, and policy suggestions for altering or circumventing established procedures for obtaining consent to forgo life-sustaining treatments in certain circumstances.[20-30] These efforts may help to lay the ethical groundwork necessary to guide future physician practice. However, the empirical research that could help define current physician practice in this area is almost exclusively anecdotal.

The purpose of this study was to examine the withholding and withdrawing of life support by critical care physicians. We surveyed physicians practicing in adult medical and surgical intensive care units in the United States and asked them to report their experiences in withholding and withdrawing life-sustaining treatment. We focused particularly on decisions to continue life support against the wishes of patients or surrogates, and on decisions to limit treatment on the basis of medical futility.

METHODS

In February 1990, we mailed a survey to all 1,970 self-identified members of the Critical Care Section of the American Thoracic Society. The American Thoracic Society is the medical arm of the American Lung Association and represents a large professional society for physicians specializing in pulmonary and critical care medicine. The survey contained ninety-one items divided into sections soliciting professional information relating to training and practice type; information about the respondents primary hospital affiliation; clinical experience with the withholding or withdrawal of life-sustaining medical therapy; and opinions regarding professional, administrative, and educational efforts that might improve clinical practices in this area. (A copy of the survey instrument is available from the American Lung Association, Attn.: Susan Rappaport, 1740 Broadway, New York, N.Y. 10019-4374.)

One section of the survey explored subjects' clinical experience with and attitudes toward the withholding or withdrawing of life-sustaining treatment on the basis of medical futility. Because the definition of futility can be ambiguous and controversial, we provided subjects with a definition to use in this part at the questionnaire. This definition was based on a position statement from the American Thoracic Society,[4] and explicitly contrasted decisions based on medical futility from those made on the basis of requests or consent from the patient or family, as follows:

> In most cases in which life-sustaining treatment is withheld or withdrawn, it is at the request of the patient or family or with their informed consent. In other cases, the patients physician may decide to withhold or withdraw a certain treatment solely because the physician judges it to be medically futile, i.e., it provides no significant chance for survival per se or for a meaningful survival (meaningful in relation to the patient's values and life goals).

The survey was designed so that individual respondents could not be identified, and subjects were assured of the confidentiality of their responses. Surveys were sent in a single mailing, and no monetary incentive was offered.

We used logistic regression to model self-reported practices as a function of age (expressed as a continuous variable), percentage of time spent in clinical practice, whether the respondent's primary hospital affiliation was a teaching hospital, and whether it had a religious affiliation. Statistical analyses were performed using Systat version 5.2.1 for the Macintosh personal computer.

RESULTS

Of the 1,970 physicians surveyed, 1,050 (53%) responded. Of these, 74 were excluded because a portion of their practice represented pediatrics or they practiced primarily in a pediatric intensive care unit; 20 were excluded because they indicated no current clinical practice; and 77 were excluded because they practiced in non–United States hospitals. The remaining 879 respondents are the subjects of this study. Because of occasional missing data, not all totals equal 879.

Table 9-1 presents summary characteristics of the physicians as reported on the questionnaire. Respondents practiced in all states except Alaska. Table 9-2 presents summary characteristics of physicians' primary hospital affiliations.

Table 9-3 presents physicians' self-reported experience in withdrawing life-sustaining medical therapy. All but 31 respondents (4%) reported that they had discon-

Table 9-1. Characteristics of 879 Respondents

Physician Characteristic	
Mean age SD	41.8 ± 7.2
Mean distribution of professional activity	
Administration	9%
Clinical	68%
Research	9%
Teaching	13%
Board certified/eligible, n (%)	
Anesthesia	14 (1.6%)
Critical care medicine	544 (62%)
Pulmonary medicine	701 (80%)
Other	49 (6%)
None	130 (15%)
Primary intensive-care-unit practice site, n (%)	
Adult combined medical/surgical	510 (58%)
Adult medical	305 (35%)
Adult surgical	34 (4%)
Other	20 (3%)
Ever been a member of an ethics committee	189 (23%)

tinued at least one form of treatment with the expectation that the patient would die as a result. More than half had at least once discontinued artificially provided food or water. Seven hundred thirty-six physicians (85%) reported withdrawing mechanical ventilation at least once in the preceding year, 256 (29%) reported withdrawing it three to five times, and another 229 (26%) reported withdrawing it more than five times in the preceding year. Eighty-three physicians (9%) reported that they had discontinued life-sustaining mechanical ventilation in a patient not expected to die within six months otherwise, and 293 (33%) reported that they had discontinued mechanical ventilation because of what they felt to be the best interests of a patient who had neither the ability to make decisions nor a surrogate decision maker.

Although nearly all respondents had participated in the withdrawal of life-sustaining treatment, 294 physicians (34%) reported that they had declined to withdraw mechanical ventilation at least once in the preceding year despite having been asked to do so by a patient or surrogate. Table 9-4 lists the reasons given by physicians to explain these decisions. Of note, 11 of the 25 physicians who thought the withdrawal of mechanical ventilation was unethical, and 24 of the 42 physicians who thought the withdrawal of mechanical ventilation might be illegal, indicated that at other times they had participated in its withdrawal. Of the 23 physicians who indicated that they were unsure of how to proceed, 12 practiced in hospitals in which they knew there was an ethics committee or bioethicist on staff. Physicians practicing in New York State who had declined to withdraw mechanical ventilation were much more likely

Table 9-2. Characteristics of 879 Respondents' Hospitals

Hospital Chracteristic	
Hospital type, n (%)	
University teaching hospital	267 (30%)
Community hospital	516 (59%)
County or municipal hospital	43 (5%)
U.S. government hospital	53 (6%)
Hospital size, n (%)	
< 100 beds	13 (2%)
101–500 beds	564 (64%)
> 500 beds	300 (34%)
Hospital religious affiliation, n	
Catholic	126 (15%)
Jewish	37 (4%)
Protestant	68 (8%)
Other	33 (4%)
None	601 (69%)
Hospital ethics committee or bioethicist	597 (68%)

Table 9-3. Proportion of 879 Physicians Who Have Withdrawn Various Forms of Life-Sustaining Treatments

Form of Treatment	n (%)
Mechanical ventilation	786 (89%)
Intravenous vasopressors	758 (88%)
Renal dialysis	604 (71%)
Blood or blood products	687 (80%)
Artificial nutrition and/or hydration	486 (58%)
Never	31 (4%)

to report their concern that the withdrawal of mechanical ventilation was illegal in that state as a reason for their decision (12 of 26 respondents).

Tables 9-5 and 9-6 report physicians' experience in withholding and withdrawing life-sustaining therapy on the basis of medical futility. The majority of physicians reported they had done so: 726 physicians (83%) reported withholding life-sustaining treatment and 713 (82%) reported withdrawing treatment under these circumstances. Three hundred twenty physicians (37%) reported withdrawing life-sustaining treatment on the basis of medical futility from three to five times during the preceding year, and another 266 (31%) reported withdrawing it more than five times in the preceding year. Many physicians reported withholding or withdrawing life-sustaining treatment without the consent of the patient or family or without their knowledge, and some reported doing so over patients' or family members' objections.

The results of the logistic-regression modeling reveal that older physicians were

Table 9-4. Reasons Physicians (n = 294) Declined Requests to Withdraw Life-Sustaining Mechanical Ventilation in the Past Year

Reason	n (%)
Physician believed the patient still had a reasonable chance to recover	227 (77%)
Physician believed the family might not be acting in the best interest of a patient who lacked decision-making capacity	115 (39%)
Physician concerned about malpractice litigation	55 (19%)
Physician believed that the withdrawal of mechanical ventilation is or might be illegal in the state	42 (14%)
Family opposed to the withdrawal of mechanical ventilation even though it was requested by a patient capable of making decisions	33 (11%)
Physician believed that withdrawal of mechanical ventilation is unethical in general	25 (9%)
Counter to current practices at the hospital	24 (8%)
Physician unsure of how to proceed	23 (8%)
Physician advised by hospital legal counsel not to withdraw mechanical ventilation	14 (5%)

Table 9-5. Proportion of Physicians (n = 726) Who Withdraw Life-Sustaining Treatment on the Basis of Medical Futility

Consent Status	n (%)
Without the written or oral consent of the patient or family	219 (25%)
Without the knowledge of the patient or family	120 (14%)
Despite the objections of the patient or family	28 (3%)

less likely to report having withdrawn mechanical ventilation than younger physicians (odds ratio = 0.94; 95% CI 0.91 to 0.96). The odds ratio reflects a single year's difference in age, and can be interpreted to mean that if two physicians are a year apart in age, the chance the older physician has withdrawn mechanical ventilation is about 94% of the chance that the younger one has. Wider differences in age would expand differences in odds. This effect remains the same when controlling for the percentage of time spent in clinical practice, whether the hospital is a university teaching hospital, and whether it has a religious affiliation. These other variables are not independently significant and do not change the model. Age was not found to be significant in similar models of the withdrawal of intravenous vasopressors, renal dialysis, blood products, or food and water; nor was it found to be significant in models designed to analyze the withholding of resuscitation on the basis of medical futility.

DISCUSSION

Our results support several conclusions. First, the vast majority of our respondents (96%) reported that they had withdrawn or withheld medical treatments from patients with the understanding that death would follow. This finding is consistent

Table 9-6. Proportion of Physicians (n = 713) Who Withdraw Life-Sustaining Treatment on the Basis of Medical Futility	
Treatment Modality or Consent Status	**n (%)**
Mechanical ventilation	554 (63%)
Intravenous vasopressors	650 (74%)
Renal dialysis	494 (56%)
Artificial nutrition and/or hydration	405 (46%)
Without the written or oral consent of the patient or family	203 (23%)
Without the knowledge of the patient or family	105 (12%)
Despite the objections of the patient or family	23 (3%)

with those of other studies, suggesting widespread diffusion of these practices.[11,13] In aggregate, our physicians reported withdrawing a variety of forms of life-sustaining treatment, including artificially provided food and water. Although fewer physicians reported withdrawing food and water than other forms of life support, this difference may have resulted from differences in opportunity rather than attitude. Earlier studies of physician attitudes suggest that physicians are less willing to withdraw food and water than other forms of life support.[13,16]

Second, one-third of our physicians reported withdrawing life-sustaining treatment from a patient not capable of making decisions and not represented by a surrogate decision maker. We suspect that the vast majority of these decisions were made without the benefit of an advance directive or other prior communication of personal preferences between patient and physician.[17] That a third of our respondents have had to make decisions in the absence of a patient proxy identifies an extremely common problem, raises questions about how these decisions were made or evaluated, and suggests the need for guidelines to assist clinicians in these decisions.

Third, despite the growing acceptance of requests by patients or surrogates to limit medical treatment, a third of our physicians also reported refusing such requests. In most cases the reason they provided—that the patient still had a reasonable chance to recover—reveals the importance physicians place on prognosis in these decisions. Indeed, only 9% of physicians reported withdrawing life-sustaining treatment from a patient not otherwise expected to die in six months. A host of other concerns, including fears about malpractice litigation or perceptions of ethical or policy impediments, were also offered to explain why physicians might not comply with the preferences expressed by patients or their surrogates. These findings are consistent with those of other investigators,[11,31] and help to define what in practice are some of the limits of patients' autonomy. Some of these limits, such as misconceptions that the withdrawal of life-support is illegal, or personal opinions that it is unethical, might be overcome through the use of resources that already exist at the institutions in which our subjects practice.

Fourth, many of the physicians we surveyed also reported withholding or withdrawing life-sustaining treatment unilaterally because they had judged that further intervention would be futile. Some of these decisions were made without the knowledge or consent of patients or their surrogates, and some were made despite their objections. In these instances, physicians may have disagreed with patients or their surrogates on the intended goals of life support or on the possibility of achieving agreed-upon goals; we cannot tell which. Regardless of the specific circumstances in each case, such decisions exist inescapably in an area of conflict between patient or surrogate and physician.

There are no generally accepted rules of engagement for these conflicts, and the justification and appropriateness of our physician's decisions is therefore unclear. In fact, it is doubtful that ethical principles regarding the appropriate practical definition of medical futility will ever be noncontroversial. Some would argue that the goals of medicine should be set by the patient, and that the physician's responsibility is to help achieve these goals.[28] Others have argued that physicians should sometimes have the authority to determine whether life-sustaining treatment should be provided to meet patients' demands. These circumstances result because physicians require sufficient latitude in their decision making to maintain their important role as professionals and as moral agents, and also because it is inherently and unavoidably misleading to offer a futile treatment.[21] Braithwaite and Thomasma have argued more simply that in some cases a physician's assessment that life-sustaining technology would be cruel should supersede contrary decisions that might be reached by surrogate decision makers or other standards.[22]

Critics of these arguments contend that criteria for determining what is futile are ambiguous[28] and that physicians often disagree in their prognostic assessments of critically ill patients.[32] Others express concern that arguments in favor of reducing the role of patients or surrogates in decisions relating to life support are in fact excuses to avoid difficult but necessary discussions with patients,[25] or that in general, arguments on the basis of futility can too easily be used to disguise less defensible motives.[27] Regardless of ones definition of futility, the results presented in Tables 9-5 and 9-6 largely speak for themselves, and at least define physicians' decisions to forgo life-sustaining treatment without patients' or surrogates' explicit consent or request.

We believe that most decisions to limit life support on the basis of futility are of two distinct types. Sometimes, treatment is withheld or withdrawn in the final stage of a fatal illness when life cannot be sustained longer than a few hours by any intervention. For example, infusion of vasopressors might be discontinued as the blood pressure fades despite an earnest but unsuccessful attempt to reverse septic shock. Some have described lifesupporting treatment in such instances as "physiologically futile."[2,25] Clinicians may believe that technical decisions of this first type do not necessarily need the concurrence or even the awareness of the patients surrogate.

At other times, physicians may decide that life-sustaining treatment should be stopped even when death is not imminent, because further treatment is not expected to achieve a meaningful survival for the patient.[4,26] Such might be the case, for example, when a patient with widespread, untreatable cancer develops multiple organ failure: Unconscious life can be sustained for a while, but not beyond the intensive care unit. Physicians making decisions of this second type may anticipate greater conflict.

We did not determine the circumstances under which our physicians made decisions on the basis of futility. However, the distinction between the two types of decision described here may explain why more than 80% of the respondents reported that they had withheld or withdrawn therapy they judged to be futile, but fewer reported having done so unilaterally. Another possible explanation is that many physicians may limit life-supporting treatment with what they believe is tacit consent.

Still, much of the concern about unilateral decisions made on this basis is that there are few mechanisms to provide oversight. Physicians might too easily invoke this rationale as an excuse, for example, to avoid explicit discussions with patients or their surrogates—discussions that might lead them to actions supporting contrary values and goals.[27] Seen in this light, the finding that 12 to 14% of our respondents reported withdrawing or withholding life-sustaining treatment without the knowledge of a surrogate may be a disturbing sign of paternalism. We are unaware of other studies that have reported this finding.

Finally, in contrast to the findings in some previous studies,[33,34] but in accord with others,[12,35] we found that younger physicians are more likely than older physicians to report withdrawing mechanical ventilation, controlling for percentage of time spent in clinical practice and various hospital characteristics. When compared to research of twenty years ago,[33] this finding may reflect a shift in behavior among recently trained physicians. Our study has several limitations. First, we surveyed only critical care physicians, and most of our respondents were internists practicing in medical or combined medical-surgical intensive care units. The practices of these respondents may not reflect the practices in other types of intensive care units by anesthesiologists, surgeons, or cardiologists, for example. Second, we studied physicians' reported rather than observed practice. Although these might differ, we have no reason to suspect systematic errors in an anonymous and confidential survey. Third, given the response rate of less than 100% in our study, concerns might be raised about nonrespondent bias. Our response rate is comparable to that of other published surveys in similar contexts requiring physician completion.[10-13,16] Although we cannot be sure that nonrespondents do not differ from respondents in the examined domains, any differences would have to be profound in order to significantly alter our findings.

What do we learn from this study that we did not already know? First, among a national sample of critical care physicians, the practice of withholding and withdrawing life-sustaining treatment is extremely widespread. Second, physicians do not reflexively accept requests by patients or surrogates to limit treatment, but place these requests alongside a collection of other factors, including assessments of prognosis and perceptions of other ethical, legal, and policy guidelines.

Third, while debate continues on the ethical and legal foundations of medical futility, most critical care physicians are incorporating some concept of medical futility into decision making at the bedside. Life-sustaining treatment is being withheld or withdrawn on the basis that further intervention is futile, sometimes without the consent or knowledge of patients or their surrogates.

The authors are grateful to Brian L. Strom, M.D., for help with the design at this study, and to Susan Rappaport and the Epidemiology and Statistics Unit of the American Lung Association for their assistance in implementing this project.

REFERENCES

1. President's Commission for the Study of Ethical Problems in Medicine and Bioethical and Behavioral Research. *Deciding to Forego Life-Sustaining Treatment: Ethical, Medical, and Legal Issues in Treatment Decisions.* Washington, DC: US Government Printing Office; 1983.

2. Hastings Center. *Guidelines on the Termination of Life-Sustaining Treatment and the Care of the Dying.* Bloomington, IN: Indiana University Press, 1987.

3. *Current Opinions of the Council on Ethical and Judicial Affairs of the American Medical Association: Withholding or Withdrawing Life-Prolonging Treatment.* Chicago, IL: American Medical Association; 1992.

4. American Thoracic Society Bioethics Task Force. Withholding and withdrawing life-sustaining therapy. *American Review of Respiratory Disease.* 1991;144:726–731.

5. American College of Physicians. American College of Physicians ethics manual, part 2: the physician and society; research; life-sustaining treatment; other issues. *Annals of Internal Medicine.* 1989;111:327–355.

6. *Cruzan v. Director, Missouri Department of Health,* 497 U.S. 111, 110 S. Ct. 2841 (1990).

7. Omnibus Budget Reconciliation Act of 1990, P. L. 101–508 §§ 4206, 4751.

8. Greco PJ, Schulman KA, Lavizzo-Mourey R, Hansen-Flaschen J. The Patient Self-Determination Act and the future of advance directives. *Annals of Internal Medicine.* 1991;115:639–643.

9. Pearlman RA, Inui TS, Carter WB. Variability in physician bioethical decision making. *Annals of Internal Medicine.* 1982;97:420–425.

10. Von Preyss-Friedman SM, Uhlmann RF, Cain KC. Physicians' attitudes toward tube feeding chronically ill nursing home patients. *Journal of General Internal Medicine.* 1992;7:46–51.

11. Fried TR, Stein MD O'Sullivan PS, Brock DW, Novack DH. Limits of patient autonomy. Physician attitudes and practices regarding life-sustaining treatments and euthanasia. *Archives of Internal Medicine.* 1993;153:722–928.

12. Caralis PV, Hammond JS. Attitudes of medical students, housestaff, and faculty physicians toward euthanasia and termination of life-sustaining treatment. *Critical Care Medicine.* 1992;20:683–690.

13. Christakis NA, Asch DA. Biases in how physicians choose to withdraw life support. *Lancet.* 1993;342:642–646.

14. Christakis NA, Asch DA. Physician characteristics associated with decisions to withdraw life support. *American Journal of Public Health.* 1995;85(3):367–372.

15. Nightingale SD, Grant M. Risk preference and decision making in critical care situations. *Chest.* 1988;93:684–687.

16. Solomon MZ, O'Donnell L, Jennings B. Decisions near the end of life: professional views on life-sustaining treatments. *American Journal of Public Health.* 1993;83:14–23.

17. The Society of Critical Care Medicine Ethics Committee. Attitudes of critical care

medicine professionals concerning foregoing life-sustaining treatments. *Critical Care Medicine.* 1992;20:320–326.

18. Faber-Langendoen K, Bartels DM. Process of foregoing life-sustaining treatment in a university hospital: an empirical study. *Critical Care Medicine.* 1992;20:570–577.

19. Smedira NG, Evans BH, Grais LS. Withholding and withdrawal of life-support from the critically ill. *New England Journal of Medicine.* 1990;322:309–315.

20. Brett AS, McCullough LB. When patients request specific interventions: defining the limits of physicians' obligation. *New England Journal of Medicine.* 1986;315:1347–1351.

21. Tomlinson T, Brody H. Futility and the ethics of resuscitation. *JAMA.* 1990;264:1276–1280.

22. Braithwaite S, Thomasma DC. New guidelines on foregoing life-sustaining treatment in incompetent patients: an anti-cruelty policy. *Annals of Internal Medicine.* 1986;104:711–715.

23. Hackler JC, Hiller FC. Family consent to orders not to resuscitate. Reconsidering hospital policy. *JAMA.* 1990;264:1281–1283.

24. Youngner SJ. Futility in context. *JAMA.* 1990;264:1295–1296.

25. Youngner SJ. Who defines futility? *JAMA.* 1988;260:2094–2095.

26. Hansen-Flaschen J. When life support is futile. *Chest.* 1991;100:1191–1192.

27. Schneiderman LJ, Jecker N. Futility in practice. *Archives of Internal Medicine.* 1993;153:437–441.

28. Lantos JD, Singer PA, Walker RM, et al. The illusion of futility in clinical practice. *American Journal of Medicine.* 1989;87:81–84.

29. Schneiderman LJ, Jecker NS, Jonson AR. Medical futility: its meaning and ethical implications. *Annals of Internal Medicine.* 1990;112:949–954.

30. Jecker NS, Pearlman RA. Medical futility. Who decides? *Archives of Internal Medicine.* 1992;152:1140–1144.

31. Perkins HS, Bauer RL, Hazuda HP, Schoolfield JD. Impact of legal liability, family wishes, and other "external factors" on physicians' life-support decisions. *American Journal of Medicine.* 1990;89:185–194.

32. Poses RM, Bekes C, Copare FJ, Scott WE. The answer to "What are my chances, Doctor?" depends on whom is asked: prognostic disagreement and inaccuracy for critically ill patients. *Critical Care Medicine.* 1989;17:827–833.

33. Crane D. *The Sanctity of Social Life: Physicians' Treatment of Critically Ill Patients.* New Brunswick, NJ: Transaction Press; 1977.

34. Goetzler RM, Moskowitz MA. Changes in physician attitudes toward limiting care of critically ill patients. *Archives of Internal Medicine.* 1991;151:1537.

35. Neu S, Kjellstrand CM. Stopping long-term dialysis: an empirical study of withdrawal of life-supporting treatment. *New England Journal of Medicine.* 1986;314:14–20.

10

OREGON'S DEATH WITH DIGNITY ACT

The First Year's Experience

Department of Human Resources,
Oregon Health Division,
Center for Disease Prevention and Epidemiology

INTRODUCTION

On October 27, 1997, physician-assisted suicide became a legal medical option for terminally ill Oregonians. The Oregon Death with Dignity Act requires that the Oregon Health Division (OHD) monitor compliance with the law, collect information about the patients and physicians who participate in legal physician-assisted suicide, and publish an annual statistical report.[1] This report describes the monitoring and data collection system that was implemented under the law, and summarizes the information collected on patients and physicians who had participated in the act through December 31, 1998. To better understand the impact of physician-assisted suicide on the care of and decisions made by terminally ill Oregonians, we also present the results of two studies conducted by the OHD. Each study compared the characteristics of physician-assisted suicide participants with a sample of Oregon patients and physicians who did not participate in the Death with Dignity Act.

THE OREGON DEATH WITH DIGNITY ACT

The Oregon Death with Dignity Act, a citizens' initiative, was first passed by Oregon voters in November 1994 by a margin of 51 percent in favor and 49 percent opposed.

Immediate implementation of the act was delayed by a legal injunction. After multiple legal proceedings, including a petition that was denied by the United States Supreme Court, the Ninth Circuit Court of Appeals lifted the injunction on October 27, 1997, and physician-assisted suicide then became a legal option for terminally ill patients in Oregon. In November 1997, Measure 51 (authorized by Oregon House Bill 2954) was placed on the general election ballot and asked Oregon voters to repeal the Death with Dignity Act. Voters chose to retain the act by a margin of 60 percent to 40 percent.

The Death with Dignity Act allows terminally ill Oregon residents to obtain from their physicians and use prescriptions for self-administered lethal medications. The act states that ending one's life in accordance with the law does not constitute suicide.[1] However, we have used the term "physician-assisted suicide" rather than "death with dignity" to describe the provisions of this law because physician-assisted suicide is the term used by the public, and by the medical literature, to describe ending life through the voluntary self-administration of lethal medications, expressly prescribed by a physician for that purpose. The Death with Dignity Act legalizes physician-assisted suicide, but specifically prohibits euthanasia, where a physician or other person directly administers a medication to end another's life.[1]

To request a prescription for lethal medications, the Death with Dignity Act requires that a patient must be:[1]

- An adult (18 years of age or older);
- A resident of Oregon;
- Capable (defined as able to make and communicate health-care decisions);
- Diagnosed with a terminal illness that will lead to death within six months.

Patients who meet these requirements are eligible to request a prescription for lethal medication from a licensed Oregon physician. To receive a prescription for lethal medication, the following steps must be fulfilled:[1]

- The patient must make two verbal requests to their physician, separated by at least fifteen days.
- The patient must provide a written request to their physician.
- The prescribing physician and a consulting physician must confirm the diagnosis and prognosis. The prescribing physician and a consulting physician must determine whether the patient is capable. If either physician believes the patient's judgment is impaired by a psychiatric or psychological disorder, such as depression, the patient must be referred for counseling.
- The prescribing physician must inform the patient of feasible alternatives to assisted suicide including comfort care, hospice care, and pain control.
- The prescribing physician must request, but may not require, the patient to notify their next-of-kin of the prescription request.

To comply with the law, physicians must report the writing of all prescriptions for lethal medications to the OHD.[1,2] Reporting is not required if patients begin the request process but never receive a prescription. Physicians and patients who adhere to the requirements of the act are protected from criminal prosecution, and the choice of legal physician-assisted suicide cannot affect the status of a patient's health or life insurance policies. Physicians and health-care systems are under no obligation to participate in the Death with Dignity Act.[1]

THE REPORTING SYSTEM

The Death with Dignity Act requires that the OHD develop a reporting system to monitor and collect information on physician-assisted suicide.[1] To fulfill this mandate, the OHD implemented a reporting and data collection system with two components. The first involves physician prescription reports. When a prescription for lethal medication is written, the physician must submit specific information to the OHD that documents compliance with the law.[2] We review all physician reports and contact reporting physicians regarding missing or discrepant data.

The second component of the reporting system involves death certificate review. All Oregon death certificates are screened by the OHD Vital Records staff. Death certificates of all recipients of prescriptions for lethal medications are reviewed by the OHD State Registrar and matched to the prescribing physician reports. In addition, OHD Vital Records files are searched periodically for death certificates that correspond to physician reports, but that may have been missed by initial death certificate screening.

For 1998, we enlarged the scope of our data-collection system to include in-person or telephone interviews with all prescribing physicians after receipt of their patients' death certificate. Physicians were asked to confirm whether the patient took the lethal medications, and were then asked a series of questions to collect data not available from physician reports or death certificates (e.g., insurance status, end-of-life care, end-of-life concerns, medications prescribed, and medical and functional status at the time of death). In instances where the patient took the lethal medication, we collected information on the rapidity of the medication's effect and on any unexpected adverse reactions. Many terminally ill patients have more than one physician providing care at the end of life. To maintain consistency in data collection and to protect the privacy of the patient and the prescribing physician, interview data were only collected from prescribing physicians. All physician interviews were performed after the patients' death. We did not interview or collect any information from patients prior to their death, nor did we collect data from patients' families at any time. Reporting forms and the physician interview questionnaire are available at www.ohd.hr.state.or.us/cdpe/chs/pas/pas.htm.

DATA COLLECTION

Data on all recipients of prescriptions for lethal medications were collected from physician reports, death certificates, and prescribing physician interviews using the reporting system just described. We collected information on request dates and consultations from the prescription reports submitted to the OHD. Demographic data (e.g., age, place of residence, level of education) were obtained from death certificate reviews. Using physician interviews, we collected additional information about prescription recipients that was not available from either physician reports or death certificates as well as information about prescribing physician characteristics such as age, sex, number of years in practice, and medical specialty.

COMPARISON STUDIES

We collected information on all patients who received a prescription for lethal medications and died in 1998. Prescription recipients died either by ingesting their lethal medications or from their underlying illnesses. Because there may be differences in the characteristics of patients who completed the physician-assisted suicide process and those who received lethal medications but never used them, we did not classify or analyze the prescription recipients as a single group. Instead, our comparison studies focus only on those persons who chose physician-assisted suicide and died after taking their lethal medications. We did not conduct similar analyses of persons who received lethal medications, but chose not to use them, because of the small number of patients (six) in this group.

For our comparison studies, we included all persons who died between January 1, 1998, and December 31, 1998, after ingesting a lethal dose of medication prescribed under the Death with Dignity Act (no prescriptions for lethal medications were written under the act in 1997). We compared persons who chose physician-assisted suicide with two control groups. First, we compared persons who chose physician-assisted suicide with all Oregonians who died from similar underlying illnesses (e.g., lung cancer, ovarian cancer, congestive heart failure) in 1996 (the most recent year that finalized Oregon mortality data are available). Next, we compared persons who chose physician-assisted suicide with a group of matched control patients, Oregonians who died in 1998 and were similar with respect to age, underlying illness, and date of death. Matched control patients who would not have met the requirements of the Death with Dignity Act were excluded from the study (e.g., control patients who were not Oregon residents, or who were not capable of making health-care decisions). Finally, we compared the characteristics of physicians who cared for patients that chose physician-assisted suicide with the characteristics of physicians who cared for the matched control patients.

RESULTS

Results of our data collection and comparison studies are presented in two formats. In addition to this report, the results are also presented in a manuscript published in the *New England Journal of Medicine* ("Legalized Physician-Assisted Suicide in Oregon: The First Year's Experience") on February 18,1999.[3] These data are published in a peer-reviewed medical journal for two reasons. First, legalized physician-assisted suicide is unique to Oregon. As such, the reporting system implemented by the OHD under the Death with Dignity Act has no precedent. We believe that a new reporting system that is responsible for collecting data on a controversial issue, such as the Death with Dignity Act, should be subject to the scrutiny of peer review in the medical literature. Such critique may lead to future improvements in the way data are collected. Second, the data and analyses presented in these reports will be of interest and used by parties on all sides of this issue. Again, we believe that the methods, results, and analyses that we present can only benefit from the critique offered by the peer-review process.

Characteristics of Prescription Recipients

Twenty-three persons who received legal prescriptions for lethal medications in 1998 were reported to the OHD. Of these twenty-three persons, fifteen died after taking their lethal medications, six died from their underlying illness, and two were alive as of January 1, 1999. Table 10-1 presents information on the 21 prescription recipients who died in 1998 and further subdivides this information into two categories: patients who took their lethal medications and prescription recipients who died of their underlying illnesses. The median age of the 21 prescription recipients was 69 years and ranged from the third to the tenth decade of life. All 21 patients were white, 11 (52%) were male, and 11 (52%) lived in the Portland Tri-County area. Of the 21 recipients, 20 had been residents of Oregon for longer than six months when they received their prescriptions. One patient had moved to Oregon four months prior to death to be cared for by family members and not because of legalized assisted suicide. Four of the twenty-one prescription recipients had a psychiatric or psychological consultation and all patients were ultimately determined to be capable in the context of the Death with Dignity Act. All physician reports were in full compliance with the law.

Twenty (95%) of the 21 prescription recipients who died in 1998 were prescribed nine grams of a fast-acting barbiturate, either secobarbital or pentobarbital. One patient was prescribed one gram of secobarbital to be taken with an oral narcotic. Most patients also received a number of nonlethal medications to be taken in conjunction with the lethal medications. These included medications to increase stomach emptying and to prevent nausea and vomiting.

Table 10-1. Characteristics of Patients Who Received Prescriptions for Lethal Medications and Timing of Events

Demographics	Death after Lethal Medication Ingestion (N=15)		Death from Terminal Illness (N=6)		All Lethal Prescription Recipients (N=21)	
Age—median (years)	69		47		69	
Race—white	15	100%	6	100%	21	100%
Sex—male	8	53%	3	50%	11	52%
Oregon resident greater than 6 months	15	100%	5	83%	20	95%
Residence—Portland-Metro	7	47%	4	67%	11	52%
Legal Requirements						
Psychiatric/psychological consultation	4	27%	0	0%	4	19%
Full compliance	15	100%	6	100%	21	100%
Underlying Illness						
Cancer (all types)	13	87%	5	83%	18	86%
Lung, ovarian, or breast cancer	9	60%	3	50%	12	57%
Acquired Immune Deficiency Syndrome	0	0%	1	17%	1	5%
Congestive heart failure	1	7%	0	0%	1	5%
Chronic obstructive pulmonary disease	1	7%	0	0%	1	5%
PAS Lethal Prescription						
secobarbital 9 grams	13	87%	6	100%	19	90%
phenobarbital 9 grams	1	7%	0	0%	1	5%
secobarbital 1 gram/ morphine 1 gram	1	7%	0	0%	1	5%
antiemetic agent	14	93%	5	83%	19	90%
gastric promotility agent	6	40%	5	83%	11	52%
chlorpromazine	1	7%	0	0%	1	5%
beta blocker	3	20%	3	50%	6	29%
	median	range	median	range	median	range
Prescription Time Line (days)						
First and second oral requests	18	(15–68)	30	(16–83)	20	(15–83)
First oral request and death	20	(15–75)	93	(26–101)	26	(15–101)
Prescription receipt and death	1	(0–22)	28	(8–66)	4	(0–66)

Reprinted with permission *New England Journal of Medicine* 340(7):577–583.[3] Copyright 1999 Massachusetts Medical Society. All rights reserved.

The Physician-Assisted Suicide Process

Fifteen prescription recipients chose physician-assisted suicide and died after taking their lethal medications. The median time from medication ingestion to unconsciousness (available for 11 patients) was 5 minutes (range 3-20 minutes). The median time from medication ingestion to death (available for 14 patients) was 26 minutes (range 15 minutes to 11.5 hours). For 8 of the 15 persons who chose physician-assisted suicide, the prescribing physician was at the bedside when they took the lethal medications. For 6 of the 15 patients, the physician was also at the bedside when they died. In instances where the physician was not present for the medication ingestion or death, times to unconsciousness and death, as well as reports of complications, were provided to the physician by persons present at the bedside. No complications, such as vomiting or seizures, were reported by any physician.

Comparison Studies

We first compared the 15 persons who chose physician-assisted suicide with all deaths in Oregon in 1996, the latest year for which finalized mortality data are available. The 15 persons who chose physician-assisted suicide accounted for 5 of every 10,000 deaths in Oregon, based on the 28,900 deaths that occurred in 1996.[4] The 13 persons with cancer who chose physician-assisted suicide accounted for 19 of every 10,000 cancer deaths, based on the 6,784 persons who died of cancer in Oregon in 1996.[4] Next, we compared the 15 persons who chose physician-assisted suicide with the 5,604 Oregonians who died in 1996 from similar underlying illnesses. Age, race, sex, and Portland Tri-County residence status did not predict participation in physician-assisted suicide (Table 10-2). Twelve of the 15 persons who chose physician-assisted suicide had at least a high school diploma. Four of these 12 had graduated from college. The proportions of high school and college graduates were similar among persons who chose assisted suicide and the 5,604 controls. In contrast, marital status was associated with participation in physician-assisted suicide. Persons who were divorced and persons who had never married were 6.8 times and 23.7 times, respectively, more likely to choose physician-assisted suicide than persons who were married.

For our second comparison study, the matched case-control study, we identified control patients who had not participated in the Death with Dignity Act but who were similar to the persons who chose physician-assisted suicide with regard to age, underlying illness, and date of death. Using 1998 death certificates, we identified 81 potential control patients who met these criteria. Of these 81 persons, 17 were disqualified from the study because we could not contact the physician who provided end-of-life care or because we could not identify an end-of-life-care provider. We were able to obtain physician interviews for 64 potential control patients. Of these 64 persons, 21 were disqualified because they would not have been eligible for a prescription for lethal medications under the law: 10 were deemed incapable of making health-care decisions by their physicians; 2 were not Oregon residents; 2 could not take oral medications; and for 7 patients, the time between when the physician determined that the patient had less than 6 months to live and death was less than the required 15-day waiting period. Ultimately, we collected data on 43 persons to serve as controls, 3 matched controls for each of 14 persons choosing physician-assisted suicide and 1 matched control for the single remaining person.

Results of the matched case-control study are similar to the comparison with 1996 Oregon deaths just described. Persons who chose physician-assisted suicide and 1998

Table 10-2. Characteristics of Case Patients and Oregon Residents Who Died from Similar Illnesses in 1996

Demographic Characteristic	Deaths	Physician-Assisted Suicide Cases	Rate Physician-Assisted Suicides per 10,000 deaths	Risk Ratio (95% CI^)	2-tailed P value
Race*					
nonwhite	116	0	0.0	referent	
white	5450	15	27.4	undefined	1.00
Sex					
female	3026	7	23.1	referent	
male	2578	8	30.9	1.3 (0.5–3.7)	0.57
Residence					
rural	3582	8	22.3	referent	
urban (Portland-Metro)	2022	7	34.5	1.6 (0.6–4.3)	0.39
Education*					
did not graduate high school	1540	3	19.4	referent	
high school graduate	3901	12	30.7	1.6 (0.5–5.6)	0.58
college graduate	614	4	64.7	3.3 (0.8–14.8)	0.11
Marital Status at Death*					
married	2703	2	7.4	referent	
widowed	1868	5	26.7	3.6 (0.7–18.6)	0.13
divorced	789	4	50.4	6.8 (1.3–37.2)	0.03
never married	224	4	175.4	23.7 (4.4–128.9)	<0.001

	1996 Oregon Death Cohort (N=5604)	Physician-Assisted Suicide Deaths (N=15)	P value
Median Age (years)	74	69	0.40

*Of the 5,604 persons who died in 1996 from illnesses that matched the case-patients' underlying illnesses, data on race were available for 5,566; data on education were available for 5,441; and data on marital status were available for 5,584.

^CI denotes confidence intervals

matched controls did not differ statistically by race, sex, Oregon resident status (greater than 6 months), Portland Tri-County resident status, or education level (Table 10-3). Although not statistically significant, there was a trend in that persons who chose physician-assisted suicide were more likely to be divorced than controls. Persons who chose physician-assisted suicide were more likely than controls to have never married.

No patients who chose physician-assisted suicide or matched control patients voiced concern to their physician about the financial impact of their illnesses. Both groups contained similar proportions of patients insured through Medicare, Medicaid, or private insurance, or who lacked health insurance. One patient who chose physician-assisted suicide (7%) and 15 (35%) controls expressed concern about end-of-life pain, although this difference was not statistically significant. Patients who chose physician-assisted suicide and controls were equally likely to have been enrolled in hospice, to have had advance medical directives, and to have died at home. The proportion of patients in each group who expressed concerns about being a physical or emotional burden, or about the inability to participate in activities that made life enjoyable, were similar. However, patients who chose physician-assisted suicide were significantly more likely than controls to express concern to their physicians about loss of autonomy, and more likely to express concern about loss of control of bodily functions (e.g., incontinence, vomiting) due to their illness.* At death, patients who chose physician-assisted suicide were significantly less likely than controls to be completely disabled and bedridden.*

Physician Characteristics

Fourteen physicians wrote prescriptions for lethal medications for the 15 patients who chose physician-assisted suicide. Forty physicians were the end-of-life providers for the 43 control patients. The two groups of physicians were similar with respect to age, sex, specialty, and years in practice, although there was a trend for prescribing physicians to have been older and in practice longer (Table 10-4).

For some physicians, the process of participating in physician-assisted suicide had a great emotional impact. In response to general, open-ended inquiries, prescribing physicians offered comments such as, "It was an excruciating thing to do... it made me rethink life's priorities"; "This was really hard on me, especially being there when he took the pills"; and "This had a tremendous emotional impact."

Not all Oregon physicians were willing to participate in physician-assisted suicide in 1998. Six patients who chose assisted suicide had requested lethal medications from one or more providers before finding a physician who would begin the prescription process. Physicians for 67% (29/43) of control patients would have refused to write a prescription for lethal medications had the patient asked; physicians for 21% (9/43) of control patients would have provided prescriptions; and physicians for 12% (5/43) of control patients were unsure. Six control patients (14%) had discussed physician-assisted suicide with the physician we interviewed, but none had begun the formal request process.

---

*This sentence contained an error in the original manuscript dated February 18, 1999. The sentence was edited and corrected on March 15, 1999.

Table 10-3. Characteristics of Case Patients and Matched Controls

Demographics	Case Patients (N=15) N	%	Control Patients (N=43) N	%	Matched Odds Ratio	95% Confidence Interval	2-tailed P value
race—white	15	100%	43	100%			
sex—male	8	53%	15	35%	4.5	0.6–32.1	0.30
Oregon resident >6 months	15	100%	43	100%			
Portland-Metro resident	7	47%	16	37%	1.4	0.4–4.9	0.87
Education*							
did not graduate high school	3	20%	11	27%	referent		
high school graduate	12	80%	30	73%	1.4	0.3–9.7	0.90
college graduate	4	27%	7	17%	undefined		1.00
Marital Status at Death							
married	2	13%	20	47%	referent		
widowed	5	33%	14	33%	1.7	0.1–24.7	0.93
divorced	4	27%	7	16%	7.5	0.7–354.5	0.12
never married	4	27%	2	5%	undefined		0.04
Insurance Coverage at Death							
private insurance	8	53%	28	65%	referent		
Medicare only	4	27%	7	16%	6.0	0.3–288.4	0.41
Oregon Medicaid	2	13%	7	16%	0.8	0.1–7.7	0.81
no insurance	1	7%	0	0%	undefined		0.56
unknown	0	0%	1	2%	undefined		0.56
Hospice/Advance Directives at Death							
enrolled in hospice†	10	71%	32	74%	0.8	0.2–4.2	1.00
written advance directives	11	79%	37	93%	0.4	0.1–3.3	0.55
Place of Death							
private home	12	80%	29	67%	3.5	0.4–29.7	0.55
Patient End-of-Life Concerns							
Financial cost of treating/prolonging illness	0	0%	0	0%			
Burden on family/friends/caregivers	2	13%	15	35%	0.2	0.0–1.5	0.21
Inability to participate in activities	10	67%	26	60%	1.2	0.3–4.3	1.00
Inadequate pain control	1	7%	15	35%	0.2	0.0–1.4	0.10
Loss of autonomy due to illness	12	80%	17	40%	7.3	1.5–35.9	0.01
Loss of control of bodily function	8	53%	8	19%	9.0	1.6–51.4	0.02
Functional Status at Death							
completely disabled	3	21%	32	84%	0.1	0.0–0.4	<0.001

	median	range	median	range	P value
Age (years)	69		74		0.70
Patient-physician relationship (days)	69	15–3780	720	35–7284	0.03

*Education data were available for 15 case patients and 41 controls
†Hospice data were available for 14 case patients and 43 controls
‡Advance directives data were available for 14 case patients and 40 controls
§Functional status data were available for 14 case patients and 38 controls
¶Column totals may not sum to 100% due to multiple responses for a single patient
Reprinted with permission: *New England Journal of Medicine* 340(7):577–583.[3] Copyright 1999 Massachusetts Medical Society. All rights reserved.

Table 10-4. Characteristics of Physicians Who Prescribed Lethal Medications and Physicians Who Provided Care at the End of Life for Controls

	Case Physicians (N=14)		Control Physicians (N=40)		O.R.	95% Confidence Interval	2-tailed P value
Sex—male	11	79%	35	88%	0.5	0.1–3.4	0.41
Specialty—primary care*	9	64%	22	55%	1.5	0.4–6.6	0.55
Median age—years (range)	51	(37–69)	44	(30–62)			0.07
Median years in practice —years (range)	18	(1–45)	12	(1–36)			0.11

*Primary care specialities defined as family practice, internal medicine, obstetrics and gynecology
Reprinted with permission: *New England Journal of Medicine* 340(7):577–583.[3] Copyright 1999 Massachusetts Medical Society. All rights reserved.

DISCUSSION/CONCLUSIONS

Currently, Oregon is the only place in the world where physician-assisted suicide is legal. Physician-assisted suicide was briefly legalized in the Northern Territory of Australia between July 1996 and March 1997.[5] In the Netherlands, physician-assisted suicide has been practiced for many years; although technically illegal, it has been rarely prosecuted.[6]

The Death with Dignity Act continues to be the focus of highly charged ethical, legal, and medical debates.[7-13] The role of the Oregon Health Division is neither to take sides nor to settle these controversies; however, we believe that the data collected on 1998 participants in the Death with Dignity Act and on patients who chose physician-assisted suicide are important to all concerned parties. Among the important findings from our 1998 data collection and comparison studies are:

- Physician-assisted suicide accounted for approximately 5 of every 10,000 deaths in Oregon in 1998. Patients with cancer who chose physician-assisted suicide accounted for 19 of every 10,000 cancer deaths in Oregon in 1998.
- Patients who chose physician-assisted suicide in 1998 were similar to all Oregonians who died of similar underlying illnesses with respect to age, race, sex, and Portland residence.
- Patients who chose physician-assisted suicide were not disproportionately poor (as measured by Medicaid status), less educated, lacking in insurance coverage, or lacking in access to hospice care.
- Fear of intractable pain and concern about the financial impact of their illnesses were not disproportionately associated with the decision to choose physician-assisted suicide.
- The choice of physician-assisted suicide was most strongly associated with concerns about loss of autonomy and personal control of bodily functions.

- In 1998, many hospitals and physicians in Oregon were unable or unwilling to participate in physician-assisted suicide.
- Physicians who wrote prescriptions for lethal medications for patients who chose physician-assisted suicide represented a wide range of specialties, ages, and years in practice.

Considerable debate has focused on the characteristics of terminally-ill patients who choose physician-assisted suicide. Some feared that patients who were minorities, poor, or uneducated would more likely be coerced into choosing physician-assisted suicide. Others feared that terminally ill persons would feel pressured, either internally or through external forces (e.g., family members or health-care systems), to choose physician-assisted suicide because of the financial impact of their illnesses.[9–11,14,15] To date, the Oregonians who have chosen physician-assisted suicide have not had these characteristics. Patients who chose physician-assisted suicide and our two comparison groups were similar with respect to age, sex, race, education level, and health insurance coverage. No person who chose physician-assisted suicide expressed a concern to their physician about the financial impact of their illness. The proportion of patients with private insurance and Medicaid were similar among those who chose physician-assisted suicide and among controls. This provides some evidence that socioeconomic status was not associated with the decision to take lethal medications.

End-of-life care has made great strides in Oregon in recent years. Oregon ranks third, nationally, in the rate of hospice admissions.[15] More than two-thirds of the patients who chose physician-assisted suicide were enrolled in a hospice program when they died. A similar proportion of control patients were also enrolled in hospice. Of the four patients who chose physician-assisted suicide, but who were not receiving hospice care, three had repeatedly refused enrollment offers. To date, lack of access to hospice care has not been associated with the decision to take lethal medications. Fear of intractable pain was also an end-of-life care issue not associated with physician-assisted suicide. Only one person who chose physician-assisted suicide expressed concern to her physician about inadequate pain control at the end of life (compared with 15 of 43 control patients). This may reflect confidence in one's end-of-life care. Alternatively, recipients of lethal medications may not have been concerned about end-of-life pain because physician-assisted suicide offered them the option of avoiding intractable pain.

The primary factor distinguishing persons in Oregon selecting physician-assisted suicide is related to the importance of autonomy and personal control. Patients who chose physician-assisted suicide were more likely to be concerned about loss of autonomy and loss of control of bodily functions than control patients.* Autonomy was a prominent patient characteristic in physicians' answers to open-ended questions about their patients' end-of-life concerns. Many prescribing physicians reported that their patients decision to request a lethal prescription was consis-

---

*This sentence contained an error in the original manuscript dated February 18, 1999. The sentence was edited and corrected on March 15, 1999.

tent with a long-standing philosophy about controlling the manner in which they died. The fact that 79% of persons who chose physician-assisted suicide did not wait until they were bedridden to take their lethal medication provides further evidence that controlling the manner and time of death were important issues to these patients. Thus, in Oregon the decision to request and use a prescription for lethal medications in 1998 appears to be more associated with attitudes about autonomy and dying, and less with fears about intractable pain or financial loss.

There are several limitations that are important to consider when interpreting these results. First, the number of patients who chose physician-assisted suicide in 1998 was relatively small. This limits our ability to detect, from a statistical stand-point, small differences between the characteristics of persons who chose physician-assisted suicide and control patients. Second, the possibility of physician bias must be considered. Physicians prescribing lethal medications may have spent more time exploring end-of-life concerns and care options with patients who requested lethal medications. Because of the unique nature of lethal prescription requests, physicians may have recalled their conversations and interactions with requesting patients in greater detail than physicians of terminally ill patients who did not request such pre-scriptions. Finally, the Death with Dignity Act requires the OHD to collect data on patients and physicians who participate in the act.[1,2] However, the OHD must also report any noncompliance with the law to the Oregon Board of Medical Examiners for further investigation.[16,17] Because of this obligation, we cannot detect or collect data on issues of noncompliance with any accuracy. A 1995 anonymous survey of Oregon physicians found that 7% of surveyed physicians had provided prescriptions for lethal medications to patients prior to legalization.[18] We do not know if covert physician-assisted suicide continued to be practiced in Oregon in 1998.

Considerable debate has also surrounded the interpretation of very limited data on the medications prescribed for physician-assisted suicide and the rapidity of their effects.[19-22] With one exception, all of the lethal prescriptions were similar. This may reflect information available from Oregon physician-assisted suicide advocacy groups. Although all patients were unconscious within 20 minutes of medication ingestion, the time from ingestion to death ranged from 15 minutes to 11.5 hours. In four instances, patients died more than 3 hours after taking the medications, including the one patient who died 11. 5 hours afterward. The last patient fell asleep 5 minutes after taking all 9 grams of barbiturate, the same prescription given to 14 of the 15 persons who chose physician-assisted suicide. Physicians, patients, and their families should be aware that the time from medication ingestion to death is not always rapid or predictable.

In 1998, not all hospital systems or physicians in Oregon participated in physician-assisted suicide. Federal law prohibits participation by patients or physicians within federal health-care systems such as Veterans Administration Hospitals and Indian Health Service clinics.[23] Some health-care systems, including at least one Catholic medical system in Oregon, have placed similar restrictions on patients and staff within their facilities. Although some physicians are unable to participate in the Death with

Dignity Act because of restrictions by their employers, other physicians have chosen not to participate in physician-assisted suicide because of other concerns. Six of the patients who chose physician-assisted suicide had to approach more than one physician before finding one that would start the prescription process. Two-thirds of otherwise eligible control patients, had they asked, would not have received such prescriptions from the physicians that we interviewed. Both findings provide evidence that a substantial proportion of Oregon physicians are not willing to participate in legalized physician-assisted suicide.

Physicians who wrote prescriptions for lethal medications for those patients who chose physician-assisted suicide represented a wide range of medical specialties, ages, and years in practice and were similar to physicians for control patients with respect to these characteristics. Several Oregon physicians have publicly acknowledged their participation in the Death with Dignity Act, but the majority of prescribing physicians have remained anonymous. Several physicians commented that despite the emotional impact of participating in a physician-assisted suicide, they were unwilling to share their experience with others because they feared repercussions from colleagues or patients if they did not keep their identities as Death with Dignity Act participants anonymous.

In publishing this report, we recognize that the Death with Dignity Act has been and remains a focal point for ethical, legal, and medical debate. As required by the act, we will continue to collect information regarding compliance with the statute, and we emphasize that our role is to do so as a neutral party. In accordance with the act, we will make available to the public an annual statistical report of the information collected. Future reports may not, however, contain the level of detail provided in this first study.

REFERENCES

1. Oregon Death with Dignity Act, Oregon Revised Statute 127.800-127.897.

2. Oregon Administrative Rules 333-009-0010.

3. Chin AE, Hedberg K, Higginson GK, Fleming DW. Legalized physician-assisted suicide in Oregon—the first year's experience. *New England Journal of Medicine.* 1999;340:577–583.

4. Centers for Health Statistics—Oregon Health Division. Oregon vital statistics county data 1996. Portland, OR: Oregon Department of Human Resources; 1997.

5. Kissane DW, Street A, Nitschke P. Seven deaths in Darwin: case studies under the Rights of the Terminally Ill Act, Northern Territory, Australia. *Lancet.* 1998;352:1097–1102.

6. van der Maas PJ, van der Wal G, Haverkate I, et al. Euthanasia, physician-assisted suicide, and other medical practices involving the end of life in the Netherlands, 1990–1995. *New England Journal of Medicine.* 1996;335:1699–1705.

7. Angell M. The Supreme Court and physician-assisted suicide—the ultimate right. *New England Journal of Medicine.* 1997;336:50–53.

8. Foley KM. Competent care for the dying instead of physician-assisted suicide. *New England Journal of Medicine.* 1997;336:54–57.

9. OKeefe M. The pursuit of liberty and death. *Oregonian.* October 19,1997:Al.

10. Bachman JG, Alcser KH, Doukas DJ, Lichtenstein RL, Coming AD, Brody H. Attitudes of Michigan physicians and the public toward legalizing physician-assisted suicide and voluntary euthanasia. *New England Journal of Medicine*. 1996;334:303–309.

11. Annas GJ. Death by prescription—the Oregon initiative. *New England Journal of Medicine*. 1994;331:1240–43.

12. Burt RA. The Supreme Court speaks—not assisted suicide but a constitutional right to palliative care. *New England Journal of Medicine*. 1997;337:1234–1236.

13. Orentlicher D. The Supreme Court and physician-assisted suicide—rejecting assisted suicide but embracing euthanasia. *New England Journal of Medicine*. 1997;337:1236–1239.

14. Pellegrino ED. The false promise of beneficent killing. In: Emanuel LL (ed.). *Regulating How We Die*. Cambridge, MA: Harvard University Press; 1998:71–91.

15. Tolle SW. Care of the dying: clinical and financial lessons from the Oregon experience. *Annals of Internal Medicine*. 1998;128:567–568.

16. Hedberg K. Oregon Health Division reporting. In: Haley K, Lee M (eds.). *The Oregon Death with Dignity Act—A Guidebook for Health-Care Providers*. Portland, OR: Center for Ethics in Health Care, Oregon Health Sciences University, 1998:43–45.

17. Haley K, Tolle S. Responding to professional non-compliance. In: Haley K, Lee M (eds.). *The Oregon Death with Dignity Act—A Guidebook for Health-Care Providers*. Portland, OR: Center for Ethics in Health Care, Oregon Health Sciences University, 1998:40–41.

18. Lee MA, Nelson HD, Tilden VP, Ganzini L, Schmidt TA, Tolle SW. Legalizing assisted suicide—views of physicians in Oregon. *New England Journal of Medicine*. 1996;334:310–315.

19. O'Keefe M. Dutch Researcher warns of lingering deaths. *Oregonian*. December 4,1994:Al.

20. Drickamer, MA, Lee, MA, Ganzini L. Practical issues in physician-assisted suicide. *Annals of Internal Medicine*, 1997;126:146–151.

21. Long L. Basics on Ballot Measure 51. Salem, OR: Oregon Legislative Policy and Research Office; 1997:1–6.

22. Preston TA, Mero R. Observations concerning terminally ill patients who choose suicide. *Journal of Pharmaceutical Care in Pain and Symptom Control* 1996;4:183–192.

23. Assisted Suicide Funding Restriction Act of 1997, H. R. 1003, 105th Congress, 1st Sess. (1997).

11

OREGON'S DEATH WITH DIGNITY ACT

The Second Year's Experience

Department of Human Services
Oregon Health Division
Center for Disease Prevention and Epidemiology

INTRODUCTION

When voters approved the Death with Dignity Act in November 1997, Oregon became the only state allowing legal physician-assisted suicide.[1] The Oregon Death with Dignity Act requires that the Oregon Health Division (OHD) monitor compliance with the law, collect information about the patients and physicians who participate in legal physician-assisted suicide, and publish an annual report. Information about participating patients and physicians helps in evaluating concerns that physician-assisted suicide might be forced onto poor, uneducated or uninsured patients; or that it might be disproportionately sought by patients with inadequate end-of-life care.[2,3]

We previously reported that during 1998, the first year of the act's implementation, fifteen Oregonians used physician-assisted suicide.[4] Their participation was not associated with low education level, lack of health insurance, or poor access to hospice care. Physician interviews indicated that patients requested lethal medication because of concerns over losing autonomy and control of bodily functions, not worsening pain or financial loss.

This report reviews the monitoring and data collection system that was implemented under the law, and summarizes the information collected on patients and physicians who participated in the act in the second year of the act's implementation (January 1, 1999, to December 31, 1999). We compare patients who participated in

1999 to those who participated in 1998 and to other Oregonians who died of similar diseases. To better understand why some patients choose physician-assisted suicide, we also present information from interviews with family members of patients who participated in the Death with Dignity Act.

THE OREGON DEATH WITH DIGNITY ACT

The Oregon Death with Dignity Act was a citizen's initiative first passed by Oregon voters in November 1994 by a margin of 51 percent in favor and 49 percent opposed. Implementation of the act was delayed by a legal injunction. After legal proceedings, including a petition that was denied by the United States Supreme Court, the Ninth Circuit Court of Appeals lifted the injunction on October 27, 1997, and physician-assisted suicide became a legal option for terminally ill Oregonians. In November 1997, a measure asking Oregon voters to repeal the Death with Dignity Act was placed on the general election ballot (Measure 5 1, authorized by Oregon House Bill 2954). Voters rejected this measure by a margin of 60 percent to 40 percent, thereby retaining the Death with Dignity Act.

The Death with Dignity Act allows terminally ill Oregon residents to get and use prescriptions from their physicians for self-administered, lethal medications. Under the act, ending one's life in accordance with the law does not constitute suicide. However, we use the term "physician-assisted suicide" in this report because this is the term used by the medical literature to describe ending life through the voluntary self-administration of lethal medications prescribed by a physician for that purpose. The Death with Dignity Act legalizes physician-assisted suicide, but specifically prohibits euthanasia, where a physician or other person directly administers a medication to end another's life.[1,5]

To request a prescription for lethal medications, the Death with Dignity Act requires that a patient must be:

- An adult (18 years of age or older)
- A resident of Oregon
- Capable (defined as able to make and communicate health care decisions)
- Diagnosed with a terminal illness that will lead to death within six months

Patients meeting these requirements are eligible to request a prescription for lethal medication from a licensed Oregon physician. To receive a prescription for lethal medication, the following steps must be fulfilled:

- The patient must make two verbal requests to their physician, separated by at least fifteen days.
- The patient must provide a written, witnessed request to their physician.
- The prescribing physician and a consulting physician must confirm the diagnosis and prognosis.

- The prescribing physician and a consulting physician must determine whether the patient is capable.
- If either physician believes the patient's judgment is impaired by a psychiatric or psychological disorder, such as depression, the patient must be referred for a psychological examination.
- The prescribing physician must inform the patient of feasible alternatives to assisted suicide including comfort care, hospice care, and pain control.
- The prescribing physician must request, but may not require, the patient to notify their next-of-kin of the prescription request.

To comply with the law, physicians must report to the OHD all prescriptions for lethal medications.[5,6] Reporting is not required if patients begin the request process but never receive a prescription. In the summer of 1999, the Oregon legislature added a requirement that pharmacists must be informed of the prescribed medication's ultimate use. Physicians and patients who adhere to the requirements of the act are protected from criminal prosecution, and the choice of legal physician-assisted suicide can not affect the status of a patient's health or life insurance policies. Physicians and health-care systems are under no obligation to participate in the Death with Dignity Act.[1,5]

THE REPORTING SYSTEM

The Death with Dignity Act requires the OHD to develop a reporting system to monitor and collect information on physician-assisted suicide.[1] To fulfill this mandate, the OHD uses a system involving physician prescription reports and death certificate reviews.

When a prescription for lethal medication is written, the physician must submit to the OHD information that documents compliance with the law. We review all physician reports and contact physicians regarding missing or discrepant data. OHD Vital Records files are searched periodically for death certificates that correspond to physician reports. These death certificates allow us to confirm patients' deaths, and provide patient demographic data (for example, age, place of residence, level of education).[4]

For this report, we also included telephone interviews with all prescribing physicians after receipt of their patients' death certificate. Each physician was asked to confirm whether the patient took the lethal medications. We also collected data not available from physician reports or death certificates—including insurance status, end-of-life care, and medical and functional status at the time of death. We asked why the patient requested a prescription, specifically exploring concerns about the financial impact of the illness, loss of autonomy, decreasing ability to participate in activities that make life enjoyable, loss of control of bodily functions, and uncontrollable pain. If the patient took the lethal medication, we collected information on the time to unconsciousness and death, and asked about any unexpected adverse reactions. Many terminally ill patients have more than one physician providing care at the end of life: To maintain consistency in data collection, we only interviewed prescribing physicians. Information about prescribing physicians—such as age, sex, number of years in practice, and medical specialty—were collected during the interviews. We do not interview or collect any information from patients prior to their death. Reporting forms and the physician questionnaire are available at www.ohd.hr.state.or.us/cdpe/chs/pas/pas.ht.[4]

DATA COLLECTION AND ANALYSIS

Using physician reports, death certificates, and prescribing physician interviews from the reporting system described, we collected information on all patients who received a prescription for lethal medications and died in 1998 and 1999. Prescription recipients died either by ingesting their lethal medications or from their underlying illnesses. Because of possible differences between patients who used the lethal medication and patients who received lethal medications but never used them, we looked at these two groups separately. Our report focuses on patients who chose physician-assisted suicide and died after taking their lethal medications.

Comparison to 1998 Participants and All Oregonian Who Died of Similar Diseases

The comparisons presented here include all patients who died in 1999 (January 1, 1999, through December 31, 1999) after ingesting a lethal dose of medication prescribed under the Death with Dignity Act. These patients were compared with those who died in 1998 after ingesting a lethal dose of medication (for 1998 patients, see the first-year report at http://www.ohd.hr.state.or.us/cdpe/chs/pas/ ar-index.htrrL). We also compared patients who chose physician-assisted suicide in 1999 with all Oregonians who died from similar underlying diseases in 1998 (the most recent year that finalized Oregon mortality data were available). The proportion of deaths resulting from legal physician-assisted suicide were calculated for 1998 and estimated for 1999 using total and disease-specific 1998 deaths in the denominator.

Interviews with Family Members

We interviewed close relatives or friends (subsequently referred to as "family") of patients who participated between September 15, 1998, and October 15, 1999. We selected this period to minimize recall inaccuracies, conducting interviews within approximately one year of death, and to allow families a mourning period for deaths occurring in late 1999. Physicians, or other providers involved in the patient's terminal health care, identified the most appropriate family member to interview (one per patient). Each family member knew of the patient's request for and use of lethal medication and was involved in the patient's health-care decisions. Patients were excluded if no family familiar with their illness and death could be identified, or if the family member declined the interview. Oral informed consent was obtained from all family members interviewed.

Most questions on the family interview were analogous to those asked of participating physicians, including questions probing specific concerns that may have contributed to the patients' requests for lethal medication. Additional questions were asked regarding physical suffering, finances, and hospice care. Some family members had difficulty separating pain from other aspects of physical suffering (for example, difficulty breathing, difficulty swallowing, and medication side effects), so we did not distinguish pain from physical suffering in assessing family responses. Consequently, physician responses about pain are not directly comparable to family responses about physical suffering.

Statistical Methods

Proportions were compared using Pearson's chi-square test and Fisher's exact test. Continuous variables were compared using Wilcoxon Rank Sum test. Unadjusted relative risks with 95% confidence intervals (CIs) were calculated when comparing participating patients to the 1998 death cohort. Physician and family responses were compared using a corrected McNemar's chi-square test for paired proportions. Two-tailed P values ≤0.05 were considered statistically significant. Statistical calculations were performed using SAS.[8]

RESULTS

The results from our report are presented in two formats. In addition to this report, the results are presented in a manuscript published in the *New England Journal of Medicine* ("Legalized Physician-Assisted Suicide in Oregon—The Second Year") on February 24, 2000.[9]

Year Two Patients and Physicians Participating in the Death with Dignity Act

In 1999, 33 prescriptions for lethal doses of medication were written, compared to 24 prescriptions written in 1998. Ten (30%) of the 33 prescriptions were written in the last two months of the year. Five 1999 prescription recipients died from their underlying disease; two were alive at the end of the year. In total, 27 patients died after ingesting the medication in 1999: 26 of the 1999 prescription recipients and one of the 1998 prescription recipients. The one other 1998 prescription recipient alive on December 31, 1998, died in 1999 from their underlying disease. (In our 1998 report we included 23 prescription recipients and 15 physician-assisted suicide deaths. A twenty-fourth 1998 prescription recipient participated late in that year and was not reported until 1999. This individual ingested the medication, bringing the total number of physician assisted suicide deaths in 1998 to 16.)

The median age of the 27 patients participating in 1999 was 71 years. They were similar to the 16 patients participating in 1998 with respect to demographic characteristics, underlying illness, hospice use, and health insurance coverage (Table 11-1), although a higher proportion of patients participating in 1999 were married (44% versus 13%, P = 0.05). Sixty-three percent of 1999 patients had end-stage cancer—most commonly lung cancer—and 78% were in hospice before death (Table 11-1).

In 1999, the median time between first requesting physician-assisted suicide and ingesting the lethal medication was 83 days, longer than the 22 days observed in 1998 (P = 0.006; Table 11-2). One patient used the prescription more than 6 months after it was written (247 days). Twenty-six participating patients were prescribed >9 grams secobarbitol, usually in conjunction with antiemetics; one patient was prescribed 6 grams of phenobarbitol. The median time between ingestion and unconsciousness was 10 minutes (range: 1 to 30 minutes); and between ingestion and death, 30 minutes (range: 4 minutes to 26 hours). Twenty-four patients died within four hours, and three after 11 hours. Two of the latter three ingested the entire dose, and one ingested two-thirds of the dose before becoming unconscious after 13 minutes and dying 26 hours later.

In 1999, 22 physicians legally prescribed the 33 lethal doses of medication. Six of them also prescribed in 1998. Fourteen of the 22 physicians were in family practice or internal medicine, five were oncologists, and three were in other subspecialties. Their median age was 52 years (range 30 to 78 years) and the median number of years they had been in practice was 20 years (range 1 to 48 years). According to physician reports, eight (31 %) participating patients received a prescription from the first physician they asked (data unavailable for one patient; Table 11-2). Of the remaining 18 participating patients, 10 (56%) asked one other physician and eight (45%) asked two to three physicians.

Comparison with the 1998 Oregon Death Certificate Cohort

During 1998, a total of 29,281 Oregonians died; 6,994 died of cancer and 76 died of amyotrophic lateral sclerosis (ALS). Using these 1998 values for comparison, patients who ingested lethal medications in 1999 represented an estimated 9 out of 10,000 total Oregon deaths and 39 out of 10,000 Oregon cancer deaths. Patients participating in 1998 represented 6 out of 10,000 total and 20 out of 10,000 cancer deaths. The four participating 1999 patients with ALS represented approximately 5% of ALS deaths (no 1998 participants had ALS). Participating 1999 patients resembled a cohort of 6,901 Oregonians who died from similar underlying illnesses with respect to age, race, and residence (Table 11-3). However, as education increased so did likelihood of participation (chi-square test for linear trend, P<0.001), and college graduates were more likely to participate than people without a high school education (Relative Risk = 12.1; 95% Confidence Interval [3.8–38.7]; P<0.001).

**Table 11-1. Characteristics of 43 Patients Who Died
after Ingesting a Lethal Dose of Medication—Oregon, 1998 and 1999**

Characteristics	1999 (N = 27)	1998 (N = 16)[a]	Total (N = 43)
Age—Median, years (range)	71 (31–87)	70 (25–94)	70 (25–94)
Race—White (%)	26 (96)	16 (100)	42 (98)
Sex—Male (%)	16 (59)	8 (50)	24 (56)
Marital status			
Married (%)*	12 (44)	2 (13)	14 (33)
Widowed (%)	6 (22)	5 (31)	11 (26)
Divorced (%)	8 (30)	5 (31)	13 (30)
Never married (%)	1 (4)	4 (25)	5 (13)
Education			
Less than high school graduate	2 (7)	3 (19)	5 (12)
High school grad./some college (%)	12 (44)	9 (56)	21 (49)
College graduate (%)	13 (48)	4 (25)	17 (40)
Residence			
Portland metropolitan area (%)	10 (37)	7 (44)	17 (40)
Other Oregon	17 (63)	9 (56)	26 (60)
Underlying Disease			
Cancer (%)	17 (63)	14 (88)	31 (72)
Lung	5 (18)	5 (31)	
Colon	3 (11)	0—	
Ovarian	0—	3 (19)	
Other cancer	9 (33)	6 (38)	
Other diseases (%)	10 (37)	2 (12)	12 (28)
Acquired Immune Deficiency Syndrome	1 (4)	0—	
Amyotrophic lateral sclerosis	4 (15)	0—	
Congestive heart failure	0—	1 (6)	
Chronic obstructive pulmonary disease	4 (15)	1 (6)	
Multisystem organ failure	1 (4)	0—	
Hospice[b]			
When sought prescription (%)	12 (44)	10 (67)	22 (52)
Immediately prior to death (%)	21 (78)	11 (73)	32 (76)
Advance medical directives[c] (%)	25 (96)	14 (93)	39 (95)
Insurance[d]			
Private (%)	18 (69)	9 (56)	27 (64)
Medicare only (%)	4 (15)	4 (25)	8 (19)
Oregon Medicaid (%)	4 (15)	2 (13)	6 (14)
None (%)	0—	1 (6)	1 (2)
Mobility before Death[b]			
good (%)	7 (26)	4 (27)	11 (26)
poor (%)	10 (37)	7 (47)	17 (40)
none (%)	10 (37)	4 (27)	14 (33)

[a]The sixteenth 1998 patient was not included in 1998 report[4] as the death was not reported until late in 1998.

*Significantly more participants were married than not married (including widowed, divorced and never married) in 1999 compared to 1998, P=0.03

[b]For 1998, n = 15; for total, n=42 (1 respondent did not know)

[c]For 1999, n = 26; for 1998, n=15; for total, n = 41 (2 respondents did not know)

[d]Insurance coverage for the patient's terminal illness. For 1999, n = 26, for total, n = 42 (1 respondent did not know)

Adapted with permission: *New England Journal of Medicine* 342:598–604 Copyright © 2000 Massachusetts Medical Society. All rights reserved.

Table 11-2. Death with Dignity Act Utilization Characteristics for 43 Patients Who Died after Ingesting a Lethal Dose of Medication—Oregon, 1998 and 1999

Characteristics	1999 (N = 27)	1998 (N = 16)[a]	Total (N = 43)
First physician approached wrote prescription[b] (%)	8 (31)	8 (53)	16 (39)
Referred for psychiatric evaluation (%)	10 (37)	5 (31)	15 (35)
Prescribed ≥ 9 grams secobarbitol (%)	26 (96)	14 (88)	40 (93)
Died at home (%)	25 (93)	13 (81)	38 (88)
Physician present when patient ingested medication (%)	16 (59)	8 (50)	24 (56)
Physician present when patient died (%)	13 (48)	6 (38)	19 (44)
Vomited or had seizures after ingesting medication[b] (%)	0—	0—	0—
Emergency medical services called after ingestion	0—	0—	0—
End-of-Life Concerns Expressed to Physician			
Financial implications of treatment	0—	0—	0—
Burden on friends and family (%)	7 (26)	2 (13)	9 (21)
Losing autonomy[c] (%)	21 (81)	12 (75)	33 (79)
Decreasing ability to participate in activities that make life enjoyable (%)	22 (81)	11 (69)	33 (77)
Losing control of bodily functions (%)	16 (59)	9 (56)	25 (58)
Worsening pain (%)	7 (26)	2 (13)	9 (21)
Timing of events			
Duration (weeks) of patient-physician relationship			
Median	22	11	22
Range	2–817	2–540	2–817
Days between first and second oral requests			
Median	21	19	20
Range	14–96	14–68	14–96
Days between first oral request and death			
Median*	83	22	45
Range	15–289	15–75	15–289
Days between prescription receipt and death			
Median	7	2	3
Range	0–247	0–22	0–247
Minutes between ingestion and unconsciousness[d]			
Median	10	5	5
Range	1–30	3–20	1–30
Minutes between ingestion and death[e]			
Median	30	22	30
Range	4–1560	10–690	4–1560

[a]The sixteenth patient in the first year was not included in the first annual report due to the late date of that death in that year.

[b]For 1999, n = 26; for 1998, n=15; for total, n = 42 (1 respondent did not know)

[c]For 1999, n = 26; for total, n=42 (1 respondent did not know)

*Significantly greater in year two (1999) than year one (1998), P=0.006

[d]For 1999, n = 24; for 1998, n = 12; for total, n = 36 (7 respondents did not know)

[e]For 1999, n = 25; for 1998, n = 15; for total, n = 40 (3 respondents did not know)

Concerns Contributing to Requests for Lethal Medication

Physician Interviews

Based on 1999 physician interviews, multiple end-of-life concerns contributed to patient prescription requests. Eighteen (68%) of 27 patients discussed three or more concerns with their physicians; 13 of these patients included among these concerns loss of autonomy, decreasing ability to participate in activities that make life enjoyable, and loss of control of bodily functions. In 1998, only seven (44%) of 16 physicians included three or more reasons for patient prescription requests. The most frequently cited patient concerns in both years were loss of autonomy (1999, 81%; 1998, 75%; Table 11-2) and decreasing ability to participate in activities that make life enjoyable (1999, 81%; 1998, 69%; Table 11-2). In 1999, seven (26%) of 27 patients expressed concern about worsening pain as their illness progressed, compared with two (13%) of 16 in 1998, though this difference was not statistically significant (P = 0.30). The financial implications of treating or prolonging the illness were not reported to be a concern for any patient.

Family Interviews

Of the 24 participating patients who died after ingesting a lethal dose of medication between September 15, 1998, and October 15, 1999, family members of 19 (79%) were interviewed: eight spouses, two siblings, seven children, one parent, and one close friend. Eighteen interviews included discussions beyond what was explored in the structured instrument. Two patients had been married for over 45 years to the spouses who were present at their deaths. Family interviews were not done for five patients because the contact was overwrought (n = 1) or had no current telephone number (n = 2); or the provider could not identify an appropriate contact (n = 2).

Similar to physicians, family members often cited multiple concerns contributing to the patient's decision to request the prescription (Table 11-4). Twelve (63%) of the 19 family members noted at least three concerns. Overall, the most frequently cited reasons identified for patient participation were concern about loss of control of bodily functions (68%), loss of autonomy (63%), and physical suffering (53%). Nine family members (47%) included concern about decreasing ability to participate in activities that make life enjoyable. Ten family members (53%) included patient concern about both loss of control of bodily functions and loss of autonomy. All of eight family members (47%) who believed the patient was concerned about being a burden also reported that the patient was concerned about loss of autonomy and/or loss of control of bodily functions. (Two family members did not know if concern about becoming a burden on family and friends was an issue for the patient.) Four of 10 patients who were concerned about physical suffering were not reported by family to be suffering when use of the lethal medication was first discussed. The one patient who expressed concern to a family member about the financial impact of

Table 11-3. Characteristics of Patients Participating in 1999 and Oregon Residents Who Died from Similar Disease in 1998

Demographic Characteristic	Participating Estimated 1999 Patients (N=27)	Oregon Deaths, Similar Diseases (N=6901)	Estimated Proportion of Participating 1999 Patients (per 10,000)	Risk Ratio (95% CI)[a]
Mean age, years (SD)	68 (14)	73 (14)	—	—
Race				
White	26	6686	39	1.0[b]
Nonwhite	1	198	50	0.7 (0.1–5.6)
Sex				
Female	11	3481	32	1.0[b]
Male	16	3420	47	1.5 (0.7–3.2)
Residence				
Other Oregon	17	4405	38	1.0[b]
Portland metropolitan	10	2496	40	1.0 (0.4–2.3)
Education[c]				
Did not graduate high school	2	1701	12	1.0[b]
High school graduate/ some college	12	4121	29	2.3 (0.5–9.8)
At least college graduate	13	899	143	12.1 (3.8–38.7)
Marital Status at Death				
Married	12	3386	35	1.0[b]
Widowed	6	2231	27	0.8 (0.3–2.0)
Divorced	8	976	81	2.3 (1.0–5.5)
Never married	1	290	34	1.0 (0.1–7.5)

a CI denotes confidence intervals
b Reference category
c $P<0.001$ for chi-square test for trend
Adapted with permission: *New England Journal of Medicine* 342:598–604 Copyright © 2000 Massachusetts Medical Society. All rights reserved.

the illness was concerned about all issues except physical suffering. This patient was privately insured and spent only a "little bit" of money on health-related expenses. One spouse did not believe that any of the concerns we explored in the structured interview contributed to the patient's request.

Overall, physician responses for these 19 patients were similar to those of family ($P = 0. 15$ to 0.34) for all concerns except physical suffering. Physicians cited concern about loss of autonomy (83%) and decreasing ability to participate (78%) more often than families (63% and 47%, respectively). Concern about loss of control of bodily functions was mentioned by 61% of physicians. Physicians reported patient concerns about pain (32%) less frequently than families reported the more broad concerns about physical suffering.

During the interviews, families raised additional patient concerns not explicitly addressed in the structured interview. Fourteen of 19 family members volunteered that

Table 11-4. Patient Characteristics and Concerns Reported by Family Members of 19 Patients Who Died after Ingesting a Lethal Dose of Medication between September 15, 1998 and October 15, 1999

Characteristics	Family Reporting (N=19)
Had difficulty identifying a physician to write prescription[a] (%)	4 (24)
Enrolled in hospice (%)	17 (89)
Number of weeks patient was in hospice before death[b]	
Median	7
Range	2–25
Physical suffering present day before death (%)	13 (68)
Medication controlled physical suffering on day before death[c]	
Completely (%)	5 (33)
Somewhat (%)	7 (47)
Not at all (%)	3 (20)
Insurance[d]	
Private (%)	15 (79)
Medicare only (%)	1 (5)
Oregon Medicaid (%)	3 (16)
Spent money on illness-related expenses (%)	16 (84)
End-of-life concerns expressed to family[e]	
Financial implications of treatment N	1 (5)
Burden on friends and family[a] (%)	8 (47)
Losing autonomy (%)	12 (63)
Decreasing ability to participate in activities that make life enjoyable (%)	9 (47)
Losing control of bodily functions (%)	13 (68)
Physical suffering[f] (%)	10 (53)

a n = 17 (Two family members did not know)
b n = 16 (Three family members did not know)
c Includes two patients with surgical intervention for pain; n= 15 (four family members could not evaluate the level of pain control)
d Insurance coverage for the patient's terminal illness
e Includes responses coded as "Yes, likely" and "Yes, definitely."
f Includes pain, difficulty breathing, difficulty swallowing, side effects of pain medication. Not comparable to the more narrowly defined concern about pain cited by physicians.

the patients were determined to control the circumstances of their death. Eleven of these 14 and three other family members mentioned the patient's wish to avoid a prolonged death, with four specifically noting the patient's fear of ending life comatose on a respirator despite having advance medical directives. Many family members noted improved pain management after patients initiated hospice. In addition, six family members mentioned how difficult it was fulfill the requirements of the act.

DISCUSSION

In 1999, the second year of legal physician-assisted suicide in Oregon, the number of patients choosing this option increased compared to 1998, but remained small compared to the overall number of deaths in Oregon. Although concern about possible abuses persists,[10-12] information on participating patients indicates that poverty, lack of education or insurance, or poor end-of-life care are not important factors influencing patient decisions to use the Death with Dignity Act. Physician and family interviews suggest that the concerns contributing to patient requests for prescriptions relate to losing autonomy, losing control of bodily functions, decreasing ability to participate in activities that make life enjoyable, physical suffering, and a determination to control the timing and manner of death.

Compared with Oregonians dying from similar diseases, participating patients were better educated but otherwise alike with respect to age, race, and other demographic factors. The relative underrepresentation of married persons in 1998[4] was not seen in 1999. Although most patients spent out-of-pocket money on medical expenses (for example, on prescription drugs) all participants were insured for most other major medical expenses, often through a combination of Medicare and private supplemental policies.

The family members we interviewed reported that the majority of participating patients did not have difficulty identifying a physician willing to write the prescription for lethal medication. However, half of these patients asked more than one physician, indicating that not all Oregon physicians are willing to participate in physician-assisted suicide. This finding is consistent with reports on the attitudes of Oregon physicians and medical students toward physician-assisted suicide.[13,14] Some physicians who refused to prescribe lethal medication acted as consulting physicians.

As best we could determine, all participating physicians complied with the provisions of the act. Although the Health Division is not a regulatory agency for physicians, it does report to Oregon's Board of Medical Examiners any cases of noncompliance. Under reporting and noncompliance is thus difficult to assess because of possible repercussions for noncompliant physicians reporting to the division. In an independent anonymous survey, Oregon physicians reported writing 29 legal prescriptions for lethal doses of medication from December 1997 through August 1999.[15] All but one physician had reported to the Health Division by the time they completed the survey (the status of one report was undetermined).

Responses from both physician and family interviews indicate that patients' decisions to request PAS were motivated by multiple interrelated concerns. Physical suffering was discussed by several families as a cause of loss of autonomy, inability to participate in activities that made life enjoyable, or a "nonexistent" quality of life. For example, "She would have stuck it out through the pain if she thought she'd get better ... [but she believed that] when quality of life has no meaning, it's no use hanging around." For another participant, a feeling of being trapped because of ALS contributed to concern about loss of autonomy. Family members frequently commented on loss of control of bodily functions when discussing loss of autonomy. Those reporting patient concern about being a burden on friends and family also reported concern about loss of autonomy and control of bodily functions. Reasons for requesting a prescription were sometimes so interrelated they were difficult to categorize. According to one family member being asked to distinguish reasons for the patient's decision, "It was everything; it was nothing; [he was suffering terribly]."

Difficulty categorizing and differences in interpreting the nature of the concerns made physician and family member responses hard to compare quantitatively. Nonetheless, family interviews corroborate physician reports from both years[4] that patients are greatly concerned about issues of autonomy and control. In addition, responses of both physicians and family consistently pointed to patient concerns about quality of life and the wish to have a means of controlling the end of life should it become unbearable. As one family member said, "She always thought that if something was terminal, she would [want to] control the end. . . . It was not the dying that she dreaded, it was getting to that death."

Initially, we also wanted to compare responses of family members we interviewed to family members of other Oregonians who died of similar causes but did not use the Death with Dignity Act. We identified patients by randomly selecting death certificates. We then contacted the physicians on the death certificates to see if the patients would have been eligible to use PAS (if they had chosen to) and to identify an appropriate family member to interview. One in four physicians contacted did not identify a family member; one in three patients were not eligible or had no family who knew about their illness and death. Of 12 eligible patients initially identified, three family members were too overwrought to be interviewed, two who had consented to be interviewed stopped the interview because of overwhelming emotion, and four had had limited discussion with patients on the end-of-life issues we raised. We stopped these interviews because of difficulties in identifying patients and family members, and in conducting the interviews.

When family members of the patients who used PAS discussed patient's concerns about physical suffering, they included concerns about difficulty breathing and difficulty swallowing, as well as pain. Some patients were concerned that to adequately control pain, the side effects of the medication would render quality of life meaningless. A previous study found that physical factors, especially difficulty breathing, became important predictors of decreasing will to live as death drew near.[16] However, it is important to note that among patients here, concern about physical suffering was not always equivalent to experiencing it. End-of-life care was available to participating patients, and three quarters of them were in hospice before dying. Family members noted improved pain management for the patients after entering hospice. Physician reports did note a slight increase in the number of patients concerned about pain, but this is consistent with hospital-based reports from Oregon wherein an overall increase in pain has been reported among terminally ill patients.[17]

Oregonians choosing physician-assisted suicide appeared to want control over how they died. One woman had purchased poison over a decade before her participation, when her cancer was first diagnosed, so that she would never be without the means of controlling the end of her life should it become unbearable. Like many others who participated, she was described as "determined" to have this control. Another woman was described as a "gutsy woman" who was " . . . determined in her lifetime, and determined about [physician-assisted suicide]." Family members expressed profound grief at losing a loved one. However, mixed with this grief was great respect for the patient's determination and choice to use physician-assisted suicide. As one husband said about his wife of almost 50 years, "She was my only girl; I didn't want to lose her . . . but she wanted to do this."

The authors would like to thank Dr. Susan Tolle of Oregon Health Sciences University for her comments on the family interview instrument, and Dr. Thomas Torok of the Centers for Disease Control and Prevention for his comments on the manuscript. We thank staff at Kaiser Permenente Northwest and the Oregon Health Sciences University, as well as participating physicians, for helping us identify family members. We also sincerely thank the family members who spoke with us for sharing their thoughts on this very personal subject. This study was conducted as part of the required surveillance and public health practice activities of the Oregon Health Division and was supported by Division funds.

REFERENCES

1. Oregon Death with Dignity Act. Oregon Revised Statute 127.800-127.995. Available at: www.ohd.hr. state. or.us/cdpe/chs/pas/ors.htm.

2. Gianelli D. Oregon suicide report contains some surprises. *American Medical News.* March 8, 1999.

3. Drickamer M, Lee M, Ganzini L. Practical issues in physician-assisted suicide. *Annals of Internal Medicine.* 1997;126:146–151.

4. Chin G, Hedberg K, Higginson G, Fleming D. Legalized physician-assisted suicide in Oregon—the first year's experience. *New England Journal of Medicine.* 1999;340:577–583.

5. Haley K, Lee M (eds.). *The Oregon Death with Dignity Act—A Guidebook for Health-Care Providers.* Portland, OR: Oregon Health Sciences University; 1998.

6. Oregon Administrative Rules 333-009-000 to 333-009-0030. Available at: www. ohd.hr. state. or.us/cdpe/chs/pas/oars.htm.

7. Oken M, Creech R, Tormey D, et al. Toxicity and response criteria of the Eastern Cooperative Oncology Group. *American Journal of Clinical Oncology.* 1982;5:649–655.

8. SAS Version 6.12. 1995. SAS Institute Inc. Cary, North Carolina.

9. Sullivan AD, Hedberg K, Fleming DW. Legalized physician-assisted suicide in Oregon—the second year. *New England Journal of Medicine.* 2000;342:598–604.

10. Tolle SW. Care of the dying: clinical and financial lessons from the Oregon experience. *Annals of Internal Medicine.* 1998;128(7):567–568.

11. Foley K, Hendin H. The Oregon report: don't ask, don't tell. *Hastings Center Report.* 1999; 20:37–42.

12. Quill T, Meier D, Block S, et al. The debate over physician-assisted suicide: Empirical data and convergent views. *Annals of Internal Medicine.* 1998;128:553–558.

13. Lee M, Nelson H, Tilden V, Ganzini L, Schmidt T, Tolle S. Legalizing assisted suicide views of physicians in Oregon. *New England Journal of Medicine.* 1996;334:310–315.

14. Mangus R, Dipiero A, Hawkins C. Medical students' attitudes toward physician-assisted suicide. *JAMA* 1999;282:2080–2081.

15. Ganzini L, Nelson HD, Schmidt TA, et al. Physicians' experiences with the Oregon Death with Dignity Act. *New England Journal of Medicine.* 2000;342:557–563.

16. Chochinov H, Tataryn D, Clinch J, Dudgeon D. Will to live in the terminally ill. *Lancet.* 1999;354:816–819.

17. Tolle SW, Tilden VP, Rosenfeld A, Hickman SE. Family reports of barriers to optimal care of the the dying. *Nursing Research.* In press.

Part 4

PATIENTS, FAMILIES, AND HEALTH-CARE DECISIONS

❧

Over the past five decades we have seen patient autonomy go from being almost unheard of to being paramount. Unfortunately, in all our zeal to develop our current patient-centered decision-making process, we ignored something very crucial: how we *actually go about* making major life decisions. Consequently, we now have a process in which patients have many rights, but lack the support and resources necessary to make decisions that have the best chance of promoting their interests as they see them.

Consider the process of buying a home: You go to an open house. You come back a few times to look the house over some more. Your family looks it over and gives you their thoughts. You have it inspected. You shop around for low interest rates. All required documents are reviewed by probably a dozen people before you sign them. Only after all of that do you make your decision by signing on the dotted line.

Now consider the process of making a health-care decision: You are probably wearing a paper gown while sitting in an exam room. You are most likely anxious and under a great deal of stress. You could be in pain or have difficulty breathing or walking. According to some studies, you will have ten to twelve minutes with your physician. Within these ten to twelve minutes you must find out your treatment options, their benefits and burdens, the likelihood of those benefits and burdens actually occurring, how the various treatments might effect your quality of life, and what your physician recommends and why. Armed with this overwhelming amount of information, you go home to your family and attempt to tell them everything you remember. You might hop on the Web to see what you find about your diagnosis and treatment. You may make another ten- to twelve-minute appointment with their physician to ask follow-up questions. In the end, your decision will result from what you remember of your physician's appointment (the accuracy of which is questionable), what your family thinks (based on your questionable recollection), and what you found on the Web. By creating a decision-making process that does not reflect how people actually go about making major life decisions, we basically force patients into a lottery—a lottery in which half-blindfolded patients reach into a bowl and hope their decision is the one with the best chance of promoting their interests.

Conversely, a decision-making process that reflects how we make major life decisions would take into account how people take in information, process it, weigh it, seek counsel from those they trust, reconsider information in light of such counsel, ask for clarification from experts and reconsider again. The first two articles in this section speak to some of these needs, particularly the need to have the active involvement of those the patient trusts, typically family. In "Reconceiving the Family: The Process of Consent in Medical Decision Making," Mark Kuczewski walks us through a framework of informed consent as a patient-as-part-of-a-family process, as opposed to a patient-as-an-island process. With this information, health-care providers and ethics committees can work to incorporate this richer conception into their institution's policies and procedures. The Joint Commission on Accreditation of Healthcare Organizations (JCAHO) provides a good incentive to pursue this change, as their Patients Rights and Organizational Ethics standard RI.1.2.2 states: "The family participates in care decisions."[1]

The second article, by Rebecca Dresser and Peter Whitehouse, is titled "The Incompetent Patient on the Slippery Slope." By taking us through the issues a surrogate decision maker needs to consider, the authors make clear the necessity of including the family in this process. If family members are excluded from discussions until called upon to be surrogates (or proxies), how can we possibly expect them to appreciate how the patient would have weighed the benefits and burdens? Only by including the family throughout the health-care decision-making process can we ensure that the voice of the patient will be heard long after he has lost the ability to communicate.

At this point it is important to mention a fairly common source of confusion. The terms *incompetent* and *incapacity* tend to be used interchangeably, but they do not mean the same thing. Lack of decision-making capacity is a medical judgement reserved for physicians, nurses, paramedics, and the like. When patients are asked the standard "alert and oriented" questions, it is their decision-making capacity that is being assessed—if he can answer the questions then he has it, all things being equal. Competency, on the other hand, is a judgement reserved solely for the judicial process. Only after a hearing can a judge deem a patient to be incompetent.

This section ends with "A Chronicle: Dax's Case As It Happened," by Keith Burton. In just about every introductory medical ethics course, students are forced (in the weak sense) to view a video in which some of the most excruciating medical treatments imaginable are forced (in the strong sense) upon a patient. That patient was Don Cowart, who later came to refer to himself as "Dax." Dax's story is probably the original "right-to-die" situation, preceding Karen Ann Quinlan's case by several years. Although Dax's situation never culminated in a trial, it gave the patient's rights movement its first poster child.

In essence, Dax was as severely burned as a person can probably be and still live. During his fourteen-month hospital stay, along with numerous other treatments and surgeries, he was continually debrided and put into sulfa baths. Throughout these horrific treatments Dax loudly and consistently made it known that he did not want to be treated and that he wanted to die. His mother, his attorney, and his physician decided to ignore his preferences—even though a psychiatrist determined he had complete decision-making capacity.

Dax's struggle against this paternalism took place during a pivotal time in America. As a result of the protests and counterculture surrounding the Vietnam War, authority of all kinds was under siege, including the medical profession. It was also around this time that a new multidisciplinary field known as medical ethics (aka bioethics, health-care ethics, or biomedical ethics) came into being as the Hastings Center was established in 1969. From these social, political, and historical antecedents came the philosophy of patient autonomy. Now, almost thirty years removed from this transformation, we have the hindsight to see that neither framework truly serves the patient's interests. Patients are not served when their preferences are ignored (paternalism-based model) or when they are left to themselves (autonomy-based model).

The solution lies in providing a mean to these two extremes. This mean takes the patient's preferences to be fundamental in all health-care decisions, while situating these preferences within the context of family relationships, recognizing that it is through these relationships that the patient is supported and taken care of during diagnosis, treatment, and recovery. By bringing the patient's family into this matrix we will finally have a process that reflects how we actually live our lives.

REFERENCE

1. Joint Commission on Accreditation of Healthcare Organizations. *2000 Hospital Accreditation Standards*. Oakbrook, IL: JCAHO; 2000:77.

12

RECONCEIVING THE FAMILY

The Process of Consent in Medical Decision Making

Mark G. Kuczewski, Ph.D.

✧

M edical ethics has rediscovered the family. At least two factors have contributed to widening the focus from the individual. There has been a general revival of communitarian rhetoric in the United States that, of course, brings the role of social relations to the fore. Similarly, we should not underestimate the natural progression and development of medical ethics. Having focused on the rights of the patient for so long, it follows that ethicists now wish to map the relationships surrounding the individual that may affect medical decision making. Because this interest in the family is a concern with the significant relationships that surround the patient, the family is described in terms of "closeness," not biology. This way of describing the family is commonplace in medical ethics and is a meritorious convention.[1(p127), 2(p136)] Thus, when John Hardwig asks, "What about the Family?"[3] he asks whether there is any role in medical decision making for those close to the patient. This is *the* question, because our thinking about medical decisionmaking is entirely patient-centered. This patient-centered ethic is systematized as the doctrine of informed consent.

Without much exaggeration it can be said that all of medical ethics is but a footnote to informed consent. It is the concept that first called medicine out of its paternalistic slumber and into the open light of public scrutiny. Informed consent serves as

M. Kuczewski. "Reconceiving the Family: The Process of Consent in Medical Decision-making." *Hastings Center Report.* 1996;26(2):30–37. Reproduced by permission. © The Hastings Center.

the foundation upon which answers to new questions and problems are constructed. Informed consent is a kind of doctrine, that is, an amalgam of legal and philosophical reasoning with a conceptual framework and a number of specific prescriptions. This framework entails a few basic actions and presupposes certain conditions. At the heart of the doctrine is the legal principle that "the right of a competent person to refuse medical treatment is virtually absolute."[4(p319)] The exercise of this right presupposes that the patient must receive all information relevant to the decision to undergo or forgo a proposed treatment and that he or she must comprehend the information. The legal principle indicates that the patient needs to be competent and it is also implicit that the choice is relatively freely made. Although influence is acceptable, all forms of coercion are beyond the pale.[5(p274)]

The individualistic nature of this line of thought is clear. The person is conceptualized as possessing a sphere of protected activity or privacy free from unwanted interference. Within this zone of privacy, one is able to exercise his or her liberty and discretion. Within this protected sphere take place disclosure, comprehension, and choice, which express the patient's right of self-determination over her body.[5(p123)] Of course, these are legal formulations. The philosophical justification for them draws on egalitarian or democratic intuitions regarding personhood.

The person is opaque to others and therefore the best judge and guardian of his or her own interests. Although the physician may be the expert on the medical "facts," the patient is the only individual with genuine insight into his private sphere of "values." Because treatment plans should reflect personal values as well as medical realities, the patient must be the ultimate decision maker.[6(p74)] Once we sketch the person in this way, the problem for ethicists is obvious. The doctrine of informed consent is based on an individual profile rather than a family portrait. The individual is outlined first, and only then do we ask where close others may be added to the picture. Because the philosophical and legal premises of the doctrine leave few other reasonable options, the family is usually conceived as comprising competing interests. Such a result is not adequate to our ordinary intuitions regarding the relationship of the patient to the family. Furthermore, these premises limit ethicists to arguing about the relative merits of these rival bundles of interests.

Once we understand the relationship between the doctrine of informed consent and the inability of medical ethicists to adequately describe the role of the family in medical decision making, the tasks become clear. To follow the communitarian impulse and characterize the family in a way that transcends an atomistic view of human relations will require a several-part investigation. First, I must critique the traditional doctrine of informed consent and show how it has "hijacked" what questions can be asked about the role of the family. By examining the doctrine's major assumptions and fixing the limits of its application, we can find room for the family in situations where such legalistic thought is inappropriate. Second, I shall explain how several promising "process" models of informed consent better describe the role of the family in medical decision making. Finally, I shall apply these process models to a case and show how they also demand a different role for the physician in the decision-making process. Only by exploring the traditional doctrine of informed consent and escaping its individualistic and legalistic assumptions can we hope to enrich the theoretical picture of the family in the decision-making process.

SUBVERTING INDIVIDUALISM
IN MEDICAL ETHICS

The communitarian impulse that has revived inquiry into the family represents a dissatisfaction with the "rugged individualism"[7(p7)] that a patient-centered ethic implies. Medical ethicists sometimes investigate the family in the hope of finding a way to place the interests of the patient in proper perspective. Of course, the only way to describe the role of the family is in terms of the doctrine of informed consent, since it is the foundation of medical decision making. In addition to the patient, each member of the family also has his or her sphere of privacy, values, and interests. The obvious question follows: What are the family's rights? Another way of formulating the same question is to ask how we should balance the rights of the individual patient and those of the family when they conflict. This is the framework that virtually every medical ethicist investigating the family has accepted. As a result, the answers vary little in substance even though, at first glance, there seems to be wide disagreement. In this kind of rights-based investigation, the family usually loses to the patient.

John Hardwig advances the most radical view by advocating that we abandon our current patient-centered ethic in favor of a presumption of the equality of interests, both medical and nonmedical, of each family member. This presumption can and usually will be overridden by the patient's interests in optimal health and a longer life.[3(p7)] On some occasions, however, the family's interests may outweigh those of the patient and should receive preference. Hardwig's essay is paradigmatic in a number of ways for those which have followed. All agree that the patient is usually vulnerable and in need of advocacy and protection. Therefore, they begin with a strong presumption in favor of the patient's right to be the primary decision maker. However, the advance these authors make is that they do not characterize the patient's rights as a trump card. Instead, they model their arguments on a scale of justice. The patient's claims are usually weighty compared to the side of the balance on which family rights rest. On occasion, however, the interests of the patient are not very compelling while the family may have a great stake, financially or emotionally, in what course is followed. All argue that family interests should hold sway to some extent under such circumstances.

Jeffrey Blustein sums up this position when he says, "because treatment decisions often do have a dramatic impact on family members, procedures need to be devised, short of giving family members a share of decisional authority, that acknowledge the moral weight of their legitimate interests."[8(p11)] Blustein argues that patients be encouraged to include the interests of family members in thinking about choices but that the choice per se belongs to the patient. James Nelson tilts the scales slightly more in favor of the family. He argues that we should begin with a presumption that the competent patient is the decision maker, but acknowledge that this presumption is rebuttable by showing that family interests are sufficiently compelling to override the patient's wishes. Hardwig's position can be interpreted as virtually identical with Nelson's. These arguments are framed in terms of a conflict between the interests of the patient and those of the family. With some exceptions, most such conflicts must be settled in favor of the patient.[9] This is hardly a satisfactory outcome for these inquiries.

Hardwig's essay is, at first glance, provocative and radical because he argues that morality requires heeding family interests. Unfortunately, he asks questions of individual and group rights that must be answered in either/or terms. But it is the dissatisfaction with this kind of rights-oriented individualism that revived discussion of the family in the first place. Furthermore, it is not obvious that the role of the family in decision making is exhausted by discussions of such conflicts. The profundity of the links and bonds between family members is hidden from view in these legalistic discussions of interests and rights. This failure to escape the limitations of rights-based thinking clearly emanates from the acceptance of the doctrine of informed consent. While trying to subvert individualism in medical ethics, these ethicists remain trapped by the individualism implicit in the doctrine. To overcome such individualism, informed consent will have to be rethought. We must also be clear regarding the question to which the doctrine is the answer.

THE FAMILY: WHAT'S THE QUESTION?

We can see that there is an ambiguity regarding the question medical ethicists ask about the family. Is the question, Whose interests and wishes should take precedence when those of the patient and family conflict? or What are the respective roles of the patient, family, and physician in medical decision making? In other words, are we asking what to do in a particular event, such as when wishes irresolubly conflict, or are we sketching the process of decision making? The question of unresolvable conflict has an initial attraction because of its clarity and practicality. Its answer is also clear. The patient's wishes and interests must take priority, but there can be exceptions. This conclusion follows from the legalistic aspect of the doctrine of informed consent. Persons are defined in terms of rights and interests and so conflicts must be resolved in such terms. Answering this question, however, does not explain the more general phenomenon of the family's place in medical decision making, such as in the vast majority of cases that lack an unresolvable conflict.

We noted at the outset that informed consent is not only a legal doctrine, but also includes certain philosophical justifications. The legal doctrine is supported by philosophical notions of self-determination and the opacity of an individual's values. These notions, however, are usually considered tenets of political philosophy. That political philosophy should supply the justifications is natural because the legal notion of informed consent is, in large part, an outgrowth of the right to be free from unwanted government interference in one's affairs.[5(p40)] Political philosophy is thereby called upon to justify an essentially political doctrine. The political notions of liberty and the right to base decisions on one's private values also do important philosophical work in cases of unresolvable conflict because these are instances in which the state must adjudicate claims. However, when recourse to the conflict-resolution mechanisms of the state is not necessary, these conceptions of liberty and privacy seem out of place.

Most major writers on the family in medical decision making implicitly accept the political view of the person contained in the legalistic aspect of the doctrine of informed consent. The competent adult person has developed values and preferences. Informed consent involves a conference in which the physician discloses treatment options along with risks, costs, and benefits to the patient or to the patient and family. A calculation is made regarding what is in the patient's best interest or in the interest of the family unit and the treatment is thereby chosen. When illness transforms a person into a patient, his autonomy is compromised and needs to be restored. Jeffrey Blustein suggests that this is a temporary situation caused by the emotionally traumatic nature of illness and the need to cognize the situation, the treatment opdons, and the interests of all those affected. Thus, the family can primarily assist with the patient's "thinking" and thereby help to "restore" the patient's autonomy.[8(p12)] According to this view, the family's role when there is no unresolvable conflict is trivial and uninteresting.

In sum, certain presuppositions of the traditional legalistic vision of informed consent have caused the dialogue to focus on familial conflict and prevented the question of the family's role in medical decision making from being addressed. These assumptions are that the person is mainly a cognitive animal in need of information and, perhaps, assistance due to impairment in mental functioning and has a developed set of private and opaque values from which the patient's treatment preferences readily flow. These assumptions not only emphasize the legalistic aspects of the doctrine of informed consent, but lead to conceiving consent as an event. Consent takes place during a conference when information is exchanged and comprehended, and the patient makes a choice evidenced in the signing of the consent form. We see that the legalistic, event model of informed consent and its implicit notion of the person is preventing us from seeing the family in all its richness. Fortunately, as we move away from the literature on the family and examine recent scholarship on informed consent, we find resources on which to draw. Rugged individualism is not the only conception of consent in contemporary bioethics.[10(p31)]

RECONCEIVING INFORMED CONSENT

Bioethicists such as Charles Lidz,[11] Howard Brody,[12] and Ezekiel and Linda Emanuel[13] have developed models of informed consent and the physician-patient relationship that do not assume patients have a developed set of private values.

Instead, they see informed consent as a process of shared decision making in which the thinking and values of the patient and physician gradually take shape. The legalistic, event model of informed consent conceived the patient and physician as experts over their distinctly private realms with the patient reigning over his or her private values. Process models view the physician and patient as each having access to interrelated and evolving facts and values. They mutually monitor each other in order that their thinking and evaluations become transparent. Once informed consent is conceived in this manner, more integral roles for the physician and for others close to the patient are apparent. Let us illustrate this with a case.

> Mrs. L. was a fifty-year-old female who was transferred to this tertiary care facility from a primary care hospital. Her husband visited daily. She also had several brothers and sisters but no children. Mrs. L.'s recent problem concerned multiple external lacerations on her hands, chest, and groin area as well as kidney failure. These health problems are related to her long-term insulin-dependent diabetes. She had suffered from diabetes since childhood, but the complications and consequences of this illness have increased recently with a leg amputation being necessary about a year ago. Shortly thereafter, dialysis was begun.
>
> The patient was transferred to the tertiary care facility to have her lesions biopsied for diagnostic purposes. These were open, draining, and very painful to the patient. Initial work-up ruled out vasculitis as the causal agent. Finding the source of the lesions proved difficult and the hospitalization became prolonged as other complications developed. Mrs. L. was in great pain and was placed on a sand bed and given a patient-controlled analgesia machine to help provide relief. Despite these measures, pain continued to be a factor in the slow process of diagnostic testing.
>
> Mrs. L. began to ask the nurses to stop dialysis. These requests began about one month into this hospitalization and continued at intervals. Each time the requests became frequent, a discussion would be held with Mrs. L., her husband, and the attending physician. In these meetings, Mr. L. would often ask Mrs. L. to change her mind regarding the dialysis or other tests she was resisting "for him." Each time, this request was granted by the patient after some resistance. On a couple of occasions, the patient agreed to further diagnostic work if her husband would be able to be with her through the test. The nursing staff became increasingly unnerved by the situation as Mrs. L. would often continue to tell the nurses that she "really" wished to stop and "just wanted to die in peace." This particular wish was always superseded by the results of the patient-husband-physician conferences. Eventually it seemed that the patient's husband also grew tired of the long hospital stay.
>
> About eight weeks into her hospitalization, Mrs. L. remained adamant in her treatment refusals during a conference with her husband and physician. Mr. L. then agreed to accept her wishes and agreed to stay by her during her death. The physician wrote a DNR order on the chart along with orders to discontinue dialysis. Palliative care continued to be provided. The patient died within forty-eight hours accompanied by her grieving husband.[14]

This case is likely to be reported to an ethics consultation service as involving a familial conflict. Such conflicts are supposedly what the literature on the family analyzes. Nevertheless, these analyses cannot help because a legalistic, event model of informed consent does not explain the difficulties between Mr. and Mrs. L. Any view of informed consent or the family premised upon a patient with a sturdy set of interests and values must necessarily be beside the point. Mrs. L.'s wishes and values are not clear or are somewhat inaccessible to her.

The legalistic view of the doctrine of informed consent tells us that a competent patient has a right to refuse treatment and therefore counsels that we call for a determination of the patient's decision-making capacity or competence to give consent. If the patient is competent, then we should stand by her wishes (of course, with some occasional exceptions). Competence typically requires that the patient understand the situation, base her choices on relatively stable values, and be able to communicate her wishes. Unfortunately this means we must determine which utterances represent fleeting whims and which disclose underlying values. To verify when Mrs. L. is "being herself" requires input from someone who knows her well and can place the current episode in a larger context. This role, as the verifier of the patient's competence, has been the most widely accepted role accorded the family. Nevertheless, this approach makes us nervous. Even if we discount selfish motives on the part of family members, it is difficult to know if Mrs. L. really has a single set of preferences or values to be verified. Thus, we must take a different, process-oriented approach.

We can view the process of informed consent in cases like the one at hand in one of two related ways. Each emphasizes a different element of the patient's decisional capacity and undermines slightly different assumptions of the event model of informed consent. We can take a clue from event models of informed consent that emphasize the patient's cognitive nature. We then advance the suggestion that the role of the family is to assist the patient's "thinking." This approach is sometimes called the *interpretive model*[13(p2221)] because the physician and family assist the patient in interpreting her values and translating them into treatment preferences. This process model allows that the patient has relatively well-developed and stable values but stresses that they may not only be opaque to others, but can also be unclear to the patient. Thus, translating values into treatment choices is not merely logical "thinking" but is a process of self-discovery.

A more radical process model of informed consent is required in those cases, perhaps including that of Mrs. L., where the fundamental layer of necessary values is lacking and needs to be developed. This process of value development is the *deliberative model*. Which of these two process models is more applicable in a given case can be difficult to know. It is seldom clear whether we are helping a patient to uncover her values and translate them into preferences or to develop new values. Thus, these two ways of viewing the process of informed consent, two types of process models, are complementary aspects of one and the same theory of consent.

AN INTERPRETIVE PROCESS OF CONSENT: RESTORING "THINKING"

The interpretive model of consent starts from the assumption that there is a gap between the fundamental core of a human being that we call her values and her "preferences" that are relatively transient, circumstantial expressions of her personality. In many common situations, our preferences reflect no more than taste or whimsy. In choices of gravity, we wish our preferences to reflect who we are, that is, to follow from the values at our core. Sometimes people come to situations with their values and preferences already developed and in harmony. Nevertheless, to assume that this is generally the case in clinical situations is not plausible. Why think a patient has preferences applicable to situations that are rather new? Her prognosis changes, new treatment choices are presented, and the relative merits of ongoing treatments may change. Additionally, the patient gains new appreciation for various treatments as she accumulates experiential information from undergoing them. This continuous refinement of knowledge and development of preferences are important aspects of process approaches to consent.

The interpretive approach focuses on the articulation of preferences from the patient's underlying values. The patient may possess stable values, for example, love of her husband, desire to be relatively pain free, and so on, but not yet know how to apply these values to particular treatment choices. Hence, as she gains experience with the treatment and refines her understanding of her illness, the choices follow. This *interpretive process* model differs from an *event* model of informed consent in two ways. First, the process model sees the family's role in restoring the patient's thinking as primarily one of providing the appropriate surrounding and context through presence and interaction. "Restoring the patient's thinking" is an experiential and interactive process of which the cognitive deduction from values to preferences is a small moment. Second, the idea that the patient's values and preferences are opaque to others while the patient has privileged access is rejected.

Interpreting our values usually involves the feedback of those close to us and often the advice of persons with professional expertise. Just as we are uncomfortable with the idea that a family member can gain access to the patient's real values and definitively say when she is being herself, so too there is something unrealistic in thinking that the patient has private and privileged access to her values. The feedback of others is necessary to one's reality testing and the construction of an interpersonal narrative that forms the framework for choices. Thus, the process of decision making is interpretive in nature.

Although Blustein recognized the need for family to help patients with their thinking, we see that a process model of consent goes beyond this in making "thinking" a metaphor. Though the patient may be quite capable of a syllogistic deduction of treatment choices from her values, illness somehow distances her from her identity and causes a loss of touch with her everyday values. Family members do not merely help the patient to clarify his or her thinking. They take part in the patient's narrative self-discovery that helps her to reconnect with her values and give them meaning as expressed in choices. This self-discovery is not prior to the event of giving consent, but, in a sense, is the process of informed consent.

Our initial hope in cases like Mrs. L.'s is that matters unfold as the interpretive model suggests: A changing prognosis and new treatment options will interact over time with a relatively stable set of values to produce rational treatment preferences. Values, however, do not always prove to be the kind of unchanging thing that can serve as such an Archimedean point. Mrs. L.'s values or vision of the good may not be sufficiently developed to make the choices confronting her. In other words, her values are also in process. The patient is not only uncovering values; she is also creating them. For instance, one may never have developed values or virtues relating to extreme pain or never needed to develop more than the sketchiest concept of personal dignity. Perhaps such dispositions and character traits exist but are undergoing radical shifts. If so, the justification for family involvement becomes all the dearer. When values must be constructed, this construction process is unlikely to be an individual affair.

A DELIBERATIVE PROCESS OF CONSENT: DEVELOPING VALUES

Ezekiel and Linda Emanuel explore the process of choosing oneself and one's values, that is, the deliberative model of physician-patient encounters.[19(p2222)] In this model, the physician assists the patient by elucidating the values embodied in the different treatment options. Because the patient's values are not fixed, the physician is free, even obligated, to advocate certain values. He is helping to shape the patient's values through his recommendations. The Emanuels do not mention the family in this process, but the justification for familial involvement flows from the same sources. Because we discover our values in dialogue with those closest to us, the family is naturally an integral part of this process. In Mrs. L.'s encounter with her physician and husband, she is coming to choose her values over time.

If we assume that values do not simply emanate from some ineffable core within us but take shape through interaction with our environment, the family is a natural part of this process. Much of our youth is spent internalizing the values of close others. In adult life our values usually are not acquired through mere passive internalization, but this process has a dialectical character. Furthermore, we seldom decide our values in a single, irrevocable act of will. Instead, values must become sturdy and defined if they are to form the foundation for our preferences. They must take shape and concretize. By "trying out" expressions of these developing values with close others, they begin to take shape and become firm. There is still a further reason for including the family. As in Mrs. L.'s case, these values are often about them. In part, the values Mrs. L. is developing or reranking are about her love for and relationship to her husband. To truly know whether she has arrived at the proper ordering may require testing them together with him. Similarly, his values may also be developing and changing, and these values are about her.

In an ongoing dialogue between intimates, there will be a mutual discovery and shaping of values. In the particular case at hand, Mr. L. may simply have the more stable values, or his are challenged less by the present situation. For whatever reason, he does not seem to experience the vacillation that his wife undergoes. This is merely the fact of this case. Nevertheless, a family member, especially one who is often the patient's primary caregiver, may undergo a process of self-discovery and adoption of a new value structure in the same way that patients often do. In this particular case, Mr. L. eventually tires from the prolonged course and then supports his wife's treatment refusal. We do not know whether this is adapting his same long-held values to a changing situation (the interpretive model) or a fundamental reordering of priorities (the deliberative model). Either way, informed consent is a process of mutual self-discovery. Family does not simply provide the context for the patient's thinking in the way a familiar object would. In the process of decision making, the context is also dynamic.

In sum, we see that process models of informed consent are comfortable with active roles for physicians and families in the medical decision-making process. This comfort with collaborative decision making grows from the assumption that values are not the hidden and privileged property of the individual. They take shape publicly, and when they are opaque or absent their discovery or construction is also a communal process. Nevertheless, several questions may trouble us. On what basis might the physician legitimately advocate certain values? Should the physician advocate these values only to the patient or also to the family, since the family's values are also in process? Is the physician simply one more person in the process of informed consent or does he occupy a particular role in the relationship between the patient and family? In other words, the process models of informed consent suggest active roles for the physician and family and we must more clearly define and circumscribe these roles. In cases like the one at hand, these are not abstract questions. There is something about Mr. L.'s behavior that makes us uneasy and raises the question of the physician's obligation to the patient and to him.

RECONCEIVING THE ROLES OF THE PHYSICIAN AND FAMILY

The physician's role requires justification for two reasons. First, the physician is being characterized as an advocate of certain values, and we must provide appropriate content and reasons for this advocacy. Second, we have allowed a much greater role for the family, and we need a counterweight to prevent the family's role from becoming a coercive one. We must be careful to avoid justifying unbridled paternalism in the name of family values. Ezekiel and Linda Emanuel propose that the physician's advocacy is legitimate because she only advocates health-related values. Certain of these are deemed more worthy than others. It is easy to imagine that health is more worthwhile than sickness, and therefore good eating, hygiene, and exercise habits can uncontroversially be advocated. But what should the physician advocate in Mrs. L.'s case? How can the doctor avoid his professional bias to treat this patient as long as there is a medical treatment at hand? Perhaps we can take a cue from the literature on patient competency and suggest a sliding scale or risk-related standard of advocacy.[2,15,16]

In assessing patient capacity to give informed consent, the standard of competence is based upon the risks and benefits of a proposed course of treatment. When patients wish to consent to a treatment that poses few risks and whose benefits are considerable and clear, they do not need great comprehension of the situation. Mere awareness will justify allowing the patient to make this decision. However, to refuse this same treatment, especially if the refusal will place the patient in great jeopardy, we need to be sure the patient truly appreciates the ramifications of her choice. As the risks of a treatment increase and the benefits become more dubious, one again relaxes the standard of competence needed to refuse. The physician need only require that the patient understands what she is being told. This same schema may be transposed upon the present case. Instead of focusing on the patient's cognitive capacity, we can apply this scale to the relative stability of her values. For instance, to refuse a dearly beneficial treatment that poses few burdens, the decision must represent rather stable values of the patient. If the refusal does not, the physician is justified in more strenuously advocating for the treatment. Thus, by advocating "health-related values only," we are talking about common notions of clear benefits to health. When such benefits are not so dear, advocacy recedes. This same schema can guide the physician in deciding how intense to allow the family's persuasive efforts to become.

Mrs. L.'s case reflects this sliding-scale model of decision making. Early in the patient's treatment course, it was thought that diagnostic work would reveal the cause of her lesions. The caregivers hoped that once the etiology was revealed, the lesions could be treated and the patient restored to a more comfortable state. Refusals of treatment and diagnostic work at that point would have run counter to a commonsense notion of a risk/benefit calculation. Thus, the physician was justified in further investigating the strength of the patient's views and whether this refusal was "in character," that is, reflective of relatively stable values. In this kind of investigation, the family can be helpful. If the refusal was firm enough to stand up to the influence of the physician and husband, of course, the refusal should have been honored. But it was not.

As the course of diagnostic work and treatment grew longer, the expected benefits of the medical interventions declined in value. At the same time, the persistence of Mrs. L.'s requests to stop dialysis indicated that this desire reflected a new value that was becoming stable or that she was interpreting this treatment refusal as indicative of her long-held values. Thus, the exertion of influence to persuade the patient differently became less and less justified. Fortunately, the influencing family member also came to discover and hold the same values or same reinterpretation of old values as the patient. He engaged in the process of mutual self-discovery with her. Had Mr. L. failed to evolve in the way Mrs. L. did, the sliding-scale approach would have justified the physician's influencing Mr. L. to acquiesce to his wife's wishes and persuading Mr. L. to be supportive of her desires in the conferences. If this effort had failed, the physician should have sought formal institutional mechanism to protect the patient from her husband's influence. In other words, although Mr. L.'s behavior might have remained the same, the changing clinical situation and the development of stable wishes or values in the patient meant that his persistence would no longer be seen as influence, but as coercion.

The physician remains the patient advocate. He tries to relieve the patient's pain and suffering and restore her to health. To actually determine the means of doing this, and to be sure that such means do not violate the patient's autonomy, the physician must engage in the process of informed consent with the patient. In some cases, the family will provide assistance merely by verifying the patient's competence by vouching for the stability of the patient's values and wishes. In other cases, these values may be below the surface and need to emerge to meet the weighty challenges posed by the illness and choices that must be made. The family provides a kind of personal and social context for the exploration of the meaning of values for the present situation. Sometimes, however, the situation requires that new values be chosen or developed because there are none available that adequately address the changing situation. In these situations, the physician is truly "treating the family" because they are the soil out of which the patient's values and preferences grow.

As we have noted, the physician must be careful to monitor the emergence of such values in both the patient and family and to assess their relative stability. In doing this, he is doing no more than has traditionally been seen as assessing competence to give informed consent. In these assessments, he must muddle through with his professional and commonsense evaluations of the merit of proposed treatments and the rationality of choices that are made. Ultimately, he must be willing to engage in a process that strains the limits of his clinical judgment.

RECONCEIVING THE FAMILY

Clinicians may be running well ahead of medical ethicists in dealing with families. This is a surprising situation for bioethics because of clinicians' initial resistance to the development of informed consent procedures. However, when it comes to the role of the family in medical decision making, ethicists have fallen prey to "either/or" thinking; for example, the patient's wishes versus the family's.

Bioethicists argue that either the patient must make the decision or the family must make it. This disjunction is resolved in the patient's favor, relegating the family to an afterthought in the process. This argument is sound but limited in its range of application. Arguments that affirm patient rights are important mainly in cases in which the patient has developed and stable views. In such cases of unresolvable conflict between patient and family, a legalistic, event model of consent is appropriate. In the cases that demand more profound self-discovery, the family should be described in a more nuanced manner.

When the values, wishes, preferences, and thoughts of the persons involved are in transformation, only the family truly can be said to exist. The previously existing individuals have metaphorically dissolved into this group due to crisis—but also are in the process of emerging from the unit with developed and stable values. In other words, they will again become individuals. Then, communitarian formulations should recede as interests and rights can be identified and become weightier considerations. This process of vacillation between identity and difference makes the family a meta-physically mysterious entity that has eluded capture by legalistic models. In sum, I am advocating that we view the development of patient autonomy as the goal of the process of informed consent rather than as something given or in need of restoration. The family, as those who have been reciprocal participants in the attainment of the patient's personhood,[17] have a natural place in the ongoing process.

I would like to thank Bob Arnold, William Gardner, Sandy Janaszak, and Mark R. Wicclair for their suggestions on earlier versions of this manuscript.

REFERENCES

1. President's Commission for the Study of Ethical Problems in Biomedical and Behavioral Research. *Deciding to Forego Life-Sustaining Treatment.* Washington, DC: U.S. Government Printing Office; 1983.

2. Buchanan AE, Brock DW. *Deciding for Others: The Ethics of Surrogate Decision Making.* New York, NY: Cambridge University Press; 1989.

3. Hardwig J. What about the family? *Hastings Center Report.* 1990;20(2):5–10.

4. Meisel A. The legal consensus about forgoing life-sustaining treatment: its status and prospects. *Kennedy Institute of Ethics Journal.* 1992;2(4):309–345.

5. Faden RR, Beauchamp TL. *A History and Theory of Informed Consent.* New York, NY: Oxford University Press; 1986.

6. Pellegrino EG, Thomasma D. *The Virtues in Medical Practice.* New York, NY: Oxford University Press; 1993.

7. Nelson JL. Taking families seriously. *Hastings Center Report.* 1992;22(4):6–12.

8. Blustein J. The family in medical decision making. *Hastings Center Report.* 1993;23(3):6–13.

9. Strong C. Patients should not always come first in treatment decisions. *Journal of Clinical Ethics.* 1993;4(1):63–65, 75.

10. Mappes TA, Zembary JS. Patient choices, family interests, and physician obligations. *Kennedy Institute of Ethics Journal.* 1994;4(1):27–46.

11. Lidz CW, Appelbaum PS, Meisel A. Two models of implementing informed consent. *Archives of Internal Medicine.* 1988;148:1385–1389.

12. Brody H. Transparency: informed consent in primary care. *Hastings Center Report.* 1989;19(5):5–9.

13. Emanuel EJ, Emanuel LL. Four models of the physician-patient relationship. *JAMA.* 1992;267:2221–2226.

14. Kuczewski MG, Lynn R (eds.). *An Ethics Casebook for Community Hospitals.* Unpublished.

15. Drane JD. Competency to give informed consent. *JAMA.* 1984;252:925–927.

16. The many faces of competency. *Hastings Center Report.* 1985;15(2):17–21.

17. Kuczewski MG. Whose will is it, anyway? A discussion of advance directives, personal identity, and consensus in medical ethics. *Bioethics* 1994;8(1):27–48.

13

THE INCOMPETENT PATIENT
ON THE SLIPPERY SLOPE

Rebecca Dresser, J.D., and
Peter J. Whitehouse, M.D., Ph.D.

꿎

Nearly three decades of analysis and debate have produced the contemporary legal and ethical standards governing life-sustaining treatment for incompetent patients. According to the widely accepted view, the premier goal of treatment decision making is to choose as the patient would if she were competent and aware of her current circumstances. Relatives and other proxy decision makers are to be guided by evidence concerning the patient's former treatment preferences; if this evidence is unavailable, they are to choose according to the patient's more general values and attitudes toward life and illness. Only when evidence concerning the patient's former beliefs is completely absent or inconclusive are proxy decision makers to direct their full attention to the incompetent patient now before them. The best-interests standard, also known as the objective, benefit-burden, or "reasonable person" standard, is thus accorded secondary status in treatment decision making.

We discern three major reasons for the disproportionate attention devoted to the patient's former competent concerns as opposed to her experiential interest as an incompetent patient. First, the currently preferred model was developed by competent persons, understandably preoccupied by the threats that unwanted future treatment or nontreatment pose to their interests as presently conceived. In consequence, the model tends to overlook the substantial changes in interests that could accompany the onset

R. Dresser, P. Whitehouse. "The Incompetent Patient on the Slippery Slope." *Hastings Center Report.* 1994;24(4):6–12. Reproduced by permission. © The Hastings Center.

of incompetency and impaired mental status. The second source of the imbalance is a legitimate desire to avoid the dangers arising whenever healthy persons assign qualitative value to the life experiences of impaired individuals. Once we move away from relying on the patients themselves for answers about the treatment they should receive, we risk unjustifiably undervaluing the lives of these vulnerable individuals who impose such substantial emotional and financial burdens on others. Also responsible for the existing imbalance are lurking epistemological doubts many people have about any observer's ability to judge accurately the subjective state of patients who cannot talk about their experiences in the usual way. It seems that such judgments will inevitably be sufficiently indeterminate to allow third parties to base treatment choices on their own concerns and needs, as opposed to those of the patients.

Yet the current subordination of the incompetent patients' experiential interests is unsatisfactory on several scores. The ethicists' and policymakers' near-obsession with defending the competent person's right to control her future treatment has left the best-interests standard inadequately developed and subject to widely varied interpretation. As a practical matter, this omission leaves proxy decision makers and clinicians with insufficient guidance about how to resolve the vast majority of real cases, for it is rare that an incompetent patient leaves a comprehensive and unambiguous indication of her former competent treatment preferences.[1]

In a recent issue of the *Hastings Center Report* Dr. Denise Niemira powerfully describes the bedside dilemmas of physicians now caring for incompetent elderly patients. Society, through its law and institutional policies, offers little guidance to physicians struggling with the question of what constitutes appropriate care for their fragile elderly patients whose consciousness is impaired. In confronting the spectrum of treatment options ranging from the most to the least aggressive, Dr. Niemira and her colleagues are left to muddle through, "do [ing] what feels right in the context of our beliefs about what it means to be a good physician."[2] It is generally agreed that patients' families and other proxy decision makers should be given some discretion to determine the outcome in these cases, but how extensive should their discretion be? When does a proxy's decision constitute the "exploitation" or "abuse" that demands intervention. by hospital and legal officials?[3] The failure to develop a robust and principled approach to best-interests decision making has left a moral vacuum for those who must respond to this question.

The current ambiguities regarding the appropriate treatment of conscious, incompetent patients is especially disturbing in light of our country's growing population of persons with Alzheimer's disease and other forms of dementia. Modern medicine and other health-related interventions are enabling an increasing number of people to live into their eighth decade and beyond. With the aging of the Baby Boom generation, these numbers are expected to escalate drastically. Dementia is estimated to affect from 7 to 20 percent of persons between the ages of seventy-five and eighty-four, and 25 to 47 percent of persons above that age.[4]

Patients with dementia experience excessive memory loss and decreased general intellectual functioning. Most forms of dementia are incurable, progressive, and lethal, although the period of decline can be as long as twenty years. During this time, the patient's mental capacities gradually diminish, but there can be much variation in the experiential course of dais process, both among different patients and within the same patient at different times. Until the final stages of their illnesses, these patients are awake and aware, but unable to process information or communicate in the customary way.[5] Questions as to whether they should receive life-sustaining interventions, particularly nutritional support, antibiotics, and cardiopulmonary resuscitation, frequently arise while they are still conscious and before they are terminally ill in any narrowly defined sense of the term.

The vast majority of dementia patients have an experiential world. Unlike Nancy Cruzan and Karen Quinlan, most dementia patients are subjects with their own thoughts, perceptions, emotions, and perspectives. These patients are themselves affected by the medical interventions they receive—they subjectively experience the consequences of the treatment decisions made on their behalf. Yet the subjectivity of the dementia patient is often overlooked in treatment decision making. The increasing number of treatment dilemmas involving patients with dementia challenges clinicians and policy makers to develop a more principled approach to evaluating "what it is like" to be the particular patient whose treatment is at issue. In this article, we elaborate on the need for this approach and offer our thoughts on how it should be constructed and implemented.

OBJECTIVE TREATMENT STANDARDS

Objective treatment standards are premised on society's ethical responsibility to protect the welfare of vulnerable individuals who cannot make their own choices about whether life-sustaining treatment would be worthwhile for them. The objective approach seeks to identify the basic features of conscious experience that affect human welfare.[6] In essence, its goal is to ascertain which treatment option would be preferable from the patient's point of view. It focuses on the incompetent patient's current condition (as opposed to prior preferences), and requires an evaluation of the benefits and burdens that administering or forgoing treatment would entail for that particular patient.[7] This emphasis on the experiential welfare of the individual patient gives the "objective" approach an essential subjective component.

Despite its importance, the objective approach remains insufficiently developed. Existing analyses and applications of the approach emphasize the patient's physical sensations, particularly any pain the patient might experience. This was the focus of the *Conroy* decision, which set forth two versions of objective treatment standards. Under the "limited objective" test, which applies when there is "some trustworthy evidence" but no clear proof that the incompetent patient would have refused life-sustaining measures, treatment may be forgone if

> patient is suffering, and will continue to suffer throughout the expected duration of his life, unavoidable pain, and... the net burdens of... prolonged life (the pain and suffering of life with the treatment less the amount and duration of pain that the

patient would likely experience if the treatment were withdrawn) markedly out-weigh any physical pleasure, emotional enjoyment, or intellectual satisfaction that the patient may still be able to derive from life.[8]

If no evidence is available regarding the patient's former treatment preferences, *Conroy* held that treatment may be forgone if "the recurring, unavoidable, and severe pain of the patient's life [is] such that the effect of administering lifesustaining treatment would be inhumane."

As the *Conroy* analysis reveals, formulating and applying an objective treatment approach involves multiple epistemic and moral judgments. These include: (1) determining which positive and negative experiences (burdens and benefits) are relevant to the decision; (2) measuring the burdens and benefits experienced by an individual incompetent patient; and (3) deciding what balance of burdens and benefits indicates that continued life would confer sufficient benefit to mandate life-sustaining treatment. There is also a fourth consideration (often left unspoken), which involves balancing any benefit the incompetent patient would gain from continued life against the burdens such life imposes on others, including the patient's family and a society confronting the need to allocate scarce health-care resources.

WHAT EXPERIENCES SHOULD COUNT IN OBJECTIVE WELFARE TESTS?

The objective approach to treatment decision making raises one of the most fundamental moral questions: What makes life a "good" for people? Although some members of our society believe that biologic human life is a good that must be maintained whenever possible, the more common view is that life is valuable because it allows us to have the rich variety of conscious experiences that constitute human life. Thus, consciousness is a prerequisite for patients to benefit directly from, or to have an interest in, continued life.[9]

What is it about conscious life that matters? What capacities and experiences should be considered in determining whether conscious individuals have an interest in having life maintained? This obviously is a complex subject, debated at length by bioethicists and other moral philosophers. Besides pain and suffering, *Conroy* refers to "physical pleasure, emotional enjoyment, and intellectual satisfaction"; in a subsequent case, the same court listed as burdens "embarrassment, frustration, helplessness, rage, and other emotional pain" and as benefits "enjoyable feelings like contentment, joy, satisfaction, gratitude, and well-being."[10] Others have focused on underlying capacities, including sentience, thought, memory, self-consciousness (the conception of oneself as a continuing subject of experience over time), relational capacity (the ability to interact with other persons and the environment), and the capacity to have plans and desires about the future.[11] These abilities, and the experiences they make possible, are representative of what makes people care about and benefit from continued life. Incorporating such factors into a workable objective treatment assessment requires translating these abstract terms into a concrete evaluation process. In the next section, we discuss how this task might be approached.

ENTERING THE WORLD OF THE INCOMPETENT PATIENT

Fundamental to the objective treatment approach is the need to gain access to the consciousness of another human being whose cognitive capacities depart from those of the "normal" observer performing the welfare assessment. It is indisputably difficult for the competent observer to step into the shoes of a cognitively impaired individual. Frequently, patients are unable to communicate by using language. The worlds of those who can speak can be especially difficult to interpret. In such cases, observers are left to rely on behavioral and physiological data as the basis for attempting to understand how incompetent patients experience their lives. Again, problems of interpretation will be common; observers will be unsure how various objective data relate to the patient's subjective experience.

These difficulties have led some commentators to express doubts about the legitimacy of the objective approach. In their view, consciousness is in principle subjective, phenomenological, irreducible, and impossible to understand from the outside. Though it may be possible for similarly situated individuals to "know or say what the quality of the other's experience is," the greater the difference between the experiencer and her observer, the less it is possible for the observer to adopt the experiencer's point of view.[12] Such attitudes give rise to statements such as the following: "We cannot approximate the severely demented person's point of view, and we cannot assess the quality of her life,"[13] and "We cannot enter [dementia patients'] world to know their pleasure and their pain. Once like us, they have crossed a threshold, never to return."[14]

While we acknowledge the pitfalls inherent in objective welfare assessments, we believe that they are a necessary element in morally defensible decision making about life-sustaining treatment. First, we are less dubious than these commentators about the prospects for obtaining a reasonably accurate picture of the incompetent patient's subjective situation. Of course, it is always possible to question one person's ability to "know" the mind of another—the so-called problem of other minds remains fertile ground for philosophical debate after hundreds of years of analysis. Yet we do in fact engage in mind-reading every day: Our social and biological survival requires us to be fairly successful at this task.[15] The process becomes more challenging when we are asked to evaluate the mental states of nonspeaking creatures, but parents and pet owners usually become rather skilled at doing so. We see no compelling basis for excluding dementia patients and other incompetent people from the realm of subjects whose mental lives can be studied "from the outside." The endeavor simply requires observers to develop a more specialized understanding of how patients' brain damage or other physical impairments affect their information processing capacities, sensations, perceptions, short- and long-term memory, and so on.

We also believe that careful, systematic objective welfare assessments are a prerequisite for meeting our societal obligations to protect these vulnerable patients. If we took the position that comprehending the mental lives of incompetent patients is beyond our grasp, then we would be precluded from appealing to their experiential welfare as the basis for decisions about when life-sustaining treatment must be administered. As Grant Gillett put it, "If there is nothing it is like to be a thing of a certain type then our treatment of that thing does not directly matter in a way that counts morally."[16] If we adopted the skeptical position regarding our access to impaired patients' subjectivity, then no one could argue for or against a particular treatment action on grounds of its effect on the patients themselves. If, on the other hand, we accept that incompetent patients can be directly harmed and benefited, then we are obligated to attempt to understand as best we can their subjective experiences. The challenge is to develop sensitive and systematic measures of benefits and burdens that minimize the effect of any hostility, self-interest, or other bias on the observer's part.

TOOLS FOR EXPERIENTIAL ASSESSMENT

To evaluate the incompetent patient's experiential interests, we must explore the workings of her mind. This is not as radical a proposal as it might initially appear. A variety of tests have been developed to assess the cognitive processes and characteristics of individuals with dementia and other conditions producing mental impairment. The most commonly used assessment technique applied to dementia patients is the mental status examination. During this examination the clinician evaluates a variety of the patient's cognitive abilities, including perception, memory, language comprehension and usage, concentration, and orientation. Noncognitive symptoms such as agitation, anxiety, depression, and psychosis are also assessed. Once this screening mechanism identifies deficits associated with dementia, standardized interviews are conducted to assess more precisely the nature of the patient's impairments. These include the Folstein Mini-Mental State and the Dementia Rating Scale. Also available are standardized instruments designed to elicit information on the patient's abilities to engage in the activities of daily living.[17]

Other assessment tools may be used to delineate the approximate stage of the patient's dementing illness. There are a number of staging instruments, including the Global Deterioration Scales and Clinical Dementia Rating, that integrate cognitive, noncognitive, and functional dimensions into a series of progressive levels of disease.[18] In common clinical parlance, dementia patients are staged as mild, moderate, and severe. Mild dementia patients' difficulties are usually limited to memory and a few other symptoms; they are able to handle most of their activities of daily living without encountering serious problems. Moderate patients have more serious and generalized cognitive impairments and require assistance with the more complex activities of daily living such as shopping, financial transactions, and using the telephone. Severely impaired patients often cannot participate in cognitive testing because of communication difficulties; they typically require help with even the most basic activities of daily living.

Quality of life is a complex concept that includes features such as cognitive abilities, functional abilities, social relationships, and a subjective component of well-being. It is this last element that is difficult to assess in dementia patients, because the disease itself impoverishes patients' ability to communicate their sense of personal well-being. With mildly and moderately impaired patients, however, it is usually possible to obtain some form of linguistic report of their subjective well-being. The attempt to communicate with the patient, in a manner and setting most suited to her capacities, is crucial. Even moderately advanced patients "have windows of clarity which open and close irregularly," and which offer opportunities for observers to explore the patients' subjective states.[19]

In patients with severely limited ability to communicate, nonverbal tests may be used in the attempt to discern their states of mind. Facial expressions and other behaviors often provide clues to what the patient is experiencing. Techniques used to measure intellectual abilities in infants can also be applied to assess patients with severe dementia. For example, it has been demonstrated that the amount of time infants spend looking at novel objects correlates with their level of intelligence; the technique can also be used to measure their degree of interest in different stimuli— for instance, human faces. It would be possible to design similar tests to evaluate the dementia patient's awareness of an interest in her environment as well.[20]

Although these assessment techniques have been used primarily for diagnostic evaluations, they could be adapted for use in the treatment decision-making setting. Properly designed, they could both enrich and systematize the benefit-burden assessment conducted on incompetent patients when life-sustaining treatment becomes an issue. Instituting a more rigorous, thorough approach to this inquiry would reduce the possibility that patients would be denied or given treatment based on unfounded, intuitive judgments about the nature and complexity of their experiential worlds.

Moreover, there is much room for improvement in assessing the experiences of incompetent patients. Dementia patients' families and other caregivers have contributed rich accounts of the experience of dementia, based on their observations of and interactions with patients.[21] Also available are interviews with, videotapes of, and written descriptions of patients at earlier stages of the condition expressing their own views of what is happening to them.[22] Other resources include literary accounts, such as the Dutch novelist J. Bernlef's first-person description of dementia's clinical course.[23] With some imagination and creativity, competent people can devise ways to have some of the dementia patient's experiences themselves, such as through assuming the role of nursing home resident for a period of time, and even using psychoactive substances to simulate the experience of mental confusion that patients are enduring.[24] Little has been written about dementia as people subjectively experience it, in part because its relevance to treatment decision making and other aspects of dementia patients' care has not been explicitly recognized. If patients' experiences were to become a more direct focus of inquiry, we predict that clinicians, researchers, philosophers of mind, and ethicists would put more effort into investigating this topic, which would result in an improved knowledge base for treatment decision making.

BALANCING BENEFITS AND BURDENS: THE INTRAPERSONAL LEVEL

Performing a detailed individual assessment yields a picture of the benefits and burdens life holds for the incompetent patient. But what balance of burdens and benefits gives a patient a positive interest in receiving life-sustaining treatment? Besides the patient's present state, the calculation must also include a prediction of the patient's future with and without treatment. This requires clinicians to evaluate the proposed intervention's positive and negative effects on the patient's subjective experience, as well as the kind of death that would follow the failure to administer treatment.

It is an intimidating, indeed, frightening responsibility to calculate the overall value of life for another human being. Both history and current practice reveal too many examples of its abuse. It is understandable that some would prefer to avoid the calculation, erring on the side of treating all who cannot decide for themselves. Yet this "solution" would expose incompetent patients to unjustified experiential burdens; it would also impose severe burdens on patients' families and others without countervailing benefit to the patients themselves.

Although the benefit-burden calculus inevitably confronts a conflict of values in our pluralistic society, reasonable consensus is apparent on some points. Perhaps the clearest agreement exists regarding the situation *Conroy* describes: The only life that can be sustained is one of overriding pain and suffering. A persuasive case against this "anticruelty" position is difficult to imagine.[25]

The *Conroy* pain standard would support nontreatment of some dementia patients. Although impaired consciousness, analgesics, and sedatives spare most advanced dementia patients the pain and suffering *Conroy* contemplates, a few such patients may be in this category. Certain forms of life-sustaining treatment would probably inflict severe pain on frail advanced dementia patients, including the chest compression necessary to perform cardiopulmonary resuscitation, the effects of major surgery, and the side effects and complications resulting from various cancer treatments. Another possible source of severe distress is the restraints put on many advanced dementia patients to prevent them from removing their feeding tubes. Although their physical resistance to the tubes may indicate that these patients are experiencing discomfort and panic at being deprived of physical freedom, their behavior could also be a more primitive, less conscious reflex response.[26] These patients may be sedated to decrease their agitation; however, one must question the benefit this action confers, since it substantially reduces any remaining awareness possessed by the patients.[27] The experiential significance of these patients' physical resistance is a question that merits deeper investigation, for the number of advanced dementia patients who are restrained so that nutritional support can be delivered is reportedly quite high.[28]

The second group of dementia patients who might experience the severe burdens *Conroy* describes includes patients with higher levels of consciousness. Such patients appear capable of a wider array of subjective experiences, both positive and negative, than the dementia patients whose consciousness is substantially reduced. For example, because of the motor impairment sometimes associated with their condition, patients with multi-infarct dementia may become bedridden earlier than patients with other forms of dementia. Patients in this situation at times remain extremely sensitive to pain and other forms of discomfort, but lack the ability to appreciate why caregivers are imposing therapeutic burdens on them. Even simple hygienic care can inflict "considerable pain and exhaustion" on them. According to one clinician, "It is often impossible to feed, move, or lift such patients without unintentionally torturing them."[29] If these patients stop eating or develop an acute illness, the *Conroy* nontreatment standard could justify the decision to forgo life-sustaining treatment, assuming that the decision could be implemented without exposing them to additional discomfort, distress, or other experiential burdens.

The *Conroy* standard could also apply to some ambulatory dementia patients. In some patients, dementia produces persistent and untreatable paranoia and hallucinations. Many dementia patients appear capable of experiencing fear, terror, panic, anxiety, and like emotions. When life-sustaining treatment requires them to be immobilized or otherwise restricted for long periods, or exposes them to pain, distress, or other experiential burdens, the justification for such treatment should be carefully examined. As one physician cautions, "patients who lack the ability to envision goals cannot comprehend why they should cooperate when treatment is onerous. Such patients may be baffled by their perception of the caring milieu turning on them. They feel fear and terror, and their remaining days may be darkened by distrust."[30] For life-sustaining treatment to be appropriate, it must confer a substantial enough benefit to outweigh both its customary risks and the distinctive experiential burdens it poses for dementia patients unable to fathom its purpose.

The appropriate balance regarding other groups of dementia patients is more controversial and unsettled. Some patients are "barely conscious," "stuporous . . . with negligible awareness of self, other, and the world."[31] Their capacity for sentience gives such patients an interest in avoiding pain and other unpleasant physical sensations, which justifies the administration of pain-relieving medication and other palliative measures. It is questionable, however, that such individuals retain any direct interest in having their lives continued.[32] *Conroy* implicitly adopts an opposing view, for the court's objective tests would mandate life-sustaining treatment for this group of patients, as long as severe pain could be avoided. We join others, however, in questioning whether preserving life as a "repository . . . of physical sensations"[33] is required to protect these patients' welfare. When the ability to communicate, respond, or otherwise interact with people and objects in the world is lost, how can continued life, even in the absence of severe pain, constitute a benefit of any significance to these patients themselves? Of course, a decision to mandate treatment for these patients could be made on other grounds such as to preserve the general social value of respect for human life. This is a separate issue, however, that merits debate on its own terms.

Many mentally impaired patients do not fit the previous categories. Instead, these moderately impaired patients are capable of simple relationships, retain some memory of the past and concept of the future, can initiate purposeful movement, or are otherwise able to participate in the lives they are living. A substantial number are also responsive to rehabilitative and other positive efforts to improve their quality of life. Although their existence may strike observers as "degrading" or "undignified," these patients typically are not concerned about such matters. Many fail to exhibit signs of distress, and caregivers frequently note that patients' families seem to suffer much more than the patients themselves.[34] In balancing the burdens and benefits treatment could confer on this group, observers must be especially careful to identify and keep separate their personal discomfort about aging and mental decline from the patient's own subjective reality. As others have warned, such feelings can too easily shape the perceptions of those observing the cognitively impaired patient, yielding a flawed judgment that treatment should be forgone for the patient's "own good."

Most moderately impaired patients have an interest in receiving life-sustaining treatment, for they appear to obtain an overall benefit from life in that state. At least some of these patients, however, have a degree of insight into their problems and as a result of this awareness suffer greater burdens than patients who deny or are unable to recognize or to remember their impairments.[35] Certainly caregivers must do everything they can to offer comfort and reassurance to such patients. For those patients who exhibit persistent and severe distress that cannot be ameliorated by therapeutic measures, however, life-sustaining treatment might not confer a benefit—indeed, such treatment might be "inhumane" according to the *Conroy* objective tests.

BALANCING BENEFITS AND BURDENS: THE INTERPERSONAL LEVEL

It would be disingenuous to discuss decisions regarding life-sustaining treatment in isolation from the implications such decisions hold for others. These treatment decisions occur in a social context of concern over allocation of scarce health-care resources and burdens felt by patients' families and caregivers. We ought to be honest in acknowledging that these economic and social concerns can influence our views about when incompetent patients ought to receive life-sustaining treatment. For example, the current discussions on treatment "futility" implicitly assume that life-sustaining treatment should be withheld when it is insufficiently beneficial to justify the expenditure of monetary and professional resources.[36] Conversely, other considerations external to the patient, such as the preservation of respect for human life in our society, are often cited as reasons to adopt a policy in which all or nearly all incompetent patients are treated aggressively.[37]

How these and other considerations external to the patient should affect decisions and policy on life-sustaining treatment for incompetent patients is a controversial and complicated matter, one likely to be debated extensively in the foreseeable future. Much of the argument will center on whether particular approaches are sufficiently protective of incompetent patients' welfare. We hope that in the coming years at least some of the effort will be concentrated on improving our ability to take the patient's perspective in responding to this question. We simply cannot make a defensible judgment about when life-sustaining treatment would advance an incompetent patient's interest without attempting to ascertain that patient's subjective reality. We encourage clinicians, bioethicists, and policy makers to develop more sensitive approaches to understanding this reality.

REFERENCES

1. For instance, see Gamble ER, McDonald PJ, Lichstein PR, "Knowledge, attitudes, and behavior of elderly persons regarding living wills," *Archives of Internal Medicine*, 1991;151:277–280, reporting on a survey of seventy-five elderly persons, which found that none had completed a living will.

2. Niemira D, "Life on the slippery slope: a bedside view of treating incompetent patients," *Hastings Center Report*, 1993;23(3):14–17. See also Solomon M et al., "Decisions near the end of life: professional views on life-sustaining treatment," *American Journal of Public Health*, 1993;83(1):14–23, reporting on a survey in which a substantial number of health professionals expressed concern about giving patients inappropriate, overly burdensome care.

3. These phrases are used in Capron AM, "Where is the sure interpreter?" *Hastings Center Report*, 1992;22(4):26–27; and King PA, "The authority of families to make medical decisions for incompetent patients after the *Cruzan* decision," *Law, Medicine & Health Care*, 1991;19(1–2):76–79.

4. See generally Larson EB, "Illnesses causing dementia in the very elderly," *New England Journal of Medicine*, 1993;328:203–205; Selkoe DJ, "Aging brain, aging mind," *Scientific American*, 1992;267(3):134–140.

5. For general discussion of dementia's characteristics, see Office of Technology Assessment, *Confronting Alzheimer's Disease and Other Dementias* (New York, NY: Harper & Row; 1988): 59–83; Jacques A, *Understanding Dementia*, 2d ed. (Edinburgh: Churchill Livingstone; 1992); Whitehouse PJ, "Dementia: the medical perspective," in: Binstock RH, Post S, Whitehouse PJ (eds.), *Dementia and Aging: Ethics, Values, and Policy Choices* (Baltimore, MD: Johns Hopkins University Press; 1992):21–29.

6. See Rhoden NK, "Litigating life and death," *Harvard Law Review*, 1988;102(2):375–446.

7. See Buchanan AE, Brock D, *Deciding for Others* (New York, NY: Cambridge University Press; 1989): 122–126.

8. In re Conroy, 486 A.2d 1209 (N.J. Sup. Ct. 1985).

9. See Buchanan and Brock, n. 7, pp. 126–132; Arras JD, "The severely demented, minimally functional patient: an ethical analysis," *Journal of the American Geriatrics Society*, 1988;36(10):938–944.

10. In re Peter, 529 A.2d 419 (N.J. Sup. Ct. 1987).

11. See Steinbock B, *Life before Birth* (New York: Oxford University Press; 1992): 9–24; Macklin R, "Personhood in the bioethics literature," *Milbank Quarterly*, 1983;61:35–57; Loewy EH, "Treatment decisions in the mentally impaired," *New England Journal of Medicine*, 1987;317(23):1465–1469; Rango N, "The nursing home resident with dementia," *Annals of Internal Medicine*, 1985;102(6):835–841.

12. See, for example, Nagel T, "What is it like to be a bat?" in: *Mortal Questions* (Cambridge: Cambridge University Press; 1979):165–180.

13. Battin MP, "Euthanasia in Alzheimer's disease?" in: Binstock RH, Post S, Whitehouse

PJ (eds.), *Dementia and Aging: Ethics, Values, and Policy Choices* (Baltimore, MD: Johns Hopkins University Press; 1992): 118–137.

14. Niemra, n.2, p. 15.

15. See Dennett DC, *The Intentional Stance* (Cambridge, MA: MIT Press; 1987): 7–35; Smith P, Jones OR, *The Philosophy of Mind* (Cambridge: Cambridge University Press; 1986): 165–176. For more extensive analysis of how the "other minds" problem affects treatment decision making on behalf of incompetent patients, see Dresser R, "Missing persons: legal perceptions of incompetent patients," *Rutgers Law Review*, 1994;46(2):609–719.

16. Gillett G, "Consciousness, the brain, and what matters," *Bioethics*, 1990;4:181–198.

17. See Mayeux R et al., "The clinical evaluation of patients with dementia," in: Whitehouse P (ed.), *Dementia* (Philadelphia, PA: F. A. Davis; 1993):92–129; Folstein MF, Folstein SF, McHugh PR, "'Mini-Mental State': a practical method for grading the cognitive state of patients for the clinician," *Journal of Psychiatric Research*, 1975;12:189–98; Vitaliano P et al., "The clinical utility of the dementia rating scale for assessing Alzheimer patients," *Journal of Chronic Diseases*, 1984;37:743–753; Lawton MP, Brody EM, "Assessment of older people: self-maintaining and instrumental activities of daily living," *Gerontologist*, 1969;9:179–186.

18. See Reisberg B, "Clinical presentation, diagnosis, and symptomatology of age-associated cognitive decline and Alzheimer's disease," in: *Alzheimer's Disease* (New York, NY: Free Press; 1983):173–187; Hughes CP et al., "New clinical scale for the staging of dementia," *British Journal of Psychiatry*, 1982;140:566–572.

19. See Foley JM, "The experience of being demented," in: Binstock RH, Post S, Whitehouse PJ (eds.), *Dementia and Aging: Ethics, Values, and Policy Choices* (Baltimore, MD: Johns Hopkins University Press; 1992):30–43.

20. See Fagan J, Corrigan P, Layton B, "Selective visual attention to novel targets predicts severity of brain damage and level of cognitive function in neurologically impaired adults," *Journal of Clinical and Experimental Neuropsychology*, 1992;14:36. For additional discussion, see Hurley AC et al., "Assessment of discomfort in advanced Alzheimer patients," *Research in Nursing & Health*, 1992;5:369–377.

21. Some examples include Jacques, n. 5, pp. 171–202; Sabat SR, Harré R, "The construction and deconstruction of self in Alzheimer's disease," *Ageing and Society*, 1992;12:443–461; Buchanan J, *Patient Encounters* (Charlottesville, VA: University of Virginia Press; 1989):35–50.

22. See Lerner AB, "I've lost a kingdom: a victim's remarks on Alzheimer's disease," *Journal of the American Geriatrics Society*, 1984;32(12):935; Foley, n. 19, pp. 33–36. Two insightful and haunting accounts by patients are McGowin DF, *Living in the Labyrinth* (New York, NY: Delacourt Press; 1993); and Davis R, *My Journey into Alzheimer's Disease* (Wheaton, IL: Tyndale House; 1989).

23. Bernlef J, *Out of Mind* (Boston, MA: David R. Godine; 1989). For another account of dementia from the patient's point of view, see Quisenberry EM, "What are we going to do about Mother?" *JAMA*, 1990;263:232.

24. See Malcolm AH, "Nurses taste what it's like when you're elderly and in the hospital," *New York Times*, October 20, 1992. Owen Flanagan offers creative approaches to the task of understanding what it is like to be another subject of experience in *Consciousness Reconsidered* (Cambridge, MA: MIT Press; 1992):103–107.

25. See Braithwaite S, Thomasma D, "New guidelines on foregoing life-sustaining treatment in incompetent patients: an anti-cruelty policy," *Annals of Internal Medicine*, 1986;104(5):711–715. See also Steinbock, n. 11, pp. 23–24, arguing that pain is "objectively bad."

26. See Lo B, Dornbrand L, "Understanding the benefits and burdens of tube feedings," *Archives of Internal Medicine*, 1983;149:1925–1926.

27. Lynn J, Childress JF, "Must patients always be given food and water?" *Hastings Center Report*, 1983;13(5):17–21.

28. In a recent survey of patients in a community-based teaching hospital, Timothy Quill found that restraints were used in 63 percent of chronically ill, elderly incompetent patients with nasogastric feeding tubes. Quill T, "Utilization of nasogastric feeding tubes in a group of chronically ill, elderly patients in a community hospital," *Archives of Internal Medicine*, 1989;149:1937–1941.

29. Rango, n. 11, p. 838.

30. Loewy, n. 11, p. 1468.

31. Rango, n. 11, p. 838.

32. See Arras, n. 9, p. 941; Brock DW, "Justice and the severely demented elderly," *Journal of Medicine and Philosophy*, 1988;13(1):75–99.

33. Rhoden, n. 6, p. 406.

34. See, for example, Goodwith JS, "Mercy killing: mercy for whom?" *JAMA*, 1991;265:326; Meier DE, Cassel C, "Nursing home placement and the demented patient," *Annals of Internal Medicine*, 1986;104:98–105. For an example of a dementia patient whose mental deterioration left her "carefree, always cheerful," see Firlik A, "Margo's logo," *JAMA*, 1991;265:201.

35. See Foley, n. 19, pp. 30–31.

36. See Truog RD, Brett AS, Frader J, "The problem with futility," *New England Journal of Medicine*, 1992;326:1560–1564.

37. See Dresser R, "Life, death, and incompetent patients: conceptual infirmities and hidden values in the law," *Arizona Law Review*, 1986;28(3):397–99.

14

A CHRONICLE

Dax's Case As It Happened

Keith Burton

꧁꧂

When I was a boy, death was not an enemy. Its presence brought peace and new beginnings—feelings I still connect with when remembering my grandfather's death twenty-five years ago: He was buried on a cold November day. A bitter wind forced us to huddle closely together near the casket. The preacher comforted us with final remarks at the open grave. In the winter sky, the setting sun bathed wispy clouds in crimson red. Grief gave way to a peaceful release. These are the images remembered.

My own feelings about death occupied me as I drove on toward the causeway bridge linking Galveston Island to Texas. The date was April 19, 1980. Five months earlier, in a bioethics course at Southern Methodist University, I had viewed a videotape about a man named Donald Cowart who had been severely burned in a 1973 propane gas explosion in East Texas. Cowart had sought to refuse the medical treatment that saved his life. The videotape, *Please Let Me Die*, had become a living record of this man's struggle for release from pain and despair. But the videotape left me wondering whatever happened to that man. My journey in search of Cowart had taken me to Galveston, where I would meet him for the first time.

The story of Don Cowart is remarkable in some ways but commonplace in

---

K. Burton. "A Chronicle: Dax's Case As It Happened." In *Dax's Case: Essays in Medical Ethics and Human Meaning*, ed. Lonnie D. Kliever. Dallas, TX: Southern Methodist University Press; 1989: 1–12. Reprinted by permission.

others. A man's wish to die is rather extraordinary in and of itself; but the pattern of events that shape such a wish often is woven of the fabric of life's everyday occurrences. Such is the case with Cowart.

Ray and Ada Cowart moved their family from the Rio Grande Valley to the small East Texas town of Henderson in the sixties. Ray prospered over the years as a rancher and real estate agent. Ada became a teacher in the Henderson school district. Their three children—Don, Jim, and Beth—were no different from other kids reared in a close-knit community. In fact, they were ordinary people living ordinary lives.

"Donny Boy," as he came to be called by his father, was popular in school and excelled in athletics. He was captain of his high school football team and performed in rodeos. He liked to take risks, a trait that often dismayed his mother. It was risk taking that would later lure him to skydiving, surfing, and other sports of chance.

Don Cowart left Henderson in 1966 to attend the University of Texas at Austin. He had planned to return home at his graduation three years later to join his father in business; however, when notified of his military draft selection, Cowart instead elected to join the U.S. Air Force. He became a pilot and served in Vietnam. He married a high school sweetheart in 1972, but they divorced eight months later. In May 1973 he was discharged from active duty and returned to Henderson, where he began working with his father in real estate.

Life back in East Texas brought Cowart warmth and new independence in the summer of 1973. It was a quiet summer. Now twenty-five years old, he had returned home to decide the future course of his career. He had several options—to become a commercial airline pilot, to join his father as a real estate broker, or to attend law school. And he was dating again after having endured the breakup of his first marriage. The new relationship seemed promising.

July 23, 1973, seemed no different to Cowart from any other Wednesday. It was hot and sultry as the afternoon sun slipped low along the pine trees in the countryside near Henderson. Ray and Don had driven out to a ranch to look over some property being offered for sale by the owner. They parked their car on a bridge over a dry creek and took off by foot. They talked and laughed together as they surveyed points of interest on the land. Their business completed, the Cowarts then returned to their car to go home for dinner.

Ada Cowart didn't think it odd that her husband and son were late arriving home. Sometimes Ray's business dealings delayed him in the evenings. She went about preparing the meal and sat down with her daughter to eat. They turned on the radio to catch the news. Ada remembers hearing a report of an explosion and fire in the oil fields which had injured two men outside Henderson. The names of the injured had not been given. All that was known was one man was critically injured, the other seriously injured.

Wednesday was church night for the Cowarts. Though Ray and Don still hadn't arrived home, Ada went on to services without them. She was in class studying a Bible lesson when the police chief and Ray Cowart's secretary arrived at the door asking for her. There had been an explosion, Ada was told, and Ray and Don were badly hurt. The extent of their injuries remained unknown. It was then that the earlier radio report flashed back into her mind in horrifying fashion.

The accident happened with no warning. The Cowart men had returned to their car but had not been able to start the engine. Ray had lifted the hood and removed the air cleaner from the engine. He primed the carburetor by hand and instructed Don to try the ignition. Several tries failed. It seemed to Don that the battery was near exhaustion. A final attempt proved fateful, however, as a blue flame shot from the carburetor and ignited a terrible explosion and fire.

Ray Cowart was hurled into heavy underbrush by the force of the explosion. The blast rocked the car and showered window glass over Don's body. Around them, the fireball spread quickly, consuming pine trees and the scrub vegetation in the area. Don reacted quickly. He climbed from the burning car and began running toward the woods. But he was forced to stop by a fear that he would become entangled in the underbrush and slowly burn to death.

Don wheeled about and decided to chance the dirt road on which they had driven in. He ran through three walls of fire, emerged into a clearing, then fell to the ground and rolled his body to extinguish the flames. He got back to his feet and resumed running in search of help for his father.

It all seemed dreamlike. Don noticed his vision was blurred as though swimming under water. His eyes had been badly burned. Now the pain was coming in waves, and he knew it was real. He kept running.

Loud voices filtered through the woods. Don collapsed at the roadside as help arrived. He heard the footsteps of a man and then the exclamation, "Oh, my God!" when a farmer found him. Don sent the man after his father and lay wondering how badly he was burned. When the man returned, Don asked him to bring a gun—a gun he would use to kill himself. The farmer refused.

In shock, Don assumed he and his father had caused the explosion by igniting gasoline from the car's engine. Later he would learn that the explosion actually had been caused by a leaking propane gas transmission line in the area where they had parked. It was a freak event. A pocket of propane gas had formed in the dry creek bed. When the carburetor flamed up, it had ignited the gas.

Rescuers took the Cowart men to a hospital in nearby Kilgore. There, a decision was made to transport them by ambulance to a special burn unit at Dallas's Parkland Hospital. Ray Cowart died en route to Dallas. Don Cowart remembers incredible pain, his begging for pain medication, and the paramedic's refusal to administer drugs prior to their arrival in Dallas. By this time, Ada Cowart, too, was on her way to Dallas. She had returned home first to pack several changes of clothes. The radio had said the men were badly hurt. She didn't expect to return to Henderson any time soon.

Even as the ambulance sped the 140 miles from Kilgore to Dallas, Don Cowart's treatment regimen had begun. By telephone, Dr. Charles Baxter, head of Parkland's burn unit, had directed fluid therapies to help in preventing shock to vital organs. On examination in Dallas, Baxter found Cowart had severe burns over 65 percent of his body. His face suffered third-degree burns and both eyes were severely damaged. His ears and hands were also deeply burned. Fluid therapies continued and were aided by several other measures: the insertion of an intertracheal tube to control the airway, catheters placed in every body opening, treatment with antibiotics, cleansing the wounds with antibacterial drugs, and tetanus prophylaxis. Heavy doses of narcotics were given for the pain.

In the early days of Don's 232-day hospitalization at Parkland, doctors could not predict whether he would survive. It was touch and go for many weeks. Ada Cowart felt helpless; she could do little more than sit in the waiting area outside the intensive care unit with relatives of other burn victims, where she prayed and hoped for the best. Doctors permitted only short visits with her son. Don had given his mother power of attorney in the Parkland emergency room, and she in turn deferred to the medical professionals on treatment decisions.

For Cowart, there were countless whirlpool tankings in solutions to cleanse his wounds, procedures to remove dead tissue, grafts to protect living tissue, the amputation of badly charred fingers from both hands and the removal of his right eye. The damaged left eye was sewn shut. And there was terrible pain.

Through it all, Don had remained constant in his view that he did not want to live. His demands to die had started with the farmer at the accident site. They had continued at the Kilgore hospital, in the ambulance, and now at Parkland. He didn't want treatment that would extend his misery and he made this known to his mother and family, Dr. Charles Baxter, a nurse named Leslie Kerr, longtime friend Art Rousseau, attorney Rex Houston, and many others.

Baxter remained undaunted by Don's pleas to stop treatment, dismissing them at first as the typical response of burn victims to the pain of their wounds and treatment. In time, however, he openly discussed Cowart's wish to die with Don, his mother, and lawyer, considering all the medical and legal ramifications. Failing to get Ada Cowart's and Rex Houston's consent to the withdrawal of treatment, Baxter continued to deliver it.

For her part, Ada Cowart understood her son's pain and anguish. She was haunted, nonetheless, by these thoughts: What if treatment were ceased and Don changed his mind in a near-death state? Would it be too late? Furthermore, her religious beliefs simply made mercy killing or suicide deplorable options. These religious constraints were reinforced by her fear that her son had not yet made his "peace with God."

Rex Houston also had mixed feelings about Don's wishes. On the one hand, he sympathized with Cowart's condition—being unable to so much as take medication to end his life without the assistance of others. On the other hand, it was Houston's duty to reach a favorable resolution of a lawsuit filed against the pipeline owners for Ray Cowart's death and for Don Cowart's disability. With regard to the latter, he needed a living plaintiff to achieve the best damage award for the Cowart family. Moreover, Houston believed that such an award would provide the financial means necessary for Don Cowart's ultimate rehabilitation. He therefore encouraged Cowart to see the legal proceedings through.

In February 1974, the lawsuit was settled out of court—one day prior to trial. Almost immediately, Don's demands to die quickened. There had been talk before with Art Rousseau of getting a gun. Don had asked Leslie Kerr if she would help him by injecting an overdose of medication. Now Cowart even talked with Houston about helping him get to a window of his sixth-floor hospital room, where presumably he would leap to his death. All listened but none agreed to help.

On March 12, 1974, Don was discharged from Parkland. He, his family, and doctors agreed that his condition had improved sufficiently to warrant his transfer to the Texas Institute for Research and Rehabilitation in Houston. Nine months removed from his medical residency, Dr. Robert Meier of TIRR found Cowart to be a passive recipient of medical care, although the philosophy of treatment in this rehabilitation center encouraged patient involvement in treatment decisions. Previously Don had no say in his care; now he would be offered choices in his own treatment.

All seemed to go well during the first three weeks of his stay, until Cowart realized the pain he had endured might continue indefinitely, thanks to a careless comment by a resident plastic surgeon that his treatment would be years in completion. Faced with that prospect, Cowart refused treatment for his open burn areas and stopped taking food and water. In a matter of days, Cowart's medical condition deteriorated rapidly. Finding his patient in serious condition, Dr. Meier was deeply perplexed about what do do next. He believed it his duty to help Cowart achieve the highest measure of rehabilitation, but he was not inclined to force upon the patient care he did not wish to receive. Faced with this dilemma, he called for a meeting with Ada Cowart and Rex Houston to discuss with Don the future course of his treatment.

Ada Cowart was outraged by Don's condition. She had been discouraged from staying with her son at TIRR, and in her absence his burns had worsened. He was again near death, due to his refusal of whirlpool tankings and dressing changes. It was agreed in the meeting that Cowart would be transferred to the burn unit of John Sealy Hospital of the University of Texas Medical Branch in Galveston, where his injuries could again be treated by bum specialists.

On April 15, 1974, Don was admitted to the Galveston hospital, in chronic distress from infected wounds, poor nutrition, and severe depression. His right elbow and right wrist were locked tight. The stubs of his fingers on both hands were encased in grotesque skin "mittens." There was practically no skin on his legs. His right eye socket and closed left eye oozed infection. And excruciating pain remained his constant nemesis.

Active wound care was initiated immediately and further skin grafts were advised by Dr. Duane Larson to heal the open wounds on Cowart's chest, legs, and arms. But Cowart bitterly protested the daily tankings and refused to consent to surgery. One night he even crawled out of bed, hoping to throw himself through the window to his death, but he was discovered on the floor and returned to bed.

Frustrated by Cowart's behavior, Dr. Larson consulted Dr. Robert White of psychiatric services for an evaluation of Don's mental competency. White remembers being puzzled by Cowart: Was he a man who tolerated discomfort poorly or perhaps was profoundly depressed? Or was this an extraordinary man who had undergone such an incredible ordeal that he was frustrated beyond normal limits? White concluded, and a colleague confirmed, that Cowart was certainly not mentally incompetent. In fact, he was so impressed with the clarity of Cowart's expressed wish to die that he asked permission to do a videotape interview for classroom use in presenting the medical, ethical, and legal problems surrounding such cases. That filmed interview, which White entitled *Please Let Me Die*, eventually became a classic on patient rights in the field of medical ethics.

Having been declared mentally competent, Cowart still found it difficult to gain control over his treatment. He and his mother argued constantly over treatment procedures. Rex Houston helped get changes in his wound care but turned a deaf ear to Cowart's plea to go home to die from his wounds or to take his own life. In desperation, Cowart turned to other family members for assistance in securing legal representation, but without success. Finally, with White's help, Cowart reached an attorney who had represented Jehovah's Witnesses in their efforts to refuse medical treatment, but he was not optimistic that a lawsuit would free him from the hospital.

Rebuffed on every hand, Cowart reluctantly became more cooperative. White secured changes in Don's pain medication before and after the daily tankings, making treatments more bearable. Psychotherapy and medication helped improve his overall outlook by relieving his depression and improving his sleep. Encouraged that he might still regain sight in his left eye, Don more or less accepted his daily wound care and even agreed to surgical skin grafts early in June 1974. By July 15, his physical condition had improved enough to allow him to transfer out of the burn unit of the John Sealy Hospital to the psychiatric unit of the Jennie Sealy Hospital in the University of Texas Medical Branch under White's direct care while his wounds continued to heal.

Amid these changes there were still periodic conflicts between Cowart and those around him over his confinement in the hospital. There were reiterated demands to die and protests against treatment. A particularly explosive encounter between Cowart and Larson occurred on the day preceding his second and last major surgical procedure in the Galveston hospital. Cowart had agreed to undergo surgery to free up his hands, but the night before he changed his mind. The next morning, Larson angrily confronted Cowart with the challenge that, if he really wanted to die, he would agree to the surgery that would enable him to leave the hospital and go home where he could take his own life if he wished. Anxious to do exactly that, Cowart consented to the surgery, which was performed on July 31.

Don Cowart's stormy stay at Galveston finally ended on September 19, 1974. He had been hospitalized for a total of fourteen months, but at last he was going home. His prognosis upon dismissal was listed simply as "guarded."

Cowart was glad to be back in Henderson. The little things counted the most—sleeping in his own bed, listening to music, visiting with friends. But it was different for him than before the accident. He was totally blind, his left eye having failed to recover. His hands and arms remained useless. He was badly scarred. A dropped foot now required that someone assist him in walking. Some of his burn sites still were not healed.

Everything he did required the help of others. Someone had to feed him, bathe him, and help with personal functions. The days seemed endless. He tried to find peace in sleep, but even this dark release was impossible without drugs. While he couldn't see himself, Don knew his appearance drew whispers and stares in restaurants.

He had his tapes, talking books, television, and CB radio. He could use his sense of hearing, though not as well as before due to the explosion and burns. And he could think. For a while, he could see in his mind's eye the memories of earlier times. Then the memories started to fade.

Ada Cowart had lost much, but she never lost her religious faith. There had been times when even she had admitted that maybe it would have been best if Don had died with her husband. She reconciled her doubt with the thought that no mother can give up the life of a son. Ada never gave up hope that Don could find new faith in God.

Homecoming brought peace for a time. As Don's early excitement for returning home gave way to deep depression and despair, however, conflict returned to their lives. They argued about how he could occupy himself, how he dressed, his personal habits, and his future. Frustration led to a veiled suicide attempt, Don stealing away from the house during the night to try throwing himself in the path of trucks hauling clay to a brick plant. The police found him and brought him home quietly.

For the next five years, Cowart lived in a shadow world of painful rehabilitation, chronic boredom, and failed relationships. His difficulties were not for want of trying. With Rex Houston's encouragement and assistance he tried pursuing a law degree. Fortunately, his legal settlement with the pipeline company provided the financial means for the nursing care and tutorial assistance which would be required because of his massive handicaps.

Cowart tested out his abilities as a blind student in two undergraduate courses at the University of Texas in Austin during the fall of 1975. He spent the spring at home in Henderson preparing for the tests that were required for admission to law school. In the summer of 1976, he enrolled for a part-time course load in Baylor University's School of Law.

Don handled his studies at Baylor in fine fashion despite his handicaps, but the strain was tremendous. He was forced to live with other people, his independence was limited, and his sleep problems persisted. When a special relationship with a woman ended abruptly in the spring of 1977, his life caved in. He tried to commit suicide by taking an overdose of pain and sleep medications, but he was discovered in time to have his stomach pumped at the hospital emergency room. He had trouble picking up his studies again, so he dropped out before the spring quarter was completed.

Cowart returned home defeated and discouraged, living with his mother for the next half year. He resumed his studies at Baylor in the spring of 1978, only to drop out again before he had completed the third quarter in the fall of 1979. He again retreated to his mother's home, filled with doubts that he would ever be able to pass the bar. By the spring of 1980, he was ready for another try at schooling, this time in a graduate program in building construction at Texas A&M University. Once again, the old patterns of sleepless nights and boring days got the best of him and he made a halfhearted effort at slashing his wrists with a razor blade.

Looking back, Cowart saw his futile efforts to take his own life as a bitter human comedy. The doctors in Galveston had encouraged him to accept treatment that would free him of hospitalization and permit him to end his life, if that was his wish.

But he found it difficult to find a way of killing himself without bringing further misery on himself—brain damage or further hospitalization. Ironically, he realized that he was no more successful in ending his life than in making his life work.

As a last resort, Cowart contacted White for help and was voluntarily readmitted under White's care to the Jennie Sealy Hospital on April 12, 1980. During his month-long stay, he met with White for psychotherapy treatments daily. Even more important, his sleep problems were finally resolved by weaning him away from the heavy sleep medications that he had taken for years. Cowart describes that experience as being like "coming out of a fog." For the first time since his harrowing burn treatment ordeal, his sleep became normal and his depression lifted.

It was during this stay that I met Don Cowart and we began early discussions of a film that would eventually come to be known as *Dax's Case*. I still call him Don because that is how I know him, but he legally changed his name to Dax in the summer of 1982. Some commentators on the film speculate that this change of name reflects some personal metamorphosis that Cowart went through during his lengthy rehabilitation period. But Cowart offers a simpler explanation. As a blind man with impaired hearing, he often found himself responding to comments addressed to others bearing the name of Don. I accepted his reasons for changing his name but asked him not to think the poorer of me for persisting in calling him Don.

It would be easy to believe that *Dax's Case*, more than five years in the making, served as a crucible for Don Cowart's rehabilitation. During this time, new hope and independence came into his life. He started a mail-order specialty foods business in Henderson using his creative powers. He moved into his own house. He became an articulate spokesperson for "the right to die" under auspices of Concern for Dying. And he married a former high school classmate in February 1983.

There is always another chapter, however. Even now, Don's life continues to shift. His first venture in business did not succeed financially. His second marriage ended unhappily. Amid failure has also come achievement. He returned to law school at Texas Tech University in Lubbock, where he completed his law degree in May and passed the bar in the summer of 1986. He set up a small law practice in Henderson and has recently taken in his first partner. He continues to represent his views on patient rights at educational symposiums and public forums. In time, he hopes to become a specialist in personal injury cases.

The film project was a crucible to Don Cowart in that it helped him reshape his life in dramatic ways. This retelling of the Cowart story has played a key role in his own reconstruction of a personal and public identity. His achievements in this regard have surpassed anything he, his family, or his physicians dared imagine. But this process of making a new life for himself is far from over. Only time will tell if *Dax's Case* is a heroic story with a happy or a tragic ending.

Part 5

PAIN MANAGEMENT AND PALLIATIVE CARE

❦

As a rule, Western medicine does not treat pain. And, as a rule, it addresses suffering even less. Although the line between pain and suffering is sometimes thin, there is a line. The distinction between the two can be thought of in terms of tangible versus intangible. Pain is something you can point to; for example, "It hurts right there." Patients can describe it in precise detail, as patients with angina can characterize their pain as burning, heaviness, crushing, or stabbing. Patients with pain from an aortic aneurysm can describe it as ripping, shearing, or tearing. They can also state the exact time it starts and stops. If the pain radiates, they can draw you a line. The severity of the pain can also be rated on a scale of 1 to 10, with patients stating, with a sense of exactness, when their pain is a 7 and when it is a 6.5.

Suffering, on the other hand, is more diffuse and less definable, but it can certainly be just as devastating as pain. It can arise directly from pain or the anticipation of being in pain, or it can be completely independent of pain. Suffering can be expressed in a multitude of ways, such as the sense of loss and anger that comes from a child asking her cancer-ridden father why he can no longer come to her soccer games or ride bikes with her. It can come about when a family matriarch who was once vigorous and proud must now have her diapers changed by those who only a short while ago came to her for strength and guidance.

With this somewhat fuzzy dichotomy in mind, this section takes on the meaning of pain and suffering, the ways health-care providers can recognize when a patient is experiencing them, and the duty and obligtion of a health-care provider to assuage the resulting harms. The first article, by Linda Farber-Post and colleagues, is titled "Pain: Ethics, Culture, and Informed Consent to Relief." The authors raise an extremely important issue when considering pain: people experience, respond to, and gain relief from pain in very different ways. Culture, ethnicity, social standing, gender roles, and individual life experiences all play a part. All or any one of these attributes can drastically affect a patient's pain-related signs and symptoms.

Just as importantly, a health-care provider's culture, ethnicity, professional standing, gender role, and individual life experiences can play a large part in the recognition and response, or lack thereof, to a patient's pain. The authors also take issue with the meaning of informed consent within the context of pain management. Can a patient who is racked with pain truly appreciate the consequences of her options, even when she possesses decision-making capacity? From this they expand their discussion to the crosscultural issues that arise from encapsulating everyone within the autonomy-driven American informed-consent paradigm.

If there were one article that every health-care provider was required by law to read, it would be this next one. Eric Cassel's "The Nature of Suffering and the Goals of Medicine" is one of the most important articles ever written on patient care. Cassel uses a case study to explain how suffering can come about, as well as how a patient's interactions, relationships, goals, sense of future, and identity, as conceived by herself and by others, can be completely consumed by her suffering. From there Cassel goes on to consider how some of these patients change the meaning of their suffering in response to their inability to extinguish its cause. Thus, their suffering is transformed from a source of agony and despair to a sense of salvation or existential/spiritual fulfillment.

Pain and suffering are issues about which individual health-care providers and ethics committees can do something. Health-care providers can look more carefully for those cues that might indicate a patient is in pain. They can work at better understanding how pain and its treatment should be differently addressed depending on the patient's (and sometimes the family's) worldview. Health-care providers can also consider the meaning of pain for themselves and how that can affect, positively and negatively, their patients. Ethics committees can begin to work on institutional policies that promote aggressive pain management and palliative care, particularly in preparation for the JCAHO's soon-to-be-required standard on pain management (RI.1.2.8: "Patients have the right to appropriate assessment and management of pain").[1] Furthermore, suffering can be addressed through the educational activities of ethics committees by providing the staff with the opportunity to devise strategies for reformulating how medications, tests, procedures, and treatments are provided in order to ameliorate, instead of contribute to, a patient's suffering.

REFERENCE

1. Joint Commission on Accreditation of Healthcare Organizations. *2000 Hospital Accreditation Standards.* Oakbrook, IL: JCAHO; 2000:79.

15

PAIN

Ethics, Culture, and Informed Consent to Relief

Linda Farber Post, J.D., Jeffrey Blustein, Ph.D.,
Elysa Gordon, and Nancy Neveloff Dubler, LL.B.

❧

As medical technology becomes more sophisticated, the ability to manipulate nature and manage disease forces the dilemma of when *can* becomes *ought*. Indeed, most bioethical discourse is framed in terms of balancing the values and interests and the benefits and burdens that inform principled decisions about how, when, and whether interventions should occur. Yet, despite advances in science and technology, one caregiver mandate remains as constant and compelling as it was for the earliest shaman—the relief of pain. Even when cure is impossible, the physician's duty of care includes palliation. Moreover, the centrality of this obligation is both unquestioned and universal, transcending time and cultural boundaries.

Although universally acknowledged, pain is a complex phenomenon for both the patient and the caregiver, influenced as much by personal values and cultural traditions as by physiological injury and disease. The multiplicity of factors that influence the perception and expression of pain take on special importance in the health-care setting, where pain becomes an interpersonal experience between the sufferer and the reliever. How pain is signified by the patient and understood by the provider determines in large measure how it is valued and, ultimately, how it is treated.

L. Farber Post, J. Blustein, E. Gordon, N. Dubler. "Pain: Ethics, Culture and Informed Consent to Relief." *Journal of Law, Medicine & Ethics.* 1996;24(4):348–359. ©1996. Reprinted with the permission of the American Society of Law, Medicine & Ethics. All rights reserved.

If the perception of and response to pain are to be understood in a useful way, they must be examined in the context of culture, gender, imbalances of power, morality, and myth. This paper will not address the anthropological dimensions of pain—how patients of different cultural and ethnic backgrounds experience and express pain.[1] Rather, we focus on professional attitudes toward pain management, and we suggest there is a moral imperative for relieving pain that transcends (1) the expressed wish to be treated, and (2) the informed consent process. Even though informed consent has become the lens for viewing the doctor-patient relationship, it is not a singularly useful model in the treatment of pain. We argue that the ethical duty of beneficence is sufficient justification for providers to relieve the pain of those in their care absent rejection of analgesia by a capacitated patient.

Accordingly, this discussion will be framed by the following questions:

- What is the philosophical significance of pain and how is it reflected in the physician's obligation to relieve pain?
- Do ethnicity, gender, age, and race make a significant difference in how people perceive, experience, and react to pain?
- Do the differing values placed on the expression and relief of pain affect the interaction between patients and providers, or the effectiveness of care giving?
- How are the ethical principles of autonomy and beneficence implicated in the pain experience?
- How is the process of informed consent changed by incorporating issues of pain?

THE MORAL IMPERATIVE TO RELIEVE PAIN

Pain, Suffering, and Choice

During the past thirty years, the ethic of medical care in the United States has changed radically. The traditional paradigm was largely paternalistic—the doctor would decide what was medically appropriate and present it to the patient, not for consent, but for assent. Today, the governing ethic is antipaternalistic. Bioethicists, philosophical and legal scholars, physicians, and judges all have made a powerful case for patient autonomy and have objected to paternalistic medicine on the grounds that it supplants patient values and preferences with those of the provider.

Given personal idiosyncrasies, frequent denial of reality, and greater or lesser dependence on others for strength and direction, autonomy becomes very complex. Because it focuses primarily on self-determination and liberty, with less attention to the needs for support, autonomy alone cannot provide a sufficiently rich doctrine to inform the doctor-patient relationship. In defining the moral framework for this relationship, we must consider other values.

Principled analyses of the doctor-patient relationship suggest that it is the dual obligation of physicians to respect and promote the autonomy of their patients *and* to protect and enhance their well-being. This obligation of beneficence requires physicians to do good and prevent harm, the list of goods typically including prolongation of life, restoration of function, and relief of pain and suffering.[2] Whether something is counted as a good or a harm depends on the specific circumstances, the patient's values, and some shared notions of suffering and well-being.

Despite its subjective quality, the experience of pain is both real and reverberating. As one writer describes it:

> Pain is dehumanizing. The severer the pain, the more it overshadows the patient's intelligence. All she or he can think about is pain: there is no past pain-free memory, no pain-free future, only the pain-filled present. Pain destroys autonomy: the patient is afraid to make the slightest movement. All choices are focused on either relieving the present pain or preventing greater future pain, and for this, one will sell one's soul. Pain is humiliating: it destroys all sense of self-esteem accompanied by feelings of helplessness in the grip of pain, dependency on drugs, and being a burden to others. In its extreme, pain destroys the soul itself and all will to live.[3]

The lay, medical, and bioethics literatures tend to equate pain and suffering, and most people assume that the greater the pain, the greater the suffering. However, as Dr. Eric Cassell[4] points out, pain and suffering are, in fact, distinct phenomena. He gives as an example childbirth: although the pain can be extreme, many women regard the experience as joyous and life-enhancing.[5] Conversely, some people may suffer greatly even when they are not in great (physical) pain, perhaps in anticipation of pain.

When pain and suffering *are* closely related, Cassell claims, it is for one or more of the following reasons: the pain is overwhelming; the patient does not believe the pain can be controlled; the source of the pain is unknown; or the pain is apparently without end. Suffering is preeminently a threat to the personhood of patients—a threat not merely to their lives, but also to "their integrity as persons."[6] Only when one's continued existence is threatened in this way can the experience of pain properly be said to cause suffering. Thus, when patients are told their pain cannot be managed, diminished, or controlled, they frequently experience suffering because they believe their personal intactness is jeopardized. In some instances, emotional isolation adds to patients' suffering, as when the physician suggests that the pain is only imagined.[7]

Common parlance often distinguishes among physical, spiritual, or emotional pain, that is, between pain that is physiological or psychological in origin. But, whether we speak of different kinds of pain or of pain and suffering, the relief of physical pain is regarded as a primary moral goal of medicine because of its intimate connection with patient well-being.

As a threshold matter, then, it is necessary to understand this relationship between pain and well-being, and why the obligation to serve patient well-being encompasses the obligation to relieve pain. "No one wants to be in pain," is a rather careless way of expressing a commonly shared assumption. It is important to distinguish between (1) wanting to live a life that is free of pain, and (2) wanting to be relieved of the pain one is currently experiencing. Given a choice between living pain-free and living with some admixture of pain and pleasure, it would not seem wise to choose the former. A life without pain would be rather shallow and uninteresting, and would leave one vulnerable to the injury and disease that pain often signals.

The obligation of physicians to relieve pain is what moral philosophers call a prima facie or conditional obligation, something physicians ought to do unless some other duty or moral consideration takes precedence. One such consideration is the refusal of a decisionally capacitated patient to have her pain relieved. Pain control may be welcomed by some who are capable of choosing, while others may view it as yet another instance of unwarranted physician paternalism. For example, if a patient with the capacity to make health-care decisions says she wants the pain to continue because for her it has redemptive meaning, then the obligation to relieve pain is overridden. The patient is saying that, although in pain, she is not suffering or that the suffering is chosen and accepted.

A more common reason for electing to experience pain is the choice of cognition and affective response over relief. Many patients refuse higher doses or more potent pain medication because they do not want chemically to compromise their intellectual and emotional awareness. For these individuals, the choice is a deliberate and delicate value-based balance between relief of pain and erosion of personality.

But suppose a patient is incapacitated and clearly in pain. Should efforts always be made to provide relief? Does the incapacity automatically abrogate choice? Although honoring the wishes of a capable individual shows respect for the person, withholding relief from one who cannot decide or communicate is a form of abandonment, indefensible for caregivers. Compassion, then, is the basis of a moral presumption favoring pain relief. It will always tip the balance in favor of pain relief if the patient can no longer choose or if the patient's intent is in question. Pain is not always devalued, but it is something we need a compelling reason not to treat. The most humane approach, and the one to which caring physicians are disposed, is to relieve pain until evidence of patient refusal is forthcoming.

The Response of Caregivers to Patients' Pain Behaviors

Just as patients' attitudes about and responses to pain are affected by their personal and cultural values,[8] so are those of their caregivers.[9] For example, physicians' clinical judgments about pain are influenced by group-based factors, including age, gender, race, and ethnicity,[10] as well as physical appearance, with the more attractive patients perceived as experiencing less pain than those who are physically unattractive.[11]

The effect of age and gender stereotyping on how patients are medicated for pain was studied by Karen Calderone.[12] Because physicians and nurses saw women as more emotionally labile and prone to exaggerating pain complaints, they were given analgesia less frequently and sedatives more frequently than male patients. These gender distinctions were not related to the patients' sensory perceptions, only to their overt expressions of pain, with women seen as more expressive. Both men and women under sixty-one years of age received more frequent pain medication than their elders; younger men were medicated most frequently and older women least frequently.[13]

A 1993 study by Knox Todd et al.[14] of patients treated for long-bone fractures at the UCLA Emergency Medicine Center found that Hispanics were twice as likely as non-Hispanic whites to receive no medication for pain. Todd et al. explain the distinction as (1) culturally influenced expressions of pain, and (2) the failure of health-care professionals to recognize the presence of pain in patients whose cultural backgrounds differ from their own. The study suggests that the difference in how doctors managed the two groups may occur either when pain is assessed or when analgesia is ordered. A subsequent study of the same population found that, although physicians did not assess pain differently in the two groups, their estimates of pain in both were consistently lower than those of the patients themselves.[15] The ethnically based inequity in pain treatment was found again in the follow-up study, with Hispanics receiving analgesia less often than non-Hispanic whites. Nevertheless, Todd et al. reject the notion that cultural bias among physicians aware of similar pain in two patient groups could account for their undertreating one group.[16]

The balance of power between provider and patient is yet another theme in the pain management interaction. So long as therapeutic control is vested in the caregiver, the patient remains the passive victim of pain. In examining the "regularly and systematically inadequate" treatment of severe pain in hospitalized patients, Dr. Marcia Angell[17] asserts that the standard "prn" (administer as needed[18]) regimen makes patients powerless supplicants, forcing them to endure pain until the next scheduled opportunity to ask for medication. Even then, she concedes, the request might be inhibited by the patient's "desire to please the medical staff and not be a nuisance."[19] The result is an adversarial, rather than a therapeutic, relationship. Dr. Angell suggests a more flexible regimen, which prevents rather than treats pain and better balances the treatment benefits and risks.

Caregivers' responses to their patients' pain are also shaped by their understanding—often misunderstanding—of pain and the agents for its relief. Numerous studies have demonstrated that inadequate professional education and the susceptibility of health-care providers to misconceptions and unfounded fears about opioid addiction and related regulation undermine effective analgesia.[20] These misconceptions are also shared by the lay public. A 1993 survey[21] found that 92 percent of Americans accept pain as an inevitable part of life, with most having either experienced severe pain or observed it in someone close to them. Even so, most Americans were found to reject what they believe to be effective medicinal pain relief because they fear overreliance and/or addiction. These fears, plus concerns about legal liability, are reflected in the stringent laws regulating drug prescription and the suspicion of health-care providers who see patient requests for pain relief as drug-seeking behavior related to addiction. The unsurprising result is the routine undermedication of even terminally ill patients.[22]

These interesting and counterintuitive findings may have their roots in beliefs that are not peculiarly American, but common to Western cultures generally. Commenting on the Agency for Health Care Policy and Research practice guidelines on pain,[23] Patricia Crowley[24] asserts that the current health-care standard of treating acute pain retroactively rather than preventively stems from two well-established myths of Western culture: (1) enduring pain is a character-building, moral-enhancing endeavor, and (2) patients who receive pain medication will become addicted to the drugs.

Pain, Suffering, and Death

An article by Dr. Timothy Quill[25] presents the obligation of health-care providers to help terminally or severely ill patients achieve a "good death." He focuses on the needless suffering of those whose experiences have left them terrified of a bad (painful, prolonged, lonely) death. He argues that it is the provider's duty to relieve pain, suffering, terror, and fear of abandonment. Dr. Quill notes that, given data that 50 to 100 percent of pain can be effectively relieved, dying patients must be reassured and then provided effective pain control while being helped to remain as alert as possible.

An oft-quoted article by Dr. Sidney Wanzer et al.[26] about the care of hopelessly ill patients examines an array of accepted treatment policies, their implementation and deficiencies, including pain management. Dr. Wanzer et al. assert that not only should patients be treated aggressively with pain medication, as much and as often as necessary, but they must also be reassured early in the terminal disease process that they will not be allowed to suffer.[27]

Physician-assisted suicide, a subject of growing concern within the lay, medical, and legal communities, also has implications for any discussion of pain attitudes, behavior, and management. A substantial body of evidence indicates that many, if not most, people who request assistance in ending their lives are really seeking their doctors' help in ending their pain,[28] and that what patients fear more than the prospect of death is the prospect of life with unrelieved pain. The clear implication is that severe and unremitting pain may make even death seem preferable, and that such a request may in fact signal the need for more aggressive palliation rather than assisted suicide.[29]

DECISION MAKING, INFORMED CONSENT, AND PAIN

Autonomy, Beneficence, and Consent to Pain Relief

The ethical principles that classically inform a bioethical analysis are autonomy (respecting the privacy and self-determination of the individual), beneficence (providing benefits and balancing risks or burdens against those benefits), nonmaleficence (avoiding harm), and justice (fairly distributing the risk, burdens, and benefits).[30] Pain and its relief implicate especially autonomy and beneficence, and discussions of pain management and informed consent highlight the tension between the two principles.

Autonomy underlies decision making that gives priority to the values and wishes of the individual when they are not legitimately restricted by the rights of others. It is only when the individual's wishes are obscure, inaccessible, or overridden by competing principles that the judgment of others is substituted. This concept of the individual and independent self is accorded near reverence in Western cultures.[31] Indeed, commentators challenge the attempt of American bioethics to define its concepts and frame its discourse in terms so unbiased and culturally neutral as to create the impression of universality. In fact, its principles reflect mainly Western values[32] and it is asserted that patient autonomy is almost exclusively a product of the Western preoccupation with individuality and self-control.[33]

The principle of beneficence underlies obligations to benefit others and the ways in which these obligations are fulfilled. These behaviors include actions that defend, prevent harm, and rescue those in danger. Beneficence is the principle with arguably the greatest resonance for caregivers, whose mission is to provide patients with therapeutic benefit and shelter from harm. These notions of nurturing and protecting reach fullest expression in caring for those who are the most vulnerable, conferring a special responsibility on those who care for the very young, the very old, those who are suffering, and those who are incapable of looking after themselves.

In the health-care setting, autonomy is reflected most prominently in the doctrine of informed consent. This paradigm of self-determination is the process of knowledgeable and expressed choice whereby a decisionally capacitated individual, who has been apprised of the risks and benefits of a proposed treatment, grants explicit permission for or rejects a particular intervention.[34] It is by now well-established theory, although not always well-established practice,[35] that the contemporaneous or prior expression of treatment wishes by a capacitated individual controls the health-care decision.[36] The doctrine of informed consent represents the legal embodiment of the right to self-determination in health care.[37] In addition, it guides the process of medical decision making by defining the parameters of the patient-physician dialogue.

The Roots of Informed Consent

The ethical and legal roots of informed consent provide the basis for its power. The notion of informed consent was initially grounded in the law of assault and battery, holding that any unconsented-to touching constituted an unlawful act.[38] The subsequent trend toward negligence rather than battery reflected judicial dissatisfaction with the artificial notion that consent either did or did not happen.[39] The doctrine of negligence permits a nuanced examination of whether the discussion reflected the risks and benefits that were material to this patient. Although modern law treats failure to disclose as an action in negligence, the patient's right to make knowledgeable health-care decisions has expanded the focus to make the informed consent process act as a protection of privacy and autonomy,[40] rather than as a barrier to negligent failure of a "duty to warn."[41] Finally, in the current climate of malpractice, cost containment, and managed care, informed consent has become a defensive weapon of risk management.

Courts hearing negligence cases based on absence of informed consent tend to rely on an objective reasonable-person standard, which assumes that the reasonable person is one holding Western values and favoring Western-defined approaches to medical decision making.[42] In contrast, a subjective standard requires physicians to disclose information relevant to the particular patient and judges whether that individual would have reached the same decision absent disclosure. Ultimately, a subjective standard evokes a richer notion of informed consent by considering the diverse ways and the different contexts in which patients and physicians communicate and make decisions. Although courts have not adopted a pure subjective standard,[43] recent statute and case law have considered the importance of patients' particular values in making medical decisions and suggest a trend toward a more patient-centered notion of informed consent.[44]

During the past thirty years since the explosion of the various rights movements, the ethical principle of autonomy has become the major support for individual empowerment and self-determination. In virtually every social sphere, the aim has been to level the playing field by eliminating power imbalances caused by race, gender, class, and education.[45] In the health-care setting, the twin notions of patient as partner in medical decision making and patient as informed health-care consumer reflect patient autonomy as the controlling principle. Simultaneously, malpractice litigation involving informed consent placed the wishes of the patient, rather than the conventions of physician practice, at the core of possible liability for negligent disclosure. In time, patients came to see informed consent as their offensive security against physician overreaching, while doctors perceived it as their defensive protection against charges of malpractice—the medical equivalent of a prenuptial agreement. The unfortunate result is an adversarial rather than therapeutic climate, with informed consent as the weapon of choice.

Because of its ethical and legal supports, informed consent is now broadly accepted as indispensable to patient rights, the violation of which essentially invalidates the legal and ethical propriety of medical treatment. However, autonomy itself is a doctrine that may be imposed on individuals whose values support a more communally experienced ethic. The elevation of patient autonomy to its preeminent position has increased the potency of explicit patient permission to the point where it effectively trumps all other avenues for determining and implementing what is in the patient's best interests. Exalting the patient's right to exercise autonomy has correspondingly restricted the doctor's discretion and opportunities for therapeutic intervention. Ironically, the pursuit of greater patient power has actually devalued the physician's duty of beneficence. The obsession with autonomy has led to a fetish of informed consent that substitutes delivery of consumer-chosen health care for the provision of patient-oriented health *caring*.

Barriers to a Universal and Inflexible Informed Consent Requirement

Although the principle of autonomy, manifested through knowledgeable consent, is routinely required for therapeutic interventions, we argue that, for at least two reasons, informed consent should not be invoked in decisions about pain management. Substantial evidence confirms that the key elements in the pain experience (the perception and expression of pain; the relief-seeking behavior and response to it; and the capacity or willingness to assume decisional responsibility) are highly complex and dependent on numerous variables. The informed-consent doctrine depends entirely on the elevation and expression of self-determination. Under these conditions, requiring that pain management rely exclusively on or be constrained by an affirmative act of patient consent threatens to undermine the very foundations of the caregiver duty of beneficence.

Legally valid informed consent can only be provided by a decisionally capable[46] individual. The presence or absence of decisional capacity is evaluated according to the specific decision under consideration, with a higher level of capacity generally required for those decisions carrying greater risks.[47] If a person clearly has the capacity to understand and process his situation, reference values, consider the consequences, and make his wishes known, then his decision should control and his consent is required.[48]

This analysis does not apply to the formerly capable and communicative individual. Often, when choices must be made, age or illness has destroyed the abilities of reasoning and expression. If this incapacitated individual, while still capable, had articulated treatment wishes prospectively through advance directives (by appointing a health-care proxy agent, by executing a living will, or by leaving explicit oral instructions), those directions should be respected and implemented even though capacity has lapsed.

Likewise, people unable to grant informed consent either because they have lost capacity through age or infirmity and left no advance directives, or because they never were capacitated (such as newborns, children, and mentally retarded adults) are excluded from the requirement to provide consent. Their health-care decisions must be made by surrogates using substituted judgment (based on what is known about the patient's values and preferences) or the best-interest standard (based on the surrogate's evaluation of the patient's welfare). For these individuals, many of whom require pain control, the informed consent requirement is fulfilled by others acting on their behalf, although some notion of their assent may be important. In these situations, surrogate refusal of pain treatment is ethically problematic, especially if it is based on fear of addiction. Consider, for example, the young man who is dying of end-stage AIDS. He is wasted, obtunded, and writhing in pain. His mother, who cannot accept either his diagnosis or his prognosis, refuses to allow him to be given pain medication because she does not want him to become addicted. In this instance, the caregivers would have to overrule a mother's misplaced attempt to protect her son in order to do what is, in fact, in his best interests.

The second reason why informed consent cannot always frame health-care determinations about pain is that individual autonomy is not the universal paradigm for decision making. The architecture of informed consent represents a legal attempt to find and secure the patient's voice in medical deliberations and to equalize the balance of power between patients and their physicians. It is also increasingly a risk-management strategy to protect the institution from later liability by demonstrating that the risk of negative outcomes was known and accepted by the patient. The patient voice sought, however, echoes a notion of autonomy based on Western cultural values that favor the individual over the community, self-reliance over dependence, action over passivity, scientific rationality over spirituality, and forthrightness over harmony. This doctrine focuses on the right—often, it seems, the obligation—of the individual to make decisions concerning medical treatment. In addition, it advocates candor and assertiveness regarding the disclosure of medical prognosis, treatment options, and their risks and benefits. Finally, it promotes the active participation of the individual patient, rather than family, community, or other surrogates, in medical treatment decisions.

It is important to bear in mind that this preoccupation with patient autonomy does not apply universally. Western values often clash with worldviews held by non-Western cultures that may place greater emphasis on spirituality, family and community, or authority and social stratification. These communitarian ethics may value less assertive decision-making processes and encourage deference to physician judgment. By mechanically applying narrow Western-defined doctrines of autonomy and informed consent, American law deprives non-Western cultures of their proper position of power and actually devalues the notion of autonomy.[49] The very meanings of health, illness, and healing are shaped by cultural values. Sensitivity to these distinctions encourages critical thinking about how they affect medical-care discussions and decisions, as well as the experience and expression of illness, disability, and discomfort—issues that form the essential background for considerations of pain control.

Finally, it has been suggested that when a person is in extreme pain, truly informed consent may not be possible. Caregivers have an ethical obligation to inform the capacitated patient about the salient effects and side effects, benefits and risks of pain management options, especially those related to use of narcotics, to help the patient to reach an informed decision about treatment. But, despite the best efforts to provide relevant information and elicit the patient's values and wishes, severe pain may erode an individual's cognition and autonomy. A patient suffering such pain often can think of nothing except relief and will agree to anything that will provide it. For such patients, truly free and informed consent may be an illusion.[50]

Exceptions to Informed Consent

Inevitably, the rigid express permission requirement has necessitated the invention of ways to get around it in order to provide patients with the care they need. These loopholes are embodied in three well-established exceptions to the informed-consent requirement: medical emergency, therapeutic privilege, and waiver.

In an emergency, the patient might be precluded from consenting because of unconsciousness or incapacity, and life-saving treatment delay or failure would result in harm so grave as to outweigh any potential harm of a proposed treatment.[51] Under these critical conditions, courts agree that physicians may dispense with informed consent, so long as they conform to practices customary in such emergencies. Some courts even hold that in emergencies, consent is implied.[52]

The second exception falls within therapeutic privilege, under which information may be withheld from the patient when, in the physician's judgment, disclosure of the information "would itself be harmful to the patient." Some commentators strongly criticize this exception, arguing that it risks destroying the theory of informed consent and signals a return to medical paternalism.[54]

The third recognized exception, waiver,[55] provides either statutory[56] or judicial[57] support for patients to give up their right to receive and to act on medical information. The notion of waiver acknowledges that some patients lack the confidence to analyze risk data or prefer to depend on their physician's professional judgment; others simply prefer not to hear adverse information, or choose to depend on family judgment.[58] Patients may waive their right to receive relevant information, and they may also waive the right to make a specific decision or any decision at all.[59] As a result, the waiver mechanism accommodates diverse cultural values by respecting alternative approaches, such as family-centered decision making and deference to physician authority. Because the patient remains in control of the decision-making process by choosing when to allow others to make the actual treatment decision, the waiver also upholds the value of self-determination. In theory, then, the law allows patients who understand their right of waiver to relinquish their right to grant informed consent so long as the waiver is given with full information and without coercion.[60] In fact, in the health-care setting, waiver is rarely used because risk-management concerns require the patient's expressed consent to protect the institution from liability.

In addition to these customary exceptions, it has been necessary to create other varieties of nonexpressed consent to validate the notion that treatment has been authorized. Most relevant are *presumed consent*, derived from a general theory about the way rational people behave, and *implied consent*, inferred from the actions of a particular individual in a specific circumstance.[61] The presumption underlying both exceptions appears to that, because people will invariably opt for treatment to restore health, individuals who are physically or cognitively incapacitated can also be presumed to prefer health and would consent to therapeutic intervention if they were able to do so. Thus freed from the need to obtain expressed informed consent, the physician's twin duties of beneficence and nonmaleficence trigger a default posture that supports treatment.

Informed Consent and the Management of Pain

Predating the current emphasis on patient autonomy, the duty of beneficence has been a core value of the healing professions, incorporating the relief of pain as well as the promotion of healing. It has been claimed that relieving pain is a "moral duty, based on both beneficence and respect."[62] And yet, despite this ethical mandate, it has been repeatedly demonstrated that caregivers routinely, often deliberately, undermedicate patients in pain.[63]

Aside from the few exceptions noted, informed consent is required for most treatment interventions, especially those that are invasive or carry more than minimal risk. It is interesting, therefore, that pain control interventions are traditionally exempt from this requirement. As a matter of practice, physicians are expected to ask patients about drug allergies and inform them about the proper dosages and potential side effects of prescribed pain medications, and pharmacists are required to enclose warning labels and information about synergistic effects; but there is no formal requirement that patients give informed consent for analgesia.[64] It is true that pain medication is routinely given on a prn basis, which requires patients to request the medication and thereby affirmatively signal their consent to receive it. Recently, patients have also been given the option of patient-controlled analgesia, whereby they actively participate in the decisions about and administration of their own pain medication, usually through a self-regulated intravenous pump.[65] Finally, it is certainly plausible that a patient who does not want pain medication at all and is able to communicate that preference would have that refusal honored. The crucial point here is that these circumstances apply only to patients who are decisionally capacitated or at least alert and articulate enough to determine and communicate whether they want pain relief.

The more challenging situation involves those patients who are decisionally incapacitated or unable to communicate, and who require surrogate decision makers to authorize treatment interventions. Perhaps an individual has left an advance directive stating that, should he become incapacitated and be in pain, no analgesia is to be administered. Even in the absence of contemporaneous refusal or explicit advance instructions, enough may be known about him, about his values and beliefs, to determine that he is or was the sort of person who finds meaning in pain.

However, the duty to honor the refusal of analgesia issued prospectively by a currently incapacitated patient is significantly weaker than the duty to honor the contemporaneous refusal of a capacitated patient. It has even been argued that the currently incapacitated patient may be so different from the formerly capacitated one that they are in effect two distinct people with different interests.[66] However, when there is no advance directive and inferences must be drawn about what the patient would want, not making an effort to relieve the patient's current pain is even more ethically problematic than proceeding without expressed instructions. It would be both irrational and inhumane to withhold relief because of inability to request it. Analgesia is routinely given when patients are *understood* to be in pain. Physicians and nurses, using their well-developed skills of observation and clinical judgment, evaluate patients' body language, cardiac and respiratory function, facial expressions, emotional signals, and verbal and nonverbal cues, and do what they believe their patients would want done for them.

Applying the primacy of patient autonomy to the issue of pain management, one could argue for yet another exception to the informed consent requirement that would be applicable to an incapacitated patient in pain. It is generally acknowledged that, except for the rare instances when pain is believed to have some character-building or redemptive quality, people desire to be rid of the pain they are currently experiencing, even though some may choose to endure it as the only alternative to diminished consciousness. If *presumed consent* is that which can be expected of most people, then the incapacitated postoperative, terminally ill, or grievously wounded person can be presumed to consent to pain relief intervention. Likewise, if *implied consent* is that which can be inferred from an individual's conduct, then the incapacitated person writhing and moaning in pain certainly can be believed to consent to the administration of analgesia. It is a short step from there to the concept of an implied waiver by which an incapacitated patient in pain is understood to delegate decisional authority regarding analgesia. It could even be argued that an individual who seeks medical attention is, by definition, seeking relief of the presenting pain and/or implying consent to the relief of any pain resulting from treatment.

Although it is tempting to subscribe to these arguments and suggest that pain management requires no expressed informed consent because the patient is believed to have given presumed or implied consent, or waived consent altogether, we decline the opportunity to use such flimsy contrivances. Rather, we submit that providing relief from pain is central to the very notion of healing and, for that reason alone, it requires no exceptions or intellectual artifice for its validity. Indeed, we agree with the following sentiments regarding implied consent:

> [I]t is quite obvious that implied consent is a legal fiction. Clearly there is no consent in this [emergency medical] situation. Rather, the law gives physicians a privilege to provide treatment in emergencies, even in the absence of consent, in order to promote other important societal goals besides individual choice—namely, the preservation of life or the restoration of health.... [I]n such a situation a physician has an obligation to do what is best for the patient.[67]

We do not accept the proposition that the caregiver's twin duties of respect for persons and beneficence are mutually exclusive in the realm of pain management or even necessarily conflicting. Rather, we argue that principled and compassionate caring embraces both the respect for and the protection of persons.[68] It has been claimed that beneficence can legitimately outweigh autonomy when it is clearly in the best interests of the patient and, especially, when the treatment interventions are consistent with the patient's own therapeutic goals.[69] We would go further and argue that the current obsession with patient autonomy risks courting a form of patient abandonment in which healers are prevented from healing, and those in pain are denied relief because expressed consent is lacking. To succumb to such reasoning demonstrates a lack of respect for patients and places caregivers in danger of sacrificing beneficence on the altar of autonomy.

The persuasive argument that the individual's diminishing cognitive capacity changes her needs and goals[70] carries the implicit notion that decisions, such as advance health-care directives, made by a formerly capacitated person are not necessarily appropriate for the now incapacitated person, and caregivers should not be bound to honor these directives if they are clearly contrary to the patient's current best interests. The implications for pain management are compelling. The person who, never having experienced severe pain, says, "No matter what happens, I do not want pain medication," may feel very different about the need for analgesia when experiencing an attack of renal colic. The caregiver might well be justified in giving more weight to the individual's current relief-seeking behavior than any prior theoretical statements. Likewise, an incapacitated patient's signals of pain can and should speak as clearly as any articulated request for relief.[71]

CONCLUSION

Pain, although universally acknowledged, is experienced in ways that vary with ethnicity, gender, age, class, and condition. The implications for health care are obvious. If culture is a lens through which the world is perceived and understood, each refraction will depend on the particular prism employed. People bring their culturally determined values and behaviors to all consequential experiences, especially interpersonal encounters. The meaning pain holds for sufferers and the person(s) attending them determines the intensity with which it is perceived and the response it calls forth. Substantial differences among patients, families, and caregivers in their perceptions of and reactions to pain can affect significantly the ways in which pain is expressed, the ways in which relief is requested, and how it is administered.

The importance of decision making is nowhere more striking than in the healthcare setting. Issues of control and choice, influenced by cultural background, current illness, and perceived obligations, are brought into sharp focus as people from different vantage points grapple with complex and emotion-laden dilemmas. The twin duties of autonomy and beneficence assume special significance in this context. Self-determination, valued most highly in Western cultures, is articulated in the doctrine of informed consent, required for almost every therapeutic intervention. Yet, the duty of beneficence, reflected in the caregiver mandate to relieve pain, can be seen to transcend boundaries of culture and even selfdetermination. Ultimately, compassion speaks in the most forceful and universal tongue to relieve pain.

REFERENCES

1. It is beyond the scope of this paper to discuss the considerable research that has been devoted to the effects of culture, ethnicity, gender, and age on the perception, expression, and signification of pain, and the ways in which people make health-care decisions. See, for example, Morris DB, *The Culture of Pain* (Berkeley, CA: University of California Press; 1991); Helman C, "Pain and culture," in: *Culture, Health, and Illness: Introduction for Health Professionals* (Oxford: Butterworth Heinemann; 1994); Spector R, *Cultural Diversity in Health and Illness*, 3rd rev. ed. (East Norwalk, CT: Appleton-Century-Crofts; 1985); Pellegrino ED et al. (eds.), *Transcultural Dimensions in Medical Ethics* (Frederick, MD: University Publishing Group; 1992); Henderson G, Primeaux M, *Transcultural Health Care* (Philippines: Addison-Wesley Publishing; 1981); Villarruel AM, de Mantellano BO, "Culture and pain: a Mesoamerican perspective," *Advanced Nursing Science*, 1992;15:21–32; Zatzick DF, Dimsdale JE, "Cultural variations in

response to painful stimuli," *Psychosomatic Medicine*, 1990;52:544–557; Pfefferbaum B, Adams J, Aceves J, "The influence on pain in Anglo and Hispanic children with cancer," *Journal of the American Academy of Child and Adolescent Psychiatry*, 1990;29:642–647; Bates MS, "Ethnicity and pain: a biocultural model," *Social Science and Medicine*, 1987;24:47–50; Greenwald HP, "Interethnic differences in pain perception," *Pain*, 1991;44:157–163; Lipton J, Marbach JJ, "Ethnicity and the pain experience," *Social Science of Medicine*, 1984;19:1279–1298; Thomas VJ, Rose FD, "Ethnic differences and the experience of pain," *Social Science and Medicine*, 1991;32:1063–1066; Honeyman PT, Jacobs EA, "Effects of culture on back pain in Australian aboriginals," *Spine*, 1996;21:841–843; Stein JA, Fox SA, Murata PJ, "The influence of ethnicity, socioeconomic status, and psychological barriers on use of mammography," *Journal of Health and Social Behavior*, 1991;32:101–113; Jackson JJ, "Urban Black Americans," in: Harwood A (ed.), *Ethnicity and Medical Care*, (Cambridge, MA: Harvard University Press; 1981):37–129; de Rios MD, Achauer BM, "Pain relief for the Hispanic burn patient using cultural metaphors," *Plastic and Reconstructive Surgery*, 1991;88:161–164; Kodiath MF, Kodiath A, "A comparative study of patients who experience chronic malignant pain in India and the United States," *Cancer Nursing*, 1995;18(3):189–196; Koopman C, Eisenthal S, Stoeckle JD, "Ethnicity in the reported pain and emotional distress requests of medical outpatients," *Social Science and Medicine*, 1984;18:487–490; Beyer JE, Wells N, "Assessment of cancer pain in children," in: Patt RB (ed.), *Cancer Pain* (Philadelphia, PA: J. B. Lippincott; 1993):57–84; Bucklew SP, et al., "Health locus of control, gender differences and adjustment to persistent pain," *Pain*, 1990;42:287–294; Bates MS, Edwards WT, Anderson KO, "Ethnocultural influences on variation in chronic pain perception," *Pain*, 1993;52:101–112; Bates MS, Rankin-Hill L, "Control, culture, and chronic pain," *Social Science and Medicine*, 1994;39:629–645; Dane JR, Kessler RS, "A matrix model for the psychological assessment and treatment of acute pain," in: Hamill RJ, Rowlingson JC (eds.), *Handbook of Critical Care Pain Management* (New York, NY: McGraw-Hill; 1994):53–81; Jecker NS, Carrese JA, Pearlman RA, "Caring for patients in cross-cultural settings," *Hastings Center Report*, 1995;25(1):6–14; Blackhall LJ et al., "Ethnicity and attitudes toward patient autonomy," *JAMA*, 1995;274:820–825; Murphy ST et al., "Ethnicity and advance care directives," *Journal of Law, Medicine, & Ethics*, 1996;24:108–117; Carrese J, Rhodes LA, "Western bioethics on the Navajo reservation," *JAMA*, 1995;247:826–829; Daley A et al., "Effective coping strategies of African Americans," *Social Work*, 1995;40:240–248; Ewalt PL, Mokuau N, "Self-determination from a Pacific perspective," *Social Work*, 1995;40:168–174.

2. According to the official policy of the American Medical Association, "the social commitment of the physician is to prolong life and relieve suffering." Council on Ethical and Judicial Affairs, American Medical Association, *Code of Medical Ethics: Current Opinions* (Chicago, IL: American Medical Association; 1989). Likewise, the American Nurses Association's position is that "[n]ursing encompasses the ... promotion of health; the prevention of illness; and the alleviation of suffering in the care of clients." American Nurses Association, *Code for Nurses* (Kansas City, MO: American Nurses Association; 1985).

3. Lisson EL, "Ethical issues related to pain control," *Nursing Clinics of North America*, 1987;22:654.

4. Cassell E, *The Nature of Suffering and the Goals of Medicine* (New York, NY: Oxford University Press; 1991):35–37.

5. Ibid., p. 35.

6. Ibid., p. 36.

7. Ibid.

8. See n. 1.

9. In addition to research on professional caregivers' responses to patients' pain, the

influence of family caregivers' attitudes on the perception and treatment of pain has received attention. See, for example, Ferrell BR et al, "Pain as a metaphor for illness, part II: family caregivers' management of pain," *Oncology Nursing Forum*, 1991;18:1315–1321.

10. See Lopez SR, "Patient variable biases in clinical judgment: conceptual overview and considerations," *Psychological Bulletin*, 1989;106:184–203.

11. Hadjistavropolous HD, Ross M, von Baeyer CL, "Are physicians' ratings of pain affected by patients' physical attractiveness?" *Social Science and Medicine*, 1990;31:69–72; Hadjistavropoulos T, Hadjistavropoulos HD, Craig KD, "Appearance-based information about coping with pain: valid or biased?" *Social Science and Medicine*, 1995;40:537–543.

12. Calderone KL, "The influence of gender on the frequency of pain and sedative medication administered to postoperative patients," *Sex Roles*, 1990;23(11/12):713–725.

13. See also a discussion of "learned inhibitors" to nurses' appropriate decision making regarding treatment of pain. Greipp MA, "Undermedication for pain: an ethical model," *Advanced Nursing Science*, 1992;15:44–53; Ferrell BR, "When culture clashes with pain control," *Nursing*, 1995;25(5):90.

14. Todd KH, Samaroo N, Hoffman JR, "Ethnicity as a risk factor for inadequate emergency department analgesia," *JAMA*, 1993;269:1537–1539.

15. In a study that has received considerable attention, poor physician assessment of pain was cited as one reason patients too often suffer at the end of life. SUPPORT Principal Investigators, "A controlled trial to improve care for seriously ill hospitalized patients," *JAMA*, 1995;274:1591–1598. See also Foley KM, "Misconceptions and controversies regarding the use of oploids in cancer pain," *Anti-Cancer Drugs*, 1995;6(supp. 3):4–13.

16. Recognizing the impact of these factors, researchers have developed ethical approaches to cross-cultural encounters and decision making in the health care setting. See, for example, Jecker, Carrese, and Pearlman, n. 1.

17. Angell M, "The quality of mercy," *New England Journal of Medicine*, 1982;306:98–99.

18. Abbreviation for the Latin *pro re na'ta*, "according as circumstances require." *Dorland's Illustrated Medical Dictionary* (Philadelphia, PA: W. B. Saunders; 1985):1355.

19. See Angell, n. 17, p. 98. See also Gail Davis, suggesting that the patient should be an active participant pant in, rather than a recipient of, the pain management process. Davis GC, "The meaning of pain management: a concept analysis," *Advanced Nursing Science*, 1992;15:77–86.

20. See, for example, Mananey FX Jr., "Proper relief of cancer pain is worldwide concern," *Journal of the National Cancer Institute*, 1995;87:481–483; Foley, n. 15, p. 13; Foley KM, "Pain and America's culture of death," *Wilson Quarterly*, 1994 (autumn):20–21; McIntosh H, "Regulatory barriers take some blame for pain undertreatment," *Journal of the National Cancer Institute*, 1991;83:1202–1204; Doyl D, "Morphine: myths, morality, and economics," *Postgraduate Medicine Journal*, 1991;67(supp. 2):S70–S73; Zenz M, "Morphine myths: sedation, tolerance, addiction," *Postgraduate Medicine Journal*, 1991;67(supp. 5):S100–S102; Porter J, Jick J, "Addiction rate in patients treated with narcotics," *New England Journal of Medicine*, 1980;302:123; Portenoy RK, "Opioid therapy for chronic nonmalignant pain: a review of the critical issues," *Journal of Pain and Symptom Management*, 1996;11:203–217.

21. Mellman, Lasarus, Lake, Inc., Presentation of Findings: Mayday Fund (September 1993), reporting results of a national public opinion survey (on file with the authors); See also Rouse F, "Decision making about medical innovation: role of the advocate," *Albany Law Review*, 1994;57:607–616.

22. See Rouse, n. 21.

23. Agency for Health Care Policy and Research, *Clinical Practice Guidelines, Acute Pain*

Management: Operative or Medical Procedures and Trauma 2 (Rockville, MD: Department of Health and Human Services, Pub. No. 92-0032; 1992).

24. Crowley PC, "No pain, no gain? The Agency for Health Care Policy and Research's attempt to change inefficient health care practice of withholding medication from patients in pain," *Journal of Contemporary Health Law and Policy,* 1993;10:383–403.

25. Quill T, "You promised me I wouldn't die like this!" *Archives of Internal Medicine,* 1995;155:1250–1254.

26. Wanzer SH et al. "The physician's responsibility toward hopelessly ill patients, a second look," *New England Journal of Medicine,* 1989;320:844–849.

27. "The proper dose of pain medication is the dose that is sufficient to relieve pain and suffering, even to the point of unconsciousness." Ibid., p. 847.

28. Foley KM, "Pain, physician-assisted suicide and euthanasia," *Pain Forum,* 1995;4:163–178; Quill TE, "When all else fails," *Pain Forum,* 1995;4:189–191; Berde CB et al., "Proper palliative care should reduce requests for euthanasia and physician-assisted suicide," *Pain Forum,* 1995;4:195–196; Foley, n. 20; Breitbart W, "Suicide risk and pain in cancer and AIDS patients," in: Chapman CR and Foley KM (eds.), *Current and Emerging Issues in Cancer Pain: Research and Practice* (New York, NY: Raven Press, 1993): 49; Quill TE, "Death and dignity: a case of individualized decision making," *New England Journal of Medicine,* 1991;324:691–694; Quill, n. 25.

29. Quill TE, Cassel CK, Meier DE, "Care of the hopelessly ill: proposed clinical criteria for physician-assisted suicide," *New England Journal of Medicine,* 1992;327:1380–1383. William Breltbart asserts that "[p]ersistent pain and terminal illness are the most common reasons for euthanasia or physician-assisted suicide." Breitbart, n. 28, p. 49 (citations omitted).

30. See generally Beauchamp TL, Childress JF, *Principles of Biomedical Ethics,* 4th ed. (New York, NY: Oxford University Press; 1994).

31. See, for example, Warren HS, "Unlimited human autonomy—a cultural bias?" *New England Journal of Medicine,* 1997;336:954–956.

32. See Jecker, Carrese, and Pearlman, n. 1.

33. Pellegrino ED, "Patient and physician autonomy: conflicting rights and obligations in the patient-physician relationship," *Journal of Contemporary Health Law and Policy,* 1993;10:47–86. Dr. Edmund Pellegrino also argues that this biased view of autonomy prevents care providers from recognizing that some patients may not want to make health-care decisions and that beneficence and respect include adapting to multicultural considerations and not imposing an unwanted burden of autonomous decision making. See Pellegrino ED, "Prologue: intersections of Western biomedical ethics and world culture," in: Pellegrino ED et al. (eds.), *Transcultural Dimensions in Medical Ethics* (Frederick, MD: University Publishing Group; 1985): 13–19.

34. See Beauchamp and Childress, n. 30, p. 128.

35. See, for example, a study by Dr. Joan Teno and Dr. Joanne Lynn recently asserted that, in spite of substantial publicity and educational efforts, very few people at the end of life have advance directives and, when they do exist, these prospective instructions have little effect on medical care. Kolata G, "Documents like living wills are rarely of aid, study says," *New York Times,* April 8, 1997: A12.

36. See, for example, *Mohr v. Williams,* 95 Minn. 261 (1905) (holding that "the free citizen's first and greatest right, which underlies all others—the right to himself—"precludes even the most skillful medical or surgical intervention without patient consent); *Pratt v. Davis,* 224 Ill. 300 (1906) (holding that, unless there is an emergency or a circumstance where disclosure would be harmful to the patient, a capable individual must be consulted and must give consent before surgery can be performed); *Natanson v. Kline,* 86 Kan. 393 (1960) (upholding the neces-

sity for physicians to employ discretion in disclosure of information to patients); *Salgo* v. *Leland Stanford University Board of Trustees*, 154 Cal. App. 2d 560 (1970) (introducing the term "informed consent," and holding that the physician is under an affirmative duty to disclose the risks, benefits, and alternatives to the proposed treatment intervention); *Canterbury* v. *Spence*, 464 F.2d 772 (D.C. Cir.), cert. denied, 409 U.S. 1064 (1972) (holding that the physician is obliged to provide sufficient information about a procedure's risks so that a reasonable patient can make an informed decision); *Moore* v. *Regents of the University of California*, 51 Cal. 3d 120 (1990) (holding that informed consent requires physician disclosure of "personal interests unrelated to the patient's health" but potentially affecting medical judgment); and *Arato* v. *Auedon*, 5 Cal. 4th 1172 (1993) (holding that the duty to obtain informed consent does not require a physician to disclose a patient's statistical life expectancy).

37. Presently, each of the fifty states and the District of Columbia have legally recognized patient rights by adopting an informed consent doctrine.

In addition, the U.S. Congress has expressly legislated patients' rights to individualized medical decision making. The Patient Self-Determination Act (PSDA) (42 U.S.C.A. S 1395cc(f) [1992]) advocates patients expressing their wishes about future treatment in the event they become incapacitated. PSDA requires all health-care facilities funded by Medicare or Medicaid to inform patients on admission of their right to execute advance directives under the laws of the respective states. Although most people use these written instruments prospectively to *refuse* care, advance directives are value neutral and can be used to *request* care as well.

38. See, for example, 95 Minn. 261; and 224 Ill. 300. See also A. Kiev, "A history of informed consent doctrine," *Applied Clinical Trials*, 1993;2:61; Katz J, "Informed consent: ethical and legal issues," in: Arras JD, Steinbock B (eds.), *Ethical Issues in Modern Medicine* (Mountain View, CA: Mayfield Publishing; 1995): 88–91; President's Commission for the Study of Ethical Problems in Medicine and Biomedical and Behavioral Research, *Making Health Care Decisions: A Report on the Ethical and Legal Implications of Informed Consent in the Patient-Practitioner Relationship* (1982): 18–20. The question in a battery action is whether the physician informed the patient of the nature of the procedure and whether the patient consented to the intervention. Proponents of the battery theory argue that its purpose is to protect bodily integrity, thus linking informed consent to the principle of personal autonomy. See Faden R, Beauchamp T, *A History and Theory of Informed Consent* (New York, NY: Oxford University Press; 1986): 26–27. Critics counter that the theory is useful only when a physician intentionally withholds information or acts beyond the scope of the patient's consent. Ibid., pp. 29–30. Battery law is also criticized as limiting physicians to a single defense, that of having obtained explicit consent or, in an emergency situation, presumed consent. See Pellegrino, n. 33, p. 78. Others maintain that battery theory disadvantages the patient because many courts are reluctant to view physicians as acting in bad faith or in an antisocial manner. See, for example, Faden and Beauchamp, *History and Theory of Informed Consent*, pp. 29–30, 127–28. Currently, Pennsylvania is the only state that characterizes the lack of informed consent as battery. See *Gray* v. *Grunnagle*, 223 A.2d 663 (1966), *on reh'g*, 228 A.2d 735 (1967) (finding that, based on a battery analysis, consent to treatment must be knowledgeable and informed). All jurisdictions, however, permit a battery approach when consent is absent or is determined to be absent for a particular procedure. Rosovsky FA, *Consent to Treatment: A Practical Guide*, 2d ed. (Boston: Little Brown, 1990: sec. 1.3.

39. In contrast to the battery analysis, the negligence theory of liability examines the defendant's unintended harmful act or failure to act. The elements required to establish negligence include the presence of a legal duty, the breach of that duty, measurable injury, a direct causal link between the breach and the injury, and a proximate causal relation between the act and the injury. Thus, to win the case, the patient must prove physical injury. See Rosovsky, *Consent to Treatment*, §51.3. Advocates of negligence theory applaud its allowing physicians to

invoke many defenses and acknowledging that most physicians act in good faith. Opponents argue that negligence theory reduces the informed consent doctrine to a "failure to warn law," based more on professional liability and the expectations of the medical profession than on patient decision making and self-determination. See Katz J, "Informed consent: a fairy tale? Law's vision," *University of Pittsburgh Law Review*, 1977;39:139. Other commentators argue that the negligence theory's emphasis on proving physical harm ignores the rights-based aspects of informed consent. See Dworkin R, "Medical law and ethics in the post-autonomy age," *Indiana Law Journal*, 1996;68:729. ("The loss of dignity, autonomy, free choice, and bodily integrity that is so exalted in the rhetoric of informed consent is worth nothing at judgment time.").

40. See, for example, *Canterbury*, 464 F.2d 772 (D.C. Cir), cert. denied, 409 U.S. 1064; and *Wilkinson v. Vesey*, 295 A.2d 6769 (R.I. 1972). See also Kiev, n. 38, p. 62.

41. *Making Health Care Decisions*, n. 38, p. 20.

42. See Beauchamp and Childress, n. 30, pp. 147–48, 142. For an analysis of informed consent as upholding patient choice and a proposal for refraining the doctrine as a constitutional right to patient choice in medical decision making, see Schultz MM, "From informed consent to patient choice: a new protected interest," *Yale Law Journal*, 1985;95:219–299.

43. This judicial reluctance may reflect fears that the patient, in retrospect, will decide that the information not disclosed was material to the decision and that, with full disclosure, she/he would have declined treatment. See *Canterbury v. Spence*, 464 F.2d 772, 790-91 (D.C. Cir. 1972) ("It places the physician in jeopardy of the patient's hindsight and bitterness, thus an objective test is preferable).

44. *Arato v. Avedon*, 858 P.2d 598, 606 (Cal. 1993) (finding that "the contexts and clinical settings in which physician and patient interact and exchange information material to therapeutic decisions are so multifarious, the informational needs and degree of dependency of individual patients so various, and the professional relationship itself such an intimate and irreducibly judgment-laden one that we believe it is unwise as a matter of law that a particular species of information be disclosed.").

45. Note the civil rights and feminist movements in general, with examples from education (the de jure and de facto integration of religious and ethnic minorities into educational institutions; the admission of women into formerly all-male schools); art (serious artistic criticism of the highly suggestive, and to some offensive, art; greater acceptance of homosexuality as an artistic subject and homosexuals as actors in drama); sports (the acceptance and success of athletes from ethnic minorities and alternative sexual orientation); professions (women and [religious and ethnic] minorities increasing their presence in medicine, law, and academic faculties). Note the parallel consumer movement awakening the buying public to its right to full disclosure as a prerequisite to informed purchasing.

46. Mental capacity or competence has been defined as "[s]uch a measure of intelligence, understanding, memory, and judgment relative to the particular transaction (e.g., making of will or entering into contract) as will enable the person to understand the nature, terms, and effect of his or her act." *Black's Law Dictionary*, 6th ed. (St. Paul, MN: West; 1990): 986. Although the terms *capacity* and *competence* are often used interchangeably, for bioethics purposes there are important distinctions that go beyond semantics. *Competence* is technically a legal designation made only by a court, whereas health-care decisions are a matter of medical determination. Because the legal system is rarely involved in decision making in the clinical setting, it has become customary to refer to the patient's *capacity* to make health-care decisions, and to refer to the clecisionafly *capacitated* or *capable* individual. See Lo B, "Assessing decision-making capacity," *Law, Medicine & Health Care*, 1990;18:196–197; see also Warizer et al., n. 26, p. 845.

47. See Beauchamp and Childress, n. 30, pp. 138–39.

48. According to the President's Commission for the Study of Ethical Problems in Medicine and Biomedical and Behavioral Research, capacity to make health care decisions requires "(1) possession of a set of values and goals; (2) the ability to communicate and to understand information; and (3) the ability to reason and to deliberate about one's choices." *Making Health Care Decisions*, n. 38, p. 57 (footnote omitted).

49. For example, a study found that traditional Navajo culture includes the belief that reality, rather than being reflected in language, is shaped by language. Because great importance is placed on avoiding negative thoughts or speech, policies requiring discussion of end-of-life issues in compliance with PSDA become ethically problematic in the Navajo community. See Carrese and Rhodes, n. 1. Likewise, attitudinal variations have been found toward disclosure of diagnosis and prognosis of terminal illness and end-of-life decision making among elderly subjects from different ethnic backgrounds. Although European Americans and African Americans preferred the patient autonomy model, Korean Americans and Mexican Americans preferred that family members deal with medical information and decision making. See Blackhall et al., n. 1; and Murphy et al., n. 1.

50. John D. Arras, interview with Ronald Kaplan, M.D., Department of Anesthesiology, Montefiore Medical Center, Bronx, NY, 1992.

51. See Beauchamp and Childress, n. 30, pp. 147–48, 142. For an analysis of informed consent as upholding patient choice and a proposal for refraining the doctrine as a constitutional right to patient choice in medical decision making, see Shultz, n. 42.

52. See Furrow BR et al., *Health Law*, 2d ed. (St. Paul, MN: West; 1991): 435.

53. See Kiev, n. 38, p. 104; and Beauchamp and Childress, n. 30, p. 150.

54. Patterson E, "The therapeutic justification for withholding medical information: what you don't know can't hurt you, or can it?" *Nebraska Law Review*, 1985;64:721–771.

55. The U.S. Supreme Court defines *waiver* as the voluntary and intentional relinquishment of a known right. See *Miranda* v. *Arizona*, 384 U.S. 436, 475-76 (1966); and *Johnson* v. *Zerbst*, 304 U.S. 458, 464 (1938).

56. See, for example, Alaska Stat. § 09.-55.556(b)(2) (Supp. 1989); Ark. Code Ann. § 16-114-206(b)(2)(c) (Michie 1987); Del. Code Ann. tit. 18, § 6852(b)(2) (Supp. 1994); N.H. Rev. Stat. Ann. § 507-C:2(II)(b)(3) (1983); Utah Code Ann. § 78-14-5(2)(c) (Supp. 1995); and Vt. Stat. Ann. tit. 12, §1909(c)(2) (Supp. 1990).

57. See, for example, *Arato*, 858 P.2d 598 Cal. (holding that a patient may validly waive the right to be informed); *Holt* v. *Nelson*, 523 P.2d 211, 219 (1974) (holding that "a physician need not disclose the hazards of treatment when the patient has requested she not be told about the danger"); and *Cobbs* v. *Grant*, 502 P.2d, 112 (1972) (holding that "a medical doctor need not make disclosures of risks when the patient requests that he not be so informed").

58. Lawrence Gostin proposes that the conflict between the patient autonomy-based informed consent doctrine and the family-centered model of caring may require legal reform to promote cultural diversity in health-care decision making. He suggests a standard of disclosure based on patient values, including the right to decide *whether* to receive medical information. Gostin LO, "Informed consent, cultural sensitivity and respect for persons," *JAMA*, 1995;274:844–845.

59. See Meisel A, "The 'exceptions' to the informed consent doctrine: striking a balance between competing values in medical decision making," *Wisconsin Law Review*, 1979:413–488. See also Carrese and Rhodes, n. 1 (discussing the importance of respecting an individual's culturally based need not to know and adopting a more communal style of decision making).

60. Some commentators frame patient waivers in terms of patient self-determination. See Meisel A, "Entrapment, informed consent, and the plea bargain," *Yale Law Journal*, 1975;84:694.

It has been suggested, however, that legal precedent and the litigious nature of contemporary medical practice require framing the issue as one of "informed" waiver, obligating physicians to alert patients to their right to waive, as well as to the consequences of forgoing knowledge of the medical risks and benefits. For a more complete discussion of informed waiver, see Gordon E, "Multiculturalism in medical decision making: the notion of informed waiver," *Fordham Urban Law Journal*, 1996;23:1321–1362.

61. For a description of the several types of nonexpressed consent, see Beauchamp and Childress, n. 30, p. 128.

62. See Schoene-Seifert B, Childress JF, "How much should the cancer patient know and decide?" *CA—A Cancer Journal for Clinicians*, 1986;36(2):90.

63. See nn. 20–29 and accompanying text.

64. It is important to distinguish between *anesthesia* ("loss of the ability to feel pain, caused by administration of a drug or by other medical interventions"), which requires informed consent, and *analgesia* ("absence of sensibility to pain . . . designating particularly the relief of pain without loss of consciousness"), which does not require informed consent. See *Dorland's Illustrated Medical Dictionary*, n. 18, pp. 79, 70.

65. It is interesting to note that patients using patient-controlled analgesia not only have a greater sense of control over their pain and its relief, they often use less analgesic medication. Telephone Interview, Dr. Carole W Agin, Director, Pain Management Service, Dept. of Anesthesiology, Montefiore Medical Center, Bronx, NY, 1997.

66. See Dresser R, Robertson J, "Quality of life and non-treatment decisions for incompetent patients," *Law, Medicine & Health Care*, 1989;17:234–244.

67. Abramson NS et al., "Consent: informed, implied, and deferred," *JAMA*, 1986;256:1892 (footnote omitted).

68. "The principle of respect for persons incorporates at least two ethical tenets: first, that individuals should be treated as autonomous agents; and second, that persons with diminished autonomy (including minors) are entitled to protection. . . . [B]eneficence is the obligation to secure the well-being of persons by acting positively on their behalf and maximizing the benefits obtained." Leikin S, "The role of adolescents in decisions concerning their cancer therapy," *Cancer Supplement*, 1993;71:3342.

69. See Levendusky P, Pankratz L, "Self-control techniques as an alternative to pain medication," *Journal of Abnormal Psychology*, 1975;84:165–168; see also Schulte PA, Ringen K, "Notification of workers at high risk: an emerging public health problem," *American Journal of Public Health*, 1984;74:485–491.

70. See n. 67 and accompanying text; and Dresser R, Whitehouse PJ, "The incompetent patient on the slippery slope," *Hastings Center Report*, 1994;24(4):6–12.

71. See, for example, "Some patients are 'barely conscious,' 'stuporous . . . with negligible awareness of self, other, and the world.' Their capacity for sentience gives such patients an interest in avoiding pain and other unpleasant physical sensations, which justifies the administration of pain-relieving medication and other palliative measures." See Dresser and Whitehouse, n. 70, p. 10 (quoting Rango N, "The nursing home resident with dementia," *Annals of Internal Medicine*, 1985;1026:835–841).

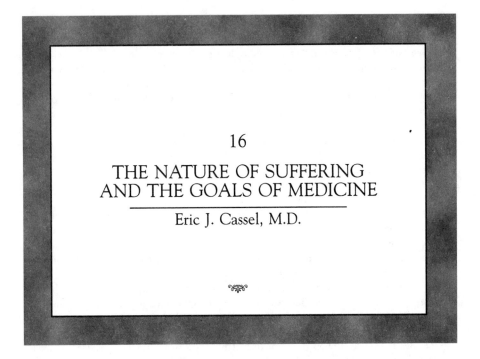

16

THE NATURE OF SUFFERING
AND THE GOALS OF MEDICINE

Eric J. Cassel, M.D.

The obligation of physicians to relieve human suffering stretches back into antiquity. Despite this fact, little attention is explicitly given to the problem of suffering in medical education, research, or practice. I will begin by focusing on a modern paradox: Even in the best settings and with the best physicians, it is not uncommon for suffering to occur not only during the course of a disease but also as a result of its treatment. To understand this paradox and its resolution requires an understanding of what suffering is and how it relates to medical care.

Consider this case: A 35-year-old sculptor with metastatic disease of the breast was treated by competent physicians employing advanced knowledge and technology and acting out of kindness and true concern. At every stage, the treatment as well as the disease was a source of suffering to her. She was uncertain and frightened about her future, but she could get little information from her physicians, and what she was told was not always the truth. She had been unaware, for example, that the irradiated breast would be so disfigured. After an oophorectomy and a regimen of medications, she became hirsute, obese, and devoid of libido. With tumor in the supraclavicular fossa, she lost strength in the hand that she had used in sculpturing, and she became

E. J. Cassel. "The Nature of Suffering and the Goals of Medicine." *New England Journal of Medicine.* 1982;306:639–645. Copyright ©1982 Massachusetts Medical Society. All rights reserved.

profoundly depressed. She had a pathologic fracture of the femur, and treatment was delayed while her physicians openly disagreed about pinning her hip.

Each time her disease responded to therapy and her hope was rekindled, a new manifestation would appear. Thus, when a new course of chemotherapy was started, she was torn between a desire to live and the fear that allowing hope to emerge again would merely expose her to misery if the treatment failed. The nausea and vomiting from the chemotherapy were distressing, but no more so than the anticipation of hair loss. She feared the future. Each tomorrow was seen as heralding increased sickness, pain, or disability, never as the beginning of better times. She felt isolated because she was no longer like other people and could not do what other people did. She feared that her friends would stop visiting her. She was sure that she would die.

This young woman had severe pain and other physical symptoms that caused her suffering. But she also suffered from some threats that were social and from others that were personal and private. She suffered from the effects of the disease and its treatment on her appearance and abilities. She also suffered unremittingly from her perception of the future.

What can this case tell us about the ends of medicine and the relief of suffering? Three facts stand out: The first is that this woman's suffering was not confined to her physical symptoms. The second is that she suffered not only from her disease but also from its treatment. The third is that one could not anticipate what she would describe as a source of suffering; like other patients, she had to be asked. Some features of her condition she would call painful, upsetting, uncomfortable, and distressing, but not a source of suffering. In these characteristics her case was ordinary.

In discussing the matter of suffering with lay persons, I learned that they were shocked to discover that the problem of suffering was not directly addressed in medical education. My colleagues of a contemplative nature were surprised at how little they knew of the problem and how little thought they had given it, whereas medical students tended to be unsure of the relevance of the issue to their work.

The relief of suffering, it would appear, is considered one of the primary ends of medicine by patients and lay persons, but not by the medical profession. As in the care of the dying, patients and their friends and families do not make a distinction between physical and nonphysical sources of suffering in the same way that doctors do.[1]

A search of the medical and social-science literature did not help me in understanding what suffering is; the word "suffering" was most often coupled with the word "pain," as in "pain and suffering." (The data bases used were *Psychological Abstracts,* the *Citation Index,* and the *Index Medicus.*)

This phenomenon reflects a historically constrained and currently inadequate view of the ends of medicine. Medicine's traditional concern primarily for the body and for physical disease is well known, as are the widespread effects of the mind-body dichotomy on medical theory and practice. I believe that this dichotomy itself is a source of the paradoxical situation in which doctors cause suffering in their care of the sick. Today, as ideas about the separation of mind and body are called into question, physicians are concerning themselves with new aspects of the human condition. The profession of medicine is being pushed and pulled into new areas, both by its technology and by the demands of its patients. Attempting to understand what suffering is and how physicians might truly be devoted to its relief will require that medicine and its critics overcome the dichotomy between mind and body and the associated dichotomies between subjective and objective and between person and object.

In the remainder of this paper I am going to make three points. The first is that suffering is experienced by persons. In the separation between mind and body, the concept of the person, or personhood, has been associated with that of mind, spirit, and the subjective. However, as I will show, a person is not merely mind, merely spiritual, or only subjectively knowable. Personhood has many facets, and it is ignorance of them that actively contributes to patients' suffering. The understanding of the place of the person in human illness requires a rejection of the historical dualism of mind and body.

The second point derives from my interpretation of clinical observations: Suffering occurs when an impending destruction of the person is perceived; it continues until the threat of disintegration has passed or until the integrity of the person can be restored in some other manner. It follows, then, that although suffering often occurs in the presence of acute pain, shortness of breath, or other bodily symptoms, suffering extends beyond the physical. Most generally, suffering can be defined as the state of severe distress associated with events that threaten the intactness of the person.

The third point is that suffering can occur in relation to any aspect of the person, whether it is in the realm of social roles; group identification; the relation with self, body, or family; or the relation with a transpersonal, transcendent source of meaning. Below is a simplified description or "topology" of the constituents of personhood.

"PERSON" IS NOT "MIND"

The split between mind and body that has so deeply influenced our approach to medical care was proposed by Descartes to resolve certain philosophical issues. Moreover, Cartesian dualism made it possible for science to escape the control of the church by assigning the noncorporeal, spiritual realm to the church, leaving the physical world as the domain of science. In that religious age, "person," synonymous with "mind," was necessarily off-limits to science.

Changes in the meaning of concepts like that of personhood occur with changes in society, while the word for the concept remains the same. This fact tends to obscure the depth of the transformations that have occurred between the seventeenth century and today. People simply are "persons" in this time, as in past times, and they have difficulty imagining that the term described something quite different in an earlier period when the concept was more constrained.

If the mind-body dichotomy results in assigning the body to medicine, and the person is not in that category, then the only remaining place for the person is in the category of mind. Where the mind is problematic (not identifiable in objective terms), its very reality diminishes for science, and so, too, does that of the person. Therefore, so long as the mind-body dichotomy is accepted, suffering is either subjective and thus not truly "real"—not within medicine's domain—or identified exclusively with bodily pain. Not only is such an identification misleading and distorting, for it depersonalizes the sick patient, but it is itself a source of suffering. It is not possible to treat sickness as something that happens solely to the body without thereby risking damage to the person. An anachronistic division of the human condition into what is medical (having to do with the body) and what is nonmedical (the remainder) has given medicine too narrow a notion of its calling. Because of this division, physicians may, in concentrating on the cure of bodily disease, do things that cause the patient as a person to suffer.

AN IMPENDING DESTRUCTION OF PERSON

Suffering is ultimately a personal matter. Patients sometimes report suffering when one does not expect it, or do not report suffering when one does expect it. Furthermore, a person can suffer enormously at the distress of another, especially a loved one.

In some theologies, suffering has been seen as bringing one closer to God. This "function" of suffering is at once its glorification and its relief. If, through great pain or deprivation, someone is brought closer to a cherished goal, that person may have no sense of having suffered but may instead feel enormous triumph. To an observer, however, only the deprivation may be apparent. This cautionary note is important because people are often said to have suffered greatly, in a religious context, when they are known only to have been injured, tortured, or in pain, not to have suffered.

Although pain and suffering are closely identified in the medical literature, they are phenomenologically distinct.[2] The difficulty of understanding pain and the problems of physicians in providing adequate relief of physical pain are well known.[3-5]

The greater the pain, the more it is believed to cause suffering. However, some pain, like that of childbirth, can be extremely severe and yet considered rewarding. The perceived meaning of pain influences the amount of medication that will be required to control it. For example, a patient reported that when she believed the pain in her leg was sciatica, she could control it with small doses of codeine, but when she discovered that it was due to the spread of malignant disease, much greater amounts of medication were required for relief. Patients can writhe in pain from kidney stones and by their own admission not be suffering, because they "know what it is"; they may also report considerable suffering from apparently minor discomfort when they do not know its source. Suffering in close relation to the intensity of pain is reported when the pain is virtually overwhelming, such as that associated with a dissecting aortic aneurysm. Suffering is also reported when the patient does not believe that the pain can be controlled. The suffering of patients with terminal cancer can often be relieved by demonstrating that their pain truly can be controlled; they will then often tolerate the same pain without any medication, preferring the pain to the side effects of their analgesics. Another type of pain that can be a source of suffering is pain that is not overwhelming but continues for a very long time.

In summary, people in pain frequently report suffering from the pain when they feel out of control, when the pain is overwhelming, when the source of the pain is unknown, when the meaning of the pain is dire, or when the pain is chronic.

In all these situations, persons perceive pain as a threat to their continued existence—not merely to their lives, but to their integrity as persons. That this is the relation of pain to suffering is strongly suggested by the fact that suffering can be relieved, in the presence of continued pain, by making the source of the pain known, changing its meaning, and demonstrating that it can be controlled and that an end is in sight.

It follows, then, that suffering has a temporal element. In order for a situation to be a source of suffering, it must influence the person's perception of future events. ("If the pain continues like this, I will be overwhelmed"; "If the pain comes from cancer, I will die"; "If the pain cannot be controlled, I will not be able to take it.") At the moment when the patient is saying, "If the pain continues like this, I will be overwhelmed," he or she is not overwhelmed. Fear itself always involves the future. In the case with which I opened this paper, the patient could not give up her fears of her sense of future, despite the agony they caused her. As suffering is discussed in the other dimensions of personhood, note how it would not exist if the future were not a major concern.

Two other aspects of the relation between pain and suffering should be mentioned. Suffering can occur when physicians do not validate the patient's pain. In the absence of disease, physicians may suggest that the pain is "psychological" (in the sense of not being real) or that the patient is "faking." Similarly, patients with chronic pain may believe after a time that they can no longer talk to others about their distress. In the former case the person is caused to distrust his or her perceptions of reality, and in both instances social isolation adds to the person's suffering.

Another aspect essential to an understanding of the suffering of sick persons is the relation of meaning to the way in which illness is experienced. The word "meaning" is used here in two senses. In the first, to mean is to signify, to imply. Pain in the chest may imply heart disease. We also say that we know what something means when we know how important it is. The importance of things is always personal and individual, even though meaning in this sense may be shared by others or by society as a whole. What something signifies and how important it is relative to the whole array of a person's concerns contribute to its personal meaning. "Belief" is another word for that aspect of meaning concerned with implications, and "value" concerns the degree of importance to a particular person.

The personal meaning of things does not consist exclusively of values and beliefs that are held intellectually; it includes other dimensions. For the same word, a person may simultaneously have a cognitive meaning, an affective or emotional meaning, a bodily meaning, and a transcendent or spiritual meaning. And there may be contradictions in the different levels of meaning. The nuances of personal meaning are complex, and when I speak of personal meanings I am implying this complexity in all its depth—known and unknown. Personal meaning is a fundamental dimension of personhood, and there can be no understanding of human illness or suffering without taking it into account.

A SIMPLIFIED DESCRIPTION OF THE PERSON

A simple topology of a person may be useful in understanding the relation between suffering and the goals of medicine. The features discussed below point the way to further study and to the possibility of specific action by individual physicians.

Persons have personality and character. Personality traits appear within the first few weeks of life and are remarkably durable over time. Some personalities handle some illnesses better than others. Individual persons vary in character as well. During the heyday of psychoanalysis in the 1950s, all behavior was attributed to unconscious determinants: No one was bad or good; they were merely sick or well. Fortunately, that simplistic view of human character is now out of favor. Some people do in fact have stronger characters and bear adversity better. Some are good and kind under the stress of terminal illness, whereas others become mean and offensive when even mildly ill.

A person has a past. The experiences gathered during one's life are a part of today as well as yesterday. Memory exists in the nostrils and the hands, not only in the mind. A fragrance drifts by, and a memory is evoked. My feet have not forgotten how to roller skate, and my hands remember skills that I was hardly aware I had learned. When these past experiences involve sickness and medical care, they can influence present illness and medical care. They stimulate fear, confidence, physical symptoms, and anguish. It damages people to rob them of their past and deny their memories, or to mock their fears and worries. A person without a past is incomplete.

Life experiences—previous illness; experiences with doctors, hospitals, and medications; deformities and disabilities; pleasures and successes; miseries and failures—a form the nexus for illness. The personal meaning of the disease and its treatment arises from the past as well as the present. If cancer occurs in a patient with self-confidence from past achievements, it may give rise to optimism and a resurgence of strength. Even if it is fatal, the disease may not produce the destruction of the person but, rather, reaffirm his or her indomitability. The outcome would be different in a person for whom life had been a series of failures.

The intensity of ties to the family cannot be overemphasized; people frequently behave as though they were physical extensions of their parents. Events that might cause suffering in others may be borne without complaint by someone who believes that the disease is part of his or her family identity and hence inevitable. Even diseases for which no heritable basis is known may be borne easily by a person because others in the family have been similarly afflicted. Just as the person's past experiences give meaning to present events, so do the past experiences of his or her family. Those meanings are part of the person.

A person has a cultural background. Just as a person is part of a culture and a society, these elements are part of the person. Culture defines what is meant by masculinity or femininity, what attire is acceptable, attitudes toward the dying and sick, mating behavior, the height of chairs and steps, degrees of tolerance for odors and excreta, and how the aged and the disabled are treated. Cultural definitions have an enormous impact on the sick and can be a source of untold suffering. They influence the behavior of others toward the sick person and that of the sick toward themselves.

Cultural norms and social rules regulate whether someone can be among others or will be isolated, whether the sick will be considered foul or acceptable, and whether they are to be pitied or censured.

Returning to the sculptor described earlier, we know why that young woman suffered. She was housebound and bedbound, her face was changed by steroids. She was masculinized by her treatment, one breast was scarred, and she had almost no hair. The degree of importance attached to these losses—that aspect of their personal meaning—is determined to a great degree by cultural priorities.

With this in mind, we can also realize how much someone devoid of physical pain, even devoid of "symptoms," may suffer. People suffer from what they have lost of themselves in relation to the world of objects, events, and relationships. We realize, too, that although medical care can reduce the impact of sickness, inattentive care can increase the disruption caused by illness.

A person has roles. I am a husband, a father, a physician, a teacher, a brother, an orphaned son, and an uncle. People are their roles, and each role has rules. Together, the rules that guide the performance of roles make up a complex set of entitlements and limitations of responsibility and privilege. By middle age, the roles may be so firmly set that disease can lead to the virtual destruction of a person by making the performance of his or her roles impossible. Whether the patient is a doctor who cannot doctor or a mother who cannot mother, he or she is diminished by the loss of function.

No person exists without others; there is no consciousness without a consciousness of others, no speaker without a hearer, and no act, object, or thought that does not somehow encompass others.[6] All behavior is or will be involved with others, even if only in memory or reverie. Take away others, remove sight or hearing, and the person is diminished. Everyone dreads becoming blind or deaf, but these are only the most obvious injuries to human interaction. There are many ways in which human beings can be cut off from others and then suffer the loss.

It is in relationships with others that the full range of human emotions finds expression. It is this dimension of the person that may be injured when illness disrupts the ability to express emotion. Furthermore, the extent and nature of a sick person's relationships influence the degree of suffering from a disease. There is a vast difference between going home to an empty apartment and going home to a network of friends and family after hospitalization. Illness may occur in one partner of a long and strongly bound marriage or in a union that is falling apart. Suffering from the loss of sexual function associated with some diseases will depend not only on the importance of sexual performance itself but also on its importance in the sick person's relationships.

A person is a political being. A person is in this sense equal to other persons, with rights and obligations and the ability to redress injury by others and the state. Sickness can interfere, producing the feeling of political powerlessness and lack of representation. Persons who are permanently handicapped may suffer from a feeling of exclusion from participation in the political realm.

Persons do things. They act, create, make, take apart, put together, wind, unwind, cause to be, and cause to vanish. They know themselves, and are known, by these acts. When illness restricts the range of activity of persons, they are not themselves.

Persons are often unaware of much that happens within them and why. Thus, there are things in the mind that cannot be brought to awareness by ordinary reflection. The structure of the unconscious is pictured quite differently by different scholars, but most students of human behavior accept the assertion that such an interior world exists. People can behave in ways that seem inexplicable and strange even to themselves, and the sense of powerlessness that the person may feel in the presence of such behavior can be a source of great distress.

Persons have regular behaviors. In health, we take for granted the details of our day-to-day behavior. Persons know themselves to be well as much by whether they behave as usual as by any other set of facts. Patients decide that they are ill because they cannot perform as usual, and they may suffer the loss of their routine. If they cannot do the things that they identify with the fact of their being, they are not whole.

Every person has a body. The relation with one's body may vary from identification with it to admiration, loathing, or constant fear. The body may even be perceived as a representation of a parent, so that when something happens to the person's body it is as though a parent were injured. Disease can so alter the relation that the body is no longer seen as a friend but, rather, as an untrustworthy enemy. This is intensified if the illness comes on without warning, and as illness persists, the person may feel increasingly vulnerable. Just as many people have an expanded sense of self as a result of changes in their bodies from exercise, the potential exists for a contraction of this sense through injury to the body.

Everyone has a secret life. Sometimes it takes the form of fantasies and dreams of glory; sometimes it has a real existence known to only a few. Within the secret life are fears, desires, love affairs of the past and present, hopes, and fantasies. Disease may destroy not only the public or the private person but the secret person as well. A secret beloved friend may be lost to a sick person because he or she has no legitimate place by the sickbed. When that happens, the patient may have lost the part of life that made tolerable an otherwise embittered existence. Or the loss may be only of a dream, but one that might have come true. Such loss can be a source of great distress and intensely private pain.

Everyone has a perceived future. Events that one expects to come to pass vary from expectations for one's children to a belief in one's creative ability. Intense unhappiness results from a loss of the future—the future of the individual person, of children, and of other loved ones. Hope dwells in this dimension of existence, and great suffering attends the loss of hope.

Everyone has a transcendent dimension, a life of the spirit. This is most directly expressed in religion and the mystic traditions, but the frequency with which people have intense feelings of bonding with groups, ideals, or anything larger and more enduring than the person is evidence of the universality of the transcendent dimension. The quality of being greater and more lasting than an individual life gives this aspect of the person its timeless dimension. The profession of medicine appears to ignore the human spirit. When I see patients in nursing homes who have become only bodies, I wonder whether it is not their transcendent dimension that they have lost.

THE NATURE OF SUFFERING

For purposes of explanation, I have outlined various parts that make up a person. However, persons cannot be reduced to their parts in order to be better understood. Reductionist scientific methods, so successful in human biology, do not help us to comprehend whole persons. My intent was rather to suggest the complexity of the person and the potential for injury and suffering that exists in everyone. With this in mind, any suggestion of mechanical simplicity should disappear from my definition of suffering. All the aspects of personhood—the lived past, the family's lived past, culture and society, roles, the instrumental dimension, associations and relationships, the body, the unconscious mind, the political being, the secret life, the perceived future, and the transcendent dimension—are susceptible to damage and loss.

Injuries to the integrity of the person may be expressed by sadness, anger, loneliness, depression, grief, unhappiness, melancholy, rage, withdrawal, or yearning. We acknowledge the person's right to have and express such feelings. But we often forget that the affect is merely the outward expression of the injury, not the injury itself. We know little about the nature of the injuries themselves, and what we know has been learned largely from literature, not medicine.

If the injury is sufficient, the person suffers. The only way to learn what damage is sufficient to cause suffering, or whether suffering is present, is to ask the sufferer. We all recognize certain injuries that almost invariably cause suffering: the death or distress of loved ones, powerlessness, helplessness, hopelessness, torture, the loss of a life's work, betrayal, physical agony, isolation, homelessness, memory failure, and fear. Each is both universal and individual. Each touches features common to all of us, yet each contains features that must be defined in terms of a specific person at a specific time. With the relief of suffering in mind, however, we should reflect on how remarkably little is known of these injuries.

THE AMELIORATION OF SUFFERING

One might inquire why everyone is not suffering all the time. In a busy life, almost no day passes in which one's intactness goes unchallenged. Obviously, not every challenge is a threat. Yet I suspect that there is more suffering than is known. Just as people with chronic pain learn to keep it to themselves because others lose interest, so may those with chronic suffering.

There is another reason why every injury may not cause suffering. Persons are able to enlarge themselves in response to damage, so that instead of being reduced, they may indeed grow. This response to suffering has encouraged the belief that suffering is good for people. To some degree, and in some persons, this may be so. If a leg is injured so that an athlete cannot run again, the athlete may compensate for the loss by learning another sport or mode of expression. So it is with the loss of relationships, loves, roles, physical strength, dreams, and power. The human body may lack the capacity to gain a new part when one is lost, but the person has it.

The ability to recover from loss without succumbing to suffering is sometimes called resilience, as though nothing but elastic rebound were involved, but it is more as though an inner force were withdrawn from one manifestation of a person and redirected to another. If a child dies and the parent makes a successful recovery, the person is said to have "rebuilt" his or her life. The term suggests that the parts of the person are structured in a new manner, allowing expression in different dimensions. If a previously active person is confined to a wheelchair, intellectual pursuits may occupy more time.

Recovery from suffering often involves help, as though people who have lost parts of themselves can be sustained by the personhood of others until their own recovers. This is one of the latent functions of physicians: to lend strength. A group, too, may lend strength: Consider the success of groups of the similarly afflicted in easing the burden of illness (e.g., women with mastectomies, people with ostomies, and even the parents or family members of the diseased).

Meaning and transcendence offer two additional ways by which the suffering associated with destruction of a part of personhood is ameliorated. Assigning a meaning to the injurious condition often reduces or even resolves the suffering associated with it. Most often, a cause for the condition is sought within past behaviors or beliefs. Thus, the pain or threat that causes suffering is seen as not destroying a part of the person, because it is part of the person by virtue of its origin within the self. In our culture, taking the blame for harm that comes to oneself because of the unconscious mind serves the same purpose as the concept of karma in Eastern theologies; suffering is reduced when it can be located within a coherent set of meanings. Physicians are familiar with the question from the sick, "Did I do something that made this happen?" It is more tolerable for a terrible thing to happen because of something that one has done than it is to be at the mercy of chance.

Transcendence is probably the most powerful way in which one is restored to wholeness after an injury to personhood. When experienced, transcendence locates the person in a far larger landscape. The sufferer is not isolated by pain but is brought closer to a transpersonal source of meaning and to the human community that shares those meanings. Such an experience need not involve religion in any formal sense; however, in its transpersonal dimension, it is deeply spiritual. For example, patriotism can be a secular expression of transcendence.

WHEN SUFFERING CONTINUES

But what happens when suffering is not relieved? If suffering occurs when there is a threat to one's integrity or a loss of a part of a person, then suffering will continue if the person cannot be made whole again. Little is known about this aspect of suffering. Is much of what we call depression merely unrelieved suffering? Considering that depression commonly follows the loss of loved ones, business reversals, prolonged illness, profound injuries to self-esteem, and other damages to personhood, the possibility is real. In many chronic or serious diseases, persons who "recover" or who seem to be successfully treated do not return to normal function. They may never again be employed, recover sexual function, pursue career goals, reestablish family relationships, or reenter the social world, despite a physical cure. Such patients may not have recovered from the nonphysical changes occurring with serious illness. Consider the dimensions of personhood described above, and note that each is threatened or damaged in profound illness. It should come as no surprise, then, that chronic suffering frequently follows in the wake of disease.

The paradox with which this paper began—that suffering is often caused by the treatment of the sick—no longer seems so puzzling. How could it be otherwise, when medicine has concerned itself so little with the nature and causes of suffering? This lack is not a failure of good intentions. None are more concerned about pain or loss of function than physicians. Instead, it is a failure of knowledge and understanding. We lack knowledge, because in working from a dichotomy contrived within a historical context far from our own, we have artificially circumscribed our task in caring for the sick.

Attempts to understand all the known dimensions of personhood and their relations to illness and suffering present problems of staggering complexity. The problems are no greater, however, than those initially posed by the question of how the body works—a question that we have managed to answer in extraordinary detail. If the ends of medicine are to be directed toward the relief of human suffering, the need is clear.

I am indebted to Rabbi Jack Bemporad; to Drs. Joan Cassell, Pew Diann, Nancy McKenzie, and Richard Zaner; to Ms. Dawn McGuire; to the members of the Research Group on Death, Suffering, and Well-Being of the Hastings Center, for their advice and assistance; and to the Arthur Vining Davis Foundations for support of the research group.

REFERENCES

1. Cassell E. Being mad becoming dead. *Soc Res.* 1972;39:528–542.

2. Bakan D. *Disease, Pain, and Sacrifice: Toward a Psychology of Suffering.* Chicago: Beacon Press; 1971.

3. Murks RM, Sachar EJ. Undertreatment of medical inpatients with narcotic analgesics. *Annals of Internal Medicine.* 1973;78:173–181.

4. Know RM, Foley KM. Pains of narcotic drug use in a cancer pain clink. *Annals of the New York Academy of Science.* 1991;362:161–172.

5. Goodwin JS, Goodwin JM, Vold AV. Knowledge and use of placebos by house officers and mum. *Annals of Internal Medicine.* 1979;91:106–110.

6. Zaner R. *The Context of Self: A Phenomenological Inquiry Using Medicine As a Clue.* Athens, OH: Ohio University Press; 1981.

Part 6

THE ROLE
OF RELATIONSHIPS
IN HEALTH CARE

꧁꧂

E laborate tests, grand technologies, and cutting-edge procedures have long defined our health-care system. Yet even with the multitude of dilemmas these advances have brought about, it is the relationships among patients, proxies, and health-care providers that create the most problems. This could not be otherwise, as even within our own families misunderstandings and conflicts easily arise, and it is our families with whom we have deeply personal bonds. Now consider an intensive care setting where there are no preexisting personal bonds: complete strangers are forced into intimate circumstances, those involved have no sense of each other's values, and every decision has the potential to cause serious harm. It is undeniable that these factors impede the development of good relationships in the intensive care setting, but they can be worked through. In this section, Nancy Neveloff Dubler and Mary Corley provide us with two important insights: First, they help us understand the complexity, magnitude, and consequences of these factors; then, they help us develop a framework to establish and maintain good relationships with proxy decision makers and fellow health-care providers.

Nancy Neveloff Dubler begins this section with "The Doctor-Proxy Relationship: The Neglected Connection." A proxy is someone who has been designated by a patient to make health-care decisions should the patient lose decision-making capacity. Depending on the language used in a state's advance directive legislation, the terms "surrogate" or "agent" may be used in place of proxy; for our purpose they are interchangeable. Proxies typically are designated though a Durable Power of

Attorney for Health Care, but they do not have to be. Many states have created a hierarchy of decision makers in the event that a patient loses capacity without having designated a proxy. The hierarchy usually flows from guardian to spouse to adult child to parent to adult sibling to adult grandchild to close friend.

Throughout her article, Dubler helps us to understand how important it is for health-care providers to seek out and connect with a proxy, if at all possible while the patient still has capacity. Through making an effort to create a relationship between patient, proxy, and health-care provider, the patient and proxy will be able to trust the health-care team as well as feel cared for, supported, and respected as a "couple." By "couple," I mean that the proxy's place in the patient's life is acknowledged and honored. Forming this kind of relationship also affords the opportunity to gain insight into the proxy: How will the patient's death affect the proxy's everyday life? What are the emotional needs of the proxy? How is the proxy likely to respond if the patient's condition worsens? What is the best way to provide this particular proxy with information? What additional circumstances or family dynamics might make the proxy's role more difficult? The benefits derived from such information are obvious.

When three-way relationships are not established, harm is caused by a lack of support, as the first case study in this article makes clear. The theme of this case study is by many accounts the status quo—proxies are recognized as such only when the question of withdrawing or withholding treatment arises. Situate yourself as the proxy in a similar situation: You are grieving and you have been alienated from your grandmother's care. You are unsure of the severity of her condition as well as what she would want done. Your grandmother's prognosis then becomes grim enough that the health-care team, with whom you have no relationship, wants to include you in a discussion of treatment options. Unfortunately, "a discussion of treatment options" is actually a euphemism for "we are going to take one of most difficult decisions someone can make, and dump it in your lap."

On the contrary, if the proxy has an established, supportive relationship with the health-care team, the decision to withhold or withdraw treatment is not so stark; nor does it feel like a bomb has been dropped. Dubler attempts to foster this kind of relationship by helping us think about the proxy's practical and emotional needs; what his role ought to be; and how health-care providers can facilitate, encourage, and support his attempt to speak for the patient.

There is an important side issue that needs to be briefly discussed regarding the distinction between having an alternative and having a choice. Returning to the scenario above, if your grandmother's condition has deteriorated to the point where the health-care team has initiated a "discussion of treatment options," it is a matter of debate whether the options (or alternatives) presented truly constitute a choice. Where is the choice in this: "If your grandmother dies, do you want us to try to save her or do you want us to let her to die?" This question does in fact offer two courses of action, but it would be naive to think that the question itself is anything but coercive.

The next article takes us from health-care provider–proxy relationships to relationships among the health-care team. In "Ethical Dimensions of Nurse-Physician Relations in Critical Care," Mary Corley carefully considers one of the most troubling moral dilemmas for health-care providers: how to respond to other health-care providers whose actions are perceived as unprofessional or unethical. Corley begins by making explicit what is at stake. It has been shown that when poor relationships between physicians and nurses are present, patient mortality increases. Conversely, studies have shown a correlation between good relationships among health-care providers and shorter hospital stays and better care for patients and their families. Importantly, even though Corley's article was written about physician-nurse conflicts, the issues raised and the conflict resolution strategies discussed are certainly relevant to other combinations of health-care providers—physician–social worker, nurse-para-medic, nurse-nurse, and so on.

Interprofessional relationships can be overtly and subtly affected by a variety of factors. For instance, gender roles, experience, socioeconomic status, "uniforms," phi-losophy of care, and ethnicity all have the potential to bring about misunderstandings, distrust, and conflicts as well as camaraderie, respect, and collaboration. Corley takes on some of the more difficult dynamics that can cause concerns and conflicts to arise between health-care providers, such as differing values, communication obstacles, willingness to trust, and various institutional impediments. With this understanding in hand we now have a grounding from which to build conflict resolution strategies. A significant first step in a relationship-improvement process would be for ethics com-mittees to review their institutions' policies and procedures in order to incorporate these strategies where appropriate.

17

THE DOCTOR-PROXY RELATIONSHIP

The Neglected Connection

Nancy Neveloff Dubler, LL.B.

꽃

Advance directives are touted by some as the "magic bullets" of bioethics. They are expected to vanquish the anguish and angst that always accompany the intractable dilemmas of decision making for incapacitated and incompetent patients. The argument goes like this: If people, when competent, execute documents attesting to their specific desires for future medical care or appoint decision makers anointed with the legal and moral authority to make future care decisions, then the ethical problems of deciding for incapacitated patients will be solved.

This enthusiasm for advance directives has infected scholars in medicine and bioethics.[1-3] There is now a vast literature that surveys which sorts of patients execute advance directives and how we can encourage more to do so.[4] Despite some critiques[5] and concerns,[6-8] professional organizations, including the American Medical Association, the American College of Physicians, and the American Nursing Association, have endorsed advance directives and urged members of their associations to pay attention to this aspect of patient discussion and care.[9-11] Citizens groups, lay bioethics councils, and organizations such as the American Association of Retired Persons (AARP), have staged community education campaigns to encourage their members to

N. Dubler. "The Doctor-Proxy Relationship: The Neglected Connection." *Kennedy Institute of Ethics Journal.* 1995;5(4):289–306. © The Johns Hopkins University Press.

This article is based on the 1995 Isaac Franck Distinguished Memorial Lecture at the Kennedy Institute of Ethics.

"sign up" their health-care agents. Indeed, the AARP has had more than 800,000 requests for the pamphlet "Health Care Powers of Attorney."[12] Editors of peer review journals continue to publish articles on the topic despite the sizeable number of articles already in existence. Both the Congress of the United States (in the passage of the Patient Self-Determination Act of 1990 [PSDA], sections 4206 and 4751 of Omnibus Reconciliation Act of 1990, Pub L No. 101-508 [November 5, 1990]) and the United States Supreme Court (in *Cruzan* v. *Director, Missouri Department of Health*, 110 S. Ct. 2841 [1990]) have endorsed the expanded use of these instruments and their constitutionality. Support for advance directives is strong and growing.

Indeed, the PSDA[13] now makes it mandatory to ask all patients in hospitals, nursing homes, and HMOs (receiving federal funds) whether they have an advance directive or wish to complete one.[14,15] And, in the *Cruzan* case, the United States Supreme Court upheld the constitutionality of a state rule that care can be discontinued from an incompetent patient only when there is clear and convincing evidence of the formerly competent patient's prior explicit directives, a standard that, in general, can only be met by the execution of an advance directive. One legal commentator noted that "the most significant impact of the *Cruzan* case is widespread advocacy for advance directives because the court decision suggests that the best protection for any person is to execute a formally written advance directive."[16]

This extensive endorsement of advance directives might make it appear as if the principled analyses of decision making and discussions of patients' rights that have occurred in the last two decades have succeeded in creating an ethically coherent universe for patient and proxy choice. We might be inclined to think that if advance directives became only a bit more widespread, we will have put to rest many of the ethical quandaries of caring for the elderly and incapacitated—a true bioethical magic bullet.

However, despite cheerleading, advocacy, and exhortation,[17-20] observations do not make one sanguine that advance directives will solve all ethical dilemmas about care and treatment of the decisionally incapacitated. The reasons for skepticism are many. First, despite education and advertisement, there are still very few patients who actually execute advance directives—somewhere between 10 and 25 percent according to the recent data.[21,22] Second, as multicultural commentaries demonstrate, willingness to talk about and plan for death is taboo in many societies.[23] In a heterogeneous population we cannot expect or require behaviors that are interdicted by religion or custom.[24] Third, the notion that advance directives serve the interests of incapacitated patients is challenged by scholars who argue that these patients are so different from their preincapacitated selves that their contemporary best interests can only be served by present analysis of their pleasures, pains, joys, and suffering.[25] And, fourth, despite the existence of advance directives, it is becoming clear that these directives have little impact on the care that is actually delivered.[26-28] An additional reason may be that proxies and health-care agents, once appointed, are either neglected or more actively excluded from the health-care decision-making process. It may be that physicians are uncertain about how to relate to proxies and are, therefore, reluctant to include them in discussions about care plans where their participation might have a real impact.

Rather than solving all problems, the use of advance directives is creating   new categories of problems: for the proxies who must face life-and-death decisions without adequate information and emotional support and for the physicians who are slipping back into decision-making patterns that revive and reinvigorate dormant paternalistic habits. Indeed, the raging debate about provision of "futile" care may reflect, in some part, the growing tension between physicians and proxies.

CASE ILLUSTRATIONS OF DILEMMAS IN THE DOCTOR-PROXY RELATIONSHIP

Proxies or health-care agents are appointed by patients when they are decisionally capable. The proxies are charged with making decisions about a patient's care. Despite the legal reality that these appointments confer broad grants of authority, the choice and powers of agents are generally, or only, invoked at the moment of deciding whether the patient should live or die. For proxies, usually loved relatives and friends of the patient, the responsibilities of deciding are awesome and the supports provided by the medical-care system are generally inadequate. Many of the problems flow from the lack of a developed ethic defining the doctor-proxy relationship. It is this relationship that I would like to explore.

Case One

A bioethics consultant was called by a surgeon—a sufficiently rare event in itself—to consult on a case under his care. The case involved an eighty-two-year-old woman, Mrs. Alba, who had been hit by a bicycle and suffered a hip fracture. The fracture had been surgically repaired; the patient had done reasonably well and had been transferred from the Surgical Intensive Care Unit (SICU). Two days after her transfer she developed internal bleeding and was returned to the SICU. Blood transfusions were started with the hope that the bleeding would cease. It did not.

Despite the fact that Mrs. Alba had lived at home before her hospitalization, she had for years suffered from hypertension, diabetes, and congestive heart failure. These chronic medical conditions had seemed under control, but as problems developed in the SICU the degree of cardiac, renal, and vascular impairment was discovered to be substantial.

Mrs. Alba deteriorated rapidly. At this point her granddaughter, who was her only living relative, was identified by the staff as the legal proxy for the patient. Despite the fact that she had come daily to the SICU and had been informed about her grandmother's progress, she had neither been engaged by the staff in an in-depth discussion of her grandmother's prognosis nor been asked to be part of decisions made about her grandmother's care plan. Care proceeded as if choices were not being made.

On the fifth day post surgical hip repair and the third day after the bleeding had begun, the surgeon met with the granddaughter and asked her if they should attempt laser surgery to stem the bleeding. The surgeon explained that there was a 50 percent chance that her grandmother would survive the surgery, but a 100 percent chance that she would die without it.

The SICU staff was far less optimistic about the patient's chance of surviving surgery. Monitored data indicated substantial multiorgan impairment and some organ failure. The SICU staff thought that the patient's chance of surviving the surgery were slim and that her chance of leaving the hospital for home was close to zero. These predictions were not shared with proxy.

The granddaughter was frightened and distraught when the ethicist met with her. She felt that she had the obligation and the power to decide if her grandmother lived or died. She felt battered by the comments of the SICU staff who joined her and the bioethics consultant for a discussion. She was dismayed by the grudging agreement of the surgeon that the patient's prospects for returning home were quite slim.

With the SICU attending physician and the surgeon in the room, the proxy began to talk about her grandmother: how she got up every day and got dressed beautifully with makeup and jewelry and made ready to face the day, shopping, visiting, and playing cards with her neighbors and friends; how she loved her apartment and valued her privacy and the control of her environment; how she had never wanted to go to a nursing home; and how fierce she was about never letting anyone see her unless she was perfectly groomed.

Gradually the granddaughter began to grope toward the conclusion that she should refuse to grant permission for the surgery because it was likely to fail and, even if it succeeded, it would place her grandmother in precisely the position that she feared most. One might think that the fact that her grandmother had told her that she would nor want to "be on machines" or ever live in a long-term care residence would have been helpful and comforting. It was not. The feelings of being alone and responsible were overwhelming.

Comment

The proxy in this case was nor involved in ongoing decisions about her grandmother's care. In many cases that involve proxies, the staff seems to view the proxy not as an extension of the patient—someone in need of information, support, and counsel—but rather as an extension of the medical team—a new sort of junior colleague to involve sporadically in the decision-making process (personal communication with Douglas Shenson, M.D., June 1995). But ambivalence about the proxy creates even more contradictions. In addition to being seen as a colleague, the proxy is also seen as a sort of superconsultant who is called in for the "really big" decision.

This represents a fundamental misunderstanding of the role and the claims of the proxy. The proxy is not only a loved and trusted relative or friend who will know and be able to apply the patient's personal values and preferences to medical choices. She is not only a convenient, legally empowered decider—although given our risk-averse medical-care environment she is that, too. The proxy is a vulnerable person who not only stands as the agent of the patient, but also stands simultaneously in the shoes of the patient and in her own shoes. In most cases the proxy is a loving relative who must make a life-and-death decision in the midst of grief. Certainly there must be obligations of support and compassion that are owed by the medical-care team to such a person. The theory of appointing an agent should lay the foundation for the notion that the proxy will inherit the persona of the patient and will be alerted to and involved in the changing medical picture. Certainly this case does not illustrate that point.

The vast literature on the doctor-patient relationship, on the appointment of proxies, and on advance directives says virtually nothing about the doctor-proxy relationship. This is so despite the fact that the underlying relationship with the patient could easily be extended to the proxy. In their discussions of doctors and patients, commentators point out that the obligations of medical professionals always extend beyond the technical aspects of truth telling and information sharing and that the demands of relationship require discussions of virtue ethics, compassion, and empathy. Doctors are urged to relate to patients with fealty and loyalty. These terms are not applied to the doctor-proxy relationship. They are, however, appropriate terms if the proxy is to inherit not only the obligation of the patient to decide, but also the right of the patient to be treated with compassion and respect.

It is even more startling, as this first case illustrates, that the staff seems not to have any conception of the role of the proxy, the place of the proxy in the decision process, the needs of the proxy, or the ability of the proxy to process adequately the information that defines and supports choice. The fact that the proxy is a person to whom obligations are owed and not just a person from whom responsibilities are demanded appears to have been overlooked.

Case Two

Mr. Morris is a seventy-six-year-old bedfast resident of a nursing home associated with a major teaching hospital. Two years prior to the events described he suffered a left brain stroke that left him with a hemiparesis. Shortly thereafter he underwent surgery for throat cancer, which left him greatly weakened and with a permanent tracheostomy. These two events, combined with chronic obstructive pulmonary disease (COPD), precluded his return home as his physical disabilities were overwhelming to his timid and very anxious wife.

In the fall of 1994, at Mr. Morris's yearly physical, the physician noticed a solitary pulmonary nodule that had not been there the year before. Given the patient's chronic alcoholism and pack year smoking history the physician suspected, with a high degree of probability, that the patient's X-ray reflected lung cancer. This would also account for the patient's recent weight loss and general weakening.

It was unclear whether the patient was capable of making health-care decisions. The stroke had clearly produced an expressive aphasia that was likely accompanied by receptive aphasia. There was clearly some cognitive compromise and some idiosyncratic presentation the meaning of which eluded the physician. These patient characteristics precluded discussion about his wishes for diagnosis and treatment.

The attending physician judged that Mr. Morris's life was not immediately threatened. He did not think the patient sufficiently strong to withstand the diagnostic tests that would confirm the diagnosis of lung cancer or sufficiently vigorous to undergo surgery or chemotherapy.

Mrs. Morris was at his bedside daily. She was anxious about his weight loss and concerned that everything be done to preserve his health and life. Whenever offered alternative options for care, Mrs. Morris, who was the legal proxy, chose the most aggressive path. The doctor decided not to tell the wife about the patient's probable condition based on her evaluation of the patient's medical condition, the likely prognosis and the impossibility of aggressive treatment, and the wife's anxiety and likely desire for aggressive care.

Comment

Under law the proxy inherits the ethical mantle and legal authority of the patient upon the patient's incapacity. Given this new status, the proxy must be treated as if she were the patient and be informed adequately and honestly about the patient's condition and prognosis. In this second case, the proxy is presented with only that information that would support her deciding as the physician thinks appropriate. It would be odd under these conditions for the physician to justify withholding information if the patient were the decider. Bur this experienced, ethically aware physician was not a bit embarrassed to recount her distorted discussion of the patient's condition with the proxy. The obligation of supportive truth telling, the backbone of the doctor-patient relationship, seems not to have survived the transition to the proxy.

As these cases demonstrate, the plight of the proxy is often to be overwhelmed and uninformed. Somehow, in the rush to urge the completion of advance directives, a notion of the obligation of others to the proxy has not emerged as a companion to the obligation of the proxy to the patient. Life-and-death decisions appear to be presented to proxies with none of the supports that we regularly expect in the doctor-patient relationship. Yet these decisions—to permit the death of another—may be even more difficult than a patient's decision to refuse care for him- or herself.

HISTORY OF THE PROXY

Technically the concept of health-care proxy or agent evolved out of the power of attorney—the basic legal instrument that permitted an adult to transfer his or her rights to another. Traditionally the appointment of an agent transferred authority over assets or property and was terminated by the incapacity of the principal. Since it was a grant of power, it ended when there was in fact no longer any power left for the person of the principal to grant. In the mid-twentieth century, however, states, by statute, made the power of attorney "durable," that is, made it able, on the election of the principal, to survive incapacity. Proxies and health-care agents are new names for this old agency appointment when the powers that are granted focus on health-care decisions and not on the management of property.

These grants of authority to specific persons have increased as the limitations of living wills in the absence of a person acting as health care proxy became more evident.[1,29,30] Living wills had a brief period of ascendance,[31,32] but the problems identified early in the history of these documents have proved to be enduring. It has remained the case that few people execute living wills, and when they do, the documents are either too vague or too specific and may have too narrow or too wide a trigger event. It is also the case that a living will is a piece of paper, which can be filed, forgotten, or lost. It is unlikely to surface, at least in an urban teaching hospital, to affect the patient's care in precisely the ways that the patient might have wished. In many cases, what is needed is not a piece of paper, but rather an advocate who can interpose, investigate, argue, cajole, and, even then, struggle to achieve the outcome that she believes the patient would have wanted. Despite the appearance of certainty that derailed, intervention-focused advance directives offer, they may actually shift attention away from overall treatment goals or request inappropriate care.[29] Such documents require a patient to predict in advance the future medical interventions that may be used to postpone death; they also require physician interpretation and may even discourage discussions with the proxy.[33]

In clinical practice, advance directives are not always important determinants of treatment decisions. Physicians may lack familiarity with and interest in these documents; they may rarely encounter them in practice; and they may very well not alter treatment decisions because of them. Instead, physicians often rely on the traditional bases for decision making: physician-patient-family consensus, medical and ethical values, their own perception of potential civil or criminal liability, and their personal moral and ethical beliefs.[34] All of these recognized limitations of living wills provide the impetus for appointing proxies.

Thus the need for a new and more effective extension of patient choice grew out of experience with the limitations of living wills as effective instruments for guiding and restraining interventions at the end of life. Perceptions of the need for change and the clever identification of the durable power of attorney as an available legal route for empowerment led to the development of health-care agent or proxy appointment. Forty-nine states now have legislation permitting these grants of authority.[35]

The durable power of attorney provides a route by which persons when capable can empower another to act for them in their future incapacity. Moreover, this agent can be a real advocate for the patient and can interpret the patient's wishes through the lens of probability of outcome. Those are the possible benefits of this appointment for the patient and for the physician. But there are also burdens and obligations that flow from the arrangement.

PROBLEMS WITH THE DOCTOR-PROXY RELATIONSHIP

A number of court decisions fueled the development of advance directives. In 1976, the Supreme Court of New Jersey decided the *Quinlan* case (In re Quinlan, 70 N.J. 10, 35S A.2d 664, *cert denied sub nom*, *Garger* v. *New Jersey*, 429 U.S. 922 [1976]), and states began to experience experiment with common law rules and statutes that would address the complex of problems that surround decisions to permit death for incapacitated patients.

The *Quinlan* case focused the public's attention on the fact that, increasingly in modern medicine, decisions must be made to permit death. The moral hazards of decisions about death were immediately apparent to physicians, to judges, and to the public. Such decisions are sufficiently grave when the patient and physician jointly assess the future and choose death. They are potentially more anguishing and certainly more legally and morally complex when the decision to facilitate death rests with someone other than the patient. Since *Quinlan*, it has become commonly accepted that a vast number of deaths, especially in hospitals, are negotiated. In an only slightly exaggerated recent statement, the medical director of an intensive care unit said to me that "no one dies in the ICU unless someone makes the decision." How these decisions will be made, with what authority, governed by what standards, and protected by what procedures and possibilities of review still remain among the important questions that engage citizens, patients, physicians, bioethicists, legislators, judges, and patient advocates.

Some of the problems now visible in the doctor-proxy relationship have their origin in early cases about surrogate decision making, such as *Quinlan*, *Saikewicz*, and *Eichner* (*Saikewicz* v. *Superintendent of Belchertown State School*, 373 Mass. 728, 370 N.E.2d 417 [1977]; In re Eichner (In re Storar), 52 N.Y.2d 363, 438 N.Y.S.2d. 266, *cert. denied*, 454 U.S. 858 [1981]). Although most commentators have seen the role of these cases as setting the substantive standards and procedural guidelines for planning care of the incapacitated, they may also be described as cases that seek to protect the patient from the decisions of the natural surrogates—the natural proxies—such as close family and friends, who traditionally made these decisions in the past.

The early cases in surrogate decision making search for a formula that will protect the patient from the possibly "wrong" decision of the natural proxy. The court opinions establish objective criteria and use due process to guide and constrain the choice. The assumption of the cases is that legal standards and legal process are necessary to protect the patient from the improper, misguided, conflicted, or self-interested decision of the proxy—a decision, we can assume, that may be at odds with the real interests of the patient.

This is neither to disparage nor to dismiss the legal and moral struggles of these cases. They probed the meaning of the advances in medical knowledge and technology that had occurred in the previous two decades and opened up public discussion of decisions to permit death. But they also challenged the authority of the previously accepted decision makers, who, prior to these cases, had been turned to for moral authority and medical choice. This suspicion of the previously accepted "natural proxy" has, I would argue, formed the historical foundation for the present problems in the doctor-proxy relationship. The fact that natural proxies were to be supervised and their decisions circumscribed diminished the stature of such persons; these same persons now appear as legally appointed proxies, but carry with them the suspicion of their role.

A second reason that the proxy may be ignored by physicians and others in the health-care team is that the proxy is a bother. Providing care to incapacitated patients is medically and ethically complex. It presents a challenge to the reflexive medical model of "do everything." It requires, or should require, the physician to engage in an ongoing benefit/burden analysis in the process of deciding about appropriate care. It requires, or should, a continuing calculus to decide whether a specific intervention is in the best interest of the patient. This most cerebral practice of medicine contrasts markedly with customary, protocol-driven approaches to practice. It also encourages physicians to decide on their own as the deliberative and cooperative modes of physician-patient decision making are impossible.

A third reason proxies may be ignored relates to the myths of proxy behavior.[36] These include the received wisdom that proxies want everything done even when it is clear that the patient would choose to refuse care; that proxies are indecisive; and that proxies do not engage in a process with other family members and thereby leave the staff to deal with unresolved conflict and discomfort.

A fourth reason physicians may nor involve proxies is that published literature on the degree of agreement between proxy and patient with respect to any individual decision has been shown to be no greater than chance. Why should persons be treated with deference when their task is so poorly performed? There are increasing numbers of studies in which nursing home patients and their proxies lacked concordance regarding the patients' wishes with regard to hospitalization, cardiac surgery, CPR, mechanical ventilation, intravenous antibiotic therapy, intravenous fluid therapy, and tube feeding.[37-40] In some cases, proxies described patient preferences for medical intervention that were contrary to the wishes of the patient when interviewed, while in other cases, the proxy believed the patient wanted nothing done when life-sustaining measures were actually desired.[41] Comparison of estimates by patients and proxies of patient health and functional status showed a tendency for proxies to overestimate the negative impact of the patient's disability on decisions to provide care.[42]

While this lack of conformity between patient and proxy choices may not negatively affect outcomes,[43] the frequency with which it occurs implies the need for greater understanding of the proxy role.[44] Greater and perhaps earlier involvement of the proxy in the patient's medical affairs might promote greater understanding and enhance agreement with the patient's wishes. Appropriate choice among treatment options is best made through a dynamic exchange of information among all health care providers and the proxy.[45]

The New York State Task Force on Life and the Law, in its discussion of guidelines for surrogate decisions, recognizes that proxies have "a duty to ascertain the medical facts" so that their decisions are "based on a firm understanding of the patient's medical condition, the expected benefits and risks of treatment, and the underlying goals of medical intervention." Therefore, the task force has recommended that proxies arrive at their decisions through consultation with health-care professionals since they "should have the right to obtain all medical information necessary to make an informed decision."[46(p104)]

The New York State Health Care Agent Act is representative of all 50 state laws in that it leaves critical issues of communication both between patient and proxy and between proxy and physician open-ended and undefined. Indeed, no state law that gives legal status to proxies says anything about the doctor's relationship with or obligations to the proxy (personal communication with Charles P. Sabatino, June 1995). Without additional guidance for physicians regarding the need for timely, efficient, effective communication with and integration of the proxy into the entire medical decision-making process, these acts are likely to fall short of their intended purpose.

A final reason for physicians' reluctance to involve proxies in decision making may be related to the growing debate about futile care. Physicians fear that legally appointed proxies may have the right to demand care that the physicians deem futile or inappropriate. What better reason to exclude them from discussions?

I suggest, however, that there is a reason, other than the perversity and perfidy of the proxy, that might explain the behavior of demanding futile care. Many physicians now give patients a rather straightforward and honest presentation of the risks and benefits of interventions such as resuscitation. After many years of struggle with honesty, kindness, and a recognition of the limits of medical technology, physicians are more likely to describe resuscitation in all its brutality than to couch it in euphemism and metaphor. In years past, physicians might have asked patients, as part of a discussion about resuscitation, "If your heart stops, do you want us to try and restart it?" Now they are likely to describe in graphic and horrific derail how the organ systems and bones will disintegrate if this assault on a weakened and morbid body is attempted. This portrayal of the inability of medicine to have a beneficial effect has been key in helping the patient to acknowledge the inevitability of death and the desirability of the least-worse dying.

In my experience, no such graphic conversation is likely to occur with a proxy. Discussions with proxies seem to reflect a far less evolved level of discussion—a level at which the burdens of interventions are not adequately identified. Why should the proxy who loves this patient want to facilitate his death? If the proxy is asked, "If the patient's heart stops should we start it?" why should that proxy say, "No"?

Many proxies feel that the decision to agree to a DNR order, or to choose less than the most aggressive interventions, actually "signs the death warrant" or "causes" the death of the patient. This prospect of feeling responsible for facilitating the death of another raises another explanation for the myths of proxy intractability. Proxies have no skill in distancing themselves from the realities of death.

When physicians and patients talk about withdrawing or withholding care and the patient makes the decision to forgo life-sustaining treatment and permit death, the moral agent, the patient, acts for him- or herself and assumes responsibility for the outcome. Even under these conditions physicians are sometimes discomfited by a feeling of "responsibility" for the death. How much more difficult is it for a proxy with little information or support when that person is asked to forgo treatment and permit the death of a loved one?

There is a boundary between physicians seizing decision-making authority inappropriately and physicians accepting emotional and moral responsibility for suggested plans of care. Perhaps proxy deciders would have an easier task if they were asked to approve decisions to permit death when the onus was already shouldered by the physician.

CONCLUSION

In the vast literature on advance directives, there is barely any discussion of the relationship between doctors and nurses and proxy decision makers, the new, legally empowered persons in the decision-making picture. Physicians and nurses are exhorted to talk with their patients about the execution of living wills and about the appointment of proxy deciders. There is literature on the appropriate tenor of the discussions, the manner in which information should be presented, and the way the possible risks and benefits of future interventions should be portrayed. The jolly exhortative tone of these articles—"out there onto the field and play the game"— assumes that if these documents can only be secured—if the goal line can be breached—all decisions will be resolved under an umbrella of ethical comfort and legal protection. Granting that proxy appointments are useful support for arriving at ethically appropriate decisions, they demand a new focus on and consideration for the welfare of the proxy.

An individual patient's decision to refuse care and permit death is a reflection of many factors including the weighing of benefits and burdens in the context of the likely diagnosis and prognosis, the present and anticipated pain and suffering, the possible emotional and financial impact on family and loved ones, the prospect of companionship or isolation that the future holds, personal religious and philosophical values and commitments, and courage or fear in the face of the unknown.

For oneself, the process of arriving at an accommodation with death is likely to be as intuitive as it is cerebral. For the proxy, however, it must be a conscious process in which the various factors are considered individually and then referenced against the known preferences, assumed tendencies, and presumed best interest of the patient. This conscious process necessarily takes place simultaneously with the increasing grief that surrounds the dying of a loved one.

Thus, as difficult as the task of forgoing treatment is for a patient, it is, in many ways, more difficult for the proxy: "It is an intimidating, indeed, frightening responsibility to calculate the overall value of life for another human being."[47] A proxy's decision can only guess at the relative weight these elements would assume in the idiosyncratic calculus of the patient. If the proxy is conscientious and has a reverence for life, the decision to permit death must, perforce, weigh heavy on the mind and the soul. This burden should not be born alone. Physicians and the health-care team have the duty to provide emotional support, compassion, and guidance to proxies acting for their loved ones and friends.

REFERENCES

1. Emanuel EJ, Weinberg DS, Gonin R, et al. How is the Patient Self-Determination Act working? An early assessment. *American Journal of Medicine.* 1993;95:619–628.

2. Emanuel L, Emanuel EJ, Stoeckle JD, et al. Advance directives: stability of patients' treatment choices. *Archives of Internal Medicine.* 1994;154:207–217.

3. Joos SK, Reuler JB, Powell JL, Hickham DH. Outpatients' attitudes and understanding regarding living wills. *Journal of General Internal Medicine.* 1993;8:259–263.

4. Rubin SM, Strull WM, Fialkow MF, et al. Increasing the completion of the durable power of attorney for health care. *JAMA.* 1994;271:209–212.

5. Eisendrath SJ, Jonsen AR. The living will: help or hindrance? *JAMA.* 1983;249:2054–2058.

6. Wolf SM, Boyle P, Calahan D, et al. Sources of concern about the Patient Self-Determination Act. *New England Journal of Medicine.* 1991;325:1666–1671.

7. Pellegrino ED. Ethics. *JAMA.* 1992;268:354–355.

8. Sugarman J, Powe NR, Brillantes D, Smith MK. The cost of ethics legislation: a look at the Patient Self-Determination Act. *Kennedy Institute of Ethics Journal.* 1993;3:387–399.

9. Orentlicher D. The illusion of patient choice in end-of-life decisions. *JAMA.* 1992;267:2101–2104.

10. Orentlicher D. Advance medical directives. *JAMA.* 1990;263:2365–2367.

11. Report of the Board of Trustees of the American Medical Association. *Living Wills, Durable Power of Attorney, Durable Powers of Attorney for Health Care.* Chicago, IL: American Medical Association; 1989.

12. Sabatino CP. *Health Care Power of Attorney.* Washington, DC: American Bar Association; 1990.

13. Rouse F. Patients, providers, and the PSDA. *Hastings Center Report.* 1991;21(5):S2–S16.

14. Capron AM. The Patient Self-Determination Act: new responsibilities for health care providers. *Journal of American Health Policy.* 1992; January/February;40–43.

15. Grant KD. The Patient Self-Determination Act: implications for physicians. *Hospital Practice.* 1992:34–38.

16. The effects of the *Cruzan* case on the rights of elderly clients. *Clearinghouse Review.* 1990;24:663–670.

17. Sabatino CP. Surely the Wizard will help us, Toto? Implementing the Patient Self-Determination Act. *Hastings Center Report.* 1993;23(1):12–16.

18. Mezey M, Latimer B. The Patient Self-Determination Act: an early look at implementation. *Hastings Center Report.* 1993;23(1):16–20.

19. Lynn J, Teno JM. After the Patient Self-Determination Act: the need for empirical research on formal advance directives. *Hastings Center Report.* 1993;23(1):20–24.

20. Kapp MB. Implications of the Patient Self-Determination Act for psychiatric prac-

tice. *Hospital and Community Psychiatry.* 1994;45:355–358.

21. Gamble ER, McDonald PJ, Lichstein PR. Knowledge, attitudes, and behavior of elderly persons regarding living wills. *Archives of Internal Medicine.* 1991;151:277–280.

22. Stelter KL, Elliot BA, Bruno CA. Living will completion in older adults. *Archives of Internal Medicine.* 1992;153:954–959.

23. Pellegrino ED, Mazzarella P, Corsi P (eds.). *Transcultural Dimensions in Medical Ethics.* Frederick, MD: University Publishing Group; 1992.

24. Robinson MK, DeHaven MJ, Koch KA. Effects of the Patient Self-Determination Act on patient knowledge and behavior. *Journal of Family Practice.* 1993;37:363–368.

25. Dresser R, Robertson JA. Quality of life and non-treatment decisions for incompetent patients: a critique of the orthodox approach. *Law, Medicine & Health Care.* 1989;17:234–244.

26. Danis M, Southerland LI, Garrett JM, et al. A prospective study of advance directives for life-sustaining care. *New England Journal of Medicine.* 1991;324:882–888.

27. Lynn J. Why I don't have a living will. *Law, Medicine & Health Care.* 1991;19:101–104.

28. Schneiderman LJ, Teetzel H, Kalmanson AG. Who decides who decides? When disagreement occurs between the physician and the patient's appointed proxy about the patient's decision-making capacity. *Archives of Internal Medicine.* 1995;155:793–795.

29. Brett AS. Limitations of listing specific medical interventions in advance directives. *JAMA.* 1991;266:825–828.

30. Catalano JT. Treatments not specifically listed in the living will: the ethical dilemmas. *Dimensions of Critical Care Nursing.* 1994;13:142–149.

31. Relman AS. Michigan's sensible "living will." *New England Journal of Medicine.* 1979;300:1270–1272.

32. Steinbrook R, Lo B. Decision making for incompetent patients by designated proxy: California's new law. *New England Journal of Medicine.* 1984;310:1598–1601.

33. Annas GJ. The health care proxy and the living will. *New England Journal of Medicine.* 1991;324:1210–1213.

34. Zinberg JM. Decisions for the dying: an empirical study of physicians' responses to advance directives. *Vermont Law Review.* 1989;13:445–491.

35. Sabatino CP. *Health Care Power of Attorney Legislation as of July 1, 1995.* ABA Commission on Legal Problems of the Elderly. Unpublished data.

36. Miles SH. Informed demand for "non-beneficial" medical treatment. *New England Journal of Medicine.* 1991;325:512–515.

37. Gerety MB, Chiodo LK, Kanten DN, et al. Medical treatment preferences of nursing home residents: relationship to function and concordance with surrogate decision makers. *Journal of the American Geriatrics Society.* 1993;41:953–960.

38. Ouslander JG, Tymchuk AJ, Rahbar BB. Health care decisions among elderly long-term care residents and their potential proxies. *Archives of Internal Medicine.* 1989;149:1367–1372.

39. Seckler AB, Meier DE, Milvihill M, Cammer-Paris BE. Substituted judgment: how accurate are proxy decisions? *Archives of Internal Medicine.* 1991;115:92–98.

40. Uhlmann RF, Pearlman RA, Cain KC. Physicians' and spouses' predictions of elderly patients' resuscitation preferences. *Journal of Gerontology.* 1988;43:115–121.

41. Diamond EL, Jernigan JA, Moseley RA, et al. Decision-making ability and advance directive preferences in nursing home patients and proxies. *Gerontologist.* 1989;29:622–626.

42. Magaziner J, Simonsick EM, Kashner TM, Hebel JR. Patient-proxy response comparability on measures of patient health and function status. *Journal of Clinical Epidemiology.* 1988;41:1065–1074.

43. Lynn J. Procedures for making medical decisions for incompetent adults. *JAMA.* 1992;267:2082–2084.

44. Hardwig J. The problem of proxies with interests of their own: toward a better theory of proxy decisions. *Journal of Clinical Ethics.* 1993;4(spring):20–27.

45. Mezey M, Kluger M, Maislin G, Mittelman M. Life-sustaining treatment decisions by spouses of patients with Alzheimer's disease. Unpublished article.

46. New York State Task Force on Life and the Law. *When Others Must Choose: Deciding for Patients without Capacity.* New York: NYTF; 1992.

47. Dresser R, Whitehouse PJ. The incompetent patient on the slippery slope. *Hastings Center Report.* 1994;24(4):6–12.

18

ETHICAL DIMENSIONS OF NURSE-PHYSICIAN RELATIONS IN CRITICAL CARE

Mary C. Corley, Ph.D., R.N.

NATURE OF NURSE-PHYSICIAN RELATIONSHIPS

Nurses who work in critical care units confront many ethical issues in their daily practice. Some of these ethical issues are dramatic, whereas others are more subtle, but they all produce moral distress. The challenges of resolving these ethical issues are complicated by the chaotic health-care environment that is characterized by concern about cost containment, rationing, and resource allocation.[1] This article focuses on the ethical conflicts in nurse-physician relationships that require further elaboration. The aim is to understand why they continue to arise and to propose strategies to address these issues.

The importance of addressing these conflicts and developing more helpful approaches is highlighted by the research of Shortell et al.[2] They found that when nurse-physician interaction was of a high quality it led to improved quality of care, met family needs, and decreased length of stay. Other research identified the impact of poor nurse-physician collaboration on higher patient mortality.[3,4]

Unresolved ethical issues can affect the ability of both nurses and physicians to perform at optimal levels. The impact of moral distress on nurses is responsible for

M. Corley. "Ethical Dimensions of Nurse-Physician Relations in Critical Care." *Nursing Clinics of North America.* 1998;33(2):325–338. Reprinted by permission of W. B. Saunders Company.

13 percent of those who have left nursing positions in the past[5] and in 5 percent of those who have left the profession.[6] Eisendrath et al.[7] reported that physicians experience stress and burnout related to ethical issues. The impact of the emotional state of clinicians on patient outcomes has not been assessed and is a major need.

Jameton[8] says moral distress occurs when a person " . . . makes a moral judgment about a case in which she/he is involved and the institution or co-workers make it difficult or impossible for the nurse to act on the judgment." Experience with troubling situations may produce anguish which is defined as " . . . personal feelings of travail when involved in a situation in which they felt powerless to assist patients or practice in a fully professional manner."[9] "Moral outrage ensues when the nurse's subsequent attempts to operationalize a moral choice are thwarted by constraints. The outrage intensifies when these constraints not only block actions, but also force a course of action that violates the nurse's moral tenets."[10] Pike further identifies as an external constraint the authority and directives of physicians or hospital policy.

The nurse-physician relationship often has been adversarial with conflict around moral dilemmas.[11] Gramelspacher et al[12] found that nurses identified physicians as a source of ethical conflicts; however, physicians rarely perceived nurses as a source. Prescott and Bowen[13] observed that ethical issues comprised the majority of nurse-physician conflicts. Clinicians reported that most of their relationships were positive; however conflicts were resolved using competitive rather than more desirable collaborative approaches. However, Prescott and Bowen[13] concluded that the conflict was not always a negative factor; in fact, some nurse-physician conflict protected patients. Holly[9] identified collegial relations, including personal conflict with the physician's treatment decisions and with unethical or incompetent activities of colleagues, as an area of ethical concern. In a longitudinal study of critical care nurses, Omery et al[14] identified patient-physician-nurse relationships as one of the major ethical issues in their practice. Not only do nurses perceive conflicts with physicians over ethical issues, but Erlen and Frost[15] also found that the nurses felt powerless to affect ethical decisions.

NURSE-PHYSICIAN ETHICAL CONFLICTS

To better understand the ethical conflicts involving nurses and physicians, the following issues are addressed: values, communication, trust and integrity, role responsibilities, and organizational politics and economics.

Values

Early sources of values are family upbringing and religious training. These values are modified by education and work experience. Ethical conflicts may arise because nurses and physicians have different work experiences and values about an issue such as what comprises informed consent, extent or invasiveness of treatment, when to stop treatment, when to resuscitate,[13] how quality of life is defined, and what constitutes euthanasia and assisted suicide.[16]

Value conflicts occur frequently over what comprises informed consent. Although the physician may review a consent form for a procedure and obtain the patient's signature, the nurse may determine from the patient's comments and questions that the patient does not understand what the procedure involves in order to make an informed decision. In some instances, verbal consent is obtained without a signed consent form. The nurse perceives that the physician has filled the "letter" but not the "spirit of the law." And, the physician may not want the nurse to discuss the issue further with the patient.

Value conflicts also involve the participation of the critically ill patient in decisions about resuscitation. Nurses believe patients should be involved in these decisions. Often, the patient has discussed his or her wishes with the nurse and even may have signed advance directives; however, the physician continues the treatment that the patient would choose not to continue or discontinues treatment when the patient wished everything done.[17] Fearing a lawsuit, the physician also may accede to the family's wishes that run counter to those of a patient regarding a decision about resuscitation.

A third conflict regarding values is about the use of technology and new treatment approaches for a patient whose condition has not responded to standard approaches. The nurses may view the use of new approaches or technology as prolonging a patient's suffering unnecessarily, whereas the physician wishes to implement these new approaches to achieve improvement in a patient's condition.

A conflict in values also may occur when a nurse perceives that the physician is pursuing treatment to add to the physician's knowledge and skill, whereas the nurse perceives this approach as adding to the patient's suffering or violating the patient's dignity. This issue is exemplified by observations of medical students and residents who practice procedures on dying or dead patients. Keeping patients alive until permission is obtained to harvest an organ for transplant also falls in this category.

Nurses and physicians also may come into conflict over what constitutes quality of life for the patient. Solomon et al[18] found a discrepancy between what the clinicians believe should be done when quality of life is seriously jeopardized by the patient's deteriorating condition and their own behavior to follow this belief. This is a major source of moral distress for nurses, who recognize this discrepancy and must care for the patients. Anspach[19] found that physicians and nurses both used incomplete but different knowledge (laboratory tests for the former and the patient's ability to respond interpersonally for the latter) about the patient to assess quality of life and prognosis. The nurses may struggle to provide relief from pain and suffering, sometimes not effectively. "Because of this frequently intense experience, nurses may question the ratio of benefits and burdens the patient is feeling."[20] Physicians, however, may observe the patient on that same day for only five minutes and not realize the extent of the patient's suffering. Moreover, the physician may have known the patient when he or she was healthy and may perceive this period as an interlude before a return to health. In fact, neither may have a complete, accurate perception of the patient's quality of life.

Nurses also are caught between physicians caring for the patient with conflicting values about termination of life-sustaining treatment.[21] Cook et al[22] found criteria for withdrawing life support from the critically ill extremely variable among physicians. Conflicting orders are written and the nurse experiences ethical distress trying to protect the patient from the repercussions.

Communication

Many factors affect communication between nurses and physicians. Two interrelated ones are gender and prestige. The high percentage of female nurses affects nurse-physician communication, despite lowering of the gender barrier. Higher prestige of physicians also affects the nature and quality of communication. Although the image of the nurse as the physician's handmaiden is fading, the influence continues. The nurse's opinions are not valued; nurses are afraid to challenge a physician, who may have more power, or are hesitant to report changes in the patient's condition because of intimidation. These changes may escalate and the nurse then regrets not being more assertive or confident in communication with the physician.

The very need for communication beyond the written orders of a physician and the nurse who carries them out reflects nurse-physician differences. Physicians who perceive that this aspect of communication is all that is necessary are in conflict with the nurse's perception of what is needed. The nurse needs physician guidance in interpreting changes in the patient's condition or in knowing the details of procedures that the physician has performed in order to plan care and make appropriate observations of the patient. Because of the lack of communication, the physician may react negatively to the nurse's questions, dismiss the questions, or leave brusquely. The nurse then experiences ethical distress because she or he lacks the information needed to provide care, adding to the patient's suffering or deteriorating condition or failing to anticipate changes that in retrospect she or he should have been able to identify. Prescott and Bowen,[13] in their study of nurse-physician conflict, found that nurses could only question a physician's decision rather than challenge a physician's authority, whereas a physician questioned the nurse's authority and competence to make certain judgments.

Physicians also may not realize that the nurse must know what discussions have taken place between the physician and the patient and family. Knowing the content of these discussions can aid the nurse in answering patients' questions or clarifying misperceptions. If discrepancies occur between what the physician and patient have discussed and the care the nurse is providing, the nurse may feel ethical distress that the patient is not receiving appropriate care.

Trust and Integrity

Beauchamp and Childress[23] identify the essential role of trust and integrity in an effective nurse-physician relationship. Patient conditions may change rather quickly and unexpectedly. Although the nurse may know what interventions are necessary, the actions may require a physician's order beyond the standard protocol already in place. In navigating patients through the maze of the contemporary health-care system, nurses frequently fill the gaps by doing something they are not authorized publicly to do.[24] The nurse must trust that the physician will back this decision.

Trust is also a factor when the nurse recognizes that a physician is incompetent. The nurse may be reluctant to believe that the physician is incompetent and delays taking action. Because charging a physician with incompetence has serious repercussions, verifying the incompetence may take time. During that interval, patients may suffer, which produces an ethical dilemma for the nurse. Nurses are torn between loyalty to the physician and the patient. Because so much of the nurse-physician relationship depends on trust, violating it can create disorder in the system. Physician competence is a major concern of critical care nurses. Carson et al[25] found that nurses had greater confidence in the ability of and preferred medical supervision by physicians whose primary responsibility was for care of patients in the intensive care unit than primary admitting physicians who used the critical care specialists for consultation.

Physicians are not reluctant to identify nurses as incompetent and to report them to administration. Although the charges of incompetence may not be justified, nonetheless the nurse is required to provide proof of competence. For example, the charge of incompetence may be failure to carry out an order when the nurse has another reason for not doing it. Achieving and maintaining competence is an important professional requirement for critical care nurses. In fact, the goal of all critical care nurses should be to achieve expert status. Benner et al[26] found that the expert critical care nurse had strong negotiating skills, including the ability to make a case to the physician about the patient's response to treatment. This skill can prevent moral distress because the nurse has input into the patient-care decisions, reducing the discrepancy between what care is needed and what care is ordered.

Lack of Understanding of Each Other's Responsibilities

Although one of the nurse's major roles is to carry out physicians' orders, nurses' knowledge base and focus of care differ from that of the physician. Physicians sometimes do not realize what it entails for the critical care nurse to have major responsibility for monitoring the patient and providing early intervention as a means of averting a more serious response. Because nurses have a more intense exposure to the patient, they expect to be involved in the decision-making process about the patient's care. Physicians sometimes do not share this perspective.[27]

Physicians also do not realize the invisible work that nurses do in addition to getting clinical information. Other invisible work Jacques[28] identified includes educating patients and families, communicating information to patients from others and vice versa, communicating to establish a relationship, and performing work neither required or expected ("above and beyond").

Nursing to achieve professional status has identified patient advocacy as a unique responsibility of the profession. Most physicians know their patients before their illness and thus believe that they are the most appropriate patient advocate. In fact, they may believe that they know what is best for the patient based on this long-term knowledge of the patient, often without further consultation from the patient. With both the nurse and physician claiming this territory, conflicts are predictable and some are ethical conflicts.

Nurses recognize that writing orders is a major physician responsibility. However, they often do not realize the extent uncertainty plays in the work of the physician.[29] Osler[30] has defined medicine as the "science of uncertainty and art of probability." Although uncertainty is one of the challenges and attractions of physician practice, it also can be a source of physician stress. Factors that impact the feelings of uncertainty are the seriousness of the patient's illness, specificity of diagnoses before the acute phase, perceived control over the illness, and contact with other experts. Uncertainty is further complicated because patients or family or both advertently or inadvertently may withhold information pertinent to the acute condition. Absolute certainty can lead to boredom, whereas a moderate degree of uncertainty produces an information pattern search and pleasure.[31] Physicians, although experiencing some uncertainty, may view the nurse's questions about the patient's treatment as questioning the physician's competency.

Physicians also assume that they are responsible for making sure that the most up-to-date technology and treatment are being used. Thus they sometimes introduce these without complete knowledge of outcomes. Nurses may perceive this practice as irresponsible and unethical—practicing on the patients without their permission and at a vulnerable time. The new technologies and procedures may challenge values and create uncertainty. They can be adopted before thoughtful reflection and evaluation have taken place because of a patient's rapidly deteriorating condition. To whom does the nurse address her or his doubts about this? How are these doubts perceived by the physician?

Organizational Politics and Economics

Nurses witness incongruities between the health-care organization's stated philosophy and the actual decisions made. Marshall et al[32] found that political power, medical provincialism, and income maximization overrode medical suitability in the provision of critical care services. A physician who is a major source of income for the hospital may have ready access to the intensive care unit for his or her patients, whereas a more acutely ill patient who meets the criteria is denied admission because all the beds are taken by patients who do not meet the admission criteria. Economic factors also may affect which patients are transferred from the intensive care unit;

when a bed shortage occurs, patients who are not able to pay may be transferred to a step-down unit rather than a comparable patient who has health insurance. In addition, treatment sometimes is based on expediency rather than a plan for the patient.[9] Kollef[33] found among patients dying within a medical intensive care unit that those patients without a private attending physician and private health insurance were more likely to undergo the active withdrawal of life-sustaining interventions. This discrepancy in care can produce moral distress for nurses. Moral distress refers to uncomfortable feelings that occur when nurses cannot provide the care they believe is appropriate because of institutional constraints such as policy or more subtle administrative requirements, such as maintaining the affiliation of a physician with the hospital or meeting reengineering objectives.[5] Thus nurses become collaborators in behavior they judge to be unethical. The negative repercussions for the patient can be profound. However, the impact on the nurses' sense of trust of the physician and the organization, although subtle, may have a serious demoralizing effect.

STRATEGIES TO ENHANCE NURSE-PHYSICIAN COLLABORATION

Although administrators, nurses, and physicians realize that ethical conflicts occur, few efforts have been made to anticipate and resolve nurse-physician ethical conflicts. Strategies to address these ethical conflicts must be identified at the policy and organizational levels.

Policy

Multidisciplinary groups of health professionals, health professional organizations, ethicists, and policy makers must develop guidelines on what constitutes euthanasia, assisted suicide, do-not-resuscitate state, medical futility and informed consent, and the power of the family to make decisions beyond medical recommendations for care. Some organizations have begun to do this. For example, in 1989, the American College of Chest Physicians and the Society of Critical Care Medicine[34] in a multidisciplinary consensus conference developed ethical and moral guidelines for initiating, continuing, and withdrawing intensive care. The guidelines also included strategies to manage disagreements, including the use of increased communication and institutional dispute resolution mechanisms, such as an ethics committee. They recommended the use of the courts only as a last resort. Similar consensus conferences on informed consent, patient participation in decisions about resuscitation and use of new technologies, and the balance between patient care and development of new knowledge are needed among major organizations of nurses, physicians, other clinicians, and ethicists. Achieving total consensus is unrealistic given the multicultural society in the United States. However, a consensus statement that highlights the major issues and provides for dispute resolution would provide a basis for decision making. These consensus statements must be disseminated widely to clinicians in critical care units where they should serve as a basis for discussion of the issues involved and the development of organizational policies.

Another powerful resource to develop improved nurse-physician collaboration is the Joint Commission on Accreditation of Hospital Organizations (JCAHO). One standard, Patient Rights and Organization Ethics,[35] focuses on respecting each patient's rights and conducting business relationships in an ethical manner. However, should JCAHO expand its criteria to require that hospitals develop an ethical environment that fosters nurse-physician collaboration and ethical treatment of personnel, it is likely that greater nurse-physician collaboration would result.

Because organizations influence clinicians who work in their environments, how the administrators treat these individuals is reflected in how the clinicians treat their patients. Schmieding[36] found that how the middle manager responds to staff nurses is reflected in how the staff nurse responds to patients in terms of exploring their behavior. When the nurse manager asked staff nurses questions that encouraged their participation in problem solving rather than questions that reflected monitoring or controlling approaches, staff nurses were more likely to use that approach with their patients. It is likely that when administration demonstrates a sense of social responsibility toward the nurses, the nurses, in turn, are concerned about the ethical issues involving their patients. And when administrators are willing to reflect and establish ethical standards for the organization, the administrators are more likely to learn from their own actions.

When nurses are in ethical conflict with the legal system,[37] administrators should provide opportunities to discuss these disagreements. If the nurses have valid arguments, several strategies lend themselves: the nurses should work through the state nurses association and state board of nursing to bring about changes in the law; and the administrators in the health-care organization have a responsibility to work through their professional organization to bring these issues before legislators.

ORGANIZATIONAL STRATEGIES

Organizational Culture

Rushton and Brooks-Brunn[38] have proposed a strategy for developing environments that support ethical practice. Although they focus end-of-life care, their recommendations are pertinent for all ethical issues in a health-care environment. They propose that administrators and clinicians examine and change the organizational culture, provide guidelines for behavior and problem solving, and identify what is morally permissible. Rushton and Brooks-Brunn identified six key points to use in assessing an organization's structure to monitor ethical performance: (1) performance reporting that includes ethical behavior, (2) employees considering ethical aspects part of their job, (3) recognition of employees who provide ethical leadership, (4) procedures for dealing with ethical-code violations, (5) mechanisms for accountability to the public and patients, and (6) assessing frequency of use of conscientious objection (taking a stand on an ethical issue different than the majority). Health-care organizations can use these assessment criteria to gauge their progress in enhancing their organizational cultures to function at a higher ethical level.

Collaboration

The ethical work environment should support a collaborative team approach with a blurring of professional boundaries, clarification of clinicians' values, and processes to monitor and evaluate ethical performance. Developing protocols or critical pathways for treatment of conditions is another strategy involving consensus building between physicians and nurses. Nurses have provided leadership in this approach, but physicians are also seeing the value of these, which in turn has led to a greater willingness to collaborate. Lassen et al[39] found that developing protocols prevented nurses from being caught between the specialists and generalists, improved nurse-physician communication and patient care, and reduced cost. Nurses were already empowered to assess and treat patients independently, but improved nurse-physician communication also occurred in a renal transplant program when a time was set for communication about patient problems.[40]

When members of the organization are successful in these collaborative efforts, administration should provide recognition to the team.[41] McDaniel[42] reported that ethics is an important aspect of work satisfaction for nurses, a fact that requires that administrators develop programs that support and sustain nurses' ethics participation in patient-care deliberations. Pike's research[10] supports these strategies. She found that a patient unit designed to study and develop collaborative relationships between nurses and physicians had the unexpected outcome of decreasing moral outrage on the part of the nurses. She credited this outcome to the growth in mutual trust and respect between nurses and physicians. Furthermore, reducing the conflicts between nurses and physicians revealed previously unrecognized constraints affecting the action they collectively took. She recommended an "enriched environment"—one that provides opportunities for shared decision making and accountability between nurses and physicians in which relationships are based on equality and reciprocity. The resulting trust and respect between nurses and physicians can be synergistic, leading to better solutions than each discipline could achieve individually. Collaboration was also important in an Ontario study of clinician-managers (nurses, physicians, and other clinicians); Lemieux-Charles and Hall[43] found that they were more satisfied with consultative practices to achieve ethical decisions than when avoidance of a decision occurred or a decision was forced by the organization. Nurses and physicians who take ethical stands must be rewarded rather than being labeled as troublemakers or receiving no response to their concerns. The paramount reason is the impact on patient outcomes, but the impact on the self-worth and stress of the clinician is also important.

Relationship between Policy and Ethics

Health-care administrators must demonstrate the connections between policy making and human values in health-care organizations to eliminate the contradiction between the behaviors organizations urge and the actions they take. Reiser[44] recommends that organizations " ... introduce into policy making and interpersonal aspects of organizational life a capacity and concern for ethical analysis." Ethical analysis must be ongoing to address changes in technology and societal values. Health-care administrators must recognize the discrepancies that occur between the philosophy and policies and the decisions and care that are actually given for its impact on the ethical climate and ethical behavior of clinicians. The drive to survive economically cannot be used to justify economic over ethical rationale for action. Nor can economic survival provide an excuse for abuse of staff. After surveying nurses about abuse, Kreitzer et al.[45] initiated a strategy to create a healthy environment, one that required staff development, a major focus being conflict management. Skill in conflict management, particularly in the use of constructive confrontation rather than smoothing over or avoiding conflict, enhances nurse-physician collaboration and better unit functioning.[46] Given the major changes in health care over which nurses feel that they have no control, recognition that physicians may not have control either can contribute to improved communication.[37] Nurses must continue to seek work empowerment and administrators must continue to find ways to empower nurses because it not only decreases moral distress but also is related to occupational mental health and work effectiveness.[47]

Educational Approaches

Health-care organizations must provide educational resources to help all clinicians acquire up-to-date knowledge about values, ethics, and decision making in an interdisciplinary format. Individual clinicians also have a responsibility to update their knowledge about ethical issues and skill in ethical decision through self-guided learning. Through discussions with and observing role models, less experienced nurses gain knowledge and skill in analyzing and managing ethical dilemmas that arise in their practice.[10] Additional strategies to facilitate knowledge development, discussion, and collaboration include nursing ethics councils, unit-based ethics rounds, and nursing grand rounds on ethical issues.[9]

Communication

The educational preparation of all clinicians addresses communication skills, focusing on the patient and family. However, clinicians also need knowledge and skill in dealing with difficult people, including members of the interdisciplinary team. Learning how to communicate in an emotionally charged environment, especially with other clinicians, is a much needed skill for nurses and physicians. Two important skills are knowing how to ask questions of someone to elicit a helpful response and how to negotiate a change in the treatment plan given the implications for patient outcomes.[26]

SUMMARY

Strategies to enhance nurse-physician collaboration and reduce the ethical conflict in care of critically ill patients must be initiated at both the national policy and organizational policy level. National consensus groups on ethical issues that occur in the intensive care unit can provide an important model for changing policies in health-care organizations. The organizational culture can enhance ethical decision making by providing opportunities for values clarification of clinicians, preferably in joint discussions among them. Both administrators and clinical leaders can use research findings on collaborative efforts among nurses and physicians to improve the joint decision making. Health-care organizations must address the conflict in their mission to provide care and survive economically, and their policies need to reflect this. They can also provide education to improve the ethical knowledge and skill of the critical care clinicians. Finally, health-care organizations can encourage research that focuses on the quality of care related to ethical decision making.

REFERENCES

1. Vladeck BC. Beliefs vs. behaviors in health care decision making [editorial]. *American Journal of Public Health.* 1993;83:13–14.

2. Shortell S, Zimmerman J, Rousseau D, et al. The performance of intensive care units: does good management make a difference? *Medical Care.* 1994;32:508–525.

3. Baggs J, Schmitt M, Mushlin AL, et al. Nurse-physician collaboration and satisfaction with the decision-making process in three critical care units. *American Journal of Critical Care.* 1997;6:393–399.

4. Knaus W, Draper E, Wagner D, et al. An evaluation of outcome from intensive care in major medical centers. *Annals of Internal Medicine.* 1986;194:410–428.

5. Corley M. Moral distress of critical care nurses. *American Journal of Critical Care.* 1993;4:285.

6. Wilkinson J. Moral distress in nursing practice. *Nursing Forum.* 1988;23:16–20.

7. Eisendrath SJ, Link N, Matthay M. Intensive care unit: how stressful for physicians? *Critical Care Medicine.* 1986;14:95–98.

8. Jameton A. Dilemmas of moral distress: moral responsibility and nursing practice. *Clinical Issues in Perinatal and Women's Health Nursing.* 1993;4:611–619.

9. Holly C. The ethical quandaries of acute care nursing practice. *Journal of Professional Nursing.* 1993; 9:110–115.

10. Pike AW. Moral outrage and moral discourse in nurse-physician collaboration. *Journal of Professional Nursing.* 1991;7:351–363.

11. Yarling RR, McElmurry BJ. The moral foundation of nursing. *Advances in Nursing Science.* 1986;8:63–73.

12. Gramelspacher GP, Howell JD, Young MJ. Perceptions of ethical problems by nurses and doctors. *Archives of Internal Medicine.* 1986;146:467–474.

13. Prescott P, Bowen S. Physician-nurse relationships. *Annals of Internal Medicine.* 1985;103:127–133.

14. Omery A, Hermeman C, Billet B, et al. Ethical issues in hospital-based practice. *Journal of Cardiovascular Nursing.* 1995;9:42–53.

15. Erlen J, Frost B. Nurses' perceptions of powerlessness in influencing ethical decisions. *Western Journal of Nursing Research.* 1991;13:397–407.

16. Asch DA. The role of critical care nurses in euthanasia and assisted suicide. *New England Journal of Medicine.* 1996; 334:1374–1379.

17. The SUPPORT Principal Investigators. A controlled trial to improve care to seriously ill hospitalized patients. *JAMA.* 1995;274:1591–1598.

18. Solomon M, O'Donnell L, Jennings B, et al. Decisions near the end of life: professional views on life-sustaining treatments. *American Journal of Public Health.* 1993;83:23–25.

19. Anspach RR. *Deciding Who Lives: Fateful Choices in the Intensive-Care Nursery.* Berkeley, CA: University of California Press; 1992.

20. Redman B, Hill M. Studies of ethical conflicts by nursing practice settings or roles. *Western Journal of Nursing Research.* 1997;19:243–260.

21. Caralis P, Hammond J. Attitudes of medical students, housestaff, and faculty physicians toward euthanasia and termination of lifesustaining treatment. *Critical Care Medicine.* 1992;20:683–690.

22. Cook D, Guyatt G, Jaeschke R, et al. Determinants in Canadian health care workers of the decision to withdraw life support from the critically ill. *JAMA.* 1995;273:703–708.

23. Beauchamp T, Childress J. *Principles of Biomedical Ethics.* 4th ed. New York: Oxford Press; 1994.

24. Liaschenko J. Ethics and the geography of the nurse-patient relationship: Spatial vulnerabilities and gendered space. *Scholarly Inquiry for Nursing Practice: An International Journal.* 1997;11:45–59.

25. Carson SS, Stocking C, Podsadecki T, et al. Effects of organizational change in the medical intensive care unit of a teaching hospital. *JAMA.* 1996;276:322–328.

26. Benner P, Tanner C, Chesla J. *Expertise in Nursing Practice.* New York: Springer; 1996.

27. Baggs J, Schmitt M. Intensive care decisions about level of aggressiveness of care. *Research in Nursing and Health.* 1995;18:355.

28. Jacques R. Untheorized dimensions of caring work: caring as a structural practice and caring as a way of seeing. *Nursing Administration Quarterly.* 1993;17:1–10.

29. Hewson MG, Kindy PJ, Van Kirk J, et al. Strategies for managing uncertainty and complexity. *Journal of General Internal Medicine.* 1997;11:481–485.

30. Osler W. *Aphorism From His Bedside Teachings and Writings.* Springfield, IL: Charles Thomas; 1961.

31. Pervin L. The need to control and predict under conditions of threat. *Journal of Personality.* 1963;31:570–587.

32. Marshall M, Schwenzere K, Orsina M, et al. Influence of political power, medical provincialism and economic incentives on the rationing of surgical intensive care unit beds. *Critical Care Medicine.* 1997;20:387–394.

33. Kollef M. Private attending physician status and the withdrawal of life-sustaining interventions in a medical intensive care unit population. *Critical Care Medicine.* 1997;24:968–975.

34. ACCP/SCCM Consensus Panel. Ethical and moral guidelines for the initiation, continuation, and withdrawal of intensive care. *Chest.* 1990; 97:947–958.

35. Joint Commission on Accreditation of Hospital Organizations. *Patient Rights and Organization Ethics.* Chicago, IL: JCAHO; 1997.

36. Schmieding JJ. Relationship between head nurse responses to staff nurses and staff nurse responses to patients. *Western Journal of Nursing Research.* 1991;13:746–760.

37. Perkin RM, Young T, Freier C, et al. Stress and distress in pediatric nurses: Lessons from Baby K. *American Journal of Critical Care.* 1996;6:225–232.

38. Rushton C, Brooks-Brunn J. Environments that support ethical practice. *New Horizons.* 1997;5:20–29.

39. Lassen AA, Fosbinder DM, Minton S, et al. Nurse/physician collaborative practice: improving health care quality while decreasing cost. *Nursing Economics.* 1997;15:87–91.

40. Watts RJ, Chmielewski C, Holland MT, et al. Nurse-physician collaboration and decision outcomes in transplant ambulatory care settings. *American Nephrology Nurses Association Journal.* 1995;22:25–31.

41. King L, Lee J, Hermeman E. A collaborative practice model for critical care. *American Journal of Critical Care.* 1993;2:444–449.

42. McDaniel C. Organizational culture and ethics work satisfaction. *Journal of Nursing Administration.* 1995;25:21.

43. Lemieux-Charles L, Hall M: When resources are scarce: The impact of three organizational practices on clinician-managers. *Health Care Management Review.* 1997;22:58–69.

44. Reiser SJ. The ethical life of health care organizations. *Hastings Center Report.* 1994;24:28–35.

45. Kreitzer M, Wright D, Hamlin C, et al. Creating a healthy work environment in the midst of organizational change and transition. *Journal of Nursing Administration.* 1997;27:35–41.

46. Mitchell PH, Shannon SE, Cain KC, et al. Critical care outcomes: linking structures, processes, and organizational and clinical outcomes. *American Journal of Critical Care.* 1996;5:353–363.

47. Laschinger HKS, Havens DS. The effect of workplace empowerment on staff nurses' occupational mental health and work effectiveness. *Journal of Nursing Administration* 1997;27:42–50.

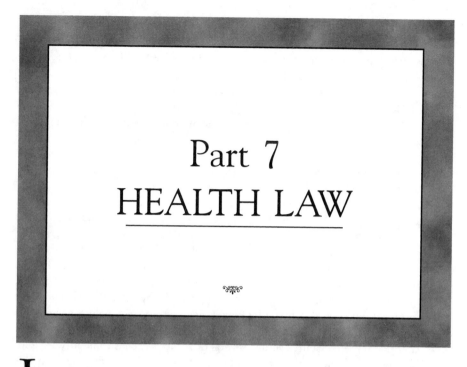

Part 7
HEALTH LAW

It has been almost twenty-five years since the New Jersey Supreme Court handed down its decision in the case of Karen Ann Quinlan; and it has been ten years since the U.S. Supreme Court handed down its decision in the case of Nancy Beth Cruzan. The issue in both cases concerned whether the parents of these two women, who were both in a persistent vegetative state, could withdraw life-sustaining treatment when their daughters' preferences were unknown. Karen's treatment was a ventilator; Nancy's was a feeding tube. The courts ultimately ruled that the treatment could be withdrawn, although each required a different process for doing so. As these cases are routinely invoked in discussions concerning either the withholding and/or withdrawing of treatment, it is important that health-care providers and ethics committees become familiar with what the courts actually held. In this section, in addition to both of these decisions, I have included their progeny, the Patient Self-Determination Act.

As you read these cases, try to see the faces through the decision. It will become apparent these cases were not really about the law or the state's interests—they were about family. The Quinlan and Cruzan families not only faced a family's worst possible tragedy, the death of a child, they actually fought their own state governments so that their children would be allowed to die. Imagine the grief from losing their daughters, the anger from having to fight their communities, and the guilt for advocating their children's death. By seeing these faces, health-care providers will gain a greater understanding of what families must endure when making decisions to withhold or withdraw treatment.

In 1976 Karen Ann Quinlan, who was twenty-one, suffered a respiratory arrest that resulted in a persistent vegetative state. After it became evident that Karen would never recover, her parents decided to take her off the ventilator; their request was refused. Her parents asked the courts to grant them the power to authorize the ventilator's withdrawal. A year later the New Jersey Supreme Court held that the state's interest in protecting Karen's life was outweighed by her right of privacy, given her poor prognosis and the invasion of her body that would be necessary to keep her alive. This decision provides a good foundation from which to explore what it means to balance the benefits and burdens of a life-sustaining treatment.

In 1983 Nancy Beth Cruzan, who was twenty-five, was found lying in a ditch after a car accident. This, too, resulted in a persistent vegetative state, but without the need of a ventilator. As with the Quinlans, Mr. and Mrs. Cruzan came to accept that Nancy would never recover. They asked her health-care providers to withdraw the feeding tube; their request, too, was refused. The Cruzans legal odyssey ended at the U.S. Supreme Court. Their decision upheld the Missouri Supreme Court's ruling, which required "clear and convincing" evidence that Nancy herself would choose to forgo artificial nutrition and hydration, given her current state, before her parents could remove the feeding tube.

After the Supreme Court's ruling, several of Nancy's friends came forward with recollections of statements that she would never want to live in that state. At this point I must clear up a very common misconception about these friends. It is widely believed that Nancy's friends fudged their testimony regarding her supposed comments on end-of-life preferences. If she really made these statements, some ask, why didn't her friends come forward years ago? Out of respect for the Cruzan family this misconception needs to be put to rest. At a conference several years ago Chris Cruzan, Nancy's sister, was on a panel discussing her family's experiences in this ordeal. In response to a question concerning these "convenient" witnesses, she quite reasonably responded that after the Supreme Court's decision newspapers all over the country carried the story. Only after that happened did some of the Nancy's friends, many of whom she had lost touch with, find out about what was going on. They then called the Cruzan family to tell them about Nancy's long-ago comments concerning end-of-life care.

After these rulings, particularly Nancy Cruzan's, the Patient Self-Determination Act (PSDA) was just a matter of time. The PSDA went into effect on December 1, 1991, and requires all hospitals, nursing homes, and hospices to provide patients, upon their admission, with information on the facility's advance directive policy. Patients are also to be provided with an advance directive upon their request.[1] The PSDA also requires these facilities to provide educational programs for their staff and surrounding communities on end-of-life issues. Ethics committees should take this opportunity to incorporate the PSDA's educational requirements into their overall educational initiatives.

As a brief review: a "Living Will" is a document that gives people the opportunity to make known what treatment they would and would not want if they were terminally ill and lost decision-making capacity, or were in a permanent vegetative state. A "Durable Power of Attorney for Health Care" is a document that allows people to designate someone (known as a proxy, agent, or surrogate) to make health-care decisions for them if they were to lose decision-making capacity. Importantly, this is a different document than a "Durable Power of Attorney for Property."

REFERENCE

1. Choice in Dying is an organization that also played a significant role in the development and dissemination of advance directives. On its Web site it has available for download the advance directive for every state. It has been very generous by doing so without charging a fee. The Web site address is www.choices.org.

19

IN THE MATTER OF KAREN QUINLAN, AN ALLEGED INCOMPETENT

Supreme Court of New Jersey
70 N.J. 10; 355 A.2d 647
January 26, 1976, Argued
March 31, 1976, Decided

❦

T he central figure in this tragic case is Karen Ann Quinlan, a New Jersey resident. At the age of 22, she lies in a debilitated and allegedly moribund state at Saint Clare's Hospital in Denville, New Jersey. The litigation has to do, in final analysis, with her life—its continuance or cessation—and the responsibilities, rights and duties, with regard to any fateful decision concerning it, of her family, her guardian, her doctors, the hospital, the State through its law enforcement authorities, and finally the courts of justice.

The issues are before this Court following its direct certification of the action under the rule, R. 2:12-1, prior to hearing in the Superior Court, Appellate Division, to which the appellant (hereafter "plaintiff") Joseph Quinlan, Karen's father, had appealed the adverse judgment of the Chancery Division.

Due to extensive physical damage fully described in the able opinion of the trial judge, Judge Muir, supporting that judgment, Karen allegedly was incompetent. Joseph Quinlan sought the adjudication of that incompetency. He wished to be appointed guardian of the person and property of his daughter. It was proposed by him that such letters of guardianship, if granted, should contain an express power to him as guardian to authorize the discontinuance of all extraordinary medical procedures now allegedly sustaining Karen's vital processes and hence her life, since these measures, he asserted, present no hope of her eventual recovery. A guardian *ad litem* was appointed by Judge Muir to represent the interest of the alleged incompetent.

By a supplemental complaint, in view of the extraordinary nature of the relief sought by plaintiff and the involvement therein of their several rights and responsibilities, other parties were added. These included the treating physicians and the hospital, the relief sought being that they be restrained from interfering with the carrying out of any such extraordinary authorization in the event it were to be granted by the court. Joined, as well, was the Prosecutor of Morris County (he being charged with responsibility for enforcement of the criminal law), to enjoin him from interfering with, or projecting a criminal prosecution which otherwise might ensue in the event of, cessation of life in Karen resulting from the exercise of such extraordinary authorization were it to be granted to the guardian.

The Attorney General of New Jersey intervened as of right pursuant to R. 4:33-1 on behalf of the State of New Jersey, such intervention being recognized by the court in the pretrial conference order (R. 4:25-1 *et seq.*) of September 22, 1975. Its basis, of course, was the interest of the State in the preservation of life, which has an undoubted constitutional foundation.[1]

The matter is of transcendent importance, involving questions related to the definition and existence of death; the prolongation of life through artificial means developed by medical technology undreamed of in past generations of the practice of the healing arts;[2] the impact of such durationally indeterminate and artificial life prolongation on the rights of the incompetent, her family and society in general; the bearing of constitutional right and the scope of judicial responsibility, as to the appropriate response of an equity court of justice to the extraordinary prayer for relief of the plaintiff. Involved as well is the right of the plaintiff, Joseph Quinlan, to guardianship of the person of his daughter.

Among his "factual and legal contentions" under such Pretrial Order was the following:

I. Legal and Medical Death

(a) Under the existing legal and medical definitions of death recognized by the State of New Jersey, Karen Ann Quinlan is dead.

This contention, made in the context of Karen's profound and allegedly irreversible coma and physical debility, was discarded during trial by the following stipulated amendment to the Pretrial Order:

Under any legal standard recognized by the State of New Jersey and also under standard medical practice, Karen Ann Quinlan is presently alive.

Other amendments to the Pretrial Order made at the time of trial expanded the issues before the court. The Prosecutor of Morris County sought a declaratory judgment as to the effect any affirmation by the court of a right in a guardian to terminate life-sustaining procedures would have with regard to enforcement of the criminal laws of New Jersey with reference to homicide. Saint Clare's Hospital, in the face of trial testimony on the subject of "brain death," sought declaratory judgment as to:

Whether the use of the criteria developed and enunciated by the Ad Hoc Committee of the Harvard Medical School on or about August 5, 1968, as well as similar criteria, by a physician to assist in determination of the death of a patient whose cardiopulmonary functions are being artificially sustained, is in accordance with ordinary and standard medical practice.[3]

It was further stipulated during trial that Karen was indeed incompetent and guardianship was necessary, although there exists a dispute as to the determination later reached by the court that such guardianship should be bifurcated, and that Mr. Quinlan should be appointed as guardian of the trivial property but not the person of his daughter.

After certification the Attorney General filed as of right (R. 2:3-4) a cross-appeal[3.1] challenging the action of the trial court in admitting evidence of prior statements made by Karen while competent as to her distaste for continuance of life by extraordinary medical procedures, under circumstances not unlike those of the present case. These quoted statements were made in the context of several conversations with regard to others terminally ill and being subjected to like heroic measures. The statements were advanced as evidence of what she would want done in such a contingency as now exists. She was said to have firmly evinced her wish, in like circumstances, not to have her life prolonged by the otherwise futile use of extraordinary means. Because we agree with the conception of the trial court that such statements, since they were remote and impersonal, lacked significant probative weight, it is not of consequence to our opinion that we decide whether or not they were admissible hearsay. Again, after certification, the guardian of the person of the incompetent (who had been appointed as a part of the judgment appealed from) resigned and was succeeded by another, but that, too, seems irrelevant to decision. It is, however, of interest to note the trial court's delineation (in its supplemental opinion of November 12, 1975) of the extent of the personal guardian's authority with respect to medical care of his ward:

> Mr. Coburn's appointment is designed to deal with those instances wherein Dr. Morse,[4] in the process of administering care and treatment to Karen Quinlan, feels there should be concurrence on the extent or nature of the care or treatment. If Mr. and Mrs. Quinlan are unable to give concurrence, then Mr. Coburn will be consulted for his concurrence.

Essentially then, appealing to the power of equity, and relying on claimed constitutional rights of free exercise of religion, of privacy, and of protection against cruel and unusual punishment, Karen Quinlan's father sought judicial authority to withdraw the life-sustaining mechanisms temporarily preserving his daughter's life, and his appointment as guardian of her person to that end. His request was opposed by her doctors, the hospital, the Morris County Prosecutor, the State of New Jersey, and her guardian *ad litem*.

THE FACTUAL BASE

An understanding of the issues in their basic perspective suggests a brief review of the factual base developed in the testimony and documented in greater detail in the opinion of the trial judge. In re Quinlan, 137 N.J. Super. 227 (Ch. Div. 1975).

On the night of April 15, 1975, for reasons still unclear, Karen Quinlan ceased breathing for at least two 15-minute periods. She received some ineffectual mouth-to-mouth resuscitation from friends. She was taken by ambulance to Newton Memorial Hospital. There she had a temperature of 100 degrees, her pupils were unreactive and she was unresponsive even to deep pain. The history at the time of her admission to that hospital was essentially incomplete and uninformative.

Three days later, Dr. Morse examined Karen at the request of the Newton admitting physician, Dr. McGee. He found her comatose with evidence of decortication, a condition relating to derangement of the cortex of the brain causing a physical posture in which the upper extremities are flexed and the lower extremities are extended. She required a respirator to assist her breathing. Dr. Morse was unable to obtain an adequate account of the circumstances and events leading up to Karen's admission to the Newton Hospital. Such initial history or etiology is crucial in neurological diagnosis. Relying as he did upon the Newton Memorial records and his own examination, he concluded that prolonged lack of oxygen in the bloodstream, anoxia, was identified with her condition as he saw it upon first observation. When she was later transferred to Saint Clare's Hospital she was still unconscious, still on a respirator, and a tracheotomy had been performed. On her arrival Dr. Morse conducted extensive and detailed examinations. An electroencephalogram (EEG) measuring electrical rhythm of the brain was performed and Dr. Morse characterized the result as "abnormal but it showed some activity and was consistent with her clinical state." Other significant neurological tests, including a brain scan, an angiogram, and a lumbar puncture were normal in result. Dr. Morse testified that Karen has been in a state of coma, lack of consciousness, since he began treating her. He explained that there are basically two types of coma, sleep-like unresponsiveness and awake unresponsiveness. Karen was originally in a sleep-like unresponsive condition but soon developed "sleep-wake" cycles, apparently a normal improvement for comatose patients occurring within three to four weeks. In the awake cycle she blinks, cries out and does things of that sort but is still totally unaware of anyone or anything around her.

Dr. Morse and other expert physicians who examined her characterized Karen as being in a "chronic persistent vegetative state." Dr. Fred Plum, one of such expert witnesses, defined this as a "subject who remains with the capacity to maintain the vegetative parts of neurological function but who ... no longer has any cognitive function."

Dr. Morse, as well as the several other medical and neurological experts who testified in this case, believed with certainty that Karen Quinlan is not "brain dead." They identified the Ad Hoc Committee of Harvard Medical School report (infra) as the ordinary medical standard for determining brain death, and all of them were satisfied that Karen met none of the criteria specified in that report and was therefore not "brain dead" within its contemplation.

In this respect it was indicated by Dr. Plum that the brain works in essentially two ways, the vegetative and the sapient. He testified:

We have an internal vegetative regulation which controls body temperature which controls breathing, which controls to a considerable degree blood pressure, which controls to some degree heart rate, which controls chewing, swallowing, and which controls sleeping and waking. We have a more highly developed brain which is uniquely human which controls our relation to the outside world, our capacity to talk, to see, to feel, to sing, to think. Brain death necessarily must mean the death of both of these functions of the brain, vegetative and the sapient. Therefore, the presence of any function which is regulated or governed or controlled by the deeper parts of the brain which in laymen's terms might be considered purely vegetative would mean that the brain is not biologically dead.

Because Karen's neurological condition affects her respiratory ability (the respiratory system being a brain stem function) she requires a respirator to assist her breathing. From the time of her admission to Saint Clare's Hospital Karen has been assisted by an MA-1 respirator, a sophisticated machine which delivers a given volume of air at a certain rate and periodically provides a "sigh" volume, a relatively large measured volume of air designed to purge the lungs of excretions. Attempts to "wean" her from the respirator were unsuccessful and have been abandoned.

The experts believe that Karen cannot now survive without the assistance of the respirator; that exactly how long she would live without it is unknown; that the strong likelihood is that death would follow soon after its removal; and that removal would also risk further brain damage and would curtail the assistance the respirator presently provides in warding off infection.

It seemed to be the consensus not only of the treating physicians but also of the several qualified experts who testified in the case, that removal from the respirator would not conform to medical practices, standards, and traditions.

The further medical consensus was that Karen in addition to being comatose is in a chronic and persistent "vegetative" state, having no awareness of anything or anyone around her and existing at a primitive reflex level. Although she does have some brain stem function (ineffective for respiration) and has other reactions one normally associates with being alive, such as moving; reacting to light, sound, and noxious stimuli; blinking her eyes; and the like, the quality of her feeling impulses is unknown. She grimaces, makes sterotyped cries and sounds and has chewing motions. Her blood pressure is normal.

Karen remains in the intensive care unit at Saint Clare's Hospital, receiving 24-hour care by a team of four nurses characterized, as was the medical attention, as "excellent." She is nourished by feeding by way of a nasal-gastro tube and is routinely examined for infection, which under these circumstances is a serious life threat. The result is that her condition is considered remarkable under the unhappy circumstances involved.

Karen is described as emaciated, having suffered a weight loss of at least 40 pounds, and undergoing a continuing deteriorative process. Her posture is described as fetal-like and grotesque; there is extreme flexion-rigidity of the arms, legs, and related muscles and her joints are severely rigid and deformed.

From all of this evidence, and including the whole testimonial record, several basic findings in the physical area are mandated. Severe brain and associated damage, albeit of uncertain etiology, has left Karen in a chronic and persistent vegetative state. No form of treatment which can cure or improve that condition is known or available. As nearly as may be determined, considering the guarded area of remote uncertainties characteristic of most medical science predictions, she can never be restored to cognitive or sapient life. Even with regard to the vegetative level and improvement therein (if such it may be called) the prognosis is extremely poor and the extent unknown if it should in fact occur.

She is debilitated and moribund and although fairly stable at the time of argument before us (no new information having been filed in the meanwhile in expansion of the record), no physician risked the opinion that she could live more than a year and indeed she may die much earlier. Excellent medical and nursing care so far has been able to ward off the constant threat of infection, to which she is peculiarly susceptible because of the respirator, the tracheal tube, and other incidents of care in her vulnerable condition. Her life accordingly is sustained by the respirator and tubal feeding, and removal from the respirator would cause her death soon, although the time cannot be stated with more precision.

The determination of the fact and time of death in past years of medical science was keyed to the action of the heart and blood circulation, in turn dependent upon pulmonary activity, and hence cessation of these functions spelled out the reality of death.[5]

Developments in medical technology have obfuscated the use of the traditional definition of death. Efforts have been made to define irreversible coma as a new criterion for death, such as by the 1968 report of the Ad Hoc Committee of the Harvard Medical School (the Committee comprising ten physicians, an historian, a lawyer, and a theologian), which asserted that:

> From ancient times down to the recent past it was clear that, when the respiration and heart stopped, the brain would die in a few minutes; so the obvious criterion of no heart beat as synonymous with death was sufficiently accurate. In those times the heart was considered to be the central organ of the body; it is not surprising that its failure marked the onset of death. This is no longer valid when modern resuscitative and supportive measures are used. These improved activities can now restore "life" as judged by the ancient standards of persistent respiration and continuing heart beat. This can be the case even when there is not the remotest possibility of an individual recovering consciousness following massive brain damage. ["A Definition of Irreversible Coma," 205 *JAMA* 337, 339 (1968)].

The Ad Hoc standards, carefully delineated, included absence of response to pain or other stimuli; pupilary reflexes; corneal, pharyngeal, and other reflexes; blood pressure; spontaneous respiration; as well as "flat" or isoelectric electro-encephalograms and the like, with all tests repeated "at least 24 hours later with no change." In such circumstances, where all of such criteria have been met as showing "brain death," the Committee recommends with regard to the respirator:

> The patient's condition can be determined only by a physician. When the patient is hopelessly damaged as defined above, the family and all colleagues who have participated in major decisions concerning the patient, and all nurses involved, should be so informed. Death is to be declared and then the respirator turned off. The decision to do this and the responsibility for it are to be taken by the physician-in-charge, in consultation with one or more physicians who have been directly involved in the case. It is unsound and undesirable to force the family to make the decision. [Ibid., p. 338]

But, as indicated, it was the consensus of medical testimony in the instant case that Karen, for all her disability, met none of these criteria, nor indeed any comparable criteria extant in the medical world and representing, as does the Ad Hoc Committee report, according to the testimony in this case, prevailing and accepted medical standards.

We have adverted to the "brain death" concept and Karen's disassociation with any of its criteria, to emphasize the basis of the medical decision made by Dr. Morse. When plaintiff and his family, finally reconciled to the certainty of Karen's impending death, requested the withdrawal of life-support mechanisms, he demurred. His refusal was based upon his conception of medical standards, practice, and ethics described in the medical testimony, such as in the evidence given by another neurologist, Dr. Sidney Diamond, a witness for the State. Dr. Diamond asserted that no physician would have failed to provide respirator support at the outset, and none would interrupt its life-saving course thereafter, except in the case of cerebral death. In the latter case, he thought the respirator would in effect be disconnected from one already dead, entitling the physician under medical standards and, he thought, legal concepts, to terminate the supportive measures. We note Dr. Diamond's distinction of major surgical or transfusion procedures in a terminal case not involving cerebral death, such as here:

> The subject has lost human qualities. It would be incredible, and I think unlikely, that any physician would respond to a sudden hemorrhage, massive hemorrhage, or a loss of all her defensive blood cells, by giving her large quantities of blood. I think that .
> . . major surgical procedures would be out of the question even if they were known to be essential for continued physical existence.

This distinction is adverted to also in the testimony of Dr. Julius Korein, a neurologist called by plaintiff. Dr. Korein described a medical practice concept of "judicious neglect" under which the physician will say:

> Don't treat this patient anymore, . . . it does not serve either the patient, the family, or society in any meaningful way to continue treatment with this patient.

Dr. Korein also told of the unwritten and unspoken standard of medical practice implied in the foreboding initials DNR (do not resuscitate), as applied to the extraordinary terminal case:

> Cancer, metastatic cancer, involving the lungs, the liver, the brain, multiple involvements, the physician may or may not write: Do not resuscitate. . . . [I]t could be said to the nurse: If this man stops breathing don't resuscitate him. . . . No physician that I know personally is going to try and resuscitate a man riddled with cancer and in agony and he stops breathing. They are not going to put him on a respirator. . . . I think that would be the height of misuse of technology.

While the thread of logic in such distinctions may be elusive to the nonmedical lay mind, in relation to the supposed imperative to sustain life at all costs, they nevertheless relate to medical decisions, such as the decision of Dr. Morse in the present case. We agree with the trial court that that decision was in accord with Dr. Morse's conception of medical standards and practice.

We turn to that branch of the factual case pertaining to the application for guardianship, as distinguished from the nature of the authorization sought by the applicant. The character and general suitability of Joseph Quinlan as guardian for his daughter, in ordinary circumstances, could not be doubted. The record bespeaks the high degree of familial love which pervaded the home of Joseph Quinlan and reached out fully to embrace Karen, although she was living elsewhere at the time of her collapse. The proofs showed him to be deeply religious, imbued with a morality so sensitive that months of tortured indecision preceded his belated conclusion (despite earlier moral judgments reached by the other family members, but unexpressed to him in order not to influence him) to seek the termination of life-supportive measures sustaining Karen. A communicant of the Roman Catholic Church, as were other family members, he first sought solace in private prayer looking with confidence, as he says, to the Creator, first for the recovery of Karen and then, if that were not possible, for guidance with respect to the awesome decision confronting him.

To confirm the moral rightness of the decision he was about to make he consulted with his parish priest and later with the Catholic chaplain of Saint Clare's Hospital. He would not, he testified, have sought termination if that act were to be morally wrong or in conflict with the tenets of the religion he so profoundly respects. He was disabused of doubt, however, when the position of the Roman Catholic Church was made known to him as it is reflected in the record in this case. While it is not usual for matters of religious dogma or concepts to enter a civil litigation (except as they may bear upon constitutional right, or sometimes, familial matters; cf. In re Adoption of E, 59 N.J. 36 [1971]), they were rightly admitted in evidence here. The judge was bound to measure the character and motivations in all respects of Joseph Quinlan as prospective guardian; and insofar as these religious matters bore upon them, they were properly scrutinized and considered by the court.

Thus germane, we note the position of that Church as illuminated by the record before us. We have no reason to believe that it would be at all discordant with the whole of Judeo-Christian tradition, considering its central respect and reverence for the sanctity of human life. It was in this sense of relevance that we admitted as *amicus curiae* the New Jersey Catholic Conference, essentially the spokesman for the various Catholic bishops of New Jersey, organized to give witness to spiritual values in public affairs in the statewide community. The *position statement of Bishop Lawrence B. Casey, reproduced in the amicus* brief, projects these views:

(a) The verification of the fact of death in a particular case cannot be deduced from any religious or moral principle and, under this aspect, does not fall within the competence of the church;—that dependence must be had upon traditional and medical standards, and by these standards Karen Ann Quinlan is assumed to be alive.

(b) The request of plaintiff for authority to terminate a medical procedure characterized as "an extraordinary means of treatment" would not involve euthanasia. This upon the reasoning expressed by Pope Pius XII in his "*allocutio*" [address] to anesthesiologists on November 24, 1957, when he dealt with the question:

Does the anesthesiologist have the right, or is he bound, in all cases of deep unconsciousness, even in those that are completely hopeless in the opinion of the competent doctor, to use modern artificial respiration apparatus, even against the will of the family?

His answer made the following points:

1. In ordinary cases the doctor has the right to act in this manner, but is not bound to do so unless this is the only way of fulfilling another certain moral duty.

2. The doctor, however, has no right independent of the patient. He can act only if the patient explicitly or implicitly, directly or indirectly gives him the permission.

3. The treatment as described in the question constitutes extraordinary means of preserving life and so there is no obligation to use them nor to give the doctor permission to use them.

4. The rights and the duties of the family depend on the presumed will of the unconscious patient if he or she is of legal age, and the family, too, is bound to use only ordinary means.

5. This case is not to be considered euthanasia in any way; that would never be licit. The interruption of attempts at resuscitation, even when it causes the arrest of circulation, is not more than an indirect cause of the cessation of life, and we must apply in this case the principle of double effect.

So it was that the Bishop Casey statement validated the decision of Joseph Quinlan:

Competent medical testimony has established that Karen Ann Quinlan has no reasonable hope of recovery from her comatose state by the use of any available medical procedures. The continuance of mechanical (cardiorespiratory) supportive measures to sustain continuation of her body functions and her life constitute extraordinary means of treatment. Therefore, the decision of Joseph ... Quinlan to request the discontinuance of this treatment is, according to the teachings of the Catholic Church, a morally correct decision.

And the mind and purpose of the intending guardian were undoubtedly influenced by factors included in the following reference to the interrelationship of the three disciplines of theology, law, and medicine as exposed in the Casey statement:

The right to a natural death is one outstanding area in which the disciplines of theology, medicine, and law overlap; or, to put it another way, it is an area in which these three disciplines convene.

Medicine, with its combination of advanced technology and professional ethics, is both able and inclined to prolong biological life. Law, with its felt obligation to protect the life and freedom of the individual, seeks to assure each person's right to live out his human life until its natural and inevitable conclusion. Theology, with its acknowledgment of man's dissatisfaction with biological life as the ultimate source of joy, ... defends the sacredness of human life and defends it from all direct attacks.

These disciplines do not conflict with one another, but are necessarily conjoined in the application of their principles in a particular instance such as that of Karen Ann Quinlan. Each must in some way acknowledge the other without denying its own competence. The civil law is not expected to assert a belief in eternal life; nor, on the other hand, is it expected to ignore the right of the individual to profess it, and to form and pursue his conscience in accord with that belief. Medical science is not authorized to directly cause natural death; nor, however, is it expected to prevent it when it is inevitable and all hope of a return to an even partial exercise of human life is irreparably lost. Religion is not expected to define biological death; nor, on its part, is it expected to relinquish its responsibility to assist man in the formation and pursuit of a correct conscience as to the acceptance of natural death when science has confirmed its inevitability beyond any hope other than that of preserving biological life in a merely vegetative state.

And the gap in the law is aptly described in the Bishop Casey statement:

In the present public discussion of the case of Karen Ann Quinlan it has been brought out that responsible people involved in medical care, patients, and families have exercised the freedom to terminate or withhold certain treatments as extraordinary means in cases judged to be terminal, i.e., cases which hold no realistic hope for some recovery, in accord with the expressed or implied intentions of the patients themselves. To whatever extent this has been happening it has been without sanction in civil law. Those involved in such actions, however, have ethical and theological literature to guide them in their judgments and actions. Furthermore, such actions have not in themselves undermined society's reverence for the lives of sick and dying people.

It is both possible and necessary for society to have laws and ethical standards which provide freedom for decisions, in accord with the expressed or implied intentions of the patient, to terminate or withhold extraordinary treatment in cases which are judged to be hopeless by competent medical authorities, without at the same time leaving an opening for euthanasia. Indeed, to accomplish this, it may simply be required that courts and legislative bodies recognize the present standards and practices of many people engaged in medical care who have been doing what the parents of Karen Ann Quinlan are requesting authorization to have done for their beloved daughter.

Before turning to the legal and constitutional issues involved, we feel it essential to reiterate that the "Catholic view" of religious neutrality in the circumstances of this case is considered by the Court only in the aspect of its impact upon the conscience, motivation, and purpose of the intending guardian, Joseph Quinlan, and not as a precedent in terms of the civil law.

If Joseph Quinlan, for instance, were a follower and strongly influenced by the teachings of Buddha, or if, as an agnostic or atheist, his moral judgments were formed without reference to religious feelings, but were nevertheless formed and viable, we would with equal attention and high respect consider these elements, as bearing upon his character, motivations, and purposes as relevant to his qualification and suitability as guardian.

It is from this factual base that the Court confronts and responds to three basic issues:

1. Was the trial court correct in denying the specific relief requested by plaintiff, i.e., authorization for termination of the life-supporting apparatus, on the case presented to him? Our determination on that question is in the affirmative.
2. Was the court correct in withholding letters of guardianship from the plaintiff and appointing in his stead a stranger? On that issue our determination is in the negative.
3. Should this Court, in the light of the foregoing conclusions, grant declaratory relief to the plaintiff? On that question our Court's determination is in the affirmative.

This brings us to a consideration of the constitutional and legal issues underlying the foregoing determinations.

CONSTITUTIONAL AND LEGAL ISSUES

At the outset we note the dual role in which plaintiff comes before the Court. He not only raises, derivatively, what he perceives to be the constitutional and legal rights of his daughter Karen, but he also claims certain rights independently as parent.

Although generally a litigant may assert only his own constitutional rights, we have no doubt that plaintiff has sufficient standing to advance both positions.

While no express constitutional language limits judicial activity to cases and controversies, New Jersey courts will not render advisory opinions or entertain proceedings by plaintiffs who do not have sufficient legal standing to maintain their actions. *Walker* v. *Stanhope*, 23 N.J. 657, 660 (1957). However, as in this case, New Jersey courts commonly grant declaratory relief. Declaratory Judgments Act, N.J.S.A. 2A:16–50 *et seq.* And our courts hold that where the plaintiff is not simply an interloper and the proceeding serves the public interest, standing will be found. *Walker* v. *Stanhope, supra*, 23 N.J. at 661-66; *Koons* v. *Atlantic City Bd. of Comm'rs*, 134 N.J.L. 329, 338–39 (Sup. Ct. 1946), aff'd, 135 N.J.L. 204 (E. & A. 1947). In *Crescent Park Tenants Ass'n.* v. *Realty Equities Corp.*, 58 N.J. 98 (1971), Justice Jacobs said:

> ... [W]e have appropriately confined litigation to those situations where the litigants concerned with the subject matter evidenced a sufficient stake and real adverseness. In the overall we have given due weight to the interests of individual justice, along with the public interest, always bearing in mind that throughout our law we have been sweepingly rejecting procedural frustrations in favor of "just and expeditious determinations on the ultimate merits." [58 N.J. at 107–08 (quoting from *Tumarkin* v. *Friedman*, 17 N.J. Super. 20, 21 (App. Div. 1951), certif. den., 9 N.J. 287 [1952])].

The father of Karen Quinlan is certainly no stranger to the present controversy. His interests are real and adverse and he raises questions of surpassing importance. Manifestly, he has standing to assert his daughter's constitutional rights, she being incompetent to do so.

I. The Free Exercise of Religion

We think the contention as to interference with religious beliefs or rights may be considered and dealt with without extended discussion, given the acceptance of distinctions so clear and simple in their precedential definition as to be dispositive on their face.

Simply stated, the right to religious beliefs is absolute but conduct in pursuance thereof is not wholly immune from governmental restraint. *John F. Kennedy Memorial Hosp.* v. *Heston*, 58 N.J. 576, 580–81 (1971). So it is that, for the sake of life, courts sometimes (but not always) order blood transfusions for Jehovah's Witnesses (whose religious beliefs abhor such procedure), Application of President & Directors of Georgetown College, Inc., 118 U.S. App. D.C. 80, 331 F. 2d 1000 (D.C. Cir.), cert. den., 377 U.S. 978, 84 S. Ct. 1883, 12 L. Ed. 2d 746 (1964); *United States* v. *George*, 239 F. Supp. 752 (D. Conn. 1965); *John F. Kennedy Memorial Hosp.* v. *Heston*, supra; *Powell* v. *Columbian Presbyterian Medical Center*, 49 Misc. 2d 215, 267 N.Y.S. 2d 450 (Sup. Ct. 1965); but see *In re* Osborne, 294 A. 2d 372 (D.C. Ct. App. 1972); In re Estate of Brooks, 32 Ill. 2d 361, 205 N.E. 2d 435 (Sup. Ct. 1965); *Erickson* v. *Dilgard*, 44 Misc. 2d 27, 252 N.Y.S. 2d 705 (Sup. Ct. 1962); see generally Annot., "Power Of Courts Or Other Public Agencies, In The Absence of Statutory Authority, To Order Compulsory Medical Care for Adult," 9 A.L.R. 3d 1391 (1966); forbid exposure to death from handling virulent snakes or ingesting poison (interfering with deeply held religious sentiments in such regard), e.g., *Hill* v. *State*, 38 Ala. App. 404, 88 So. 2d 880 (Ct. App.), cert. den., 264 Ala. 697, 88 So. 2d 887 (Sup. Ct. 1956); *State* v. *Massey*, 229 N.C. 734, 51 S.E. 2d 179 (Sup. Ct.), appeal dismissed *sub nom.*, *Bunn* v. *North Carolina*, 336 U.S. 942, 69 S. Ct. 813, 93 L. Ed. 1099 (1949); *State ex rel. Swann* v. *Pack*, Tenn. , 527 S.W. 2d 99 (Sup. Ct. 1975), cert. den., U.S. , 96 S. Ct. 1429, 47 L. Ed. 2d 360 (1976); and protect the public health as in the case of compulsory vaccination (over the strongest of religious objections), e.g., *Wright* v. *DeWitt School Dist.* 1, 238 Ark. 906, 385 S.W. 2d 644 (Sup. Ct. 1965); *Mountain Lakes Bd. of Educ.* v. *Maas*, 56 N.J. Super. 245 (App. Div. 1959), aff'd o.b., 31 N.J. 537 (1960), cert. den., 363 U.S. 843, 80 S. Ct. 1613, 4 L. Ed. 2d 1727 (1960); *McCartney* v. *Austin*, 57 Misc. 2d 525, 293 N.Y.S. 2d 188 (Sup. Ct. 1968). The public interest is thus considered paramount, without essential dissolution of respect for religious beliefs.

We think, without further examples, that, ranged against the State's interest in the preservation of life, the impingement of religious belief, much less religious "neutrality" as here, does not reflect a constitutional question, in the circumstances at least of the case presently before the Court. Moreover, like the trial court, we do not recognize an independent parental right of religious freedom to support the relief requested. 137 N.J. Super. at 267–68.

II. Cruel and Unusual Punishment

Similarly inapplicable to the case before us is the Constitution's Eighth Amendment protection against cruel and unusual punishment which, as held by the trial court, is not relevant to situations other than the imposition of penal sanctions. Historic in nature, it stemmed from punitive excesses in the infliction of criminal penalties.[6] We find no precedent in law which would justify its extension to the correction of social injustice or hardship, such as, for instance, in the case of poverty. The latter often condemns the poor and deprived to horrendous living conditions which could certainly be described in the abstract as "cruel and unusual punishment." Yet the constitutional base of protection from "cruel and unusual punishment" is plainly irrelevant to such societal ills which must be remedied, if at all, under other concepts of constitutional and civil right.

So it is in the case of the unfortunate Karen Quinlan. Neither the State, nor the law, but the accident of fate and nature, has inflicted upon her conditions which though in essence cruel and most unusual, yet do not amount to "punishment" in any constitutional sense.

Neither the judgment of the court below, nor the medical decision which confronted it, nor the law and equity perceptions which impelled its action, nor the whole factual base upon which it was predicated, inflicted "cruel and unusual punishment" in the constitutional sense.

III. The Right of Privacy[7]

It is the issue of the constitutional right of privacy that has given us most concern, in the exceptional circumstances of this case. Here a loving parent, qua parent and raising the rights of his incompetent and profoundly damaged daughter, probably irreversibly doomed to no more than a biologically vegetative remnant of life, is before the court. He seeks authorization to abandon specialized technological procedures which can only maintain for a time a body having no potential for resumption or continuance of other than a "vegetative" existence.

We have no doubt, in these unhappy circumstances, that if Karen were herself miraculously lucid for an interval (not altering the existing prognosis of the condition to which she would soon return) and perceptive of her irreversible condition, she could effectively decide upon discontinuance of the life-support apparatus, even if it meant the prospect of natural death. To this extent we may distinguish Heston, *supra*, which concerned a severely injured young woman (Delores Heston), whose life depended on surgery and blood transfusion; and who was in such extreme shock that she was unable to express an informed choice (although the Court apparently considered the case as if the patient's own religious decision to resist transfusion were at stake), but most importantly a patient apparently salvable to long life and vibrant health;—a situation not at all like the present case.

We have no hesitancy in deciding, in the instant diametrically opposite case, that no external compelling interest of the State could compel Karen to endure the unendurable, only to vegetate a few measurable months with no realistic possibility of returning to any semblance of cognitive or sapient life. We perceive no thread of logic distinguishing between such a choice on Karen's part and a similar choice which, under the evidence in this case, could be made by a competent patient terminally ill, riddled by cancer and suffering great pain; such a patient would not be resuscitated or put on a respirator in the example described by Dr. Korein, and *a fortiori* would not be kept against his will on a respirator.

Although the Constitution does not explicitly mention a right of privacy, Supreme Court decisions have recognized that a right of personal privacy exists and that certain areas of privacy are guaranteed under the Constitution. *Eisenstadt* v. *Baird*, 405 U.S. 438, 92 S. Ct. 1029, 31 L. Ed. 2d 349 (1972); *Stanley* v. *Georgia*, 394 U.S. 557, 89 S. Ct. 1243, 22 L. Ed. 2d 542 (1969). The Court has interdicted judicial intrusion into many aspects of personal decision, sometimes basing this restraint upon the conception of a limitation of judicial interest and responsibility, such as with regard to contraception and its relationship to family life and decision. *Griswold* v. *Connecticut*, 381 U.S. 479, 85 S. Ct. 1678, 14 L. Ed. 2d 510 (1965).

The Court in *Griswold* found the unwritten constitutional right of privacy to exist in the penumbra of specific guarantees of the Bill of Rights "formed by emanations from those guarantees that help give them life and substance." 381 U.S. at 484, 85 S. Ct. at 1681, 14 L. Ed. 2d at 514. Presumably this right is broad enough to encompass a patient's decision to decline medical treatment under certain circumstances, in much the same way as it is broad enough to encompass a woman's decision to terminate pregnancy under certain conditions. *Roe* v. *Wade*, 410 U.S. 113, 153, 93 S. Ct. 705, 727, 35 L. Ed. 2d 147, 177 (1973).

Nor is such right of privacy forgotten in the New Jersey Constitution. N.J. Const. (1947), Art. I, par. 1.

The claimed interests of the State in this case are essentially the preservation and sanctity of human life and defense of the right of the physician to administer medical treatment according to his best judgment. In this case the doctors say that removing Karen from the respirator will conflict with their professional judgment. The plaintiff answers that Karen's present treatment serves only a maintenance function; that the respirator cannot cure or improve her condition but at best can only prolong her inevitable slow deterioration and death; and that the interests of the patient, as seen by her surrogate, the guardian, must be evaluated by the court as predominant, even in the face of an opinion *contra* by the present attending physicians. Plaintiff's distinction is significant. The nature of Karen's care and the realistic chances of her recovery are quite unlike those of the patients discussed in many of the cases where treatments were ordered. In many of those cases the medical procedure required (usually a transfusion) constituted a minimal bodily invasion and the chances of recovery and return to functioning life were very good. We think that the State's interest *contra* weakens and the individual's right to privacy grows as the degree of bodily invasion increases and the prognosis dims. Ultimately there comes a point at which the individual's rights overcome the State interest. It is for that reason that we believe Karen's choice, if she were competent to make it, would be vindicated by the law. Her prognosis is extremely poor,—she will never resume cognitive life. And the bodily invasion is very great,—she requires 24-hour intensive nursing care, antibiotics, the assistance of a respirator, a catheter, and feeding tube.

Our affirmation of Karen's independent right of choice, however, would ordinarily be based upon her competency to assert it. The sad truth, however, is that she is grossly incompetent and we cannot discern her supposed choice based on the testimony of her previous conversations with friends, where such testimony is without sufficient probative weight. 137 N.J. Super. at 260. Nevertheless we have concluded that Karen's right of privacy may be asserted on her behalf by her guardian under the peculiar circumstances here present.

If a putative decision by Karen to permit this noncognitive, vegetative existence to terminate by natural forces is regarded as a valuable incident of her right of privacy, as we believe it to be, then it should not be discarded solely on the basis that her condition prevents her conscious exercise of the choice. The only practical way to prevent destruction of the right is to permit the guardian and family of Karen to render their best judgment, subject to the qualifications hereinafter stated, as to whether she would exercise it in these circumstances. If their conclusion is in the affirmative this decision should be accepted by a society the overwhelming majority of whose members would, we think, in similar circumstances, exercise such a choice in the same way for themselves or for those closest to them. It is for this reason that we determine that Karen's right of privacy may be asserted in her behalf, in this respect, by her guardian and family under the particular circumstances presented by this record.

Regarding Mr. Quinlan's right of privacy, we agree with Judge Muir's conclusion that there is no parental constitutional right that would entitle him to a grant of relief in propria persona. *Id.* at 266. Insofar as a parental right of privacy has been recognized, it has been in the context of determining the rearing of infants and, as Judge Muir put it, involved "continuing life styles." See *Wisconsin* v. *Yoder,* 406 U.S. 205, 92 S. Ct. 1526, 32 L. Ed. 2d 15 (1972); *Pierce* v. *Society of Sisters,* 268 U.S. 510, 45 S. Ct. 571, 69 L. Ed. 1070 (1925); *Meyer* v. *Nebraska,* 262 U.S. 390, 43 S. Ct. 625, 67 L. Ed. 1042 (1923). Karen Quinlan is a 22-year-old adult. Her right of privacy in respect of the matter before the Court is to be vindicated by Mr. Quinlan as guardian, as hereinabove determined.

IV. The Medical Factor

Having declared the substantive legal basis upon which plaintiff's rights as representative of Karen must be deemed predicated, we face and respond to the assertion on behalf of defendants that our premise unwarrantably offends prevailing medical standards. We thus turn to consideration of the medical decision supporting the determination made below, conscious of the paucity of preexisting legislative and judicial guidance as to the rights and liabilities therein involved.

A significant problem in any discussion of sensitive medical-legal issues is the marked, perhaps unconscious, tendency of many to distort what the law is, in pursuit of an exposition of what they would like the law to be. Nowhere is this barrier to the intelligent resolution of legal controversies more obstructive than in the debate over patient rights at the end of life. Judicial refusals to order lifesaving treatment in the face of contrary claims of bodily self-determination or free religious exercise are too often cited in support of a preconceived "right to die," even though the patients, wanting to live, have claimed no such right. Conversely, the assertion of a religious or other objection to lifesaving treatment is at times condemned as attempted suicide, even though suicide means something quite diferent in the law. [Byrn, "Compulsory Lifesaving Treatment For The Competent Adult," 44 *Fordham L. Rev.* 1 (1975)].

Perhaps the confusion there adverted to stems from mention by some courts of statutory or common law condemnation of suicide as demonstrating the state's interest in the preservation of life. We would see, however, a real distinction between the self-infliction of deadly harm and a self-determination against artificial life support or radical surgery, for instance, in the face of irreversible, painful, and certain imminent death. The contrasting situations mentioned are analogous to those continually faced by the medical profession. When does the institution of life-sustaining procedures, ordinarily mandatory, become the subject of medical discretion in the context of administration to persons in extremis? And when does the withdrawal of such procedures, from such persons already supported by them, come within the orbit of medical discretion? When does a determination as to either of the foregoing contingencies court the hazard of civil or criminal liability on the part of the physician or institution involved?

The existence and nature of the medical dilemma need hardly be discussed at length, portrayed as it is in the present case and complicated as it has recently come to be in view of the dramatic advance of medical technology. The dilemma is there, it is real, it is constantly resolved in accepted medical practice without attention in the courts, it pervades the issues in the very case we here examine. The branch of the dilemma involving the doctor's responsibility and the relationship of the court's duty was thus conceived by Judge Muir:

> Doctors . . . to treat a patient, must deal with medical tradition and past case histories. They must be guided by what they do know. The extent of their training, their experience, consultation with other physicians, must guide their decision-making processes in providing care to their patient. The nature, extent and duration of care by societal standards is the responsibility of a physician. The morality and conscience of our society places this responsibility in the hands of the physician. What justification is there to remove it from the control of the medical profession and place it in the hands of the courts? [137 N.J. Super. at 259].

Such notions as to the distribution of responsibility, heretofore generally entertained, should however neither impede this Court in deciding matters clearly justiciable nor preclude a reexamination by the Court as to underlying human values and rights. Determinations as to these must, in the ultimate, be responsive not only to the concepts of medicine but also to the common moral judgment of the community at large. In the latter respect the Court has a nondelegable judicial responsibility.

Put in another way, the law, equity, and justice must not themselves quail and be helpless in the face of modern technological marvels presenting questions hitherto unthought of. Where a Karen Quinlan, or a parent, or a doctor, or a hospital, or a State seeks the process and response of a court, it must answer with its most informed conception of justice in the previously unexplored circumstances presented to it. That is its obligation and we are here fulfilling it, for the actors and those having an interest in the matter should not go without remedy.

Courts in the exercise of their parens patriae responsibility to protect those under disability have sometimes implemented medical decisions and authorized their carrying out under the doctrine of "substituted judgment." *Hart v. Brown*, 29 Conn. Sup. 368, 289 A. 2d 386, 387-88 (Super. Ct. 1972); *Strunk v. Strunk*, 445 S.W. 2d 145, 147-48 (Ky. Ct. App. 1969). For as Judge Muir pointed out:

> "As part of the inherent power of equity, a Court of Equity has full and complete jurisdiction over the persons of those who labor under any legal disability. . . . The Court's action in such a case is not limited by any narrow bounds, but it is empowered to stretch forth its arm in whatever direction its aid and protection may be needed. While this is indeed a special exercise of equity jurisdiction, it is beyond question that by virtue thereof the Court may pass upon purely personal rights." [137 N.J. Super. at 254 (quoting from Am. Jur. 2d, Equity § 69 (1966))].

But insofar as a court, having no inherent medical expertise, is called upon to overrule a professional decision made according to prevailing medical practice and standards, a different question is presented. As mentioned below, a doctor is required "to exercise in the treatment of his patient the degree of care, knowledge and skill ordinarily possessed and exercised in similar situations by the average member of the profession practicing in his field." *Schueler* v. *Strelinger*, 43 N.J. 330, 344 (1964). If he is a specialist he "must employ not merely the skill of a general practitioner, but also that special degree of skill normally possessed by the average physician who devotes special study and attention to the particular organ or disease or injury involved, having regard to the present state of scientific knowledge." *Clark* v. *Wichman*, 72 N.J. Super. 486, 493 (App. Div. 1962). This is the duty that establishes his legal obligations to his patients. [137 N.J. Super. at 257–58].

The medical obligation is related to standards and practice prevailing in the profession. The physicians in charge of the case, as noted above, declined to withdraw the respirator. That decision was consistent with the proofs below as to the then existing medical standards and practices.

Under the law as it then stood, Judge Muir was correct in declining to authorize withdrawal of the respirator.

However, in relation to the matter of the declaratory relief sought by plaintiff as representative of Karen's interests, we are required to reevaluate the applicability of the medical standards projected in the court below. The question is whether there is such internal consistency and rationality in the application of such standards as should warrant their constituting an ineluctable bar to the effectuation of substantive relief for plaintiff at the hands of the court. We have concluded not.

In regard to the foregoing it is pertinent that we consider the impact on the standards both of the civil and criminal law as to medical liability and the new technological means of sustaining life irreversibly damaged.

The modern proliferation of substantial malpractice litigation and the less frequent but even more unnerving possibility of criminal sanctions would seem, for it is beyond human nature to suppose otherwise, to have bearing on the practice and standards as they exist. The brooding presence of such possible liability, it was testified here, had no part in the decision of the treating physicians. As did Judge Muir, we afford this testimony full credence. But we cannot believe that the stated factor has not had a strong influence on the standards, as the literature on the subject plainly reveals. (See note 8, *infra*). Moreover our attention is drawn not so much to the recognition by Drs. Morse and Javed of the extant practice and standards but to the widening ambiguity of those standards themselves in their application to the medical problems we are discussing.

The agitation of the medical community in the face of modern life prolongation technology and its search for definitive policy are demonstrated in the large volume of relevant professional commentary.[8]

The wide debate thus reflected contrasts with the relative paucity of legislative and judicial guides and standards in the same field. The medical profession has sought to devise guidelines such as the "brain death" concept of the Harvard Ad Hoc Committee mentioned above. But it is perfectly apparent from the testimony we have quoted of Dr. Korein, and indeed so clear as almost to be judicially noticeable, that humane decisions against resuscitative or maintenance therapy are frequently a recognized *de facto* response in the medical world to the irreversible, terminal, pain-ridden patient, especially with familial consent. And these cases, of course, are far short of "brain death."

We glean from the record here that physicians distinguish between curing the ill and comforting and easing the dying; that they refuse to treat the curable as if they were dying or ought to die, and that they have sometimes refused to treat the hopeless and dying as if they were curable. In this sense, as we were reminded by the testimony of Drs. Korein and Diamond, many of them have refused to inflict an undesired prolongation of the process of dying on a patient in irreversible condition when it is clear that such "therapy" offers neither human nor humane benefit. We think these attitudes represent a balanced implementation of a profoundly realistic perspective on the meaning of life and death and that they respect the whole Judeo-Christian tradition of regard for human life. No less would they seem consistent with the moral matrix of medicine, "to heal," very much in the sense of the endless mission of the law, "to do justice."

Yet this balance, we feel, is particularly difficult to perceive and apply in the context of the development by advanced technology of sophisticated and artificial life-sustaining devices. For those possibly curable, such devices are of great value, and, as ordinary medical procedures, are essential. Consequently, as pointed out by Dr. Diamond, they are necessary because of the ethic of medical practice. But in light of the situation in the present case (while the record here is somewhat hazy in distinguishing between "ordinary" and "extraordinary" measures), one would have to think that the use of the same respirator or like support could be considered "ordinary" in the context of the possibly curable patient but "extraordinary" in the context of the forced sustaining by cardiorespiratory processes of an irreversibly doomed patient. And this dilemma is sharpened in the face of the malpractice and criminal action threat which we have mentioned.

We would hesitate, in this imperfect world, to propose as to physicians that type of immunity which from the early common law has surrounded judges and grand jurors, see, e.g., *Grove* v. *Van Duyn*, 44 N.J.L. 654, 656-57 (E. & A. 1882); *O'Regan* v. *Schermerhorn*, 25 N.J. Misc. 1, 19-20 (Sup. Ct. 1940), so that they might without fear of personal retaliation perform their judicial duties with independent objectivity. In *Bradley* v. *Fisher*, 80 U.S. (13 Wall.) 335, 347, 20 L. Ed. 646, 649 (1872), the Supreme Court held:

> [I]t is a general principle of the highest importance to the proper administration of justice that a judicial officer, in exercising the authority vested in him, shall be free to act upon his own convictions, without apprehension of personal consequences to himself.

Lord Coke said of judges that "they are only to make an account to God and the King [the State]." 12 Coke Rep. 23, 25, 77 Eng. Rep. 1305, 1307 (S.C. 1608).

Nevertheless, there must be a way to free physicians, in the pursuit of their healing vocation, from possible contamination by self-interest or self-protection concerns which would inhibit their independent medical judgments for the well-being of their dying patients. We would hope that this opinion might be serviceable to some degree in ameliorating the professional problems under discussion.

A technique aimed at the underlying difficulty (though in a somewhat broader context) is described by Dr. Karen Teel, a pediatrician and a director of Pediatric Education, who writes in the *Baylor Law Review* under the title "The Physician's Dilemma: A Doctor's View: What The Law Should Be." Dr. Teel recalls:

> Physicians, by virtue of their responsibility for medical judgments are, partly by choice and partly by default, charged with the responsibility of making ethical judgments which we are sometimes ill-equipped to make. We are not always morally and legally authorized to make them. The physician is thereby assuming a civil and criminal liability that, as often as not, he does not even realize as a factor in his decision. There is little or no dialogue in this whole process. The physician assumes that his judgment is called for and, in good faith, he acts. Someone must and it has been the physician who has assumed the responsibility and the risk.

I suggest that it would be more appropriate to provide a regular forum for more input and dialogue in individual situations and to allow the responsibility of these judgments to be shared. Many hospitals have established an Ethics Committee composed of physicians, social workers, attorneys, and theologians, . . . which serves to review the individual circumstances of ethical dilemma and which has provided much in the way of assistance and safeguards for patients and their medical caretakers. Generally, the authority of these committees is primarily restricted to the hospital setting and their official status is more that of an advisory body than of an enforcing body.

The concept of an Ethics Committee which has this kind of organization and is readily accessible to those persons rendering medical care to patients, would be, I think, the most promising direction for further study at this point. . . .

. . . [This would allow] some much needed dialogue regarding these issues and [force] the point of exploring all of the options for a particular patient. It diffuses the responsibility for making these judgments. Many physicians, in many circumstances, would welcome this sharing of responsibility. I believe that such an entity could lend itself well to an assumption of a legal status which would allow courses of action not now undertaken because of the concern for liability. [27 *Baylor L. Rev.* 6, 8–9 (1975)].

The most appealing factor in the technique suggested by Dr. Teel seems to us to be the diffusion of professional responsibility for decision, comparable in a way to the value of multijudge courts in finally resolving on appeal difficult questions of law. Moreover, such a system would be protective to the hospital as well as the doctor in screening out, so to speak, a case which might be contaminated by less-than-worthy motivations of family or physician. In the real world and in relationship to the momentous decision contemplated, the value of additional views and diverse knowledge is apparent.

We consider that a practice of applying to a court to confirm such decisions would generally be inappropriate, not only because that would be a gratuitous encroachment upon the medical profession's field of competence, but because it would be impossibly cumbersome. Such a requirement is distinguishable from the judicial overview traditionally required in other matters such as the adjudication and commitment of mental incompetents. This is not to say that in the case of an otherwise justiciable controversy access to the courts would be foreclosed; we speak rather of a general practice and procedure.

And although the deliberations and decisions which we describe would be professional in nature they should obviously include at some stage the feelings of the family of an incompetent relative. Decision making within health care if it is considered as an expression of a primary obligation of the physician, *primum non nocere*, should be controlled primarily within the patient-doctor-family relationship, as indeed was recognized by Judge Muir in his supplemental opinion of November 12, 1975.

If there could be created not necessarily this particular system but some reasonable counterpart, we would have no doubt that such decisions, thus determined to be in accordance with medical practice and prevailing standards, would be accepted by society and by the courts, at least in cases comparable to that of Karen Quinlan.

The evidence in this case convinces us that the focal point of decision should be the prognosis as to the reasonable possibility of return to cognitive and sapient life, as distinguished from the forced continuance of that biological vegetative existence to which Karen seems to be doomed.

In summary of the present Point of this opinion, we conclude that the state of the pertinent medical standards and practices which guided the attending physicians in this matter is not such as would justify this Court in deeming itself bound or controlled thereby in responding to the case for declaratory relief established by the parties on the record before us.

V. Alleged Criminal Liability

Having concluded that there is a right of privacy that might permit termination of treatment in the circumstances of this case, we turn to consider the relationship of the exercise of that right to the criminal law. We are aware that such termination of treatment would accelerate Karen's death. The County Prosecutor and the Attorney General maintain that there would be criminal liability for such acceleration. Under the statutes of this State, the unlawful killing of another human being is criminal homicide. N.J.S.A. 2A:113-1, 2, 5. We conclude that there would be no criminal homicide in the circumstances of this case. We believe, first, that the ensuing death would not be homicide but rather expiration from existing natural causes. Secondly, even if it were to be regarded as homicide, it would not be unlawful.

These conclusions rest upon definitional and constitutional bases. The termination of treatment pursuant to the right of privacy is, within the limitations of this case, *ipso facto* lawful. Thus, a death resulting from such an act would not come within the scope of the homicide statutes proscribing only the unlawful killing of another. There is a real and in this case determinative distinction between the unlawful taking of the life of another and the ending of artificial life-support systems as a matter of self-determination.

Furthermore, the exercise of a constitutional right such as we have here found is protected from criminal prosecution. See *Stanley* v. *Georgia, supra*, 394 U.S. at 559, 89 S. Ct. at 1245, 22 L. Ed. 2d at 546. We do not question the State's undoubted power to punish the taking of human life, but that power does not encompass individuals terminating medical treatment pursuant to their right of privacy. See *id.* at 568, 89 S. Ct. at 1250, 22 L. Ed. 2d at 551. The constitutional protection extends to third parties whose action is necessary to effectuate the exercise of that right where the individuals themselves would not be subject to prosecution or the third parties are charged as accessories to an act which could not be a crime. *Eisenstadt* v. *Baird, supra*, 405 U.S. at 445-46, 92 S. Ct. at 1034-35, 31 L. Ed. 2d at 357-58; *Griswold* v. *Connecticut, supra*, 381 U.S. at 481, 85 S. Ct. at 1679-80, 14 L. Ed. 2d at 512-13. And, under the circumstances of this case, these same principles would apply to and negate a valid prosecution for attempted suicide were there still such a crime in this State.[9]

VI. The Guardianship of the Person

The trial judge bifurcated the guardianship, as we have noted, refusing to appoint Joseph Quinlan to be guardian of the person and limiting his guardianship to that of the property of his daughter. Such occasional division of guardianship, as between responsibility for the person and the property of an incompetent person, has roots deep in the common law and was well within the jurisdictional capacity of the trial judge. In re Rollins, 65 A. 2d 667, 679-82 (N.J. Cty. Ct. 1949).

The statute creates an initial presumption of entitlement to guardianship in the next of kin, for it provides:

> In any case where a guardian is to be appointed, letters of guardianship shall be granted . . . to the next of kin, or if . . . it is proven to the court that no appointment from among them will be to the best interest of the incompetent or his estate, then to such other proper person as will accept the same. [N.J.S.A. 3A:6-36. See In re Roll, 117 N.J. Super. 122, 124 (App. Div. 1971)].

The trial court was apparently convinced of the high character of Joseph Quinlan and his general suitability as guardian under other circumstances, describing him as "very sincere, moral, ethical and religious." The court felt, however, that the obligation to concur in the medical care and treatment of his daughter would be a source of anguish to him and would distort his "decision-making processes." We disagree, for we sense from the whole record before us that while Mr. Quinlan feels a natural grief, and understandably sorrows because of the tragedy which has befallen his daughter, his strength of purpose and character far outweighs these sentiments and qualifies him eminently for guardianship of the person as well as the property of his daughter. Hence we discern no valid reason to overrule the statutory intendment of preference to the next of kin.

DECLARATORY RELIEF

We thus arrive at the formulation of the declaratory relief which we have concluded is appropriate to this case. Some time has passed since Karen's physical and mental condition was described to the Court. At that time her continuing deterioration was plainly projected. Since the record has not been expanded we assume that she is now even more fragile and nearer to death than she was then. Since her present treating physicians may give reconsideration to her present posture in the light of this opinion, and since we are transferring to the plaintiff as guardian the choice of the attending physician and therefore other physicians may be in charge of the case who may take a different view from that of the present attending physicians, we herewith declare the following affirmative relief on behalf of the plaintiff. Upon the concurrence of the guardian and family of Karen, should the responsible attending physicians conclude that there is no reasonable possibility of Karen's ever emerging from her present comatose condition to a cognitive, sapient state and that the life-support apparatus now being administered to Karen should be discontinued, they shall consult with the hospital "Ethics Committee" or like body of the institution in which Karen is then hospitalized. If that consultative body agrees that there is no reasonable possibility of Karen's ever emerging from her present comatose condition to a cognitive, sapient state, the present life-support system may be withdrawn and said action shall be without any civil or criminal liability therefor on the part of any participant, whether guardian, physician, hospital or others.[10] We herewith specifically so hold.

CONCLUSION

We therefore remand this record to the trial court to implement (without further testimonial hearing) the following decisions:

1. To discharge, with the thanks of the Court for his service, the present guardian of the person of Karen Quinlan, Thomas R. Curtin, Esquire, a member of the Bar and an officer of the court.
2. To appoint Joseph Quinlan as guardian of the person of Karen Quinlan with full power to make decisions with regard to the identity of her treating physicians.

We repeat for the sake of emphasis and clarity that upon the concurrence of the guardian and family of Karen, should the responsible attending physicians conclude that there is no reasonable possibility of Karen's ever emerging from her present comatose condition to a cognitive, sapient state and that the life-support apparatus now being administered to Karen should be discontinued, they shall consult with the hospital "Ethics Committee" or like body of the institution in which Karen is then hospitalized. If that consultative body agrees that there is no reasonable possibility of Karen's ever emerging from her present comatose condition to a cognitive, sapient state, the present life-support system may be withdrawn and said action shall be without any civil or criminal liability therefor, on the part of any participant, whether guardian, physician, hospital or others.

By the above ruling we do not intend to be understood as implying that a proceeding for judicial declaratory relief is necessarily required for the implementation of comparable decisions in the field of medical practice.

Modified and remanded.

REFERENCES

1. The importance of the preservation of life is memorialized in various organic documents. The Declaration of Independence states as self-evident truths "that all men . . . are endowed by their Creator with certain unalienable Rights, that among these are Life, Liberty and the pursuit of Happiness." This ideal is inherent in the Constitution of the United States. It is explicitly recognized in our Constitution of 1947 which provides for "certain natural and unalienable rights, among which are those of enjoying and defending life * * *." N.J. Const. (1947), Art. I, par. 1. Our State government is established to protect such rights, N.J. Const. (1947), Art. I, par. 2, and, acting through the Attorney General (N.J.S.A. 52:17A-4(h)), it enforces them.

2. Dr. Julius Korein, a neurologist, testified:

A. . . . [Y]ou've got a set of possible lesions that prior to the era of advanced technology and advances in medicine were no problem inasmuch as the patient would expire. They could do nothing for themselves and even external care was limited. It was—I don't know how many years ago they couldn't keep a person alive with intravenous feedings because they couldn't give enough calories. Now they have these high caloric tube feedings that can keep people in excellent nutrition for years so what's happened is these things have occurred all along but the technology has now reached a point where you can in fact start to replace anything outside of the brain to maintain something that is irreversibly damaged.

Q. Doctor, can the art of medicine repair the cerebral damage that was sustained by Karen?

A. In my opinion, no. . . .

Q. Doctor, in your opinion is there any course of treatment that will lead to the improvement of Karen's condition?

A. No.

3. The Harvard Ad Hoc standards, with reference to "brain death," will be discussed *infra.*

3.1. This cross-appeal was later informally withdrawn but in view of the importance of the matter we nevertheless deal with it.

4. Dr. Robert J. Morse, a neurologist, and Karen's treating physisician from the time of her admission to Saint Clare's Hospital on April 24, 1975 (reference was made *supra* to "treating

physicians" named as defendants; this term included Dr. Arshad Javed, a highly qualified pulmonary internist, who considers that he manages that phase of Karen's care with primary responsibility to the "attending physician," Dr. Morse).

5. Death. The cessation of life; the ceasing to exist; defined by physicians as a total stoppage of the circulation of the blood, and a cessation of the animal and vital functions consequent thereon, such as respiration, pulsation, etc. *Black's Law Dictionary* 488 (rev. 4th ed. 1968).

6. It is generally agreed that the Eighth Amendment's provision of "[n]or cruel and unusual punishments inflicted" is drawn verbatim from the English Declaration of Rights. See 1 Wm. & M., sess. 2, c. 2 (1689). The prohibition arose in the context of excessive punishments for crimes, punishments that were barbarous and savage as well as disproportionate to the offense committed. See generally Granucci, "'Nor Cruel and Unusual Punishments Inflicted:' The Original Meaning," 57 Calif. L. Rev. 839, 844-60 (1969); Note, "The Cruel and Unusual Punishment Clause and the Substantive Criminal Law," 79 Harv. L. Rev. 635, 636-39 (1966). The principle against excessiveness in criminal punishments can be traced back to Chapters 20–22 of the Magna Carta (1215). The historical background of the Eighth Amendment was examined at some length in various opinions in *Furman* v. *Georgia*, 408 U.S. 238, 92 S. Ct. 2726, 33 L. Ed. 2d 346 (1972).

The Constitution itself is silent as to the meaning of the word "punishment." Whether it refers to the variety of legal and nonlegal penalties that human beings endure or whether it must be in connection with a criminal rather than a civil proceeding is not stated in the document. But the origins of the clause are clear. And the cases construing it have consistently held that the "punishment" contemplated by the Eighth Amendment is the penalty inflicted by a court for the commission of a crime or in the enforcement of what is a criminal law. See, e.g., *Trop* v. *Dulles*, 356 U.S. 86, 94-99, 78 S. Ct. 590, 594-97, 2 L. Ed. 2d 630, 638-41 (1957). See generally Note, "The Effectiveness of the Eighth Amendment:

An Appraisal of Cruel and Unusual Punishment," 36 N.Y.U.L. Rev. 846, 854-57 (1961). A deprivation, forfeiture or penalty arising out of a civil proceeding or otherwise cannot be "cruel and unusual punishment" within the meaning of the constitutional clause.

7. The right we here discuss is included within the class of what have been called rights of "personality." See Pound, "Equitable Relief against Defamation and Injuries to Personality," 29 Harv. L. Rev. 640, 668-76 (1916). Equitable jurisdiction with respect to the recognition and enforcement of such rights has long been recognized in New Jersey. See, e.g., *Vanderbilt* v. *Mitchell*, 72 N.J. Eq. 910, 919-20 (E. & A. 1907).

8. See, e.g., Downing, *Euthanasia and the Right to Death* (1969); St. John-Stevas, *Life, Death and the Law* (1961); Williams, *The Sanctity of Human Life and the Criminal Law* (1957); Appel, "Ethical and Legal Questions Posed by Recent Advances in Medicine," 205 *JAMA* 513 (1968); Cantor, "A Patient's Decision To Decline Life-Saving Medical Treatment: Bodily Integrity Versus The Preservation of Life," 26 *Rutgers L. Rev.* 228 (1973); Claypool, "The Family Deals with Death," 27 *Baylor L. Rev.* 34 (1975); Elkington, "The Dying Patient, The Doctor and The Law," 13 *Vill. L. Rev.* 740 (1968); Fletcher, "Legal Aspects of the Decision Not to Prolong Life," 203 *JAMA* 65 (1968); Foreman, "The Physician's Criminal Liability for the Practice of Euthanasia," 27 *Baylor L. Rev.* 54 (1975); Gurney, "Is There A Right To Die?—A Study of the Law of Euthanasia," 3 *Cumb.-Sam. L. Rev.* 235 (1972); Mannes, "Euthanasia vs. The Right To Life," 27 *Baylor L. Rev.* 68 (1975); Sharp & Crofts, "Death with Dignity and The Physician's Civil Liability," 27 *Baylor L. Rev.* 86 (1975); Sharpe & Hargest, "Lifesaving Treatment for Unwilling Patients," 36 *Fordham L. Rev.* 695 (1968); Skegg, "Irreversibly Comatose Individuals: 'Alive' or 'Dead'?," 33 *Camb. L.J.* 130 (1974); Comment, "The Right to Die," 7 *Houston L. Rev.* 654 (1970); Note, "The Time of Death—A Legal, Ethical

and Medical Dilemma," 18 *Catholic Law.* 243 (1972); Note, "Compulsory Medical Treatment: The State's Interest Re-evaluated," 51 *Minn. L. Rev.* 293 (1966).

9. An attempt to commit suicide was an indictable offense at common law and as such was indictable in this State as a common law misdemeanor. 1 Schlosser, Criminal Laws of New Jersey § 12.5 (3d ed. 1970); see N.J.S.A. 2A:85-1. The legislature downgraded the offense in 1957 to the status of a disorderly persons offense, which is not a "crime" under our law. N.J.S.A. 2A:170-25.6. And in 1971, the legislature repealed all criminal sanctions for attempted suicide. N.J.S.A. 2A:85-5.1. Provision is now made for temporary hospitalization of persons making such an attempt. N.J.S.A. 30:4-26.3a. We note that under the proposed New Jersey Penal Code (Oct. 1971) there is no provision for criminal punishment of attempted suicide. See Commentary, § 2C:11-6. There is, however, an independent offense of "aiding suicide." § 2C:11-6b. This provision, if enacted, would not be incriminatory in circumstances similar to those presented in this case.

10. The declaratory relief we here award is not intended to imply that the principles enunciated in this case might not be applicable in divers other types of terminal medical situations such as those described by Drs. Korein and Diamond, supra, not necessarily involving the hopeless loss of cognitive or sapient life.

20

CRUZAN ET UX. v. DIRECTOR, MISSOURI DEPARTMENT OF HEALTH, ET AL.

Supreme Court of the United States 497 U.S. 261
December 6, 1989, Argued
June 25, 1990, Decided

❧

Petitioner Nancy Beth Cruzan was rendered incompetent as a result of severe injuries sustained during an automobile accident. Copetitioners Lester and Joyce Cruzan, Nancy's parents and coguardians, sought a court order directing the withdrawal of their daughter's artificial feeding and hydration equipment after it became apparent that she had virtually no chance of recovering her cognitive faculties. The Supreme Court of Missouri held that because there was no clear and convincing evidence of Nancy's desire to have life-sustaining treatment withdrawn under such circumstances, her parents lacked authority to effectuate such a request. We granted *certiorari*, 492 U.S. 917 (1989), and now affirm.

On the night of January 11, 1983, Nancy Cruzan lost control of her car as she traveled down Elm Road in Jasper County, Missouri. The vehicle overturned, and Cruzan was discovered lying face down in a ditch without detectable respiratory or cardiac function. Paramedics were able to restore her breathing and heartbeat at the accident site, and she was transported to a hospital in an unconscious state. An attending neurosurgeon diagnosed her as having sustained probable cerebral contusions compounded by significant anoxia (lack of oxygen). The Missouri trial court in this case found that permanent brain damage generally results after 6 minutes in an anoxic state; it was estimated that Cruzan was deprived of oxygen from 12 to 14 minutes. She remained in a coma for approximately three weeks and then progressed to an unconscious state in which she was able to orally ingest some nutrition. In order to ease feeding and further the recovery, surgeons implanted a gastrostomy feeding and hydration tube in Cruzan with the consent of her then husband. Subsequent rehabilitative efforts proved unavailing. She now lies in a Missouri state hospital in what is commonly referred to as a persistent vegetative state: generally, a condition in which a person exhibits motor reflexes but evinces no indications of significant cognitive function.[1] The State of Missouri is bearing the cost of her care.

After it had become apparent that Nancy Cruzan had virtually no chance of regaining her mental faculties, her parents asked hospital employees to terminate the artificial nutrition and hydration procedures. All agree that such a removal would cause her death. The employees refused to honor the request without court approval. The parents then sought and received authorization from the state trial court for termination. The court found that a person in Nancy's condition had a fundamental right under the State and Federal Constitutions to refuse or direct the withdrawal of "death prolonging procedures." App. to Pet. for Cert. A99. The court also found that Nancy's "expressed thoughts at age twenty-five in somewhat serious conversation with a housemate friend that if sick or injured she would not wish to continue her life unless she could live at least halfway normally suggests that given her present condition she would not wish to continue on with her nutrition and hydration." *Id.*, at A97-A98.

The Supreme Court of Missouri reversed by a divided vote. The court recognized a right to refuse treatment embodied in the common-law doctrine of informed consent, but expressed skepticism about the application of that doctrine in the circumstances of this case. *Cruzan* v. *Harmon*, 760 S.W.2d 408, 416–417 (1988) (en banc). The court also declined to read a broad right of privacy into the State Constitution which would "support the right of a person to refuse medical treatment in every circumstance," and expressed doubt as to whether such a right existed under the United States Constitution. *Id.*, at 417–418. It then decided that the Missouri Living Will statute, Mo Rev. Stat. § 459.010 *et seq.* (1986), embodied a state policy strongly favoring the preservation of life. 760 S.W.2d at 419–420. The court found that Cruzan's statements to her roommate regarding her desire to live or die under certain conditions were "unreliable for the purpose of determining her intent," *id.*, at 424, "and thus insufficient to support the coguardians['] claim to exercise substituted judgment on Nancy's behalf." *Id.*, at 426. It rejected the argument that Cruzan's parents were entitled to order the termination of her medical treatment, concluding that "no person can assume that choice for an incompetent in the absence of the formalities required under Missouri's Living Will statutes or the clear and convincing, inherently reliable evidence absent here." *Id.*, at 425. The court also expressed its view that "broad policy questions bearing on life and death are more properly addressed by representative assemblies" than judicial bodies. *Id.*, at 426.

We granted *certiorari* to consider the question whether Cruzan has a right under the United States Constitution which would require the hospital to withdraw life-sustaining treatment from her under these circumstances.

At common law, even the touching of one person by another without consent and without legal justification was a battery. See W. Keeton, D. Dobbs, R. Keeton, & D. Owen, *Prosser and Keeton on Law of Torts* § 9, pp. 39–42 (5th ed. 1984). Before the turn of the century, this Court observed that "no right is held more sacred, or is more carefully guarded, by the common law, than the right of every individual to the possession and control of his own person, free from all restraint or interference of others, unless by clear and unquestionable authority of law." *Union Pacific R. Co.* v. *Botsford,* 141 U.S. 250, 251, 35 L. Ed. 734, 11 S. Ct. 1000 (1891). This notion of bodily integrity has been embodied in the requirement that informed consent is generally required for medical treatment. Justice Cardozo, while on the Court of Appeals of New York, aptly described this doctrine: "Every human being of adult years and sound mind has a right to determine what shall be done with his own body; and a surgeon who performs an operation without his patient's consent commits an assault, for which he is liable in damages." *Schloendorff* v. *Society of New York Hospital,* 211 N.Y. 125, 129-130, 105 N.E. 92, 93 (1914). The informed consent doctrine has become firmly entrenched in American tort law. See Keeton, Dobbs, Keeton, & Owen, *supra,* § 32, pp. 189–192; F. Rozovsky, *Consent to Treatment, A Practical Guide* 1–98 (2d ed. 1990).

The logical corollary of the doctrine of informed consent is that the patient generally possesses the right not to consent, that is, to refuse treatment. Until about 15 years ago and the seminal decision in In re Quinlan, 70 N.J. 10, 355 A.2d 647, cert. denied sub nom. *Garger* v. *New Jersey,* 429 U.S. 922, 50 L. Ed. 2d 289, 97 S. Ct. 319 (1976), the number of right-to-refuse-treatment decisions was relatively few.[2] Most of the earlier cases involved patients who refused medical treatment forbidden by their religious beliefs, thus implicating First Amendment rights as well as common-law rights of self-determination.[3] More recently, however, with the advance of medical technology capable of sustaining life well past the point where natural forces would have brought certain death in earlier times, cases involving the right to refuse life-sustaining treatment have burgeoned. See 760 S.W.2d at 412, n.4 (collecting 54 reported decisions from 1976 through 1988).

In the *Quinlan* case, young Karen Quinlan suffered severe brain damage as the result of anoxia and entered a persistent vegetative state. Karen's father sought judicial approval to disconnect his daughter's respirator. The New Jersey Supreme Court granted the relief, holding that Karen had a right of privacy grounded in the Federal Constitution to terminate treatment. In re Quinlan, 70 N.J. at 38-42, 355 A.2d at 662–664. Recognizing that this right was not absolute, however, the court balanced it against asserted state interests. Noting that the State's interest "weakens and the individual's right to privacy grows as the degree of bodily invasion increases and the prognosis dims," the court concluded that the state interests had to give way in that case. *Id.,* at 41, 355 A.2d at 664. The court also concluded that the "only practical way" to prevent the loss of Karen's privacy right due to her incompetence was to allow her guardian and family to decide "whether she would exercise it in these circumstances." *Ibid.*

After *Quinlan,* however, most courts have based a right to refuse treatment either solely on the common-law right to informed consent or on both the common-law right and a constitutional privacy right. See L. Tribe, *American Constitutional Law* § 15-11, p. 1365 (2d ed. 1988). In *Superintendent of Belchertown State School* v. *Saikewicz,* 373 Mass. 728, 370 N.E.2d 417 (1977), the Supreme Judicial Court of Massachusetts relied on both the right of privacy and the right of informed consent to permit the withholding of chemotherapy from a profoundly retarded 67-year-old man suffering from leukemia. *Id.*, at 737-738, 370 N.E.2d at 424. Reasoning that an incompetent person retains the same rights as a competent individual "because the value of human dignity extends to both," the court adopted a "substituted judgment" standard whereby courts were to determine what an incompetent individual's decision would have been under the circumstances. *Id.*, at 745, 752-753, 757-758, 370 N.E.2d at 427, 431, 434. Distilling certain state interests from prior case law—the preservation of life, the protection of the interests of innocent third parties, the prevention of suicide, and the maintenance of the ethical integrity of the medical profession—the court recognized the first interest as paramount and noted it was greatest when an affliction was curable, "as opposed to the State interest where, as here, the issue is not whether, but when, for how long, and at what cost to the individual [a] life may be briefly extended." *Id.*, at 742, 370 N.E.2d at 426.

In In re Storar, 52 N.Y.2d 363, 420 N.E.2d 64, 438 N.Y.S.2d 266, cert. denied, 454 U.S. 858, 70 L. Ed. 2d 153, 102 S. Ct. 309 (1981), the New York Court of Appeals declined to base a right to refuse treatment on a constitutional privacy right. Instead, it found such a right "adequately supported" by the informed consent doctrine. *Id.*, at 376-377, 420 N.E.2d at 70. In In re Eichner (decided with In re Storar, *supra*), an 83-year-old man who had suffered brain damage from anoxia entered a vegetative state and was thus incompetent to consent to the removal of his respirator. The court, however, found it unnecessary to reach the question whether his rights could be exercised by others since it found the evidence clear and convincing from statements made by the patient when competent that he "did not want to be maintained in a vegetative coma by use of a respirator." *Id.*, at 380, 420 N.E.2d at 72. In the companion Storar case, a 52-year-old man suffering from bladder cancer had been profoundly retarded during most of his life. Implicitly rejecting the approach taken in Saikewicz, *supra*, the court reasoned that due to such lifelong incompetency, "it is unrealistic to attempt to determine whether he would want to continue potentially life prolonging treatment if he were competent." 52 N.Y.2d at 380, 420 N.E.2d at 72. As the evidence showed that the patient's required blood transfusions did not involve excessive pain and without them his mental and physical abilities would deteriorate, the court concluded that it should not "allow an incompetent patient to bleed to death because someone, even someone as close as a parent or sibling, feels that this is best for one with an incurable disease." *Id.*, at 382, 420 N.E.2d at 73.

Many of the later cases build on the principles established in *Quinlan, Saikewicz,* and *Storar/Eichner.* For instance, in In re Conroy, 98 N.J. 321, 486 A.2d 1209 (1985), the same court that decided *Quinlan* considered whether a nasogastric feeding tube could be removed from an 84-year-old incompetent nursing-home resident suffering irreversible mental and physical ailments. While recognizing that a federal right of privacy might apply in the case, the court, contrary to its approach in *Quinlan,* decided to base its decision on the common-law right to self-determination and informed consent. 98 N.J. at 348, 486 A.2d at 1223. "On balance, the right to self-determination ordinarily outweighs any countervailing state interests, and competent persons generally are permitted to refuse medical treatment, even at the risk of death. Most of the cases that have held otherwise, unless they involved the interest in protecting innocent third parties, have concerned the patient's competency to make a rational and considered choice." *Id.*, at 353-354, 486 A.2d at 1225.

Reasoning that the right of self-determination should not be lost merely because an individual is unable to sense a violation of it, the court held that incompetent individuals retain a right to refuse treatment. It also held that such a right could be exercised by a surrogate decision maker using a "subjective" standard when there was clear evidence that the incompetent person would have exercised it. Where such evidence was lacking, the court held that an individual's right could still be invoked in certain circumstances under objective "best interest" standards. *Id.*, at 361–368, 486 A.2d at 1229–1233. Thus, if some trustworthy evidence existed that the individual would have wanted to terminate treatment, but not enough to clearly establish a person's wishes for purposes of the subjective standard, and the burden of a prolonged life from the experience of pain and suffering markedly outweighed its satisfactions, treatment could be terminated under a "limited-objective" standard. Where no trustworthy evidence existed, and a person's suffering would make the administration of life-sustaining treatment inhumane, a "pure-objective" standard could be used to terminate treatment. If none of these conditions obtained, the court held it was best to err in favor of preserving life. *Id.*, at 364–368, 486 A.2d at 1231–1233.

The court also rejected certain categorical distinctions that had been drawn in prior refusal-of-treatment cases as lacking substance for decision purposes: the distinction between actively hastening death by terminating treatment and passively allowing a person to die of a disease; between treating individuals as an initial matter versus withdrawing treatment afterwards; between ordinary versus extraordinary treatment; and between treatment by artificial feeding versus other forms of life-sustaining medical procedures. *Id.*, at 369–374, 486 A.2d at 1233–1237. As to the last item, the court acknowledged the "emotional significance" of food, but noted that feeding by implanted tubes is a "medical procedure with inherent risks and possible side effects, instituted by skilled health-care providers to compensate for impaired physical functioning" which analytically was equivalent to artificial breathing using a respirator. *Id.*, at 373, 486 A.2d at 1236.[4]

In contrast to *Conroy*, the Court of Appeals of New York recently refused to accept less than the clearly expressed wishes of a patient before permitting the exercise of her right to refuse treatment by a surrogate decisionmaker. In re Westchester County Medical Center on behalf of O'Connor, 72 N.Y.2d 517, 531 N.E.2d 607, 534 N.Y.S.2d 886 (1988) (*O'Connor*). There, the court, over the objection of the patient's family members, granted an order to insert a feeding tube into a 77-year-old woman rendered incompetent as a result of several strokes. While continuing to recognize a common-law right to refuse treatment, the court rejected the substituted judgment approach for asserting it "because it is inconsistent with our fundamental commitment to the notion that no person or court should substitute its judgment as to what would be an acceptable quality of life for another. Consequently, we adhere to the view that, despite its pitfalls and inevitable uncertainties, the inquiry must always be narrowed to the patient's expressed intent, with every effort made to minimize the opportunity for error." *Id.*, at 530, 531 N.E.2d at 613 (citation omitted). The court held that the record lacked the requisite clear and convincing evidence of the patient's expressed intent to withhold life-sustaining treatment. *Id.*, at 531–534, 531 N.E.2d at 613–615.

Other courts have found state statutory law relevant to the resolution of these issues. In Conservatorship of Drabick, 200 Cal. App. 3d 185, 245 Cal. Rptr. 840, cert. denied, 488 U.S. 958 (1988), the California Court of Appeal authorized the removal of a nasogastric feeding tube from a 44-year-old man who was in a persistent vegetative state as a result of an auto accident. Noting that the right to refuse treatment was grounded in both the common law and a constitutional right of privacy, the court held that a state probate statute authorized the patient's conservator to order the withdrawal of life-sustaining treatment when such a decision was made in good faith based on medical advice and the conservatee's best interests. While acknowledging that "to claim that [a patient's] 'right to choose' survives incompetence is a legal fiction at best," the court reasoned that the respect society accords to persons as individuals is not lost upon incompetence and is best preserved by allowing others "to make a decision that reflects [a patient's] interests more closely than would a purely technological decision to do whatever is possible."[5] *Id.*, at 208, 245 Cal. Rptr. at 854–855. See also In re Conservatorship of Torres, 357 N.W.2d 332 (Minn. 1984) (Minnesota court had constitutional and statutory authority to authorize a conservator to order the removal of an incompetent individual's respirator since in patient's best interests).

In In re Estate of Longeway, 133 Ill. 2d 33, 549 N.E.2d 292, 139 Ill. Dec. 780 (1989), the Supreme Court of Illinois considered whether a 76-year-old woman rendered incompetent from a series of strokes had a right to the discontinuance of artificial nutrition and hydration. Noting that the boundaries of a federal right of privacy were uncertain, the court found a right to refuse treatment in the doctrine of informed consent. *Id.*, at 43–45, 549 N.E.2d at 296–297. The court further held that the State Probate Act impliedly authorized a guardian to exercise a ward's right to refuse artificial sustenance in the event that the ward was terminally ill and irreversibly comatose. *Id.*, at 45-47, 549 N.E.2d at 298. Declining to adopt a best interests standard for deciding when it would be appropriate to exercise a ward's right because it "lets another make a determination of a patient's quality of life," the court opted instead for a substituted judgment standard. *Id.*, at 49, 549 N.E.2d at 299. Finding the "expressed intent" standard utilized in O'Connor, supra, too rigid, the court noted that other clear and convincing evidence of the patient's intent could be considered. 133 Ill. 2d at 50–51, 549 N.E.2d at 300. The court also adopted the "consensus opinion [that] treats artificial nutrition and hydration as medical treatment." *Id.*, at 42, 549 N.E.2d at 296. Cf. *McConnell v. Beverly Enterprises-Connecticut, Inc.*, 209 Conn. 692, 705, 553 A.2d 596, 603 (1989) (right to withdraw artificial nutrition and hydration found in the Connecticut Removal of Life Support Systems Act, which "provid[es] functional guidelines for the exercise of the common law and constitutional rights of self-determination"; attending physician authorized to remove treatment after finding that patient is in a terminal condition, obtaining consent of family, and considering expressed wishes of patient).[6]

As these cases demonstrate, the common-law doctrine of informed consent is viewed as generally encompassing the right of a competent individual to refuse medical treatment. Beyond that, these cases demonstrate both similarity and diversity in their approaches to decision of what all agree is a perplexing question with unusually strong moral and ethical overtones. State courts have available to them for decision a number of sources—state constitutions, statutes, and common law—which are not available to us. In this Court, the question is simply and starkly whether the United States Constitution prohibits Missouri from choosing the rule of decision which it did. This is the first case in which we have been squarely presented with the issue whether the United States Constitution grants what is in common parlance referred to as a "right to die." We follow the judicious counsel of our decision in *Twin City Bank* v. *Nebeker*, 167 U.S. 196, 202, 42 L. Ed. 134, 17 S. Ct. 766 (1897), where we said that in deciding "a question of such magnitude and importance . . . it is the [better] part of wisdom not to attempt, by any general statement, to cover every possible phase of the subject."

The Fourteenth Amendment provides that no State shall "deprive any person of life, liberty, or property, without due process of law." The principle that a competent person has a constitutionally protected liberty interest in refusing unwanted medical treatment may be inferred from our prior decisions. In *Jacobson* v. *Massachusetts*, 197 U.S. 11, 24-30, 49 L. Ed. 643, 25 S. Ct. 358 (1905), for instance, the Court balanced an individual's liberty interest in declining an unwanted smallpox vaccine against the State's interest in preventing disease. Decisions prior to the incorporation of the Fourth Amendment into the Fourteenth Amendment analyzed searches and seizures involving the body under the Due Process Clause and were thought to implicate substantial liberty interests. See, e.g., *Breithaupt* v. *Abram*, 352 U.S. 432, 439, 1 L. Ed. 2d 448, 77 S. Ct. 408 (1957) ("As against the right of an individual that his person be held inviolable . . . must be set the interests of society . . .").

Just this Term, in the course of holding that a State's procedures for administering antipsychotic medication to prisoners were sufficient to satisfy due process concerns, we recognized that prisoners possess "a significant liberty interest in avoiding the unwanted administration of antipsychotic drugs under the Due Process Clause of the Fourteenth Amendment." *Washington* v. *Harper*, 494 U.S. 210, 221-222, 108 L. Ed. 2d 178, 110 S. Ct. 1028 (1990); see also *id.*, at 229 ("The forcible injection of medication into a nonconsenting person's body represents a substantial interference with that person's liberty"). Still other cases support the recognition of a general liberty interest in refusing medical treatment. *Vitek* v. *Jones*, 445 U.S. 480, 494, 63 L. Ed. 2d 552, 100 S. Ct. 1254 (1980) (transfer to mental hospital coupled with mandatory behavior modification treatment implicated liberty interests); *Parham* v. *J. R.*, 442 U.S. 584, 600, 61 L. Ed. 2d 101, 99 S. Ct. 2493 (1979) ("[A] child, in common with adults, has a substantial liberty interest in not being confined unnecessarily for medical treatment").

But determining that a person has a "liberty interest" under the Due Process Clause does not end the inquiry;[7] "whether respondent's constitutional rights have been violated must be determined by balancing his liberty interests against the relevant state interests." *Youngberg v. Romeo*, 457 U.S. 307, 321, 73 L. Ed. 2d 28, 102 S. Ct. 2452 (1982). See also *Mills v. Rogers*, 457 U.S. 291, 299, 73 L. Ed. 2d 16, 102 S. Ct. 2442 (1982).

Petitioners insist that under the general holdings of our cases, the forced administration of life-sustaining medical treatment, and even of artificially delivered food and water essential to life, would implicate a competent person's liberty interest. Although we think the logic of the cases discussed above would embrace such a liberty interest, the dramatic consequences involved in refusal of such treatment would inform the inquiry as to whether the deprivation of that interest is constitutionally permissible. But for purposes of this case, we assume that the United States Constitution would grant a competent person a constitutionally protected right to refuse life-saving hydration and nutrition.

Petitioners go on to assert that an incompetent person should possess the same right in this respect as is possessed by a competent person. They rely primarily on our decisions in *Parham v. J. R., supra*, and *Youngberg v. Romeo, supra*. In *Parham*, we held that a mentally disturbed minor child had a liberty interest in "not being confined unnecessarily for medical treatment," 442 U.S. at 600, but we certainly did not intimate that such a minor child, after commitment, would have a liberty interest in refusing treatment. In *Youngberg*, we held that a seriously retarded adult had a liberty interest in safety and freedom from bodily restraint, 457 U.S. at 320. *Youngberg*, however, did not deal with decisions to administer or withhold medical treatment.

The difficulty with petitioners' claim is that in a sense it begs the question: An incompetent person is not able to make an informed and voluntary choice to exercise a hypothetical right to refuse treatment or any other right. Such a "right" must be exercised for her, if at all, by some sort of surrogate. Here, Missouri has in effect recognized that under certain circumstances a surrogate may act for the patient in electing to have hydration and nutrition withdrawn in such a way as to cause death, but it has established a procedural safeguard to assure that the action of the surrogate conforms as best it may to the wishes expressed by the patient while competent. Missouri requires that evidence of the incompetent's wishes as to the withdrawal of treatment be proved by clear and convincing evidence. The question, then, is whether the United States Constitution forbids the establishment of this procedural requirement by the State. We hold that it does not.

Whether or not Missouri's clear and convincing evidence requirement comports with the United States Constitution depends in part on what interests the State may properly seek to protect in this situation. Missouri relies on its interest in the protection and preservation of human life, and there can be no gainsaying this interest. As a general matter, the States—indeed, all civilized nations—demonstrate their commitment to life by treating homicide as a serious crime. Moreover, the majority of States in this country have laws imposing criminal penalties on one who assists another to commit suicide.[8] We do not think a State is required to remain neutral in the face of an informed and voluntary decision by a physically able adult to starve to death.

But in the context presented here, a State has more particular interests at stake. The choice between life and death is a deeply personal decision of obvious and overwhelming finality. We believe Missouri may legitimately seek to safeguard the personal element of this choice through the imposition of heightened evidentiary requirements. It cannot be disputed that the Due Process Clause protects an interest in life as well as an interest in refusing life-sustaining medical treatment. Not all incompetent patients will have loved ones available to serve as surrogate decision makers. And even where family members are present, "there will, of course, be some unfortunate situations in which family members will not act to protect a patient." In re Jobes, 108 N.J. 394, 419, 529 A.2d 434, 447 (1987). A State is entitled to guard against potential abuses in such situations. Similarly, a State is entitled to consider that a judicial proceeding to make a determination regarding an incompetent's wishes may very well not be an adversarial one, with the added guarantee of accurate factfinding that the adversary process brings with it.[9] See *Ohio v. Akron Center for Reproductive Health,* 497 U.S. 502, 515–516. Finally, we think a State may properly decline to make judgments about the "quality" of life that a particular individual may enjoy, and simply assert an unqualified interest in the preservation of human life to be weighed against the constitutionally protected interests of the individual.

In our view, Missouri has permissibly sought to advance these interests through the adoption of a "clear and convincing" standard of proof to govern such proceedings. "The function of a standard of proof, as that concept is embodied in the Due Process Clause and in the realm of factfinding, is to 'instruct the factfinder concerning the degree of confidence our society thinks he should have in the correctness of factual conclusions for a particular type of adjudication.'" *Addington v. Texas,* 441 U.S. 418, 423, 60 L. Ed. 2d 323, 99 S. Ct. 1804 (1979) (quoting In re Winship, 397 U.S. 358, 370, 25 L. Ed. 2d 368, 90 S. Ct. 1068 (1970) (Harlan, J., concurring)). "This Court has mandated an intermediate standard of proof—'clear and convincing evidence'—when the individual interests at stake in a state proceeding are both 'particularly important' and 'more substantial than mere loss of money.'" *Santosky v. Kramer,* 455 U.S. 745, 756, 71 L. Ed. 2d 599, 102 S. Ct. 1388 (1982) (quoting *Addington, supra,* at 424). Thus, such a standard has been required in deportation proceedings, *Woodby v. INS,* 385 U.S. 276, 17 L. Ed. 2d 362, 87 S. Ct. 483 (1966), in denaturalization proceedings, *Schneiderman v. United States,* 320 U.S. 118, 87 L. Ed. 1796, 63 S. Ct. 1333 (1943), in civil commitment proceedings, Addington, *supra,* and in proceedings for the termination of parental rights, *Santosky, supra.*[10] Further, this level of proof, "or an even higher one, has traditionally been imposed in cases involving allegations of civil fraud, and in a variety of other kinds of civil cases involving such issues as . . . lost wills, oral contracts to make bequests, and the like." *Woodby, supra,* at 285, n.18.

We think it self-evident that the interests at stake in the instant proceedings are more substantial, both on an individual and societal level, than those involved in a run-of-the-mine civil dispute. But not only does the standard of proof reflect the importance of a particular adjudication, it also serves as "a societal judgment about how the risk of error should be distributed between the litigants." *Santosky, supra,* at 755;

Addington, supra, at 423. The more stringent the burden of proof a party must bear, the more that party bears the risk of an erroneous decision. We believe that Missouri may permissibly place an increased risk of an erroneous decision on those seeking to terminate an incompetent individual's life-sustaining treatment. An erroneous decision not to terminate results in a maintenance of the status quo; the possibility of subsequent developments such as advancements in medical science, the discovery of new evidence regarding the patient's intent, changes in the law, or simply the unexpected death of the patient despite the administration of life-sustaining treatment at least create the potential that a wrong decision will eventually be corrected or its impact mitigated. An erroneous decision to withdraw life-sustaining treatment, however, is not susceptible of correction. In *Santosky,* one of the factors which led the Court to require proof by clear and convincing evidence in a proceeding to terminate parental rights was that a decision in such a case was final and irrevocable. *Santosky, supra,* at 759. The same must surely be said of the decision to discontinue hydration and nutrition of a patient such as Nancy Cruzan, which all agree will result in her death.

It is also worth noting that most, if not all, States simply forbid oral testimony entirely in determining the wishes of parties in transactions which, while important, simply do not have the consequences that a decision to terminate a person's life does. At common law and by statute in most States, the parol evidence rule prevents the variations of the terms of a written contract by oral testimony. The statute of frauds makes unenforceable oral contracts to leave property by will, and statutes regulating the making of wills universally require that those instruments be in writing. See 2 A. Corbin, *Contracts* § 398, pp. 360–361 (1950); 2 W. Page, *Law of Wills* §§ 19.3-19.5, pp. 61–71 (1960). There is no doubt that statutes requiring wills to be in writing, and statutes of frauds which require that a contract to make a will be in writing, on occasion frustrate the effectuation of the intent of a particular decedent, just as Missouri's requirement of proof in this case may have frustrated the effectuation of the not-fully-expressed desires of Nancy Cruzan. But the Constitution does not require general rules to work faultlessly; no general rule can.

In sum, we conclude that a State may apply a clear and convincing evidence standard in proceedings where a guardian seeks to discontinue nutrition and hydration of a person diagnosed to be in a persistent vegetative state. We note that many courts which have adopted some sort of substituted judgment procedure in situations like this, whether they limit consideration of evidence to the prior expressed wishes of the incompetent individual, or whether they allow more general proof of what the individual's decision would have been, require a clear and convincing standard of proof for such evidence. See, e.g., *Longeway,* 133 Ill. 2d at 50-51, 549 N.E.2d at 300; *McConnell,* 209 Conn. at 707-710, 553 A.2d at 604-605; *O'Connor,* 72 N.Y.2d at 529-530, 531 N.E.2d at 613; In re Gardner, 534 A.2d 947, 952-953 (Me. 1987); In re Jobes, 108 N.J. at 412-413, 529 A. 2d, [*285] at 443; *Leach* v. *Akron General Medical Center,* 68 Ohio Misc. 1, 11, 426 N.E.2d 809, 815 (1980).

The Supreme Court of Missouri held that in this case the testimony adduced at trial did not amount to clear and convincing proof of the patient's desire to have hydration and nutrition withdrawn. In so doing, it reversed a decision of the Missouri trial court which had found that the evidence "suggested" Nancy Cruzan would not have desired to continue such measures, App. to Pet. for Cert. A98, but which had not adopted the standard of "clear and convincing evidence" enunciated by the Supreme Court. The testimony adduced at trial consisted primarily of Nancy Cruzan's statements made to a housemate about a year before her accident that she would not want to live should she face life as a "vegetable," and other observations to the same effect. The observations did not deal in terms with withdrawal of medical treatment or of hydration and nutrition. We cannot say that the Supreme Court of Missouri committed constitutional error in reaching the conclusion that it did.[11]

Petitioners alternatively contend that Missouri must accept the "substituted judgment" of close family members even in the absence of substantial proof that their views reflect the views of the patient. They rely primarily upon our decisions in *Michael H. v. Gerald D.*, 491 U.S. 110, 105 L. Ed. 2d 91, 109 S. Ct. 2333 (1989), and *Parham v. J. R.*, 442 U.S. 584, 61 L. Ed. 2d 101, 99 S. Ct. 2493 (1979). But we do not think these cases support their claim. In *Michael H.*, we upheld the constitutionality of California's favored treatment of traditional family relationships; such a holding may not be turned around into a constitutional requirement that a State must recognize the primacy of those relationships in a situation like this. And in *Parham*, where the patient was a minor, we also upheld the constitutionality of a state scheme in which parents made certain decisions for mentally ill minors. Here again petitioners would seek to turn a decision which allowed a State to rely on family decisionmaking into a constitutional requirement that the State recognize such decisionmaking. But constitutional law does not work that way.

No doubt is engendered by anything in this record but that Nancy Cruzan's mother and father are loving and caring parents. If the State were required by the United States Constitution to repose a right of "substituted judgment" with anyone, the Cruzans would surely qualify. But we do not think the Due Process Clause requires the State to repose judgment on these matters with anyone but the patient herself. Close family members may have a strong feeling—a feeling not at all ignoble or unworthy, but not entirely disinterested, either—that they do not wish to witness the continuation of the life of a loved one which they regard as hopeless, meaningless, and even degrading. But there is no automatic assurance that the view of close family members will necessarily be the same as the patient's would have been had she been confronted with the prospect of her situation while competent. All of the reasons previously discussed for allowing Missouri to require clear and convincing evidence of the patient's wishes lead us to conclude that the State may choose to defer only to those wishes, rather than confide the decision to close family members.[12]

The judgment of the Supreme Court of Missouri is Affirmed.

REFERENCES

1. The State Supreme Court, adopting much of the trial court's findings, described Nancy Cruzan's medical condition as follows:

". . . (1) Her respiration and circulation are not artificially maintained and are within the normal limits of a thirty-year-old female; (2) she is oblivious to her environment except for reflexive responses to sound and perhaps painful stimuli; (3) she suffered anoxia of the brain resulting in a massive enlargement of the ventricles filling with cerebrospinal fluid in the area where the brain has degenerated and [her] cerebral cortical atrophy is irreversible, permanent, progressive, and ongoing; (4) her highest cognitive brain function is exhibited by her grimacing perhaps in recognition of ordinarily painful stimuli, indicating the experience of pain and apparent response to sound; (5) she is a spastic quadriplegic; (6) her four extremities are contracted with irreversible muscular and tendon damage to all extremities; (7) she has no cognitive or reflexive ability to swallow food or water to maintain her daily essential needs and . . . she will never recover her ability to swallow sufficient [*sic*] to satisfy her needs. In sum, Nancy is diagnosed as in a persistent vegetative state. She is not dead. She is not terminally ill. Medical experts testified that she could live another thirty years." *Cruzan v. Harmon*, 760 S.W.2d 408, 411 (Mo. 1989) (en banc) (quotations omitted; footnote omitted).

In observing that Cruzan was not dead, the court referred to the following Missouri statute:

"For all legal purposes, the occurrence of human death shall be determined in accordance with the usual and customary standards of medical practice, provided that death shall not be determined to have occurred unless the following minimal conditions have been met:

"(1) When respiration and circulation are not artificially maintained, there is an irreversible cessation of spontaneous respiration and circulation; or

"(2) When respiration and circulation are artificially maintained, and there is total and irreversible cessation of all brain function, including the brain stem and that such determination is made by a licensed physician." Mo. Rev. Stat. § 194.005 (1986).

Since Cruzan's respiration and circulation were not being artificially maintained, she obviously fit within the first proviso of the statute.

Dr. Fred Plum, the creator of the term "persistent vegetative state" and a renowned expert on the subject, has described the "vegetative state" in the following terms:

"'Vegetative state describes a body which is functioning entirely in terms of its internal controls. It maintains temperature. It maintains heart beat and pulmonary ventilation. It maintains digestive activity. It maintains reflex activity of muscles and nerves for low level conditioned responses. But there is no behavioral evidence of either self-awareness or awareness of the surroundings in a learned manner.'" In re Jobes, 108 N.J. 394, 403, 529 A.2d 434, 438 (1987).

See also Brief for American Medical Association et al. as *Amici Curiae* 6 ("The persistent vegetative state can best be understood as one of the conditions in which patients have suffered a loss of consciousness").

2. See generally Karnezis, "Patient's Right to Refuse Treatment Allegedly Necessary to Sustain Life," 93 *A. L. R.* 3d 67 (1979) (collecting cases); Cantor, "A Patient's Decision to Decline Life-Saving Medical Treatment: Bodily Integrity Versus the Preservation of Life," 26 *Rutgers L. Rev.* 228, 229, and n.5 (1973) (noting paucity of cases).

3. See Chapman, "The Uniform Rights of the Terminally Ill Act: Too Little, Too Late?" 42 *Ark. L. Rev.* 319, 324, n.15 (1989); see also F. Rozovsky, *Consent to Treatment, A Practical Guide* 415–423 (1984).

4. In a later trilogy of cases, the New Jersey Supreme Court stressed that the analytic

framework adopted in *Conroy* was limited to elderly, incompetent patients with shortened life expectancies, and established alternative approaches to deal with a different set of situations. See In re Farrell, 108 N.J. 335, 529 A.2d 404 (1987) (37-year-old competent mother with terminal illness had right to removal of respirator based on common law and constitutional principles which overrode competing state interests); In re Peter, 108 N.J. 365, 529 A.2d 419 (1987) (65-year-old woman in persistent vegetative state had right to removal of nasogastric feeding tube—under Conroy subjective test, power of attorney and hearsay testimony constituted clear and convincing proof of patient's intent to have treatment withdrawn); In re Jobes, 108 N.J. 394, 529 A.2d 434 (1987) (31-year-old woman in persistent vegetative state entitled to removal of jejunostomy feeding tube—even though hearsay testimony regarding patient's intent insufficient to meet clear and convincing standard of proof, under *Quinlan,* family or close friends entitled to make a substituted judgment for patient).

5. The *Drabick* court drew support for its analysis from earlier, influential decisions rendered by California Courts of Appeal. See *Bouvia* v. *Superior Court,* 179 Cal. App. 3d 1127, 225 Cal. Rptr. 297 (1986) (competent 28-year-old quadriplegic had right to removal of nasogastric feeding tube inserted against her will); *Bartling* v. *Superior Court,* 163 Cal. App. 3d 186, 209 Cal. Rptr. 220 (1984) (competent 70-year-old, seriously ill man had right to the removal of respirator); *Barber* v. *Superior Court,* 147 Cal. App. 3d 1006, 195 Cal. Rptr. 484 (1983) (physicians could not be prosecuted for homicide on account of removing respirator and intravenous feeding tubes of patient in persistent vegetative state).

6. Besides the Missouri Supreme Court in *Cruzan* and the courts in *McConnell, Longeway, Drabick, Bouvia, Barber, O'Connor, Conroy, Jobes,* and *Peter,* appellate courts of at least four other States and one Federal District Court have specifically considered and discussed the issue of withholding or withdrawing artificial nutrition and hydration from incompetent individuals. See *Gray* v. *Romeo,* 697 F. Supp. 580 (RI 1988); In re Gardner, 534 A.2d 947 (Me. 1987); In re Grant, 109 Wash. 2d 545, 747 P.2d 445 (1987); *Brophy* v. *New England Sinai Hospital, Inc.,* 398 Mass. 417, 497 N.E.2d 626 (1986); *Corbett* v. *D'Alessandro,* 487 So. 2d 368 (Fla. App. 1986). All of these courts permitted or would permit the termination of such measures based on rights grounded in the common law, or in the State or Federal Constitution.

7. Although many state courts have held that a right to refuse treatment is encompased by a generalized constitutional right of privacy, we have never so held. We believe this issue is more properly analyzed in terms of a Fourteenth Amendment liberty interest. See *Bowers* v. *Hardwick,* 478 U.S. 186, 194-195, 92 L. Ed. 2d 140, 106 S. Ct. 2841 (1986).

8. See Smith, "All's Well That Ends Well: Toward a Policy of Assisted Rational Suicide or Merely Enlightened Self-Determination?" 22 *U. C. D. L. Rev.* 275, 290–291, and n.106 (1989) (compiling statutes).

9. Since Cruzan was a patient at a state hospital when this litigation commenced, the State has been involved as an adversary from the beginning. However, it can be expected that many disputes of this type will arise in private institutions, where a guardian *ad litem* or similar party will have been appointed as the sole representative of the incompetent individual in the litigation. In such cases, a guardian may act in entire good faith, and yet not maintain a position truly adversarial to that of the family. Indeed, as noted by the court below, "the guardian *ad litem* [in this case] finds himself in the predicament of believing that it is in Nancy's 'best interest to have the tube feeding discontinued,' but 'feeling that an appeal should be made because our responsibility to her as attorneys and guardians *ad litem* was to pursue this matter to the highest court in the state in view of the fact that this is a case of first impression in the State of Missouri.'" 760 S.W.2d at 410, n.1. Cruzan's guardian *ad litem* has also filed a brief in

this Court urging reversal of the Missouri Supreme Court's decision. None of this is intended to suggest that the guardian acted the least bit improperly in this proceeding. It is only meant to illustrate the limits which may obtain on the adversarial nature of this type of litigation.

10. We recognize that these cases involved instances where the government sought to take action against an individual. See *Price Waterhouse* v. *Hopkins*, 490 U.S. 228, 253, 104 L. Ed. 2d 268, 109 S. Ct. 1775 (1989) (plurality opinion). Here, by contrast, the government seeks to protect the interests of an individual, as well as its own institutional interests, in life. We do not see any reason why important individual interests should be afforded less protection simply because the government finds itself in the position of defending them. "We find it significant that . . . the defendant rather than the plaintiff" seeks the clear and convincing standard of proof—"suggesting that this standard ordinarily serves as a shield rather than . . . a sword." *Id.*, at 253. That it is the government that has picked up the shield should be of no moment.

11. The clear and convincing standard of proof has been variously defined in this context as "proof sufficient to persuade the trier of fact that the patient held a firm and settled commitment to the termination of life supports under the circumstances like those presented," In re Westchester County Medical Center on behalf of O'Connor, 72 N.Y.2d 517, 531, 531 N.E.2d 607, 613, 534 N.Y.S.2d 886 (1988) (*O'Connor*), and as evidence which "produces in the mind of the trier of fact a firm belief or conviction as to the truth of the allegations sought to be established, evidence so clear, direct and weighty and convincing as to enable [the factfinder] to come to a clear conviction, without hesitancy, of the truth of the precise facts in issue." In re Jobes, 108 N.J. at 407-408, 529 A.2d at 441 (quotation omitted). In both of these cases the evidence of the patient's intent to refuse medical treatment was arguably stronger than that presented here. The New York Court of Appeals and the Supreme Court of New Jersey, respectively, held that the proof failed to meet a clear and convincing threshold. See *O'Connor*, 72 N.Y.2d at 526–534, 531 N.E.2d at 610–615; *Jobes* 108 N.J. at 442–443.

12. We are not faced in this case with the question whether a State might be required to defer to the decision of a surrogate if competent and probative evidence established that the patient herself had expressed a desire that the decision to terminate life-sustaining treatment be made for her by that individual.

Petitioners also adumbrate in their brief a claim based on the Equal Protection Clause of the Fourteenth Amendment to the effect that Missouri has impermissibly treated incompetent patients differently from competent ones, citing the statement in *Cleburne* v. *Cleburne Living Center, Inc.*, 473 U.S. 432, 439, 87 L. Ed. 2d 313, 105 S. Ct. 3249 (1985), that the Clause is "essentially a direction that all persons similarly situated should be treated alike." The differences between the choice made by a competent person to refuse medical treatment, and the choice made for an incompetent person by someone else to refuse medical treatment, are so obviously different that the State is warranted in establishing rigorous procedures for the latter class of cases which do not apply to the former class.

21

PATIENT SELF-DETERMINATION ACT

Title 42, Public Health
Chapter IV Health Care Financing Administration,
Department of Health and Human Relations
Part 489 Provider Agreement and Supplier Approval
Sec. 489.100, 102, 104
[Revised as of October 1, 1999]

SEC. 489.100 DEFINITION.

For purposes of this part, advance directive means a written instruction, such as a living will or durable power of attorney for health care, recognized under State law (whether statutory or as recognized by the courts of the State), relating to the provision of health care when the individual is incapacitated.

SEC. 489.102 REQUIREMENTS FOR PROVIDERS.

(a) Hospitals, critical access hospitals, skilled nursing facilities, nursing facilities, home health agencies, providers of home health care (and for Medicaid purposes, providers of personal care services), and hospices must maintain written policies and procedures concerning advance directives with respect to all adult individuals receiving medical care by or through the provider and are required to:
  (1) Provide written information to such individuals concerning—
    (i) An individual's rights under State law (whether statutory or recognized by the courts of the State) to make decisions concerning such medical care, including the right to accept or refuse medical or surgical treatment and the right to formulate, at the individual's option, advance directives.

Providers are permitted to contract with other entities to furnish this information but are still legally responsible for ensuring that the requirements of this section are met. Providers are to update and disseminate amended information as soon as possible, but no later than 90 days from the effective date of the changes to State law; and

(ii) The written policies of the provider or organization respecting the implementation of such rights, including a clear and precise statement of limitation if the provider cannot implement an advance directive on the basis of conscience. At a minimum, a provider's statement of limitation should:

(A) Clarify any differences between institution-wide conscience objections and those that may be raised by individual physicians;

(B) Identify the state legal authority permitting such objection; and

(C) Describe the range of medical conditions or procedures affected by the conscience objection.

(2) Document in the individual's medical record whether or not the individual has executed an advance directive;

(3) Not condition the provision of care or otherwise discriminate against an individual based on whether or not the individual has executed an advance directive;

(4) Ensure compliance with requirements of State law (whether statutory or recognized by the courts of the State) regarding advance directives. The provider must inform individuals that complaints concerning the advance directive requirements may be filed with the State survey and certification agency;

(5) Provide for education of staff concerning its policies and procedures on advance directives; and

(6) Provide for community education regarding issues concerning advance directives that may include material required in paragraph (a)(1) of this section, either directly or in concert with other providers and organizations. Separate community education materials may be developed and used, at the discretion of providers. The same written materials do not have to be provided in all settings, but the material should define what constitutes an advance directive, emphasizing that an advance directive is designed to enhance an incapacitated individual's control over medical treatment, and describe applicable State law concerning advance directives. A provider must be able to document its community education efforts.

(b) The information specified in paragraph (a) of this section is furnished:

(1) In the case of a hospital, at the time of the individual's admission as an inpatient.

(2) In the case of a skilled nursing facility at the time of the individual's admission as a resident.

(3) (i) In the case of a home health agency, in advance of the individual coming

under the care of the agency. The HHA may furnish advance directives information to a patient at the time of the first home visit, as long as the information is furnished before care is provided.

(ii) In the case of personal care services, in advance of the individual coming under the care of the personal care services provider. The personal care provider may furnish advance directives information to a patient at the time of the first home visit, as long as the information is furnished before care is provided.

(4) In the case of a hospice program, at the time of initial receipt of hospice care by the individual from the program.

(c) The providers listed in paragraph (a) of this section—

(1) Are not required to provide care that conflicts with an advance directive.

(2) Are not required to implement an advance directive if, as a matter of conscience, the provider cannot implement an advance directive and State law allows any health-care provider or any agent of such provider to conscientiously object.

(d) Prepaid or eligible organizations [as specified in sections 1833(a)(1)(A) and 1876(b) of the Act] must meet the requirements specified in Sec. 417.436 of this chapter.

(e) If an adult individual is incapacitated at the time of admission or at the start of care and is unable to receive information (due to the incapacitating conditions or a mental disorder) or articulate whether or not he or she has executed an advance directive, then the provider may give advance directive information to the individual's family or surrogate in the same manner that it issues other materials about policies and procedures to the family of the incapacitated individual or to a surrogate or other concerned persons in accordance with State law.

The provider is not relieved of its obligation to provide this information to the individual once he or she is no longer incapacitated or unable to receive such information. Follow-up procedures must be in place to provide the information to the individual directly at the appropriate time.

SEC. 489.104 EFFECTIVE DATES.

These provisions apply to services furnished on or after December 1, 1991, payments made under section 1833(a)(1)(A) of the Act on or after December 1, 1991, and contracts effective on or after December 1, 1991.

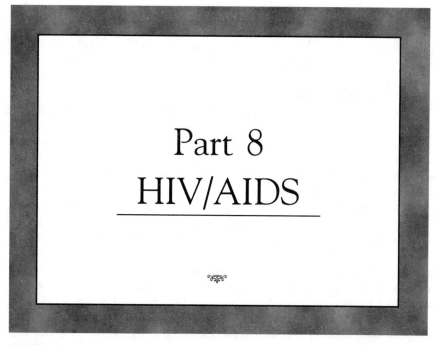

Part 8
HIV/AIDS

W hen considering how our society makes moral judgements, it seems fairly obvious that we choose to feel sympathetic or malevolent based on how responsible we perceive someone to be for his actions, particularly if those actions result in an illness or disease. So when a patient is judged to be an "innocent victim," health-care providers (as well as the public) bestow almost unlimited compassion, care, and attention. On the contrary, when a patient is judged to be responsible for his condition, he tends to be "managed" as opposed to cared for, which results in less respect, interaction, and sympathy from the health-care team. This kind of judgment also precludes any attempt to empathize with the patient. An important dichotomy does exist, however, as many see a difference between being responsible in a strong sense versus being responsible in a weak sense. A patient whose myocardial infarction (heart attack) is an indirect result of a poor diet and lack of exercise is considered responsible in the weak sense. We do not think of the patient as being a bad person, only someone with an unhealthy lifestyle. In contrast, a patient with alcohol-related cirrhosis is considered responsible in the strong sense, as he directly caused his disease and did so as a result of being a bad person. When such a judgment of strong responsibility is applied to an entire patient population there are grave consequences, as those with AIDS can attest.* The goal of this section is to explore two complex and emotionally charged AIDS-related issues—disclosure and assisted suicide—that

---

*I will use the term "AIDS" here to represent both those who are HIV-positive and those with full-blown AIDS.

have been borne of such judgements coupled with the fear of being infected, disapproval of homosexuality, and medicine's avoidance of what it cannot cure.

The first article in this section concerns not how health-care providers respond to patients with AIDS, but how patients respond to health-care providers with AIDS; or more specifically, how they respond when their tests and/or procedures are performed by a health-care provider with AIDS, without their knowledge. Even though "Nothing to Fear But Fear Itself: HIV-Infected Physicians and the Law of Informed Consent," by Kenneth DeVille, was written explicitly about physicians with AIDS, the issues he raises are certainly relevant to all health-care providers who perform invasive procedures, such as paramedics, nurses, and respiratory therapists.

Health-care providers have an intimate understanding of the stigma from which AIDS patients suffer, so it is easy to understand why they would hide their illness from patients and colleagues alike. But withholding such information raises an issue of justice (or fairness) with regard to self-determination and the opportunity to protect oneself, even from irrational fears. From the very first lecture in a health-care provider's training program she is taught, ad nauseam, to always use "universal precautions," all things being equal. Every patient is to be approached, she is told, as if he had AIDS; and if she thinks a patient really does have AIDS she should double-glove, wear eye protection, put on a gown, and perform her procedures slowly and with extreme caution. When the risk of exposure is truly present such precautions are reasonable and appropriate (e.g., in emergency settings, surgery, and so on). Health-care providers are therefore able to choose how much risk they assume by adding protective barriers as they see fit. Even when a patient denies having AIDS, an experienced health-care provider can often determine, or at least have a high index of suspicion, that the patient before her has AIDS. If a health-care provider is particularly wary of treating AIDS patients she can intentionally choose a specialty or work environment with reduced likelihood of encountering these patients.

Patients, on the other hand, do not have the ability or opportunity to choose what level of risk they are willing to assume regarding an AIDS-related iatrogenic exposure—other than never seeking medical treatment. There are no universal precautions patients can don, and they do not have the experience to determine who has, or is likely to have, AIDS. As patients do not choose what injuries or diseases befall them (at least not consciously), they cannot avoid those specialties or institutional settings that are "high risk." Therefore, a patient will only be able to minimize his risk, on par with health-care providers, if AIDS disclosures are made a part of the informed consent process.

Requiring such a disclosure is extremely controversial, with vocal advocates on both sides. Those against making this a requirement hold that their opposition is acting from fear and ignorance. They claim that the risk of actually becoming infected after an exposure is so small as to be theoretical; the Centers for Disease Control put it at less than 1 percent. Proponents of this requirement argue that it is a value, not a medical, judgment as to whether less than 1 percent constitutes something that is significant enough to mention or nothing more then theoretical. They believe that this decision ought to be left to the patient. This is the core issue that DeVille's article takes on through a discussion of the 1990 Maryland Court of Appeals ruling in *Faya* v. *Almaraz*. This case provides an excellent basis for thinking about not only the rights and interests of all concerned but how those rights and interests ought to be balanced: a health-care provider's ability to continue her career must be considered along with a patient's right to choose his risks. DeVille concludes his article by saying the cases and issues he discusses are strictly about the law, not ethics. I believe this is a bit too narrow a view of what it means to have a duty, and with a bit of digging these cases and issues are permeated with ethical issues that need to be considered and discussed by ethics committees and health-care providers.

Moving to a more somber AIDS-related issue, the authors of the next study looked at active euthanasia and assisted suicide among homosexual men dying from AIDS. "Informal Caregivers and the Intention to Hasten AIDS-related Death," by Molly Cooke and colleagues, was actually an afterthought to another study. While looking into the stress and coping skills of 253 men who were taking care of their homosexual partners who were dying from AIDS, the authors decided to also look at *how* their partners were dying. To that end, they asked the surviving partners if the patients' deaths were hastened, what factors influenced the patients' decision, and what effects that decision had on the caregivers.

Before moving forward we need to define exactly what is meant by assisted suicide and euthanasia, as some of these deaths were hastened by the former and some the latter. As commonly defined within the medical ethics literature *assisted suicide*, as opposed to *euthanasia*, is an act in which a patient is provided with something he takes himself with the intention of ending his life. Euthanasia, on the other hand, is demarcated into four subgroups. First, *active voluntary euthanasia* occurs when a patient, with his consent, is given something that ends his life (e.g., an overdose of morphine). Second, *active involuntary euthanasia* is different from the former insofar as the patient does not give his consent. Depending on the context this act can be conceived as murder or mercy killing. Third, *passive voluntary euthanasia* is the act of withdrawing or withholding life-sustaining treatment with the patient's or proxy's consent. Last, *passive involuntary euthanasia* is the same as the former but without the patient's or proxy's consent. This, too, can be conceived as either murder or mercy killing, depending on the context.

With these definitions in mind the authors made three primary observations. First, assisted suicide and voluntary active euthanasia are not uncommon among homosexual men dying from AIDS. Second, caregiver participation was grounded in care, commitment, and love, and not from depression or feelings of being burdened. This finding is quite significant, as one of the primary objections to the legalization of any kind of assisted death is the belief that patients will be coerced into accepting assisted deaths once they become a burden to their caregiver(s) whether emotionally, financially, or otherwise. And third, the caregiver was not emotionally harmed as a result of hastening his partner's death. Regardless of a health-care provider's position on hastening a patient's death, this study makes clear the importance of allowing AIDS patients and their caregivers to openly talk about all end-of-life options.

By considering the implications of the discussion in the opening paragraph, we can see the need for this study originating in many ways almost twenty years ago. Society's assignment of strong responsibility at the beginning of the AIDS epidemic created a political environment that prevented any meaningful response to the mysterious illness that, at the time, affected only homosexual men. This was clearly evident from the dearth of funding provided for research. Due to this multiyear delay in legitimate, appropriately funded research, the mode of transmission was not determined with enough certainty to bring about the necessary public-health changes that very well could have halted the spread of AIDS. This lack of certainty was used to justify a delay in the testing of our nation's blood supply, even though the test for hepatitis B was 88 percent accurate in detecting the HIV antibody.[1] This resulted in some thirty thousand patients being transfused with AIDS-infected blood. In the end, Cooke's study is both redeeming and damning. It is redeeming because it shows that many patients, caregivers, and health-care providers are talking openly about a very difficult issue in order to provide the kind of end-of-life care that promotes the patient's interests as he sees them. It is damning because without society's assignment of strong responsibility twenty years ago, the subject of this study could have possibly been moot.

REFERENCE

1. Shilts R. *And the Band Played On: Politics, People, and the AIDS Epidemic.* New York, NY: St. Martin's Press; 2000.

22

NOTHING TO FEAR BUT FEAR ITSELF

HIV-Infected Physicians and the Law of Informed Consent

Kenneth A. De Ville, Ph.D., J.D.

On March 9, 1993, in the first ruling of its kind, the Maryland Court of Appeals declared that physicians and hospitals may be sued for failing to inform patients of a practitioner's human immunodeficiency virus (HIV) status.[1] What is more significant, these suits may be pursued even in instances when the physician has followed universal precautions and the patient did not contract the virus that causes acquired immunodeficiency syndrome (AIDS). The Maryland court addressed two central questions in *Faya v. Almaraz*. First, do HIV-infected physicians have a legal duty to inform their patients of their HIV status? And, second, can patients recover damages for fear induced by a physician's conduct? While one finds numerous precedents that authorize actions to recover damages based purely on fear of disease and emotional distress, the *Faya* court's holdings on the issue significantly expand the scope of potential liability. Moreover, the court's analysis of the informed consent and HIV-infected physician issue is incomplete, inconsistent, and represents an unjustified and unwise departure from traditional informed consent theory. It, and its progeny, may have widespread and dire repercussions.

K. A. De Ville. "Nothing to Fear but Fear Itself: HIV-Infected Physicians and the Law of Informed Consent." *Journal of Law, Medicine & Ethics*. 1994;22(2):163–175. ©1994. Reprinted with the permission of the American Society of Law, Medicine & Ethics. All rights reserved.

FAYA V. ALMARAZ

Dr. Rudolf Almaraz, an oncological surgeon who practiced at the Johns Hopkins Hospital in Baltimore, was diagnosed with an HIV infection in 1986. Dr. Almaraz performed a partial mastectomy and axillary dissection on Sonia Faya in October 1998 and March 1989. In November 1989, he operated on Perry Mahoney Rossi to remove a benign lump from her breast. Both operations were successful, but Dr. Almaraz informed neither woman of his HIV infection.[2] He continued to practice until March 1990, when he informed his patients by mail that he was leaving medicine to pursue research in Texas.[3]

Almaraz died on November 16, 1990, and a newspaper report of December 2, 1990, attributed the death to AIDS-related complications. Faya and Rossi first learned of Dr. Almaraz's disease and death four days later, on December 6, 1990. Nearly twenty months had passed since Faya's last contact with Dr. Almaraz. It had been over a year since Rossi's operation. Both women immediately underwent enzyme-linked immunoabsorbent assay tests to determine their HIV status. The women received negative test results, on or about December 10, 1990, indicating a very high probability that neither had been infected.[4]

On December 11, 1990, the two women sued the Almaraz estate, his group practice, and the Johns Hopkins Hospital for damages. Faya and Rossi claimed that Almaraz had provided them with inadequate informed consent when he did not disclose his HIV status before their operations. Their suit also raised a variety of other legal claims based on the failure to inform, including: intentional infliction of emotional distress; battery; negligent misrepresentation; breach of contract, breach of fiduciary duty; and fraud.[5] Faya and Rossi argued that they were injured because: (1) they were unjustifiably exposed to a risk of HIV infection; (2) they would suffer from the fear of HIV infection for years to come; and (3) they would suffer from the pain and costs of repeated HIV testing. In addition, the women sued the hospital because Almaraz was acting as its agent, because the hospital did not investigate Almaraz's HIV status, and because the hospital failed to take proper precautions to ensure that Almaraz did not perform surgery on patients who did not know of his condition. Faya and Rossi argued that the institution either should have suspended the physician's surgical privileges or should have required that he inform every patient under his care of his health status as part of the consent process.[6] Rossi's husband also joined the suit, claiming loss of consortium and asserting that he, too, might be at risk of infection through relations with his wife.

The attorneys for Almaraz's estate and for the hospital filed a "motion to dismiss," contending that the women's suit did not state a legally justifiable claim. Almaraz's attorneys argued that the doctrine of informed consent does not require physicians to inform patients of their HIV infection, that the claim was based on a harm (seroconversion) that never materialized, and that the women had failed to allege that the virus had actually entered their bodies. In short, the Almaraz attorneys claimed that he had breached no duty and that the women had suffered no legally compensable damages.[7]

The Baltimore trial court judge dismissed the cases of both women. First, he explained that "there are no reported cases of transmission of AIDS from a surgeon to a patient, such transmission is only a theoretical possibility when proper barriers techniques are employed. . . ." Therefore, HIV-infected physicians have no duty under informed consent doctrine to warn the patients of an infinitesimal possibility of infection. Second, the judge ruled that the women had suffered no legally cognizable damage. Because both women had tested negative for HIV more than six months after their last exposure to Almaraz, it was extremely unlikely (less than 5 percent according to estimates accepted by the court[8]) that they had been infected with the virus. Because the women had not alleged any untoward contact with Almaraz's blood that could have led to infection, the court reasoned, Faya's and Rossi's supposed injuries consisted of "the fear that something that did not happen could have happened."[9] Therefore, a jury would not be allowed to decide their case.

Faya, Rossi, and their attorneys appealed the trial court dismissal to the Maryland Court of Appeals, and warned that the trial court decision "encourages physicians and surgeons in Maryland to conceal AIDS and go on treating innocent patients, spreading the disease exponentially over time. The results would be disastrous for Maryland citizens."[10]

THE COURT OF APPEALS

In *Faya* v. *Almaraz*, the court of appeals reversed the trial court's dismissal of charges. It ruled that a jury should be allowed to evaluate the appropriateness of Almaraz's actions, whether he breached his duty of informed consent, and the damages, if any, suffered by Faya and Rossi. The court of appeals explained that the trial court erred in ruling that the physician had no duty to inform his patients of his HIV status, and concluded that the women's fear of infection was not "unreasonable" and might constitute a compensable injury. The appellate ruling does not create an affirmative duty to inform, but merely allows the two women to attempt to convince a jury that such a duty exists and that Almaraz breached it. The court did not distinguish among the various legal claims made by Faya and Rossi, but recognized that the "gist of the complaints was that Almaraz acted wrongfully in operating on the two women without first telling them that he was HIV-positive."[11] The court's consolidated and generic discussion of the various legal claims is unfortunate. A more complete and careful analysis of the issues raised by the informed consent claims could have provided more insight into what potentially is a very important ruling. The court's finding on the nature of the duty to provide informed consent is problematic in several respects, and will be discussed in more detail below.

The *Faya* court began by outlining the legal standards for a viable claim of negligence. Such a claim must involve a breach of duty of care that proximately causes a legally cognizable injury.[12] The court dealt first with the existence of a duty to inform. Instead of basing its discussion primarily on Maryland informed-consent case law, the court relied on a sexually transmitted disease case which held that, because of the foreseeability of transmission, the defendant had a legal duty to refrain from sexual contact or to inform his sexual partners of his disease.[13] The court also relied heavily on a 1991 American Medical Association Council on Ethical and Judicial Affairs recommendation that HIV-infected surgeons inform their patients of their status or forgo invasive procedures. Finally, it relied on the *Restatement, Second, Torts,* § 293 (c) directive that "the seriousness of potential harm, as well as its probability, contributes to a duty to prevent it."[14] (The court mentioned only in a footnote, but did not discuss, the state's medical informed consent doctrine.[15]) Claiming that these principles applied in the *Almaraz* case, the court ruled that "we are unable to say, as a matter of law, that Dr. Almaraz owed no duty to . . . either refrain from performing the surgery or to warn them of his condition."[16] The court observed that, while the risk of transmission was admittedly quite low, the risk of death, if the patient was infected, was so severe that it was possible that the physician might owe a duty of disclosure.

The court then dealt with whether emotional distress and fear of AIDS were "legally cognizable damages" ill the absence of a positive HIV-infection test. The defendants claimed and the court recognized that a significant body of case law holds that a plaintiff cannot recover damages for fear of AIDS (or of any other disease) where no assertion or evidence exists that the plaintiffs were directly exposed to the agent that causes the disease. For example, *Burk* v. *Sage Products*[17] rejected a fear-of-AIDS claim in which Burk (the plaintiff) tested negative for HIV and could not show that he had actually been exposed to the virus. Burk worked on a hospital service that provided care for AIDS patients. He stuck his finger with a discarded needle, but could not demonstrate that the needle had been used on an AIDS patient, although it clearly could have been. In granting summary judgment for the defense, the *Burk* court noted that it had been "unable to locate a single case, from any jurisdiction, which has permitted recovery for emotional distress arising out of fear of contracting a disease when the plaintiff cannot prove exposure to the agent which has the potential to cause the disease."[18] Another case, cited by the defense and discussed by the *Faya* court, dismissed the claim of a mortician who had unknowingly embalmed an HIV-infected corpse. Because the mortician had worn proper protective gear and had not alleged a means of potential exposure, the court reasoned, he could not claim damages for the fear of disease.[19] These and other precedents[20] appear to support strongly the defendants' argument that the plaintiffs had failed to assert a legally compensable injury.[21] As the defendants' noted in their arguments, Faya and Rossi did not claim that Almaraz had cut himself, stuck himself, or bled during the surgery; that he had mixed his blood or bodily fluids with theirs; or that he had failed to adhere to standard infection-control measures.[22]

The *Faya* court, however, rejected the *Burk* line of cases; instead, it relied on the test defined in *Carroll* v. *Sisters of St. Francis Health Services, Inc.*[23] The *Faya* majority, echoing *Carroll,* abandoned the exposure requirements of *Burk,* and declared that a plaintiff could maintain an action for the fear of disease if that fear was not "unreasonable." The *Faya* court ruled that it could not say that Faya's and Rossi's initial fear was "unreasonable as a matter of law," even though they failed to allege or demonstrate "any channel of transmission" for HIV. The court reasoned that the *Burk* requirement that plaintiffs allege actual transmission "would unfairly punish them for lacking the requisite information to do so."[24] The Faya court concluded that the women could go to trial and attempt to recover damages for their fear and emotional distress that were not unreasonable.[25]

The *Faya* court's determination of which portion of the women's fear was "unreasonable," and which portion of fear a jury might find "reasonable," is curious, and it could not have entirely pleased either litigant. It is not surprising that the court ruled that Faya and Rossi could not claim damages for the emotional distress caused by fear of infection during the period in which they were unaware of Almaraz's HIV status, that is, from the time of the surgery until the time that they learned of his death of AIDS, on December 6, 1990.[26] Clearly, they could have suffered no injury for being put at a risk that did not materialize and about which they knew nothing. But, the women could go to trial and attempt to recover for the fear of AIDS suffered following their discovery of Almaraz's HIV infection on December 6, 1990.[26] While this initial fear of infection may have been reasonable and Faya and Rossi could attempt to recover damages, the court held that only a limited "window of anxiety" existed. As soon as they received information that "put that fear to rest," they were no longer suffering from legally compensable damages.

According to the *Faya* court, the women's fear should have been put to rest and was therefore legally "unreasonable" after they tested negative for HIV, several days after their discovery of their physician's illness, on or about December 10, 1990. The court noted that "there is current credible evidence of a 95% certainty that one will test positive for the AIDS virus, if at all, within six months after exposure to it." Since both women's last contact with Almaraz had been more than a year previous, the court ruled that their "continued fear" of AIDS was unreasonable as a matter of law, and that the women could not ask a jury for any damages related to emotional distress after their negative HIV test results.[27] Therefore, Faya and Rossi could ask a jury to award damages for the fear they suffered, but only for the period between December 6, 1990, and about December 10, 1990, or about four days' time.

The *Faya* approach to the issue of tort damages in fear-of-disease cases opens up new routes for litigation. Under the *Burk* line of cases, if a patient/plaintiff was able to claim a negligent surgical incident (that is, a negligently sliced finger, needle stick, and so forth) or claim that the HIV-infected physician negligently or intentionally failed to conform to universal precautions, that plaintiff might be able to defeat summary judgment and present the case to a jury. Because such a claim is not based on the individual patient's knowledge or subjective desires regarding the HIV status of the physician, but rather on the alleged negligence or wrongful intentional act of the physician, it would be equally viable if the physician informed, or did not inform, the patient of his HIV infection. This manner of claim is legitimate. If a patient was informed of a physician's HIV infection, consented to surgery, and the surgeon negligently exposed the patient to his bodily fluids, then the patient should have an opportunity to prove negligence and collect damages for related injuries that he or she suffered. If a patient was not informed of the physician's status, and the physician acted negligently, the result would be the same. In both cases, the central claim of the action is not the informed consent, but the negligent or wrongfully intentional behavior of the physician during the procedure, behavior that should be penalized if it causes an injury. The physician's defense is that he did conform to universal precautions, or that the incident that caused the exposure to body fluids was not the result of negligence.

However, *Faya's* abandonment of the *Burk* rationale amplifies the legal importance of whether the physician informed the patient of his HIV infection. Under *Faya*, no allegation of exposure to the disease-causing agent to support a claim is required. Consequently, a suit may be maintained even where no allegation of negligence or wrongful intentional[28] act during the surgical procedure exists. Under this formulation, the patient's knowledge or lack of knowledge of the physician's HIV infection suddenly becomes transcendently important because a claim of no negligence, or no exposure to the disease-causing agent, by the physician is no longer a defense. A patient can now articulate a viable cause of action merely by constructing a potential informed consent claim.

FAYA V. ALMARAZ AND THE DOCTRINE OF INFORMED CONSENT

Despite the implications of the decision for informed-consent doctrine and policy, the *Faya* court devoted only scant attention to the broad range of complex interests at stake. The court's discussion of the adequacy of Almaraz's informed consent to his patients was framed not in the context of the doctor-patient relationship, as it should have been, but was considered within the more general duty to warn of known dangers. A full and sensitive consideration of the duty to warn within the unique nature of the doctor-patient relationship could have, and should have, led to a different result.

The doctrine of informed consent for medical treatment in Maryland resembles that of many other states. According to the state's leading case, *Sard* v. *Hardy* (1977), physicians are required to inform patients of "any material risks or dangers inherent or collateral to the therapy."[29] *Sard* defined material risk as a risk that "a physician knows or ought to know would be significant to a *reasonable person* in the patient's position in deciding whether . . . to submit to a particular treatment." This material risk standard is a descendant of the famous *Canterbury* v. *Spence* (1972) decision that has served as a model for patient-centered informed consent.[30] The test, while patient-centered, is objective, not subjective. This distinction is important. The "materiality" of the risk is not judged by the subjective perception of the individual patient, but by the so-called "reasonable person." The physician is not required to inform a patient of all risks, only of those that a reasonable person would consider material. If a physician fails to inform a patient of a material risk and that risk occurs, then the physician may be liable for damages.[31]

The objective material-risk/reasonable-person standard serves several interconnected functions. Patient self-determination and bodily autonomy are important values that warrant legal protection. At the same time, the patient's right to know is balanced against both fairness to physicians and society's interest that medicine be practiced without "unrealistic and unnecessary burdens on practitioners."[32] The patient-centered characteristics of the reasonable-person test protects the interests of patients, while the objective perspective of the standard is designed to provide rationality and predictability.

Typically, a jury is permitted to decide what risks a reasonable person would consider material. The materiality of particular information depends on both the severity of the potential injury and the probability of its occurrence. As the severity of the potential injury increases, a risk becomes material at a lower level of probable occurrence.[33] However, even the risk of severe injury may be found immaterial if the probability of occurrence is so low as to be negligible.[34] As the court in *Precourt* v. *Frederick* (1985) explained:

> Regardless of the severity of a potential injury, if the probability that the injury will occur is so small as to be practically nonexistent, then the possibility of that injury occurring cannot be considered a material factor in a rational assessment of whether to engage in the activity that exposes one to the, potential injury.[35]

In *Precourt*, a patient had been given an anti-inflammatory drug (Prednisone) during eye surgery. The drug contributed to the destruction of the patient's hip. The court declared that because only a "negligible" risk of the orthopedic injury existed, the risk was not material. As a result, the appellate court reversed the jury verdict that had been rendered in favor of the patient.

Courts have been willing, in a variety of other situations, to find that a very low probability of injury is sufficient to make the risk of its occurrence immaterial and withdraw the decision from the trial jury. However, they have never provided guidelines stating specifically how remote a serious harm can be and still remain material.[36] One court, for example, held that a 1-in-100,000 chance of loss of sensation in the face following a tooth extraction was not material as a matter of law and did not require disclosure.[37] A Washington State court found that a 1-in-20,000 to a 1-in-50,000 risk of perforation of the colon during a rectal sigmoidoscopy was, as a matter of law, not material; consequently, the physician had no duty to disclose the risk to the patient.[38] The risk of a penicillin-induced anaphylactic shock death is about 1-in-100,000, similar to the risks associated with allergic reactions to local anesthetics such as lidocaine, yet many physicians do not inform patients of these arguably immaterial dangers.[39]

A strong argument could be made, on statistical grounds alone, that, contrary to the *Faya* court's ruling, the risk of transmission from HIV-infected surgeons to patients is so low as to be "immaterial" for purposes of informed consent.[40] Much of the current public concern over HIV-infected health professionals may be traced largely to the highly publicized 1990 case of Dr. David Acer, an HIV-infected dentist. Six of his patients were infected with HIV, but the exact nature of his culpability or nonculpability has yet to be resolved.[41] However, no documented account of a physician or surgeon transmitting the virus to patients is recorded. Numerous "look back" studies which screen the patients of infected physicians and surgeons have failed to uncover a single case of patient infection.[42] The studies, including one focusing on Almaraz's 1,800 patients, tested thousands of patients who had undergone procedures at the hands of HIV-infected surgeons.[43] In 1992, the National Commission on AIDS noted that studies examining the records of more than 15,000 patients treated by thirty-two health-care professionals uncovered no cases of physician-to-patient transmission. The commission rated the risk as "virtually nonexistent" if standard precautions, such as using latex gloves, were used, and it recommended against mandatory disclosure of HIV infection as part of informed consent.[44] In 1993, the Centers for Disease Control (CDC), using existing published and unpublished studies, reported that HIV tests and follow-ups on 19,036 persons treated by fifty-seven HIV-infected health care workers revealed no confirmed instances of seroconversion through health-care contacts.[45]

Because a documented account of surgeon-to-patient infection has yet to surface, statistical estimation of the likelihood of transmission during an invasive medical procedure is speculative. Nevertheless, several reputable calculations have been formulated. The CDC, in 1991, estimated that a patient undergoing a seriously invasive procedure by an HIV-infected health-care worker has between a 1-in-40,000 and a 1-in-400,000 chance of infection. Other researchers have calculated the risk of an HIV-infected surgeon infecting a patient during a one hour operation at 1-in-83,000. If an invasive procedure is performed by a surgeon of unknown HIV status, the patient's chance of infection shrinks to 1-in-20,000,000.[46]

The plaintiffs, in their brief to the Maryland Court of Appeals, argued that the *Sard* case stood for the proposition that the "materiality of risk is for the patient to decide, not the physician" and that "whether the patient's perception is reasonable is a question for the jury and not the trial judge.[47] " The plaintiffs relied on the *Behringer v. The Medical Center at Princeton*[48] court's comment that a physician's HIV infection constituted a material risk under informed-consent doctrine.[49] The plaintiffs' assertions are open to dispute. *Sard*, in fact, stands for the proposition that the "materiality" of a risk is to be judged by the reasonable-person standard. And, while *Behringer* does suggest that the risk from a HIV- infected physician may be material, that specific holding is of questionable relevance in that the case involved the permissible limitations an institution could place on a physician's practice: It was not a finding on the nature of tort damages for failure of informed consent.

But the *Faya* court did not examine the notion of the reasonable person or its importance in evaluating material risk in informed consent cases. Neither did that court consider any statistical calculations in its discussion of whether Almaraz's HIV status and the potential for transmission constituted a material risk. Instead, the court observed simply that, while the risk was very low, the result of the transmission—death—was so severe that it was possible that the physician might owe a duty of disclosure to the women. The opinion relied heavily on the AMA Council on Ethical and

Judicial Affairs' 1991 recommendation that HIV-infected surgeons inform their patients of their status or forgo invasive procedures.[50] The court's reference to the 1991 AMA recommendations is troublesome. Almaraz treated Faya and Rossi in 1988 and 1989, well before the 1991 recommendation, although a 1988 AMA recommendation advised similar disclosure. The AMA recommendation is not necessarily consistent with the appropriate legal standard in informed consent liability suits, and has since been modified. Professional guidelines, while relevant, are not conclusive, and are even more suspect when they undergo frequent (almost annual) revision. More important, under Maryland's and other states' standards, the sufficiency of the informed consent is gauged not by the profession or the AMA,[51] but by what a reasonable person would consider a material risk. The ethical standard for informed consent might be higher or lower than the standard required by law, and this standard should not serve as a substitute.

The *Faya* court's treatment of the informed-consent issue is suspect in additional respects. A suit based on lack of informed consent requires that the material risk omitted by the physician in his pretreatment discussions actually occur and injure the patient. The essence of an informed consent claim involving an HIV-infected physician would be the assertion that HIV status information was material because of the risk that the patient might become infected with the virus as a result of the treatment. But, that risk, omitted from the informed consent process in *Faya*, did not come about. Faya and Rossi may have suffered fear, but that damage is not the injury or risk that the patients would have initially considered material at the time of their surgery. To put it another way, they did not desire information about their surgeon's HIV infection because of the potential fear and emotional distress they would suffer if they later discovered his condition. Instead, their desire to know (assuming they had such a desire at the time of their treatment) was based on their concern that he might pass on the infection during a medical procedure. As the Almaraz defense team argued, "To the extent that there was any risk, whether purely theoretical or material, that Appellants could have been exposed to and contracted the AIDS virus, there is no claim by either of them that this risk materialized. Indeed, Appellants' negative HIV tests confirmed that the risk did *not* materialize."[52] The *Faya* court did not rebut this argument, which could have precluded the recovery of damages.

The *Faya* court's failure to find the extraordinarily small risk of physician-to-patient infection immaterial is inconsistent with the same court's holding on an indistinguishable issue. The *Faya* court reasoned that once the women had tested negative for HIV within a 95 percent certainty, any further fears of infection would be "unreasonable." Therefore, Faya and Rossi would not be allowed to ask a jury to award damages for any period after the negative HIV test. To rephrase, the court found that fear of a 5 percent (or a 1-in-20) chance of harm after December 10, 1990, was unreasonable as a matter of law and, therefore, not actionable. However, the court took a radically different posture when evaluating Almaraz's duty to inform the women of his HIV status. Using the CDC estimates, Faya and Rossi had between a 1-in-40,000 and a 1-in-400,000 chance of infection when undergoing invasive surgery at the hands of an HIV-Infected surgeon. However, unlike the 1-in-20 chance of harm that the court had earlier found unreasonable, the *Faya* majority refused to hold that this profoundly smaller risk represented an unreasonable fear as a matter of law. The disparity is striking. The court found that the women's fear of a 1-in-20 possibility of infection in the presence of a negative HIV test was clearly unreasonable, but it inexplicably concluded that a 1-in-40,000 to 1-in-400,000 risk of infection at the time of their initial treatment might be reasonable. It is unclear why the court used a dramatically different statistical threshold to calculate unreasonableness even though the severity of the risk, HIV infection in both instances, was the same.

MATERIAL RISK AND THE REASONABLE PERSON

The *Faya* court appears to have accepted, without explicit discussion, the plaintiffs' argument that the risk of infection from an HIV-infected physician is "material" and of a nature that a "reasonable person" would want to know. The court's approach may have been influenced by the special character of AIDS, its inexorably fatal outcome, and its ability to generate tremendous fear. The court decision also may be based on the intuitive assumption that patients want to know if their physicians have been infected by HIV. Indeed, one poll shows that over 90 percent of patients surveyed want to know if their treating physicians are HIV-infected.[53] Other surveys confirm that over 80 percent of those polled believe that controlling AIDS is more important than the protection of individual privacy, and that physicians with HIV should be required to inform their patients.[54] Even Norman Daniels, who ultimately argues against disclosure as a national policy, concedes that the demands for disclosure from the vast majority of the population are enough to suggest that such demands might not be unreasonable or irrational. Because a patient could "switch" to an uninfected physician and lower his or her already low risk to zero, Daniels reasons, the desire for such disclosure is not irrational.[55] A recent law review article, arguing in favor of an informed consent requirement and in support of the Faya decision, contends that the high percentage of individuals in favor of disclosure indicates that the risk of infection constitutes a material risk under current doctrine.[56]

Even if the polls that show an overwhelming patient desire for information about the HIV status of their physicians are correct, the statistics do not support the approach to informed consent condoned by the *Faya* court. Statistical evidence of public opinion is an improper and unwise way to determine the mind of the reasonable person. The reasonable person does not represent the subjective judgment of the majority any more than it represents the subjective judgment of one person. Therefore, the majority-rule approach to materiality, to the extent that it governs when patients can recover damages for informed consent, is flawed and inadequate.

"Material risk" to a "reasonable person" means something specific in legal contexts. The reasonable person of traditional legal doctrine represents a highly idealized being who always plays the percentages and is never influenced by personal idiosyncrasies or irrational fears. While flesh-and-blood individuals answering questions on a survey will frequently express unjustified concerns, a reasonable person will not. As a leading treatise on tort law explains:

> The courts have gone to unusual pains to emphasize the abstract and hypothetical character of this mythical person. He is not to be identified with any ordinary individual, who might occasionally do unreasonable things; he is a prudent and careful person, who is always up to standard.[57]

Restatements, Second, Torts, § 283, describes the reasonable person as a "fictitious" being who overcomes the "natural tendency" to "prefer his own interests to those of others," and who is able to "give an impartial consideration to the harm likely to be done to the interests of the other as compared with the advantages likely to accrue to his own interests."[58] Leading scholars of informed consent stress that "the reasonable person is to be distinguished both from identifiable actors and from statistical norms or averages, such as empirical findings of what the average person would do."[59]

This idealized reasonable person, one could argue, would look impartially at the scintilla of risk represented by the HIV-positive physician and conclude that it is not "material." The reasonable person might consider, for example, the extraordinarily low probability of infection, the rights and concerns of HIV-infected physicians, and the burden placed on the nation's health-care system if universal monitoring and disclosure were mandated. The fact that in excess of 90 percent of the population favor disclosure of an HIV-infected physician's status does not make their position reasonable as a matter of law, because the reasonable person is an ideal and is not necessarily synonymous with the consensus of the community.

In addition, reliance on a statistically defined reasonable person would demand that we disclose risks or alter policy in every instance that the potential injury is grave and/or a significant portion of the population desire disclosure. For example, a majority of parents probably want to be informed if an HIV-infected child is attending school with their sons and daughters—a policy that at the same time would be unreasonable, unwise, and unfair. While courts have not ruled specifically on whether parents have a right to know if one of their child's classmates is HIV-infected, existing case law has not allowed exaggerated public fears of what is a "minimal theoretical risk" to exclude infected children from schools.[60] Similarly, should physicians who treat patients with HIV inform their other patients of this practice? The statistical risk of infection to noninfected patients is minuscule, at most. But, the potential danger—death—is grave. Moreover, some studies show that much of the population wants to know if their physician is treating HIV-infected patients.[61] One survey suggested that only 40 percent of those polled believed that it was "very unlikely" that they could contract the virus through public toilets. Only 27 percent of those surveyed believed that it was very unlikely that they would contract the disease by sharing eating utensils with a person with AIDS.[62] In fact, a prisoner has filed a fear-of-AIDS suit because he had shared "a drinking fountain, toilet, towels, shower stall, bath tub, and phone booth" with two HIV-positive individuals.[63] These examples meet both tests—a grave potential danger and a significant portion of the population desires disclosure. Yet, would it be sensible to designate these situations as material risks according to the traditional reasonable-person standard? It is much more likely that the dispassionate reasonable person would weigh the probability of the risks and conclude that they do not warrant disclosure or regulation.

A NEW TREND?

Despite the arguments that the risk of infection from an HIV-positive physician does not constitute a material risk under existing informed-consent theory, it appears that courts may be moving in a different direction. At least one court has already followed the lead of *Faya*'s reasoning. In a California case, *Kerins* v. *Hartley*, a patient specifically asked her surgeon if he was infected with HIV. He assured her that he was not, and the woman consented to surgery. She later learned, through a news report, that the surgeon was already suffering from AIDS. Although she ultimately tested negative for the virus, she sued the physician's estate and the members of his group practice for the fear and anxiety she had suffered. The trial court granted summary judgment for the defendants. But the California Court of Appeals, relying heavily on *Faya*, reversed the trial court's ruling, and allowed the case to proceed to trial. As in *Faya*, the *Kerins* court held that the woman could attempt to recover damages for the "window of anxiety" from her discovery of her physician's ailment to her virtually conclusive, negative HIV tests.[64] And, in a similar case, a trial jury has awarded damages to a Jehovah's Witness patient who received a blood transfusion against his wishes. The patient complained of "AIDS phobia," even though no evidence existed that the blood had been infected with HIV.[65]

  Behringer v. *The Medical Center at Princeton* addressed an intrinsically related aspect of the informed consent and HIV-infected physician issue.[66] In it, a medical center suspended the surgical privileges of a plastic surgeon who was suffering from AIDS-related pneumonia. In addition, the hospital required that all HIV-infected surgeons inform their patients of their affliction. The plastic surgeon sued the medical center, contesting the restrictions that the hospital's requirement placed on his practice. Accepting evidence that estimated the danger of surgeon-to-patient transmission at about 1-in-130,000, the *Behringer* court concluded "that the risk of accident and implications thereof would be a legitimate concern to the surgical patient, warranting disclosure of this risk in the informed-consent setting."[67] The *Behringer* majority appeared to abandon entirely the traditional reliance on the reasonable person standard in evaluating the materiality of risks in HIV cases. In the *Behringer* court's words:

> If there is to be an ultimate arbiter of whether the patient is to be treated invasively by an AIDS-positive [*sic*] surgeon, the arbiter will be the fully informed patient. The ultimate risk to the patient is so absolute—so devastating—that it is untenable to argue against informed consent combined with a restriction on procedures which present "any risk" to the patient. . . .[68]

As a result, the court ruled that the hospital was justified in placing the restrictions on the surgeon's practice. This holding grants institutions broad authority to require informed consent of physicians who practice within their walls.

Behringer, unlike *Faya* and *Kerins*, merely upheld institutional informed consent requirements demanded by the institution. It did not consider whether the consent provided to a particular patient was sufficient or whether the patient could recover tort damages. However, the discussions are clearly interchangeable. The plaintiff's attorneys in *Faya* relied heavily on the *Behringer* court's discussion of the nature and requirements of informed consent,[69] and the *Faya* court implicitly accepted it. At the same time, other types of fear-of-HIV-infection suits are surfacing at an increasing rate.[70] For example, a Tennessee court of appeals ruled that a woman could sue a hospital for fear and anxiety, despite repeatedly testing negative for HIV during the three years after she stuck herself with a used hypodermic needle.[71] Similarly, a federal circuit court upheld a $150,000 damage award for fear and anxiety to a nurse who pricked herself with a defective needle while treating an AIDS patient. She, too, had repeatedly tested HIV-negative.[72]

Cases like *Faya*, *Kerins*, and *Behringer* may mark a significant transition in the history of informed-consent doctrine. Before the benchmark case of *Canterbury* v. *Spence*, physicians principally decided what risks were to be shared with patients during the informed consent process.[73] After *Canterbury*, jurisdictions began to require that physicians disclose all risks that would be considered material by a "reasonable" person. This standard, though patient-centered, was objective, and some risks were considered immaterial merely because they were highly unlikely to occur. Recent holdings, though, appear to require disclosure of, in the words of *Behringer*, "any risk to the patient," regardless of its unlikelihood.[74] In addition, the suggestion that the individual patient is to be the "ultimate arbiter" of what risks are material undercuts the reasonable-person standard and may allow informed consent doctrine to drift into subjective unpredictability. If this is the meaning of *Faya* and *Behringer*, it signals a new phase in informed consent development.[75] The trend, if it continues, may be at the cost of the traditional reasonable person/material risk test, and at the expense of the careers of HIV-infected physicians whose conditions appear to present virtually no danger to their patients.

As a nation, and as individuals, we are intuitively drawn toward procedures and processes that most obviously embody democratic ideals and individual rights. Medical commentators and practitioners have placed an increasing and welcome emphasis on the value of patient autonomy and self-determination. Relying on public opinion to construct the reasonable person and on juries to decide the factual issues related to informed consent appear to be consistent with these tendencies. However, while an erosion of the objective basis of the traditional reasonable person standard may be more democratic and arguably more patient-centered, the approach is neither rational, predictable, nor fair. It implies that all risks, regardless of their probability, require disclosure. In medical care, one finds hundreds of treatment-related risks with higher probabilities than HIV transmission. The disclosure of these countless, mind-numbing risks arguably would undermine the effectiveness of the consent process itself by obscuring genuine potential dangers in a cascade of highly unlikely possibilities. On the other hand, if universal disclosure of all risks is impractical, then we provide little guidance, either for physicians or for courts, as to when extraordinarily low risks warrant disclosure. Any severe risk, no matter how unlikely, can become "material" to the victim after it occurs. It will then be left subjectively to juries to decide, with virtually no consistent guide, which unlucky patients to award and which unlucky patients to ignore. The reasonable-person/material-risk standard provides both an objective guide to juries and an occasional judicial check on inflamed passions and sympathies when an extremely unlucky patient suffers a highly unexpected injury.

FAYA, BEHRINGER, AND FEDERAL CIVIL RIGHTS LEGISLATION

The *Faya, Kerins,* and *Behringer* line of cases appear to conflict with the spirit of federal civil rights legislation. The Rehabilitation Act of 1973[76] and the 1990 Americans with Disabilities Act (ADA)[77] protect persons with disabilities, and those "perceived" as disabled, including individuals infected with HIV, from discrimination. Federal case law interpreting these statutes typically has protected individuals with disabilities from the irrational fears of those around them. For example, the United States Supreme Court, in *School Board of Nassau County* v. *Arline*, ruled that a tuberculosis-infected, yet noncontagious, teacher could not be discharged from her post, despite the school board's and the parents' widespread, albeit irrational, fear of her condition.[78] Similarly, in *Chalk* v. *United States District Court*, a federal circuit court held that a school must rehire a dismissed HIV-infected teacher.[79] Neither the ADA nor the Rehabilitation Act requires that institutions, hospitals, and employers ignore risks to their clients, patients, and customers. Instead, if the disabled (infected) individual poses a "significant risk" or a "direct threat" to others in the workplace, he or she is not "otherwise qualified" for the position and not entitled to the protection of the statute. The ADA defines "direct threat" as the "high probability, of substantial harm, a speculative or remote risk is insufficient."[80] Therefore, many observers have argued convincingly that institutional practice restrictions based on the remote risk posed by the HIV-infected physicians violate the protections afforded by the Rehabilitation Act and the ADA.[81]

Health-care institutions, under the rationale of *Faya, Kerins,* and *Behringer*, may be liable if they allow their patients to be subjected to "any risk" of infection at the hands of an HIV-infected physician. Yet, prevailing interpretations of civil rights law appear to put the institutions in a double-bind by refusing to allow them to restrict the practices of infected health-care workers unless they pose a "significant risk" or a "direct threat." They may not dismiss or significantly limit the activities of the physician without risking a discrimination suit, but they may be liable for damages, even in the absence of seroconversion, if they do not. And, in the present climate, it seems clear that a requirement that HIV-infected physicians inform their patients of their status would be tantamount to ending their practice.

Article VI of the United States Constitution holds that federal statutes are the supreme law of the land and, in some instances, may preempt conflicting state law. Despite the seeming conflict between federal civil rights law and developing state tort law represented by *Faya* and *Behringer*, it is unlikely that preemption will solve the dilemma facing health-care institutions and HIV-infected health workers. Neither the ADA nor any other civil rights legislation specifically preempts any state tort law actions. And courts have outlined a legal presumption against implied federal preemption of state law, especially in issues of health and safety or where no parallel federal remedy exists.[82] Moreover, the Supreme Court has held that preemption is generally only legitimate when the state law and "the object sought to be obtained by the federal law and the character of the obligations imposed by it . . . reveal the same purpose."[83] Clearly, federal civil rights legislation and state tort actions for failure of informed consent regulate different interests, involve different parties, and provide different remedies.

However, implied preemption may sometimes be appropriate "when it is impossible to comply with both state and federal law . . . or where the state law stands as an obstacle to the accomplishment of the full purposes and objectives of Congress."[84] This approach to the preemption argument appears, on the surface, the most convincing. One might structure an argument which alleges that health institutions' fear of liability would encourage them to limit HIV-infected physicians' activity, despite the fact that such policies might violate federal discrimination law. Affected physicians would then be forced to litigate challenges to the wide array of potential HIV policies on an institution-by-institution and policy-by-policy basis. Instead of voluntary compliance by the nation's hospitals, fear of tort liability might encourage massive resistance to the ADA and endless litigation.

It is not clear, however, that compliance with both state and federal law is always impossible. The issues of informed consent and "AIDS-phobia" are currently being decided on a case-by-case basis, with no guarantee how any particular suit will be resolved. Similarly, civil rights requirements on employers under the Rehabilitation Act and the ADA are very much case- and fact-specific. It may be difficult to determine in advance which policies will meet the scrutiny of civil rights laws and which policies will yield state tort damages. Consequently, one could reasonably argue that it is not necessarily impossible to comply with both state and federal laws, and that these doctrines do not justify implied preemption. The argument against preemption seems especially strong in light of several cases that have upheld limitations placed on HIV-infected health workers. For example, in *Leckelt v. Board of Commissioners of Hospital District I*, a federal court allowed a hospital to require the HIV test results of a health-care worker. The court reasoned that patient welfare superseded the confidentiality and civil rights of the individual.[85] Similarly, a federal circuit court recently ruled that a hospital did not violate the Rehabilitation Act when the hospital transferred a surgical technician after discovering that he was infected with HIV.[86] Given these rulings, it is not foreordained that state tort law will be universally incompatible with federal civil rights law.

The rulings also demonstrate why civil rights requirements sometimes may be difficult to use as a general defense to a state tort action based on informed consent and fear of AIDS. Suppose, for example, that a hospital imposed no restrictions on its HIV-infected physicians, believing, without a specific court finding, that federal civil rights law required this policy. If the hospital was sued by patients who had been treated by an HIV-infected physician, it may not be able to claim the civil rights laws as a defense, because it had not received a ruling outlining what safeguards or policies were allowable for that physician. On the other hand, if the hospital had been required by a court to employ the physician without restrictions on his practice, it may be able to claim the common law defense of "justification" based on the court order.

IMPACT

While the initial legal impact of *Faya* and *Kerins* may be negligible, the rulings cast a very long shadow. If similar cases proceed to trial and juries find the physicians and their institutions negligent (which seems possible given public opinion), damage awards may often be quite small. The appellate court ruling only allowed Faya and Rossi to recover for the emotional distress they suffered from the time that they learned of Almaraz's HIV status until their discovery that they were not infected by the virus, perhaps four days later. However, if patients discover a physician's HIV status soon after treatment, they may be able to claim fear and anxiety damages for a lengthier portion of the so-called window of anxiety period. Under current standards, this could mean a period of up to six months—the time it takes to rule out HIV infection. These cases could yield much higher damage awards. Recall that one fear-of-infection case has already yielded $150,000 in damages. In addition, in the event that juries are allowed to assess punitive damages, total judgments could be significantly higher.

It is uncertain whether courts in other jurisdictions will follow the lead of the *Faya* and the *Kerins* opinions, but, given *Behringer*, related precedents, and the current level of public fear and understanding, it is not unlikely. Different jurisdictions have varying bodies of case law and statutes both on the duty to inform and on the fear-as-injury issues, and it is too soon to predict the course of future litigation. These cases are not indefensible. Defense attorneys may be able to keep these suits out of the hands of juries if they can focus courts' attention on the idealized "reasonable person" portion of the material risk requirement and on the statistically remote nature of the risk. Defense attorneys might also argue that, as a policy matter, it would be unreasonable to require the disclosure of all medical risks as remote as those posed by HIV-infected physicians. Finally, by scrupulously limiting damages to the "window of anxiety" between when the patients learned of their practitioners' condition and when they tested negative for the virus, defense attorneys may make future cases financially unattractive to plaintiffs' attorneys.[87]

Common law sometimes gauges the reasonableness of risk with a form of cost-benefit analysis. Requiring informed consent of HIV-infected physicians fails to meet this standard, too. According to *Restatements, Second, Torts*, § 291, a risk is unreasonable if it is of such magnitude as to outweigh the "utility of [an] act or of the particular manner in which it is done."[88] Applied to informed consent, the doctrine would require that physicians and patients exchange information and risks until the cost of further exchange of information would be greater than the benefit of the information.[89] Many writers have argued that the costs of screening, monitoring, and regulating physicians for HIV infections would far outweigh the benefits of such a policy.[90] However, the Behringer court already appears to have considered and rejected one form of cost-benefit analysis related to informed consent. Other courts may be similarly hesitant to apply cost-benefit analysis to the notion of reasonableness in the context of informed consent.[91]

Despite these observations, the *Faya* and *Kerins* decisions could have a dramatic and detrimental impact on institutional policies affecting HIV-infected physicians. Some administrators, attorneys, and risk managers undoubtedly will see these rulings as an ominous prelude to scores of potential lawsuits. In a recent case, former patients have sued an Illinois dental school clinic for the fear and mental anguish they suffered after learning that they had been treated by an HIV-infected individual.[92] And, in Minnesota, fifty-six patients have sued a clinic and the estate of a physician who died of AIDS-related complications. The state court of appeals ruled that the patients need to show only that they were in the "zone of danger," and not that they had been infected with HIV, to maintain their suit.[93] Many hospital administrations, it is fair to say, have been hesitant to risk the potential liability associated with the HIV-infected physician.[94] Before *Faya* and *Kerins*, however, it was possible to argue that these liability risks were largely illusory. An enlightened institution, in accord with CDC recommendations, might be willing to grant relatively broad practice freedom to HIV-infected health professionals, knowing that the chances of patient infection are minuscule. If the chance of infection is remote, they may reason, so, too, is the chance of liability. *Faya* dramatically undermines this reasonable justification for liberal policies regarding HIV-infected practitioners. Not only does *Faya* hold that a legal duty to inform of an infinitesimal possibility of injury may exist, but it also allows for the recovery of monetary damages even if that injury never materializes.

Consequently, institutions in jurisdictions that accept the *Faya* rationale must now concern themselves not only with those patients who contract HIV from physicians, but also with all patients who were treated by an HIV-infected health practitioner. Cases of potential injury damages and legal costs clearly will yield smaller awards than cases of actual infection, but the former will not be Inconsequential. In *Faya*, both patients had no contact with Dr. Almaraz for a period of one to two years, and each was only allowed to recover damages for the fear and anxiety they suffered over a few days, a comparatively modest amount of money. However, as noted earlier, if patients discover their physicians' HIV infection before the long incubation period has elapsed, defendants may find themselves faced with damage claims for fear, anxiety, and emotional distress stretching over several months. Finally, because the issue of materiality no longer appears precluded by even extraordinarily low statistical probabilities of occurrence, we have no way to distinguish the informed consent duties of HIV-infected physicians who do not perform invasive procedures from HIV-infected surgeons who do.

Even if damages on cases of HIV-infection fear are relatively modest, the potential number of suits will magnify their impact. Defendant institutions will have to contend with all patients treated by HIV-infected practitioners, not merely those few patients (none have been identified to date) who actually contract HIV from physicians. Almaraz, for example, treated over 1,800 individuals while at Johns Hopkins, many of whom are now potential plaintiffs. The legal and public relations cost of defending these suits alone may encourage medical institutions to take more drastic measures to ensure that HIV-infected health-care workers do not perform certain procedures on patients.

CONCLUSION

The battle over informed consent and HIV-infected physicians may ultimately be played out in other arenas. At least one court, *Behringer*, has allowed health-care institutions to bar HIV-infected physicians from surgery in the absence of informed consent from potential patients. *Leckelt* allowed a hospital to demand the HIV test results of an employee, and other rulings and statutes allow hospitals to disclose a physician's HIV status to colleagues and patients if the institution can demonstrate a "compelling need" to do so.[95] If institutions are allowed to place limits on the practice of HIV-infected physicians, they may successfully limit their and the physicians' liability. However, the extent and nature of the restrictions on the practice of infected health-care workers will continue to be tested against the equal protection clause of the Fourteenth Amendment, the Rehabilitation Act, and the ADA. While the equal protection clause may provide only limited protection against such practice restrictions,[96] federal civil rights legislation may circumscribe in a real way the number and type of limitations institutions may place on HIV-infected physicians.[97] The institutional desire to impose those restrictions, though, will be driven in part by the perception of potential liability, which in turn will depend on patients' abilities to collect damages for treatment by infected physicians who do not inform patients of their condition.

It is worth discussing whether HIV-infected physicians have an ethical, as opposed to a legal, duty to inform their patients of their status, but that is not what AIDS-phobia suits are about. Instead, the central question in fear-of-AIDS cases is whether a patient can collect damages when a physician fails to provide that information. Although powerful arguments can be made to the contrary,[98] an extralegal, ethical duty to inform patients of one's HIV status can be made. As noted earlier, the AMA once (but no longer) recommended that HIV-infected physicians either refrain from exposure-prone practices or obtain informed consent from their patients. Some commentators, discussing informed-consent theory in the abstract, argue that physicians' fiduciary relationship with their patients demands that they subject their patients to no risk, no matter how insignificant, without consent, or suggest that physicians have an ethical duty to disclose the information subjectively desired by the particular patient rather than only that information deemed objectively material by the hypothetical reasonable person.[99] I am not convinced that these arguments apply fully to HIV-infected health-care workers. But, even if an ethical duty to inform does exist, and we have no consensus for such a position, it does not establish a legal mandate to inform patients of risks that are objectively immaterial and unreasonable, and that threaten to end unnecessarily and unfairly HIV-infected physicians' ability to practice medicine.

The author thanks Nancy M. P. King, Loretta Kopelman, John Moskop, Timothy F. Murphy, Todd L. Savitt, and Mark E. Steiner, all of whom read earlier versions of this manuscript and contributed helpful editorial and intellectual suggestions. In addition, the manuscript benefited from the insights provided by the journal's two reviewers.

REFERENCES

1. *Faya v. Almaraz*, 620 A.2d 327 (Md. 1993).

2. Appellees' Brief, *Faya v. Almaraz*, 3.

3. Appellants' Brief, *Faya v. Almaraz*, 5.

4. Appellees' Brief, *Faya v. Almaraz*, 4.

5. For an excellent summary of these common law actions and their application to HIV-related cases, see Hermann DHJ, Burris S, "Torts: private lawsuits about HIV," in: Burris S, Dalton HL, Miller JL (eds.), *AIDS Law Today: A New Guide for the Public* (New Haven, CT: Yale University Press; 1993): 334–365.

6. *Faya v. Almaraz*, 330.

7. Ibid.

8. Ibid., 334.

9. Ibid., 330-331.

10. Appellants' Brief, *Faya v. Almaraz*, 34.

11. *Faya v. Almaraz*, 330.

12. Ibid., 333.

13. *Moran v. Faberge*, 332 A.2d 11, 273 Md. 538 (1975).

14. *Faya v. Almaraz*, 333.

15. Ibid., 334, n. 6.

16. Ibid., 333.

17. 747 F. Supp. 285 (E.D. Pa. 1990).

18. Ibid., 287.

19. *Funeral Services by Gregory, Inc. v. Bluefield Community Hospital*, 413 S.E.2d 79, 186 WVa. 424 (1991).

20. For example, *Doe v. Doe*, 136 Misc.2d 1015, 519 N.YS.2d 595 (Supp. 1987) (recovery denied for "AIDS-phobia" based on husband's homosexual affair, where both spouses tested negative for HIV); and *Hare v. State*, 173 A.D.2d 535, 570 N.YS.2d 125 (2 Dept. 1991) (where an employee, bitten by inmate, failed to test positive for HIV and failed to prove that the inmate was HIV-infected).

21. See Maroulis JC, "Can HIV-negative plaintiffs recover emotional distress damages for

their fear of AIDS?" *Fordham Law Review*, 1993;62:235, for a comprehensive survey and discussion of fear-of-AIDS precedents.

22. Appellees' Brief, *Faya v. Almaraz*, 6.

23. 1992 WL 276717 (Tenn. App. 1992).

24. *Faya v. Almaraz*, 337.

25. Ibid., 338–389. The *Faya* court also limited recoverable emotional damages, as do most courts, to the extent that the plaintiffs can "objectively demonstrate their existence" by physical symptoms (that is, sleeplessness, loss of appetite, depression, and so forth).

26. Ibid., 337.

27. Ibid.

28. Because intentional acts typically are excluded from coverage under medical liability insurance contracts, it is likely that plaintiffs' attorneys will plead cases under a negligence theory where possible.

29. 379 A.2d 1014 at 1020, 281 Md. 432 at 439 (1977).

30. *Canterbury v. Spence*, 464 F.2d 772, 150 A.DC 263 (1972). See Faden RR, Beauchamp TL, King NMP, *A History and Theory of Informed Consent* (New York, NY: Oxford University Press; 1986): 33–34ff., 135–137ff., for the best discussion of the theoretical and historical development of the *Canterbury* decision.

31. Pegalis SE, Wachsman HF, *American Law of Medical Malpractice*, 2d ed., vol. 1 (New York, NY: CBC, 1992): 193–202ff.

32. *Harnish v. Children's Hospital Medical Center*, 439 N.E.2d 240, 387 Mass. 152 at 156.

33. See, for example, Douthwaite G, *Jury Instructions on Medical Issues*, 4th ed. (Charlottesville, VA: Michie Co.; 1992): 319–322.

34. *Kissinger v. Lofgren*, 836 F.2d 678 (1st Cit. Mass. 1988).

35. *Precourt v. Frederick*, 481 N.E.2d 1144 at 114 (1985).

36. Gostin LO, "HIV-infected physicians and the practice of seriously invasive procedures," *Hastings Center Report*, 1989;19(1):33.

37. *Henderson v. Milobsky*, 595 F.2d 654 (D.C. Cit. 1978).

38. *Ruffer v. St. Francis Cabrini Hospital*, 7 P.2d 1288, 56 Wash. App. 625 (1990).

39. Daniels N, "HIV-infected health care professionals: public threat of public sacrifice," *Milbank Quarterly*, 1992;7(1):17.

40. This issue has been discussed most ably in Gostin, n. 36; Daniels, n. 39; Glantz LH, Mariner WK, Annas G, "Risky business: setting public health policy for HIV-infected health care professionals," *Milbank Quarterly*, 1992;70(1):43–79; Lunde JK, "Informed consent and the HIV-positive physician," *Medical Trial Quarterly*, 1991;38:186.

41. For example, see Breo DL, "The dental AIDS cases—murder or an unsolvable mystery?" *JAMA*, 1993;270:2732–2734; Barr S, "What if the dentist didn't do it?" *New York Times*, April 16, 1994: A11.

42. For example, Mishu B, Schaffnre W. Horan JM, Wood LH, Hutcheson RH, McNabb PC, "A surgeon with AIDS: lack of evidence of transmission to patients," *JAMA*, 1990;264:467–470; Danila RN, MacDonald KL, Rhame FS, et al., "A look-back investigation of patients of an HIV-infected physician," *New England Journal of Medicine*, 1991;325:1406–1411; Dickinson GM, Morhart RE, Klimas NG, Bandea CI, Laracuente JM, Bisno AL, "Absence of HIV transmission from an infected dentist to his patients: an epidemiologic and DNA sequence analysis," *JAMA*, 1993;269:1802–1806; von Reyn CF, Gilbert TT, Shaw FE, Parsonnet KC, Abramson JE, Smith MG, "Absence of HIV transmission from an infected orthopedic surgeon: a 13-year look back study," *JAMA*, 1993;269:1807–1811; Armstrong FP, Miner JC, Wolfe

WH, "Investigations of a health care worker with symptomatic human immunodeficiency virus infection: an epidemiological approach," *Military Medicine*, 1987;152:414–418; Porter JD, Cruickshank JG, Gentle PH, Robinson RG, Gill ON, "Management of patients treated by a surgeon with HIV infection," *Lancet*, 1990;335:113–114.

43. Rogers AS, Froggart JW, Townsend T, et al., "Investigation of potential HIV transmission to the patients of an HIV-infected surgeon," *JAMA*, 1993;269:1795–1801.

44. Leary WE, "Mandatory AIDS tests for doctors opposed," *New York Times*, July 31, 1992: A11.

45. CDC, "Update: investigations of persons treated by HIV-infected health care workers—United States," *MMWR*, 1993;42(17):329–331.

46. These figures are drawn from Daniels, n. 39, p. 13. Daniels's discussion of the statistical risks of physicianto-patient transmission is especially cogent and helpful (see pp. 11–17).

47. Appellants' Brief, *Faya v. Almaraz*, 14.

48. 592 A.2d 1251 (N.J. Super L. 1991).

49. Appellants' Brief, *Faya v. Almaraz*, 18.

50. *Faya v. Almaraz*, 333.

51. In those jurisdictions that adhere to the professional standard of disclosure in informed consent, plaintiffs must produce expert testimony to demonstrate that prevailing practice provided patients with information regarding the treating physician's HIV status. It is unclear how much weight an individual expert would place on the AMA recommendations.

52. Appellees' Brief, *Faya v. Almaraz*, 37.

53. Daniels N, "HIV-infected professionals, patient rights, and the 'switching dilemma,'" *JAMA*, 1992;267:1368–1371.

54. Blendon RJ, Donelan K, "Discrimination against people with AIDS," *New England Journal of Medicine*, 1988;319:1022–1026; Gerbert B, Maguire BT, Hulley SB, Coates TJ, "Physicians and acquired immune deficiency syndrome: what patients think about human immunodeficiency in medical practice," *JAMA*, 1989;262:1969–1972.

55. Daniels, n. 53.

56. Strausberg GI, Getz RD, "Health care workers with AIDS: duties, rights, and potential tort liability," *University of Baltimore Law Review*, 1993;21:302.

57. Keeton WP, Dobbs DB, Keeton RE, Owen DG, *Prosser and Keeton on the Law of Torts*, 5th ed. (St Paul, MN: West, 1984): 175.

58. *Restatements, Second, Torts*, § 293 (1965), Reporters statement (c).

59. Faden, Beauchamp, and King, n. 30, p. 46.

60. Glantz, Mariner, and Annas, n. 40, p. 61.

61. Gerbert, Maguire, Hulley, and Coates, n. 54.

62. CDC, "HIV epidemic and AIDS: trends in knowledge, United States, 1987, 1988," *MMWR*, 1989;38(20):353–358.

63. Maroulis, n. 21, p. 227 (trial judge agreed that fear was unfounded and granted the defendants motion for summary judgment).

64. *Kerins v. Hartley*, 17 Cal. App. 4th 713 (1993).

65. "Suit over AIDS fear, religious beliefs," *Medical Malpractice: Law & Strategy*, 1994;11(4):1; "Jehovah's Witness wins $500,000 on blood claim," *Medical Malpractice: Law & Strategy*, 1994;11(5):3.

66. 592 A.2d 1251 (N.J. Super L. 1991).

67. Ibid., 1280.

68. Ibid., 1283.

69. Appellants' Brief, n. 3, 17–21.

70. Maroulis, n. 21.

71. *Carroll* v. *Sisters of Saint Francis Health Services, Inc.*, 1992 WL 276717 (Tenn. App. 1992).

72. Hermann DHJ, "AIDS update: fear of infection," *Medical Malpractice: Law & Strategy*, 1992;10(1): 7.

73. See Faden, Beauchamp, and King, n. 30, pp. 114–150, especially pp. 132–137.

74. Gostin has discussed how courts in analogous circumstances have similarly misunderstood the relationship between probability and severity of risk. See Gostin LO, "The Americans with Disabilities Act and the U.S. health care system," *Health Affairs*, 1992;11(fall):255.

75. Spielman B, "Expanding the boundaries of informed consent: disclosing alcoholism and HIV status to patients," *American Journal of Medicine*, 1992;93:216–218.

76. § 504, 29 U.S.C. § 794(a) (1988).

77. 42 U.S.C. § 12101–12213 (1990).

78. 480 U.S. 273 (1987).

79. 840 F.2d 701 (9th Cir. 1988).

80. Glantz, Mariner, and Annas, n. 40, p. 63; Barnes M, Rango NA, Burke GR, Chiarello L, "The HIV-infected health care professional: employment policies and public health," *Law, Medicine & Health Care*, 1990;18(4):311–330.

81. Gostin L, "The HIV-infected health care professional: public policy, discrimination, and patient safety," *Law, Medicine & Health Care*, 1990;18(4):303–310.

82. Preuss CL, "Federal preemption of state tort actions: when and how," *Defense Counsel Journal*, 1990;57:434.

83. *Rice* v. *Santa Fe Elevator Corp.*, 331 U.S. 218, 239 (1947), quoted in ibid., p. 436.

84. Ibid.

85. 909 F.2d 820 (5th Cir. 1990).

86. *Bradley* v. *University of Texas, M.D. Anderson Center*, 3 F3d 999 (5th Cir. 1993).

87. Harrison RW, Thompson KP, "Defending practitioners who are HIV positive," *Medical Malpractice: Law & Strategy*, 1993;10(11):6–7.

88. *Restatements, Second, Torts*, § 291 (1965).

89. Fajfar M, "An economic analysis of informed consent to medical care," *Georgetown Law Journal*, 1992;80:1941.

90. Daniels, n. 53.

91. *Behringer* v. *The Medical Center at Princeton*, 592 A.2d, 1281–1282.

92. *Doe* v. *Northwestern University*, No. 92-8847, July 13, 1993.

93. "AIDS review asked," *National Law Journal*, January 31, 1994: 6.

94. Lumsdon K, "HIV-positive health care workers pose legal safety challenges for hospitals," *Hospitals*, 1992;66(18):24–32.

95. "In test of AIDS law, Pa. OK's disclosure," *Medical Malpractice: Law & Strategy*, 1993;11(1):1.

96. Doyle SD, "HIV-positive, equal protection negative," *Georgetown Law Journal*, 1992;81:375.

97. Gostin, n. 74, pp. 248–256.

98. For example, Murphy TF, "Health care workers with HIV and a patient's right to know," in: *Ethics in an Epidemic* (Berkeley, CA: University of California Press; 1994).

99. For example Brody H, "Transparency: informed consent in primary care," *Hastings Center Report*, 1989;19(5):5–9.

23

INFORMAL CAREGIVERS AND THE INTENTION TO HASTED AIDS-RELATED DEATH

Molly Cooke, M.D., Linda Gourlay, M.S.N.,
Linda Collette, M.S., Alicia Boccellari, Ph.D.,
Margaret Chesney, Ph.D., and Susan Folkman, Ph.D.

❦

The administration of medications with the intention of hastening the death of a terminally ill patient, variously termed *physician-assisted suicide, aid in dying,* and *active euthanasia,* has occasioned much public discussion during the last 7 years. However, to our knowledge, no studies document the incidence of intentionally hastened death in individuals with the acquired immunodeficiency syndrome (AIDS) or any other disease, nor are there studies that systematically describe the characteristics of the ill patient, his caregivers, and their relationship that are associated with the decision to hasten death. A number of moral,[1] legal,[2] and practical objections to the administration of aid in dying have been raised, among them are that ill individuals could be pressured or coerced into requesting assistance in dying, that provisions for aid in dying could be exploited by depressed or exhausted caregivers, and that active euthanasia may have deleterious consequences on the ill person's survivors.[3-5] Legislation intended both to restrict and to liberalize the practice has been undertaken in several states. Currently, 43 states and the District of Columbia criminalize assisted suicide.[6] Oregon and California have had ballot initiatives before the voters; Oregon's limited measure passed in November 1994 and has been reviewed in the courts and reaffirmed by the voters.[7-9] A recent editorial[10] points out that policy development

Cooke M, Gourlay L, Collette L, et al. "Informal Caregivers and the Intention to Hasten AIDS-Related Death." *Journal of the American Medical Association.* 1998;158(1):69–75. ©American Medical Asociation. Reprinted by permission.

has been compromised by the lack of information on the actual characteristics of patients, their illnesses, or their caregivers that may lead to aid in dying or the consequences for the caregiver of administering medication to hasten death.

In this article, we describe the circumstances surrounding the deaths of men ill with AIDS whose significant others provided their terminal care. We report the frequency with which narcotic analgesics and/or sedative-hypnotic medications are given to hasten death and analyze the factors, including the nature of the ill partner's illness, the caregiver's psychological status, and the quality of the relationship between the caregiver and his ill partner, that are associated with increases in the use of medications intended to hasten death. Finally, we assess the immediate and short-term effect on caregivers of increases in the use of medications intended to hasten death.

PARTICIPANTS AND METHODS

Participants

To be included in the study, caregiving men had to identify themselves as homosexual, be in a committed relationship and share living quarters with the ill partner, be willing to be tested for human immunodeficiency virus (HIV) antibodies, have no more than 2 symptoms of HIV disease, and not be an injection drug user. The partners of the caregiving men had to have a diagnosis of AIDS, need assistance with at least 2 instrumental tasks of daily living, and be living at home. Subjects were self-selected in that they were recruited through print and electronic media advertisements, as has been reported previously.[11] Subjects were told that the study was intended to elucidate the sources of stress for men caring for their partners ill with AIDS and to understand how caregivers coped with the stresses of caregiving and bereavement. All subject records were identified by code only. Caregivers were assured that any accounts of death would not be individually identifiable.

Two hundred fifty-three caregiving men enrolled in the study. During the course of the study, 156 ill partners died, their bereaved caregivers constituted the study population for the examination of terminal care and hastened death.

Design

The primary study was designed to explore the stresses of caregiving and strategies for coping used by homosexual men caring for partners dying of AIDS. Each caregiving man was interviewed bimonthly for a 2-year period between April 1990 and November 1994. This report is based on data collected in 4 of these face-to-face interviews: (1) at study entry, (2) at the last bimonthly interview before the partner died, which took place in accordance with the consent process that asked participants to notify project staff when their partner died, (3) within 2 weeks following the partner's death, and (4) at a "dying process interview" 3 months after the partner's death using a protocol developed when the study was already under way, in response to issues arising in the interviews. Both the primary study and the dying process interview were reviewed and approved by the Committee on Human Research at the University of California, San Francisco.

Measures

Characteristics of the Ill Partner

The duration of the ill partner's diagnosis of AIDS and the nature of the partner's illness and the circumstances surrounding his death were assessed at study entry; and care needs of the care recipient were assessed at entry and before the ill partner's death by asking whether the ill partner needed assistance with each of 7 daily instrumental tasks. Characteristics of the circumstances surrounding death were assessed at the interview 2 weeks following the ill partner's death.

Characteristics of the Caregiver

A Caregiver Distress Index was administered, composing of assessments of depressive mood,[12] positive and negative affect,[13] state of anxiety,[14] and state of anger.[15] Perceived social support was assessed with the Social Support Questionnaire[16] and coping was assessed with the Ways of Coping Questionnaire.[17] Caregiver burden was assessed with the Caregiver Dislocations Scale.[18] Positive meaning of caregiving was assessed with a 6-item measure.[19] All the above were administered at entry and during the month before the ill partner's death.

Characteristics of the Caregiver–Ill Partner Relationship

Years in relationship and extent of joint finances were assessed at study entry. Couple adjustment was assessed with a modified version of the Dyadic Adjustment Scale[20] at study entry and before the ill partner's death.

Medication Administered to Hasten Death

The caregiver's report in the dying process interview that an increased dose of narcotic analgesic medication and/or sedative hypnotic agent was given with the intention of hastening death was the primary dependent variable. Caregivers were asked to identify up to 2 analgesics and up to 2 sedative hypnotic agents that their ill partners were receiving at the time of death. The caregivers were then asked the following sequence of questions: "Did your partner want you to increase the dosage of (the first analgesic) beyond what was prescribed?" "Did you go ahead and increase the dosage?" occasions in which an increased dosage of medication was administered by someone other than the caregiver were ascertained through a parallel set of questions: "Did your partner want someone other than you or his physician to increase the dosage of (the first analgesic) beyond what was prescribed?" "Did someone, other than you or the patient's physician go ahead and increase the dosage?" "Who administered the increased dose?" The objective of the dose increase, whether administered by the caregiver or someone else, was assessed through 2 questions: "Was the increased dosage given to treat pain?" and "Was the increased dosage given to hasten death?" The response options for each question were no, yes, and unsure. The caregiver could answer yes to both questions, indicating that the increase in the use of medications was administered to control symptoms and to hasten death. We categorized caregivers who indicated that the use of medication was increased to hasten death and that they themselves had administered the medication as personally providing aid in dying regardless of their answer to the symptom control question.

Caregiver Comfort With Dosage Increases

The impact on the caregiver of administering an increased medication dosage before the ill partner's death was addressed in 3 questions with Likert scaled responses asked during the dying process interview: "How did you feel about administering an increased dose before you actually did it?" "How did you feel afterward?" "How do you feel now?" Possible answers were completely comfortable, somewhat uncomfortable, quite uncomfortable, and extremely uncomfortable.

Statistical Analysis

Between-group differences among the means of continuousdependent variables were examined with analysis of variance. The Pearson χ^2 nonparametric test was used when the dependent variable was categorical. The intervals between interviews varied among subjects. Therefore, time was covaried using random effects analysis of covariance for in-between group analyses, and random effects analysis of covariance with repeated measures for within-subjects analyses. These analyses were performed with the BMDP-5V[21] program for random coefficient growth curve models with variable random effect design matrixes among subjects.

Of the 156 caregivers whose partner died during the 2-year assessment period, 140 (89.7%) completed the dying process interview that provided the data about use of medications at the time of the ill partner's death. The analyses reported herein are based on the reports of these 140 bereaved caregivers.

RESULTS

Demographics

The mean age of caregivers was 38.9 years and that of ill partners was 38.8 years. Ninety percent of both caregivers and ill partners were white. Caregivers had a median education level of some college. Approximately one-third of the caregivers were seropositive for HIV. The median duration of the relationship between caregivers and their ill partners was 7.1 years. The ill partners had had a formal diagnosis of AIDS for approximately 2 years.

Decisions Regarding Terminal Care

Among the 140 bereaved caregivers who completed the dying process interview, 122 (87.5%) reported their partners had set limits on the medical treatments they would accept for their illness. The discussion about treatment limitations was initiated by the ill partner in 63% of the cases, by the caregiver in 17% of the cases, and by the partner's physician in only 11% of the cases. The caregivers were supportive of the decision to limit treatment; 83% agreed "completely," 11% agreed "quite a bit," and 6% agreed "somewhat." Sixty-two percent of the men died in their own homes; other sites of death were the hospital (25%), inpatient hospice (11%), and other (2%). Most ill partners (76%) had not wanted to be hospitalized for terminal care.

Caregivers Reporting Increased Use of Medications

Sixty-seven bereaved caregivers, (47.8%) reported that their partner had received a dosage of medication that had been increased beyond the prescribed amount. In general, this medication was a schedule II narcotic analgesic (65%), morphine sulfate being the most common example. The second most frequently used drug group was the benzodi-azepine agents (29%). Caregivers were not systematically asked to report the dosages used. The 67 caregivers who reported dosage increases did not differ from those who did not in age, employment status, income, ethnicity, HIV serostatus, religion, number of years in the relationship, and time since the ill partner's diagnosis of AIDS.

Characteristics of the Ill Partner Associated with Increased Use of Medications

Ill partners who received an increase in the use of medications beyond the prescribed amount did not differ from ill partners who did not in any of the demographic variables, disease or treatment preference characteristics, or time since a formal diagnosis of AIDS.

Objective of Increases in the Use of Medications

In 55 (82.1%) of 67 cases, the increased doses of medications were given by the care-giver himself. In 42 (62.7%) of the 67 cases, the objective of the increase in the use of medications was solely to control symptoms; however, in 17 (25.4%) of the 67 cases, increases in the use of medications were intended in part or exclusively to hasten death. In 8 cases (11.9%) the caregiver was unsure of the objective; 5 of these deaths occurred in the hospital or hospice and the caregiver may simply not have known the reason for the increase in the use of medication. Most caregivers discussed the plan to increase use of medications with the patient's physician; a similar proportion of caregivers intending to hasten death (75%) and those attempting to control symptoms alone (67%) discussed the medication increase with the physician. Of the 17 caregivers who reported increases in the use of medications intended at least in part to hasten death, 14 (82.3%) reported that they had administered the increased dosage themselves. These 14 individuals represent 10% of all bereaved caregivers who provided data about increases in the use of medications.

The site of death was specified in the caregiver's narrative for 61 ill partners. Five (21%) of the 21 caregivers whose partners died at a hospice or in the hospital were unsure of the purpose of preterminal increases in the use of medications compared with 3 (8%) of the 38 whose partners died at home. This presumably reflects the personal caregiver's greater distance from the decision to increase dosage in institutional settings. Among the 53 caregivers who reported they were sure of the objective of the increase in the use of medications, 1 (13%) of the 8 ill partners who died in a hospice received an increase in use of medications to hasten death compared with 4 (25%) of the 16 ill partners who died in a hospital and 9 (25%) of the 36 who died at home.

Characteristics of Ill Partners Who Received Increases in use of Medications to Hasten Death

Ill partners who received increases in the use of medications to hasten death did not differ from ill partners who received increases in the use of medications solely to control symptoms with respect to preferences in terminal care, the site of death, length of time since a diagnosis of AIDS was made, median number of diagnoses of AIDS, or type of diagnoses of AIDS. The median number of AIDS-related diagnoses was 2 in both groups. As would be expected, the specific diagnoses are hallmarks of advanced disease such as wasting, AIDS dementia, cytomegalovirus infection, and *Mycobacterium avium intracellulare* complex. Specific diagnoses did not distinguish the patients who received medications intended to hasten death and those receiving medications for symptom control. Likewise, the 2 groups were comparable with respect to the need for assistance both at the initial interview (scale score, 8.39 vs. 7.81) and at the interview shortly before death (scale score, 13.73 vs. 12.94).

Only the medication the ill partner received differed among patients receiving

Table 23-1. Caregiver Characteristics Associated with Increases in the Use of Medications Before Death

Characteristics	Initial Interview			Immediately Before Death		
	Symptom Control (n=36)*	Hasten Death (n=14)*	P	Symptom Control (n=36)*	Hasten Death (n=14)*	P
Psychological distress	79.61	77.85	.84	103.56	90.77	.30
Coping						
Active problem solving	8.44	8.77	.80	9.58	10.15	.55
Self-blame	1.61	1.31	.37	1.00	1.15	.72
Cognitive escape avoidance	7.14	6.77	.69	8.42	6.92	.31
Distancing	10.50	9.69	.48	10.17	8.62	.30
Positive reappraisal	10.33	10.31	.99	9.53	11.62	.22
Reflective problem solving	7.92	8.00	.93	7.25	8.38	.30
Seeking social support	6.56	9.23	.06	7.78	10.31	.01
Perceived social support	71.14	79.61	.03	70.36	83.00	.004
Caregiving experience						
Caregiver burden	33.14	33.31	.89	45.83	46.54	.92
Positive meaning of caregiving	19.61	21.38	.009	20.67	21.46	.30

*n indicates caregivers who reported they themselves administered increase in the use of medications.

medication for symptom control, those for whom the use of medication was intended to hasten death, and those for whom the caregiver was unsure of the objective of the increased use of medications. Use of benzodiazepine agents was considerably more common among ill partners receiving increases in the use of medications intended to hasten death; 8 (57%) of 14 ill partners who received medications to hasten death were given benzodiazepine agents compared with 7 (17%) of 41 of those given increases in the use of medications to control symptoms and 3 (38%) of 8 for whom the objective of the increase in the use of medications was unknown (P=.01).

Caregivers Who Administered Increased Doses to Hasten Death

Caregivers who administered increased doses of medication at least in part to hasten death differed significantly from those who used medication solely for symptom control in only 3 ways: They reported more positive meaning of caregiving at the initial interview many months before the ill partner's death; at the interview before the ill partner's death they reported seeking more social support; and they reported more perceived social support at study entry and before the partner's death (Table 23-1).

The groups were comparable in their HIV serostatus: 6 caregivers (35%) who administered increases in the use of medications to hasten death were HIV positive, compared with 14 caregivers (33%) using medications solely for symptom control. As would be expected with the progression of the ill partner's disease, all caregivers became significantly more distressed and reported greater caregiver burden between the initial interview and the last interview before the death of the ill partner, but the 2 groups did not differ on these variables at either occasion.

Relationship Characteristics Associated with Increased Dose to Hasten Death

Relationships in which medication had been administered at least in part to hasten death did not differ from those in which medication was administered solely for symptom control in the number of years in the relationship, the extent of joint financing, or the level of couple agreement at the initial interview or at the interview before the ill partner's death (Table 23-2).

Impact of Increase in the Use of Medications on Caregivers Who Administered Increased Doses

At the time of the dying process interview, 11 caregivers (69%) whose ill partners received increased medication dosages to hasten death and 28 caregivers (70%) who increased use of medications solely for symptom control described themselves as having been "somewhat," "quite," or "extremely" uncomfortable with the increases before their administration (Table 23-3). When asked how they were feeling at the

Table 23-2. Quality of Relationship and Increases in the Use of Medication Before Death*

| Relationship | Purpose of Increase in the Use of Medications | | |
	Symptom Control (n=42)	Hasten Death (n=17)	P
Mean duration of relationship, y	6.43	7.74	.09
Shared joint finances, %	79	94	.15
Mean couple agreement score at initial interview	84.60	83.13	.68
Mean couple agreement score immediately before death	86.26	86.38	.99

*Scores are based on the Likert scale.

Table 23-3. Caregiver Discomfort with Increases in the Use of Medications*

| Time | Reason for Increase in the Use of Medications, No. (%) | | |
	Symptom Control (n=40)	Hasten Death (n=16)	P
Before administration of medication	28 (70)	11(69)	.93
Immediately after administration	22 (55)	8 (50)	.73
At time of interview	11 (28)	3 (19)	.49

*Caregivers who reported they themselves administered increases in the use of medications.

time of the interview, the proportion of caregivers in the 2 groups reporting any discomfort had dropped to 3 (19%) and 11 (28%), respectively.

COMMENT

No previous studies have systematically documented the incidence of hastened death in AIDS or any other illness or characterized the psychological state of the caregivers before the decision to hasten death. This study indicates that increases in the use of medications intended to hasten death are not rare, at least in this sample of men in committed relationships dying of AIDS in San Francisco. Of those caregivers whose ill partners died during the study, 12.1% reported that narcotic or sedative hypnotic medications had been administered to hasten death. The frequency with which medications were administered to hasten death in this study is likely to be an underestimate because caregivers are presumably reticent about disclosing this objective.

The decision to increase the use of medications to hasten death was typically made by the ill partner himself and was carried out by the caregiver, after discussion with the patient's physician. As described by the caregivers in our study, the controversial practice of provision of aid in dying is both more common and more integrated into the long-term caregiving relationship than generally acknowledged. Our hypothesis that increases in the use of medications to hasten death would be more common among patients being cared for at home was not borne out; hospitalized patients were as likely to receive augmented medication doses that were perceived by the caregiver as intended to hasten death. In contrast, administration of increased narcotic and/or sedative hypnotic doses intended to hasten death was uncommon among ill partners receiving residential hospice care; this is consistent with the explicit values of hospice care.[22]

There is no evidence that the decision to increase use of narcotic or sedative-hypnotic medications to hasten death is the result of caregiver's intolerance of the burdens of caregiving; burnout, depression, or anger on the part of the caregiver; or any disturbance in the relationship between the caregiver and his ill partner. To the contrary, the higher scores of the caregivers who ultimately assist in their partners' deaths on the Positive Meaning of Caregiving scale and their comments during the interviews suggest the opposite: that the men who assist their partners in dying are especially committed to caregiving and see caring for their partners as an expression of love.

The potential for guilt, depression, and other deleterious consequences of assisting death among surviving friends and family has led some commentators to regard aid in dying as inadvisable even when both the patient and his or her loved ones request it. Again, we saw no evidence of harmful psychological repercussions in short term follow-up of the caregivers. It has been noted that inability to communicate freely about events preceding death may lead to complicated grieving after euthanasia. Interestingly, we noted an increase in social support immediately before the ill partner's death among caregivers who ultimately assisted their partners in dying. This may reflect a greater openness of communication on the part of caregivers who acknowledge using medications to hasten death and may facilitate the rapid resolution of discomfort we saw after bereavement in the caregivers who provided increases in the use of medications intended to hasten death.

Several limitations to internal validity must be acknowledged. First, the information about increases in the use of medications is based entirely on caregivers' self-report. Caregivers may not accurately represent whether increases in the use of medications were given and what the motivations were. It does not seem likely, however, that caregivers would report an intention to hasten death when, in fact, none existed. In addition, the retrospective nature of the dying process interview raises the possibility of recall bias. The interval between the ill partner's death and the interview was only a few weeks, but it is possible that the caregiver's recollection of his intentions and psychological state was affected by his assessment of the comfort and peace of the ill partner's death. Second, we cannot determine whether the dose augmentation intended to hasten the ill partner's death was likely, in fact, to have done so. However, our purpose was to examine the intention to hasten death, not whether the augmented doses actually produced this effect. Third, we have minimal information on the psychological condition of the ill partner, thus it is possible that depression, fear, inadequate treatment of physical symptoms, or some other attribute of the ill partner led to the decision to hasten death.[21-27] However, we did not see any evidence of this in the caregivers' descriptions of their partners' last days and hours. Fourth, the design of the parent study limits the information available on the exact nature of the physician's involvement. The caregivers report discussion of increase in the use of medications with the ill partner's physician but it is not clear how many practitioners proposed, endorsed, opposed, or simply permitted increases in the use of medications. Fifth, the small number of ill partners who received increased medication doses with the objective of hastening death limits the statistical power of the analyses. It is also possible that multiple comparisons have led to a type I error.

There are also limitations to the generalizability of these results to all individuals with AIDS and to persons with terminal illnesses other than HIV infection. The racial uniformity and high level of education distinguish this population from other communities with a high prevalence of AIDS.

Furthermore, the experience of dying of AIDS in San Francisco may be different than in areas where the gay community is smaller or less vocal and where AIDS predominantly affects drug users and their sexual partners. In a study[28] of physicians caring for people with AIDS in the San Francisco Bay Area, 53% reported that they had at least once acceded to a patient's request for physician-assisted suicide. In most other circumstances in which individuals with terminal illnesses are being cared for at home, the caregivers are women, usually members of the biological family. We do not know if men and women respond differently to caregiving or to the issues of hastened death. It is also noteworthy that one-third of the caregivers have the same disease of which the ill partners were dying from; this resonance undoubtedly affects the experience and possibly the decisions of the caregiver. It is, therefore, not clear that our results will extend to people with other terminal illnesses being cared for at home.

Our study has at least 2 lessons for physicians and other practitioners caring for individuals with HIV and other terminal illnesses. First, the study demonstrates that the care of people dying at home involves not just the conventional physician-patient dyad but also a triad.[29,30] From the vantage point of the bedside, the personal caregiver is a central agent. Physicians must develop skills in collaborating with caregivers, recognizing their importance as the actual agents of care, and recognizing and responding to caregivers as "hidden patients." As long as the interests of the home caregiver and the actual patient are congruent, physicians should be as attentive to their relationship with the home caregiver and as responsive to his or her questions, apprehensions, and needs as to those of the patient.

Second, concern with the issues of assisted suicide and euthanasia were virtually universal in this sample of dying patients and their caregivers. As with other preferences in late medical care,[31] these topics may be ones that worry many patients and their families but that they regard as the physician's responsibility to bring up. Physicians should be prepared to open the discussion. For example, a physician might say, "Many of my patients have asked, when they became extremely ill, if I would ever give a pill or an injection to help them die. Have you ever thought about this?" Initiating a discussion does not in itself create an obligation for the physician; in fact, the clarification of expectations may provide the physician who would never participate in physician-assisted suicide or euthanasia an opportunity to explain his or her legal constraints and moral principles to the patient.

As a corollary, clinicians typically have little appreciation for the dilemmas and, ultimately, the crisis of conscience that may be faced by personal caregivers providing terminal care at home. While some friends, lovers, and family regard the provision of terminal care as their responsibility and their right, others are deeply distressed and should not be expected to function in this role. We need to discover effective and appropriate ways to support these most qualified caregivers in their work.

This small study indicates that we have important misconceptions about the nature of assisted dying and that current policy initiatives, both those intended to liberalize and those intended to restrict the practice, may be misdirected. Despite the focus on physician-assisted suicide in policy discussions, personal caregivers played the central role in the last moments of the ill partners in our study. It did not appear that physicians were entirely uninvolved most of the time, after all, the increased medication dose was discussed with the treating physician. However, at the time of death, the physicians were not at the bedside. The control exerted over management by the personal caregivers has important implications for policy.

Hastened death in our study occurred as an exceptional act in the context of a caring, committed personal relationship, with the input from a distance of the treating physician. It was not a medical act. In contrast to hastened death as it occurred in this study, proposals to legitimize assisted suicide medicalize the act and exert control by regulating the conduct of physicians.[32,33] One class of argument against assisted suicide as public policy as currently envisioned is the profound effect it has on the nature of medicine.[34,35] Are the benefits of public policy sanctioning assisted suicide sufficient to justify the transformation of the role of the physician and the relationship of physicians to gravely ill patients that would follow? The arguments in favor of permitting physician-assisted suicide in some instances include the enhancement of patient autonomy; the minimization of abuses by increased oversight and accountability; decreased instances of failed and protracted suicide attempts; and decreased guilt and distress among friends and family, who would no longer be required to act as the agents. In 17 instances of hastened death, we saw no evidence that any of these concerns was a significant problem. Ill partners desiring increases in the use of medications obtained them. There was no evidence that the decision to act on the request of the ill patient represented anything other than an extreme of loving caregiving; as described by the caregivers, death followed within hours of the administration of medication as it did for caregivers using medication preterminally for symptom control. Finally, the caregivers who increased the use of medications to hasten death did not suffer extraordinary distress consequent to their role as agents. It may be, as suggested by Annas,[7] that the status quo of private, occasional assistance in dying accomplished by persons with loving connections to the patient, with physician input, is optimal public policy.

This work was supported by grants MH4404 5 andMH49985from the National Institutes of Mental Health, Bethesda, Md (Dr. Folkman).

REFERENCES

1. Kass LR. Is there a right to die? *Hastings Center Report.* 1993;23:34–43.

2. Kamisar Y. Are laws against assisted suicide unconstitutional? *Hastings Center Report.* 1993;23:32–41.

3. Campbell CS. "Aid-in-dying" and the taking of human life. *Journal of Medical Ethics.* 1992;18:128–134.

4. Singer PA, Siegler M. Euthanasia: a critique. *New England Journal of Medicine.* 1990;322:1881–1883.

5. Richman J. Sanctioning assisting suicide: impact on family relations. *Issues in Law and Medicine.* 1987;3:53–63.

6. Annas GJ. Physician-assisted suicide: Michigan's temporary solution. *New England Journal of Medicine.* 1993,328:1573–1576.

7. Annas GJ. Death by prescription: the Oregon initiative. *New England Journal of Medicine.* 1994;331:1240–1243.

8. Parachini A. The California humane and dignified death initiative. *Hastings Center Report.* 1989;19(supp.):10–12.

9. Alpers A, Lo B. Physician-assisted suicide in Oregon: a bold experiment. *JAMA.* 1995;274:483–487.

10. Emanuel EJ. Empirical studies on euthanasia and assisted suicide. *Journal of Clinical Ethics.* 1995;6:158–160.

11. Folkman S, Chesney M, Cooke M, Boccellari A, Collette L. Caregiver burden in partners of men with AIDS. *Journal of Consulting and Clinical Psychology.* 1994;62:746–756.

12. Radloff LS. The CES-D: a self-report depression scale for research in the general population. *Applied Psychology Measurement.* 1977;1:385–401.

13. Bradburn NM. *The Structure of Psychological Well-Being.* Chicago, IL: Aldine;1969.

14. Spielberger CD, Gorsuch RL, Lushene RE. *STAI Manual for the State-Trait Anxiety Inventory.* Palo Alto, CA: Consulting Psychologists Press; 1970.

15. Spielberger CD. *State-Trait Anger Expression Inventory.* Lutz, FL: Psychological Assessment Resources Inc; 1988.

16. O'Brien K, Wortman CB, Kessler RC, Joseph JG. Social relations of men at risk for AIDS. *Social Science and Medicine.* 1993:36:161–167.

17. Folliman S, Lazarus RS. *Ways of Coping Questionnaire.* Palo Alto, CA: Consulting Psychologists Press; 1988.

18. Gottlieb BH, Chrisjohn RC. Perceived social support and reactance as mediators of the impact of the dislocations of caregiving on depressed mood. Presented at the Consortium for Research on Stress Processes; May 18–19,1988; Toronto, Ontario.

19. Folkman S, Chesney M, Collette L, Boccellari A, Cooke M. Post-bereavement depressive mood and its prebereavement predictors in HIV+ and HIV- gay men. *Journal of Personality and Social Psychology.* In press.

20. Spanier GB. Measuring dyadic adjustment: new scales for assessing the quality of marriage and similar dyads. *Journal of Marriage and Family.* 1976;38:15–38.

21. Dixon WJ. *BMDP Statistical Software Manual.* Berkeley, CA: University of California Press; 1990:2.

22. Campbell CS, Hare J, Matthews P. Conflicts of conscience: hospice and assisted suicide. *Hastings Center Report.* 1995;25:36–43.

23. Ciesielski-Carlucci C, Kimsma G. The impact of reporting cases of euthanasia in Holland: a patient and family perspective. *Bioethics.* 1994;8:151–158.

24. Brown A Henteleff P, Barakat S, Rowe CJ. Is it normal for terminally ill patients to desire death? *American Journal of Psychiatry.* 1986;143:208–211.

25. Breitbart W. Suicide risk and pain in cancer and AIDS patients. In: Chapman CR. Foley KM (eds.). *Current and Emerging Issues in Cancer Pain.* New York, NY: Raven Press; 1993:49–65.

26. Foley KM. The relationship of pain and symptom management to patent requests for physician-assisted suicide. *Journal of Pain and Symptom Management.* 1991;6:289–297.

27. Block SO, Billings JA. Patient requests to hasten death: evaluation and management in terminal care. *Archives of Internal Medicine.* 1994;154:2039–2047.

28. Slome LR, Mitchell TF, Charlebois E, Benevedes JM, Abrams DI. Physician-assisted suicide and patients with the human immuno deficiency virus. *New England Journal of Medicine.* 1997;336:417–421.

29. Haug MR. Elderly patients, caregivers, and physicians: theory and research on health care triads. *Journal of Health and Social Behavior.* 1994;35:1–12.

30. Johnston D, Stall R, Smith K. Reliance by gay men and intravenous drug users on friends and family for AIDS-related care. *AIDS Care.* 1995;7:307–319.

31. Steinbrook R, Lo B, Moulton J, Siaka G, Hollander H, Volberding PA. Preferences of homosexual men with AIDS for life-sustaining treatment *New England Journal of Medicine.* 1986;314:457–460.

32. Miller FG, Quill TE, Brody H, Fletcher JC, Gostin LO, Meier DE. Regulating physician assisted suicide. *New England Journal of Medicine.* 1994;331:119–123.

33. Benrubi GI. Euthanasia: the need for procedural safeguards. *New England Journal of Medicine.* 1992;326:197–198.

34. Gaylin W, Kass LR, Pellegrino ED, Siegler M. Doctors must not kill. *JAMA.* 1988; 259:2139–2140.

35. Miles SH. Physician-assisted suicide and the profession's gyrocompass. *Hastings Center Report.* 1995;25:17–19.

Part 9

CARING FOR SEVERELY COMPROMISED NEWBORNS

❦

Instincts are a truly amazing part of the human condition. Among many other examples, they allow us to respond instantaneously to dire circumstances or to avoid serious injury even though we had no warning of the danger. Of all our instincts however, there is one above all others for which our response has no limit—protecting our children. Parents will rush into burning buildings, donate their organs, and spend every spare dime they have on their child's education, all without regret or hesitation. With this sense of duty to our children, how could we respond with anything other than dismay and outrage when we hear news stories about parents who refuse to allow life-sustaining treatment for their babies. Just consider the response to the 1982 "Baby Doe" case: New child abuse regulations were quickly disseminated; a toll-free number was established to allow the anonymous reporting of decisions to forgo treatment because of a newborn's actual or potential handicap(s); and special committees were created to investigate these anonymous reports. As a result of their investigations they quickly earned the moniker "god-squad"; it was not a term of endearment.

Even though these responses arose from well-intentioned instincts to protect the most vulnerable members of our society, they unfortunately created an environment that, for the parents of severely compromised newborns, has the potential to be emotionally and legally devastating. The following two articles will show us just how real and devastating this environment can be. The authors do this by recounting the stories of real families who chose to forgo life-sustaining treatment for their newborns.

The family in Susan Pierce's article withheld artificial nutrition; in the article by John Paris and Michael Schreiber, a father took his newborn son off the ventilator himself. The goals of this section are threefold: first, to provide insight into what it is to be the parent of a severely compromised newborn; second, to provide an appreciation as to why these parents respond as they do; and third, to assist health-care providers and ethics committees in addressing the suffering and uncertainty these parents endure.

With regard to the first goal it is important that we acknowledge the obvious: Even the most wonderfully caring parents make bad decisions, say hurtful things, and react poorly in stressful situations. Although this seems obvious, it is not that uncommon for parents to be labeled as "bad parents" because they made a decision, while in the worst of circumstances, that the health-care team did not agree with. Consider what parents are living through as they make these decisions: They are uncertain of who they can trust. They have a minimal understanding of what the diagnostic tests really mean. They are feeling guilty and angry for having such a critically ill baby. They are angry with God (or the world) because they were denied their "perfect baby." They resent their friends and family who have "perfect babies." They feel a complete loss of control (power) as they are little more than voyeurs in a neonatal intensive care unit. They are unsure of how this will affect the rest of their lives. And while contending with all of this, they must decide what is best for their baby. By taking all of this into account, what at first looks like an obviously bad decision made by bad parents, becomes a decision that was made by imperfect parents using imperfect information while struggling through horrific circumstances. Such empathy is at the core of this section's first reading.

In "Neonatal Intensive Care: Decision Making in the Face of Prognostic Uncertainty," Susan Pierce discusses the circumstances surrounding the birth of conjoined newborns whose life expectancy was no more than several days. With this prognosis the parents decided to withhold artificial nutrition, with the physician's agreement. The nursing staff, however, ignored the parents' decision to forgo life-sustaining treatment and fed the twins. In addition, an "anonymous" call was placed to the Child and Family Services Agency, which resulted in the parents losing custody and, along with the physician, being charged with attempted murder. In many ways this predicament was the consequence of a lack of empathy between the parents and the nurses. The author uses this incident to set out a framework (the "engagement model") for health-care providers and ethics committees to use when a newborn's condition is such that the benefits of aggressive treatment are unknown. As the name suggests, this model greatly depends on the establishment of relationships among all the stakeholders—which, of course, can only grow when we understand and connect with each other. Pierce goes on to make clear the importance of ensuring a continuity of information, so that parents do not receive conflicting information between physicians and nurses as well as between the various nursing shifts. After clearly laying out this framework she applies this to the case of the conjoined twins, providing a fuller understanding of how this can be applied in other institutions.

The last article in this section, "Parental Discretion in Refusal of Treatment for

Newborns: A Real but Limited Right," by John Paris and Michael Schreibner, makes clear that the environment has improved little since the time of the previous article. In 1995 Dr. and Mrs. Messenger were about to give birth to an extremely premature baby whose likelihood of survival was described as grim. In response, they requested that life-sustaining treatment be withheld if the baby survived delivery. Once born, their son was immediately intubated and taken to the neonatal intensive care unit. Dr. Messenger requested that the ventilator be withdrawn; however, the neonatologist believed that they should wait and see how the infant responded to the treatment. Dr. and Mrs. Messenger, while alone with their son, withdrew the ventilator themselves; Mrs. Messenger held him as he died. Dr. Messenger was charged with, and later acquitted of, manslaughter. Paris and Schreibner use this case as a starting point for a discussion of the various means that can be used to decide when to forgo life-sustaining treatment from a newborn. The different decision-making schemes include "best interests," "statistical approach," and "wait until near certainty." With these schemes clearly explained, the authors go on to apply them to the case of Dr. and Mrs. Messenger, providing an understanding for ethics committees who wish to adopt these methods as a basis for policy development in their own institutions.

24

NEONATAL INTENSIVE CARE

Decision Making in the Face of Prognostic Uncertainty

Susan Foley Pierce, Ph.D., R.N.

❦

CASE: CONJOINED TWINS

On May 5, 1981, conjoined twins were born to a physician and his wife. The twins were joined below the waist and shared the lower part of their digestive tract and three legs. Studies revealed additional internal anomalies. They suffered from respiratory distress and were not expected to survive more than a few days. A doctor's order, in the chart, written by a nurse and countersigned by the doctor, read: "Do not feed in accordance with parents' wishes." Several nurses disobeyed the order and fed the infants. An anonymous caller informed the Illinois Department of Children and Family Services that the babies were being starved to death and the parents lost custody. After four months of expensive neonatal intensive care and a charge of attempted murder against the parents and the physician (which was dismissed by the Illinois Circuit Court), it was determined that the twins could not survive surgical separation. They were returned to their parents and lived only a few months, during which time they needed twenty-four-hour nursing care.[1]

Although this situation raises many questions about whether life-saving treatment should ever be withheld from critically ill newborns, it also strikes at the very

---

S. Pierce. "Neonatal Intensive Care: Decision Making in the Face of Prognostic Uncertainty." *Nursing Clinics of North America.* 1998;33(2):287–298. Reprinted by permission of W. B. Saunders Company.

heart and nature of nursing and its covenant with society and clients. Why did nurses actively violate the known wishes of competent parents? Is such a violation of competent client/parents' wishes ever morally justified? Under what circumstances? What role should parents play? Would insurers be acting unethically if they refused to pay for experimental, marginally beneficial, expensive treatments? If parents can pay for whatever they want, should they get it?

THE NATURE OF ETHICAL DECISION MAKING

Ethics involves determining what is good, right, and fair. Nurses, particularly neonatal nurses who deal with such vulnerable lives, cannot help but be involved in daily decisions regarding the promotion of good (well-being), choosing the right path, and fairly allocating their time and their scarce resources. Moreover, as Fry[2] points out, ethics involves more than just beliefs or behavior, it also means adopting a mode of inquiry or a way of gathering, processing, and acting upon data. This article suggests a way of processing the moral dilemmas that arise from the unique and delicate role that nurses play in safeguarding the lives of critically ill neonates while supporting and respecting their families.

GUIDES TO ACTION: CODES AND PRINCIPLES

The obligation to safeguard the well-being of clients is grounded clearly in the American Nurses Association Code of Ethics for Nurses.[3] In the first tenet, the universal respect for persons is explicated as "the nurse provides services with respect for the human dignity and the uniqueness of the client." In the third tenet, "the nurse acts to safeguard the client." Moreover, the well-developed bioethical principle of beneficence delineates that, within a special relationship such as nurse-patient relationship, the nurse not only should avoid inflicting harm but also should prevent harm, remove harm, and promote the well-being of the patient.[4]

ASSESSING WELL-BEING

In order to respect the personhood of infants and safeguard their well-being, nurses must address that precise issue: the infant's well-being. What is the life of the infant like? Is it a "good" life in any respect currently or potentially in the future? Addressing the infant's well-being is much more than a mere technical assessment of the likelihood of benefit or improvement through the application of any one specific intervention or treatment. It is a total assessment of the nature of the infant's human experience. Is it, in balance, an experience of well-being?

This assessment of well-being occurs with infants who can be grouped into three separate categories: (1) infants in whom aggressive care would probably be futile; (2)

infants in whom aggressive care would probably result in clear benefit to their overall well-being, and (3) infants in whom the effect of aggressive care is mostly uncertain. Clearly, the assessment of well-being is most difficult in the last category, in instances of uncertainty and novelty, such as the opening situation with the conjoined twins.

Infants are placed in one of these three categories based on scientific and objective data. This use of scientific data, the facts, although integral to decision making, is not singularly adequate to make individual decisions about infants. Decision making, particularly ethical decision making, is a holistic process that involves not only reasoning based on scientific facts and norms but also consideration of the particularistic, contextual, and individual case affected by one's ideals, values, virtues, self-view, and worldview.[5] Nonetheless, as a first step, individual infants can be placed in one of the three categories based primarily on the accumulated scientific evidence for physiologically beneficent outcomes. Although this discussion focuses on those cases of uncertainty or novelty, a word about the first two categories is in order.

Whereas absolute prognostic certainty is elusive, most neonatology practitioners do acknowledge that futility continues to be a reality in neonatal treatment.[6] Even in the face of new technologies and therapeutics that continue to expand the definition of viability and success, cases exist in which all known evidence leads the health team to conclude that aggressive intervention is futile. In these cases of probable futility, in which the "prognosis for meaningful life is extremely poor or hopeless," as early as 1973, Duff and Campbell[7] endorsed the legitimacy of concluding to withhold aggressive treatment. In these cases of probable futility, which is recognized early in the infant's course of treatment (within the first twenty-four hours), it seems most helpful if the health team renders that as the consensus opinion. That is, rather than engage the parents in "What do you want us to do?" it is more appropriate to recommend that aggressive interventions not be pursued and that care focus on providing comfort and dignity for the infant in the time the child does have.

In contrast to futility, cases also exist in which prevailing knowledge and experience indicate excellent chances for beneficial outcomes and a life of pleasure, satisfaction, growth, development, and meaningful interaction. Again, in those cases, the primacy of preserving the infant's well-being favors aggressive intervention and the necessity of recommending such a strategy to the parents (and, potentially, even overruling them if they express a contrary wish). Clearly, this is an instance in which the nurse is morally justified in challenging the wishes of parents if those wishes do not support corrective treatments. However, the dual role of protecting the infant's well-being and supporting and respecting families calls for a dialogue among all agents involved—unlike the nurses in the opening case who covertly, without consultation, violated documented parental wishes.

ASSESSMENT IN THE FACE OF UNCERTAINTY: THE ENGAGEMENT MODEL

The previous discussion places the health professional as dominant in the treatment decision, recommending comfort care for infants in whom aggressive care would most probably be futile and aggressive care for infants when prevailing knowledge and experience indicate excellent chances for beneficial outcomes. We turn our attention to the third category, in which the effect of aggressive care is mostly uncertain. In the face of a mostly uncertain outcome, the engagement model, advocated by Hess,[8] offers a more reasonable approach to decision making than the health professional dominant approach recommended in the first two categories (see Fig. 24-1).

Hess's ethic of engagement stands in contrast both to the ethic of compliance (parents doing what health professionals recommend and prescribe) and to its opposite, an ethic of abdication (health professionals standing aside and abiding by whatever decision parents make). Basically, engagement is a thorough, philosophical description of true joint decision making. It differs from a "good discussion" in that all parties in the engagement are granted equal status and assumed to have equal decision-making capacity, although using differing data sets: health professionals principally use science, clients principally use knowledge of the self. Thus, the ethic of engagement recognizes the moral agency of all involved parties and builds on the inherent superior medical knowledge of the health professional while it defers to competent parents' autonomy, insight, and ultimate moral agency.

The idea of an ethic of engagement was first put forth by Gaddow[9] and represents a turn away from universalism. Universalism is a philosophical approach that takes the stance of detached objectivity—a right and wrong that applies to everyone, regardless of age, gender, ethnicity, or other personal characteristics or circumstances. Rather than the universal, one right answer, engagement suggests that the knowledge of the right thing to do is created in the narrative that evolves from engaging in an open dialogue. Decision options are cocreated by client or parent and the nurse. These decisions are particular and contextual to the individual case and nongeneralizable to even similar other cases. However, this cocreation of decision options is not a turn to relativism (in which no ethical theories or principles bear any weight and each moral judge renders a best decision), rather, it is the effort to work jointly to evolve how this unique case relates to what ethical theories and principles have long defined as "good" and "right" actions. However, these defined theories and principles are not the only source of moral certainty; the nurse and the client enter into a dialogue both to define the good that is mutually sought and to identify the means for best achieving that good. This model of engaging keeps the frontline participants as the actual decision makers, in contrast to a process that might defer recommendations and decisions to an ethics expert, be that a consultant or a committee.

Thus stands the model of engagement. The health professional does not simply "recommend" what to do next, because the health professional knows only the scientific, objective data and not the unique, particular views and capabilities of this infant

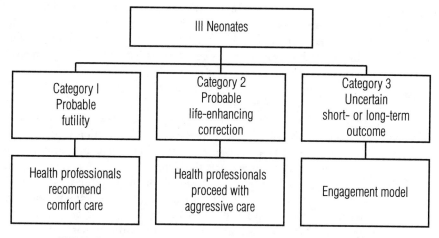

Figure 24-1. Categories of Decision Making in Neonatal Care

and his or her family. Nor is the family left to choose from myriad options that they may comprehend minimally and that may or may not take into consideration their own unique view of the world and their own sense of their infant, themselves, and their material, emotional, and spiritual resources. Rather, engagement is a holistic process of assessment and decision making. Proceeding within an ethic of engagement involves bringing all data, views, and resources of all moral agents to bear on the ongoing decisions that must be made.

These ongoing decisions revolve around the extent of treatment to provide to the critically ill infant with a continuing uncertain short- or long-term prognosis. The principle of respect for the dignity and personhood of the infant necessitates a careful assessment of both the pain and suffering of the infant as well as the potential for pleasure and satisfaction. In this assessment of the infant's well-being, utilitarian considerations, such as the emotional and financial burdens that are placed on the parents and family, do not belong.[10] Rather, assessment of the infant's well-being is a pure assessment of the worth and the goodness of the life to the child. Is the infant's current and potential life good in any respect? What is the potential for a "good life" in the future, again for the infant? Is there any reason to believe that the infant has the potential to experience any pleasure or enjoyment in life, even if it is not up to our standards of a good, quality life?

In order to make treatment decisions, the assessment of actual and potential pain and suffering versus actual and potential pleasure and satisfaction for the infant must be faced by both parents and health professionals. Respect for human dignity indicates that it is not sufficient to assess whether any given therapy has any potential for correcting or improving any given pathologic condition or instability. The overall goal, direction, and ultimate outcome of care always must be paramount in respecting the dignity of human life. Well-being is not static and must be revisited frequently and thoroughly as new treatment decisions are made. Thus, in neonatal nursing, in which a unique role exists in blending infant well-being with parents' rights to decide, the obligation is to engage continually with the parents in the assessment of possibilities and probabilities and to design what is best for this particular child given what we know at a particular point in time.

Hence, continuously involving parents in an ongoing assessment of infant well-being is critical in the ethic of engagement. Parents have important data regarding both the pain and pleasure of their neonates. Additionally, they have the unique ability and obligation to contribute to that pleasure and satisfaction in the future. However, as Mitchell[11] describes, parents of a critically ill neonate must deal with an utterly unexpected outcome of a pregnancy: the birth of a less than perfect child or worse, the imminent death of a new child. Although the neonatal nurse deals with these issues daily, for each parent this is a totally new experience. Parents' reactions are often similar to the stages of grief, shock, denial, guilt, sadness, and then, some degree of adaptation.[12] Nurses, however, must not underestimate parents' abilities, willingness, moral agency, or sense of responsibility.

The engagement approach, which recognizes the needs and responsibilities of all parties, is also comparable to Gilligan's ethic of care,[13] which also has served well as a model for nursing ethical deliberations. Like engagement, the ethic of care deals with creating and maintaining relationships based on trust and respect. In both the ethic of engagement and the ethic of care, which fully engage all parties involved in the life of the infant, it is important that the nurse remember that the stresses and unknowns of the situation may, at times, render parents vulnerable and unable to maintain full participation. Even at these times, as Hess points out, "engagement must continue to create a narrative whereby both client and nurse have a voice . . . even if the client's voice is the weaker of the two."[8]

A key element in the engagement process in neonatal nursing is keeping the parents focused on what the experience is currently and will most likely be in the future for the infant. Nurses have the great privilege of engaging intimately in patient care and thus have the unique ability to ground their assessments experientially. Nurses' well-developed senses of touch, sight, and hearing give them a rich data source for this type of pain and pleasure assessment. However, in formulating such overall assessments, it is important that the nurse project the current experiences of the neonate into the future as well. Often, infants may have to endure numerous invasive therapies in order to gain stability and comfort in the future. Again, the nurse must use both knowledge and prior experience to separate transient discomfort from a life in which pain and suffering probably will continue to outweigh pleasure, satisfaction, and meaningful human growth, development, and interaction.

The nurse must report the data and perceptions clearly to the parents and listen carefully to the parents' data and perceptions. Together, they can come to a consensus about what the experience appears to be like for the infant and a guarded judgment of what the future may hold for the child. In this exchange, the reasons behind recommendations must be rendered transparent to parents so that they have the opportunity to question the validity of assumptions and conclusions. This idea of transparency in care decisions (i.e., "sharing decision processes out loud in a language understandable to the parents"[14]) was first advanced by Brody in relation to primary care decision making and strongly endorsed by King[6] as perhaps indispensable in the neonatal intensive care unit setting.

When a nurse begins to project into what the future human experience may hold, it is important to integrate the knowledge and judgment of physician colleagues. Although parents are often more comfortable with nurses' communications,[6] parents give much credence to the opinions and recommendations of physicians. Thus, it is critical that mixed messages not be sent about either the physiologic prognosis for the future or the nature of the life that will result from whatever physiologic success can be achieved. Team conferences that involve the attending physician, the primary nurse, the parents, and the other significant family decision makers become crucial at this stage of the assessment.

As explicated earlier, in addition to reasoning and cognition, one's sense of integrity, ideals, values, and virtues, and one's self-view and worldview come into play in this complex engagement, both for the nurse and for the parents. Although it is quite complex to balance and equilibrate scientific facts with data concerning the nature of the experience for the infant as well as with ideals and values, such a rich dialogue enhances the moral adequacy of the ultimate decisions.[5] Furthermore, it is what neonatal nursing care is all about.

DECISION OUTCOMES: THE LAW AND MORAL STANDARDS

Based on this thorough assessment of actual and potential well-being, parents then have legal decision-making authority regarding which course of care to pursue. This legal right was further endorsed as a moral standard by the President's Commission for the Study of Ethical Problems in Medicine and Biomedical and Behavioral Research when they stated that "parents should be the surrogates for a seriously ill newborn unless they are disqualified by decision-making incapacity, an unresolvable disagreement between them, or their choice of a course of action that is clearly against the infant's best interests."[15] Once again, the necessity to come to a sound, deliberative judgment of what is in the infant's best interests cannot be avoided. When such a judgment is found to be particularly difficult, it is often best to engage in team discussion in addition to the process of parent engagement. In this sense, *team* refers not only to the nursing and medical staff but also to social workers, chaplains, and any other persons engaged in either the care of the infant or the support of the family.

In addition to the clear legal preference for parental decision making and the recommendation of the President's Commission, nursing's covenant with society includes a long-standing tradition of respect for client autonomy and an active stance of client advocacy. In the case of neonates, this respect for the autonomous right of individuals to make their own best decisions is transferred to the parents. According to Duff and Campbell,[7] "since families primarily must live with, and are most affected by, the decisions, it therefore appears that society and the health professions should provide only general guidelines for decision making. Moreover, since variations between situations are so great, and the situations themselves so complex, it follows that much latitude in decision making should be expected and tolerated." In summary, all else being equal (meaning there is neither a clear indication of probable futility nor a clear indication of probable success), when all the evidence for infant well-being is presented, it is the parents who have the ultimate legal right to choose a course of therapy for their child. Again, only with strong evidence of moral inadequacy (incompetence, maleficence) can that legal right be overturned.

OUTCOMES

Difficult as it may be, if the judgment is made that pain and suffering outweigh both the current good experienced by the infant and the potential for future good, the reality and necessity of facilitating a humane, dignified death then confronts parents, nurses, and others on the health-care team. Essential to assuring a humane death are exquisite relief of physical and emotional symptoms, strict limitations on aggressive therapies, and the provision of bereavement services.[16]

   This approach to safeguarding the well-being of infants also addresses the financial questions raised at the beginning of this article: Would insurers be acting unethically if they refused to pay for experimental, marginally beneficial, expensive treatments? and If parents can pay for whatever they want, should they get it? When the focus is on the well-being of the infant currently and potentially in the future, the issue of financing care becomes clearer. In the opinion of this author, if an intervention promotes actual or potential well-being or both, it should be made available to all infants, even if experimental or expensive. If the potential benefit is so marginal that it is unlikely to balance out the pain and suffering endured, then even if the finances are readily available, the infant should not be subjected to probable futile treatments. The need to advance science by piloting unknown interventions long has been reserved for those competent to give voluntary consent to being a means to someone else's gain. Infants are not in a position to give such consent and should never be regarded as a means to someone else's gain.

THE CONJOINED TWINS: A CASE ANALYSIS

So what went wrong in the opening case? This author can conceive of two potential scenarios that may have driven the nurses' actions. First, the nurses who did not follow the parental decision and acted contrary to the doctor's orders may have believed that they were not dealing with a case of uncertainty. They may have believed that the likelihood for success was probable. If their assessment of outcome stood in such sharp contrast to the clear assessment of others, step one would have been to reexamine the validity of their assessment. What evidence, facts, and information, both about con-joined twins in general and about these infants in particular, did they use? How valid, reliable, and recent was the information?

If the nurses could substantiate firmly the validity of an assessment of probable good outcome and believed that other motives were driving nontreatment, their application of the principle of beneficence (promoting good) could have driven them to action. However, the moral obligation to support and respect the autonomous wishes of parents would have necessitated dialogue with both the parents and the health-care team. Their covert actions would stand as moral violations of their covenant with society to respect legitimate autonomy. ("Baby Doe" regulations had not yet come into effect [1982] and, as we know, were quickly overturned and limited in their scope, precisely because of their violation of the covenant between health professionals and clients as well as because of the moral agency responsibilities of both caregivers and clients. Although Reiser[17] continues to call them "still unduly restrictive," the current "Baby Doe" standard in the Child Abuse Prevention and Treatment Act enlarges the medical criteria that would justify the withholding of aggressive therapeutic efforts. In the act, withholding therapies is justified if they would not be effective in correcting or ameliorating all of the baby's life-threatening conditions, if they would merely prolong dying, if they would be futile or inhumane, or if the baby is irreversibly comatose. These conditions certainly support the engaged decision making focused on infant well-being discussed in this article.)

Alternatively, the nurses who fed the infants may have believed that the situation was futile and that the parents would be making a reasonable decision to avoid aggres-sive treatment but believed that feeding was not aggressive and constituted an inter-vention to assure a humane death. Again, they acted beneficently to promote good. The obligation would then be on the nurses to be certain of the facts: Which inter-ventions provide "exquisite relief of physical and emotional symptoms at the end of life for terminal neonates"? The literature is clear that feeding and hydrating termi-nally ill persons causes more discomfort and complications.[18] What particular, con-textual data did the nurses have that feeding was producing a good outcome for these infants? Furthermore, if they had gathered information about an improvement in the current well-being as a result of feeding, they again had the obligation to share these data with the parents and to engage in a process of deciding how best to proceed.

Short of those two explanations (belief in a likelihood of successful treatment or belief that feeding improved the state of well-being for infants in their dying process; see Fig. 24-2) there appears to be no moral justification for embarking on a course that violates the legal and moral autonomy of the parents. Again, even in embarking on that course, engagement with all moral agents is the justifiable moral stance rather than covert actions. Certainly, however, should either of the explanations continue to be val-idated in the nursing data base and a situation of nonresponsiveness to that data per-sist, nurses must seek out their other institutional options. These options frequently

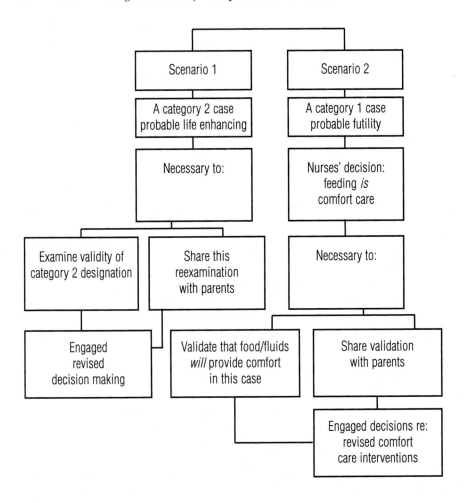

Figure 24-2. Potential Nurses' Scenarios in the Case of the Conjoined Twins

consist of an ethics committee (Joint Commission on Accreditation of Healthcare Organizations Standard 2)[19] or invoking the power structure of the institution to intervene (nursing, medical, and administrative hierarchies as well as risk-management teams). If all of these sources continue to invalidate the nurses' point of view, it seems that serious questions should be raised about either the nursing data-collection process or the viability of professional nursing practice in such an environment.

CONCLUSION

None of this engagement work is easy. However, as Brody[20] points out, moral virtue refers to "the ability of individuals to meet the moral obligations of a collectively defined role they have assumed." In taking on the role of neonatal nurse, caretaker of the most vulnerable, the nurse assumes a role of safeguarding the infant's well-being, necessitating both parental engagement and work within an interdisciplinary team. Whether the neonatal nurse has the ability to meet this moral obligation is another assessment that must be faced.

REFERENCES

1. Taub S. Withholding treatment from defective newborns. *Law, Medicine & Health Care.* 1982;10:4–10.

2. Fry S. Response to "Virtue ethics, caring, and nursing." *Scholarly Inquiry for Nursing Practice: An International Journal.* 1988;2:97–101.

3. American Nurses Association Code. *Perspectives on the Code for Nurses.* Washington, DC: American Nurses Association; 1978.

4. Beauchamp T, Childress J. *Principles of Biomedical Ethics.* New York: Oxford University Press; 1983:148–158.

5. Pierce S. A model of conceptualizing the moral dynamic in health care. *Nursing Ethics.* 1997;4:483–495.

6. King NM. Transparency in neonatal intensive care. *Hastings Center Report* 1992;22:18–25.

7. Duff R, Campbell AGM. Moral and ethical dilemmas in the special care nursery. *New England Journal of Medicine.* 1973;25:890,893.

8. Hess JD. The ethics of compliance: a dialectic. *Advanced Nursing Science.* 1996;19:18–27.

9. Gadow S. Relational ethics: mutual construction of practical knowledge between nurse and client. Presented at the Fourth Philosophy in the Nurse's World Conference; Banff, Alberta; 1995.

10. McCormick R. To save or let die: the dilemma of modern medicine. *JAMA.* 1974; 229:172–176.

11. Mitchell C. Ethical issues in neonatal nursing. In: Angelini DJ, Knapp CW, Gibes R (eds.). *Perinatal/Neonatal Nursing: A Clinical Handbook.* Boston, MA: Blackwell Scientific; 1986:429–437.

12. Fost N. Counseling families who have a child with a severe congenital anomaly. *Pediatrics.* 1981;67:321–324.

13. Gilligan C. *In a Different Voice.* Cambridge, MA: Harvard University Press; 1984.

14. Brody H. Transparency: informed consent in primary care. *Hastings Center Report.*1989; 19:59.

15. President's Commission for the Study of Ethical Problems in Medicine and Biomedical and Behavioral Research. Deciding to forego life-sustaining treatment. 1983;6:197–229.

16. Cohn F, Harrold J, Lynn J. Medical education must deal with end-of-life care. *Chronicle of Higher Education.* 1997;43:A56.

17. Reiser S. Survival at what cost? Origins and effects of the modern controversy on treating severely handicapped newborns. *Journal of Health Politics, Policy, and Law.* 1986;11:199–212.

18. Zerwekh JV. Do dying patients really need IV fluids? *American Journal of Nursing.* 1997;97:26–31.

19. Joint Commission on Accreditation of Healthcare Organizations. *Accreditation Manual for Hospitals.* Oakbrook Terrace, IL: JCAHO; 1992.

20. Brody J. Virtue ethics, caring, and nursing. *Scholarly Inquiry for Nursing Practice: An International Journal.* 1988;2:22,90.

25

PARENTAL DISCRETION IN REFUSAL OF TREATMENT FOR NEWBORNS

A Real but Limited Right

John J. Paris, S.J., Ph.D., and Michael D. Schreiber, M.D.

In a series of case studies for the *Journal of Perinatology*[1-4] we traced the decision-making process for the treatment of seriously compromised newborns. That series examined questions ranging from the medical response to lethal abnormalities, such as anencephaly or trisomy 18, through the demand that physicians terminate ventilatory support for a full-term newborn experiencing respiratory distress unless the physician could guarantee that the child would be normal.

Over the past three decades, the outer reaches of these questions have been explored and a consensus has emerged. If the burden on the infant is overwhelming or the prospects are extremely bleak, there is no obligation to subject the infant to further procedures. In such cases, the parents' decision to omit further treatment is to be respected. Alternatively, if out of ignorance, fear, misguided pessimism, or simple refusal to accept a compromised infant, parents were to decline relatively low-risk, high-benefit interventions that would save the life of a child, even if the child were to evidence some permanent handicap, there is no question that physicians would treat.

The issues raised here were first seen in the famous 1963 Johns Hopkins case in which a child with Down syndrome and a readily correctable duodenal atresia was left untreated and allowed to starve to death over an eleven-day period in a back

J. Paris, M. Schreibner. "Parental Discretion in Refusal of Treatment for Newborns: A Real but Limited Right." *Nursing Clinics of North America.* 1996;23(3):573–582. Reprinted by permission of W. B. Saunders Company.

room of the hospital. In a commentary on that case, Gustafson[5] notes that the reason the parents (the mother was a nurse, the father an attorney) refused permission for the corrective surgery was that it would be unfair to the other children of the household to raise them with a mongoloid. Further, the physicians in the Johns Hopkins case agree that in such circumstances life-saving treatment could be withheld from the infant. In their words, "When a retarded child presents us with the same [physical] problem [as a normal child], a different value system comes in." When asked why this was so, the physicians replied, "There is this tendency to value life on the basis of intelligence.... [It's] a part of the American ethic."

The physicians in the Johns Hopkins case accepted the thesis, at least in part, that newborn infants have no inherent rights or interests. Rather, the infants' claim to continued existence is conditioned on parental acceptance. Although today we might dismiss that sentiment as wholly mistaken, it is instructive to remember that in their landmark 1973 essay on moral and ethical dilemmas in the special care nursery, Duff and Campbell[6] proposed that it was the parents who should decide on the level of aggressive treatment provided to compromised infants. Their argument was much the same as that found in the Johns Hopkins case: The consequences of treatment would fall on the family.

That position, sensitive as it was to the plight of families, seemed to us to be "normless."[7] There were no guidelines, no standards, no norms on which to base the decision. It could be based as much on concerns for siblings, family convenience, or the desire for a normal child as on the best interests of the infant.

The far reach of that proposition is found in essays by Englehardt[8] and by Tooley,[9] each of whom holds that newborn infants have no interests and no independent rights. Their existence, these authors believe, is completely dependent on parental acceptance. As Englehardt writes, "While adults exist in and for themselves, as self-directive and self-conscious beings, young children, especially newborn infants, exist for their families and those who love them." The consequence of that position, Englehardt believes, is that "the decision about treatment belongs properly to the parents."

Even with his support for parental authority in decision making, Englehardt[8] argues, "Society has a right to intervene and protect children for whom parents refuse care (including treatment) when such care does not constitute a severe burden and when it is likely that the child could be brought to a good quality of life." Tooley rejects such limitations. He maintains that parents should have a reasonable amount of time, such as two weeks, to decide whether they want to keep the infant they have borne. If not, without regard to the newborn's quality of life, the infant can be killed.[9]

Despite the seemingly glaring difficulty with these proposals, there was no protest from the public or the medical community regarding the private and personal character of decision making in such cases. In fact, as the study by Shaw et al[10] indicates, an overwhelming majority of pediatricians and pediatric surgeons in the United States who were surveyed in 1977 agreed that, in a case similar to the by-then-famous Johns Hopkins case, they would abide by a parental decision to omit surgery and let the child die.

That consensus ended in 1982 with the Bloomington Baby Doe controversy in which an infant with Down syndrome and esophageal atresia was allowed to die untreated when the attending obstetrician recommended, and the family agreed to, no surgical intervention. The ensuing controversy and federal involvement culminated in the socalled Baby Doe regulations in the 1984 amendments to the Child Abuse Protection Act.[11] "Those regulations," as Fleishman[12] observes, "do not mandate unnecessary or inappropriate treatments." They allow physicians to make decisions based on a reasonable medical judgment and allow parents to have a role in the process.

The controversy, however, shifted the focus from parents to infants. Children are now seen not merely as the property of parents but as patients in their own right. In Bartholomew's[13] phrase, "The fact of a child's dependency on its parents should not be taken to mean that the child is so much chattel." The implication is that although parents may continue to be involved in decision making for their children, they do not have the sole right to demand or refuse medical interventions for the infant. It is the child's best interest, not the parents' wishes, that is to govern treatment decision.

The limits and parameters of parental discretion in refusal of treatment for a newborn were explored in a dramatic case that occurred in Lansing, Michigan, in 1995 when manslaughter charges were brought against Dr. Gregory Messenger, a local dermatologist, for removing his extremely premature infant son from a ventilator in Sparrow Hospital's neonatal intensive care unit. The newborn had been placed on mechanical life support over the explicit instructions of the parents that they did not want aggressive or resuscitative measures utilized on their 780 g, twenty-five-week gestational infant. The manslaughter charge was based on Dr. Messenger's failure to provide proper medical treatment for the infant and for gross negligence with regard to his child's care.

MESSENGER CASE

In the twenty-fifth week of her pregnancy, Mrs. Messenger was admitted for premature labor and potential rupture of membranes. Prolonged tocolytic therapy was complicated by the development of pulmonary edema necessitating discontinuation. The neonatologist counseled the parents that the mortality rate at twenty-five weeks' gestation was 50 to 70 percent. If the baby survived, the incidence of severe intracranial hemorrhage was 20 to 40 percent. They also were told of the high likelihood of respiratory distress syndrome and possible subsequent bronchopulmonary dysplasia.

In light of these grim statistics, the parents requested that no extraordinary efforts be made to resuscitate the baby. The neonatologist informed the parents that she preferred a "wait-and-see" approach and that if, once intubated, the baby took a downward course, she would remove life-sustaining technology. On leaving the hospital, the neonatologist instructed the physician's assistant that if the baby were vigorous or active at birth and needed ventilatory support, the baby should be intubated.

The baby was delivered later that evening weighing 780 g and was immediately noted to be severely hypotonic and cyanotic. The baby was immediately intubated, hand ventilated, and transported to the neonatal intensive care unit. Once there, the father questioned the decision to aggressively intervene and requested that the baby be extubated. The physician's assistant told the father that only the neonatologist could make such a decision. When the neonatologist arrived, she informed the parents that she would evaluate the baby's response to aggressive therapy before making a decision on withdrawal of life support.

The parents then requested time to be alone with their baby. Whereupon, the father extubated the baby and placed him in the mother's arms; where he died.

COMMENTARY

This case, like the earlier Linares incident[14] in Chicago in which a father brought a gun into the pediatric intensive care unit and threatened to shoot his two-year-old son, who was in a persistent vegetative condition, if anyone attempted to intervene with his removal of the ventilator, causes the hearer to gasp, "Oh, my God, you can't do that!" Although the situations of the infants were tragic, we do not want, nor could we tolerate, a system in which family members unilaterally take it upon themselves to remove life-sustaining apparatus from a patient, even one who is dying. Yet in the Linares case a grand jury refused to return an indictment against the father. In the Messenger case it took a jury less than 3 hours to return a verdict of not guilty.

An analysis of the Messenger case must begin with the medical facts and the application of the principles of bioethics to that fact pattern. The focus, as in all such cases, must be centered on the patient. It is the patient's condition and the patient's desires, not the wishes of the parents or the goals of the physician, that ought to govern these treatment decisions.

For competent adults the question is readily resolved: Ask them what they want. Even for the incompetent adult, the issue is generally resolvable by learning of their past statements or knowing their value structure.[15] For the newborn infant, however, the resolution is not so readily achieved.

The consensus in the literature seems to be that for the never competent the *best-interests* standard is the one that should be used.[16] This standard, unlike *substituted judgment* does not rest on the value of self determination but solely on the protection of the patient's welfare. That protection is particularly important with regard to infants and children because they are now seen not merely as property of parents but as patients in their own right. The implication, as we explored in the earlier essay,[1] is that although parents may continue to be involved in decision making for their children, they do not have the sole right to refuse medical treatment for their infant. It is the child's best interests that are to be the focus and goal of treatment decisions.

In the Messenger case—unlike, for example, that of a child afflicted with a lethal congenital abnormality[4]—there was not the assurance that an inevitable fatal outcome awaits. Nor was there the certainty that any and all medical interventions would prove unavailing. Here the outcome, as the neonatologist indicated to the parents, was unknown.

What were known, however, were the statistical probabilities of mortality and morbidity for this class of births. Although some might challenge the accuracy of the data given to the parents on survival rates for their baby,[17] the treating neonatologist informed the Messengers that if delivered at twenty-five weeks, their child had a 50 to 70 percent chance of dying. Further, she indicated that the comorbidities involved significant risk (20 to 40 percent) of severe intraventricular hemorrhage, as well as the likely possibility of respiratory distress syndrome.

There is no question that if the Messengers had requested aggressive treatment for their newborn of twenty-five-week gestational age, it would have been provided. The issue, in this case, is, did the information given to the parents warrant a predelivery decision to withhold resuscitation and other aggressive medical interventions? Or, as the neonatologist wanted, must the parents authorize resuscitation and the use of aggressive life-sustaining measures until it becomes clear, if not certain, that the child will not survive or, if he or she does, will be in such a devastated state as to justify removal of life-sustaining measures?[18]

A statistical approach to determine which infants should be treated based on objective criteria such as weight, gestational age, and level of severity of illness is widely used for the treatment of very premature low birthweight infants in European countries. As Dawes et al.[19] report, reliance on actuarial judgments consistently produces better overall results than does reliance on individual clinical judgments. Although such an approach reduces the problem of profoundly compromised survivors and that of parents who insist on treatments the physician judges futile, it does not take into consideration the ability of an "outlier" to survive or the willingness of some parents to cope with tragic circumstances.

Although the statistical approach does not fit with the American emphasis on individualism, it is a morally acceptable way to make treatment decisions. It is also a factor that is considered whenever a patient or proxy calculates probabilities in making an assessment of medical interventions based on burden versus benefit.

Under any schema a 50 to 70 percent risk of mortality puts a newborn into that broad area of gray in which the degree of burden and the prospects of benefit are so suffused in ambiguity and uncertainty that a decision as to whether to continue treatment properly belongs to those who bear the responsibility for the infant—the parents.[3] That stand, as the Hastings Center Project[16] on imperiled newborns reports, is contrary to the practice in the United States that responds to uncertain outcome in neonatal medicine by giving a chance to every infant who is even potentially viable. Active treatment is then continued until it is nearly certain that the particular baby will either die or be so severely impaired that, under any substantive standard, parents would legitimately opt for termination of treatment.

This *wait-until-near-certainty* approach is precisely what the neonatologist proposed to the Messengers. It is based on the belief articulated by Fleishman[12] that we as a society rank letting an infant die who could have lived a reasonable life as far worse than saving an infant who becomes devastatingly disabled. That approach is appropriate when we face complete uncertainty: that is, when decision makers have no knowledge at all about the probabilities of various outcomes, as, for example, was true in the case we described.[1] But, as the Hastings Center group put it: "It is not particularly well suited to moral situations in which there are data on which to base predictions."[16]

Dr. and Mrs. Messenger had such data. The statements of a 50 to 70 percent death rate and a 20 to 40 percent risk of severe bleeding in the brain, as well as the probability of respiratory distress syndrome, were more than sufficient evidence of the disproportionate burden that awaited this child to justify a decision to withhold resuscitation. The decision was well within the range of morally acceptable choices. It was also in conformity with widely used medical standards. It should have been respected.

The evidence supporting their decision not to resuscitate becomes more compelling when at delivery the infant was observed by the physicians present to be "lifeless," "floppy," hypotonic, hypoxic, and "purple-blue" or "black" in color with no grasp and no grimace. Had a neonatologist rather than a physician's assistant been present at birth, a judgment on the infant's medical status with regard to breathing, heart rate, color, and activity rather than a technical response to heartbeat alone should have precluded resuscitation.

Had the Messengers' request for nonresuscitation been followed—a decision that had been implemented in previous cases at Sparrow Hospital—no one would have questioned the outcome. A stillbirth or demise at delivery is a tragedy, but one that is personal to the parents involved. No public concern would have emerged from the event.

Once the infant was placed on a ventilator the dynamics changed. Although there is now universal agreement in the philosophical and legal literature that there is no moral or legal difference between withholding or withdrawing life-sustaining machinery,[20] the circumstances of this case show that psychologically and politically the gulf can be enormous.

Both the pathologist and the prosecuting attorney stated that if ventilatory support had not been initiated, they would have ruled that the infant had died of natural causes. But because the infant had been placed on a ventilator and at the time of its removal, less than an hour after its placement, was stable, "pink," and in no danger of imminent death, they held it was necessary to have objective medical data of demise or devastation before the ventilator could be removed. The neonatologist took a similar position. She was unwilling to accede to the father's request to remove the ventilator until she had reviewed the results of the blood gas tests, radiographs, and a trial of surfactant.

Lost sight of in this perception is, as the President's Commission report *Deciding to Forego Life-Sustaining Treatment* made clear, that the same justification for withholding a medical treatment applies to its withdrawal.[20] Because there was sufficient evidence to support the parents' initial decision not to intubate the infant, the child should never have been placed on a ventilator in the first place.

Given his condition, the child had a right to be free of unwanted medical interventions. His father, speaking on his behalf and acting in the infant's best interests, made a decision not to use such measures. The neonatologist disagreed with that choice.

When she failed to persuade the parents to adopt her wait-and-see approach, the neonatologist did not continue discussing the issue with the parents to learn if there could be agreement on the care of the child, nor did she offer the parents the opportunity to find another physician willing to treat their child within the ethically supportable boundaries they had chosen. Rather, she took it upon herself to instruct her physician's assistant (PA) to override the parents' instructions and intubate if the child were "vigorous" or "active."

The PA, although conceding the infant was not vigorous at delivery, intubated on the basis of heartbeat. She did this without prior discussion with the treating obstetrician or the parents, without reviewing the mother's medical records, without knowledge of the complications of the mother's labor, and without awareness that the serious medical status of the mother might have significantly compromised the fetus.

The father objected to the PA's action and was told that only the neonatologist could authorize the withdrawal of life-sustaining interventions. When the neonatologist returned to the hospital at 12:15 A.M. she continued the life-sustaining ventilation. She was determined to follow a wait-and-see approach.

Waiting for near certainty ignores information, abuses basic principles of probability, and denies the ethical complexity of these decisions. Rather than attempt to work through the complexity and make a fallible but nonetheless real human moral choice, we tend to reduce the ethical to the medical. Technology takes over and controls the choices until no choice is left. Once that tack is taken, all participants are essentially reduced to a wait-and-see stance. They cease to be active decision makers in the unfolding drama. Rather they become passive onlookers—a Greek chorus, as it were, that observes, laments, and weeps but is unable to alter the outcome.[21]

Gregory Messenger chose not to be a passive onlooker. Rather than allow the possibility that his son might die entrapped in medical technology, he placed his son in the mother's arms where for a brief moment mother and child could bond. The infant died in the mother's embrace. The jury found Gregory Messenger's actions neither grossly negligent nor a breach of his legal duty to provide proper medical treatment for his son.

POSTSCRIPT

To protect other parents who might find themselves in a similar situation, Dr. Gregory Messenger drafted "Compassion Care and Comfort Guidelines" as a standard to be used in the care and treatment of patients who face significant morbidity or death but who, such as infants and children, lack decision-making capacity.

The guidelines adopt the best interest and the proportionate burden and benefit standards articulated at his trial. They were approved and adopted as the standard of care by the Michigan State Medical Society on May 6, 1995.

REFERENCES

1. Paris JJ, Bell AJ. Guarantee my child will be normal or stop all treatment. *Journal of Perinatology.* 1993;13:469–472.

2. Paris JJ, Miles SH, Kohrman A, et al. Guidelines on the care of anencephalic infants: a response to Baby K. *Journal of Perinatology.* 1995;15:318–324.

3. Paris JJ, Newman V. Ethical issues in quadruple amputation in a child with meningococcal septic shock. *Journal of Perinatology.* 1993;13:56–58.

4. Paris JJ, Weiss AH, Soifer S. Ethical issues in the use of life-prolonging interventions for an infant with trisomy 18. *Journal of Perinatology.* 1992;12:366–368.

5. Gustafson JM. Mongolism, parental desires, and the right to life. *Perspectives in Biology and Medicine.* 1973;524:429.

6. Duff RS, Campbell AGM. Moral and ethical dilemmas in the special-care nursery. *New England Journal of Medicine.* 1973;289:890–894.

7. Paris JJ. Terminating treatment for newborns: a theological perspective. *Law, Medicine & Health Care.* 1982;2:120–124.

8. Englehardt HT. Ethical issues in aiding the death of young children. In: Kohl M (ed.). *Beneficent Euthanasia.* Amherst, NY: Prometheus Books; 1975:78.

9. Tooley M. *Abortion and Infanticide.* New York, NY: Oxford University Press; 1983.

10. Shaw A, Randolph J, Manard B. Ethical issues in pediatric surgery: a national survey of pediatricians and pediatric surgeons. *Pediatrics.* 1977;60:588–599.

11. Kopelman LM, Irons TG, Kopelman AE. Neonatologists judge the Baby Doe regulations. *New England Journal of Medicine.* 1988;318:677–683.

12. Fleishman AR. Ethical issues in neonatology: a US perspective. *Annals of the New York Academy of Science.* 1980;530:83–91.

13. Bartholomew WG. The child-patient: do parents have the right to decide? In: Spicker S, Englehardt T, Healy J, et al. (eds.): *The Law-Medicine Relation: A Philosophical Explanation.* Dordrecht: Reidal; 1981: 126–132.

14. Lantos JD, Miles SH, Cassel CK. The Linares affair. *Law, Medicine & Health Care.* 1989;17:308–315.

15. In re Conroy, 98 N.J. 321, 1985.

16. Caplan A, Cohen CB (eds.). Imperiled newborns. *Hastings Center Report.* 1987;17:5–32.

17. Allen MC, Donohue PK, Dusman AE. The limit of viability: neonatal outcome of infants born at 22 to 25 weeks' gestation. *New England Journal of Medicine.* 1993;329:1597–1601.

18. Paris JJ, O'Connell KJ. Withdrawal of nutrition and fluids from a neurologically devastated infant: the case of Baby T. *Journal of Perinatology.* 1991;11:372–373.

19. Dawes RM, Faust D, Meehl PE. Clinical versus actuarial judgement. *Science.* 1989; 243:1668–1673.

20. President's Commission for the Study of Ethical Problems in Medicine and Biomedical and Behavioral Research. *Deciding to Forego Life-Sustaining Treatment.* Washington, DC: US Government Printing Office; 1983.

21. Paris JJ, Kodish E. Ethical issues in neonatology. In: Pomerance J (ed.). *Issues in Clinical Neonatology.* Norwalk, CT: Appleton & Lange; 1993:533.

Part 10

ISSUES IN TRANSPLANTATION

❧

According to the United Network for Organ Sharing (UNOS), approximately 8,500 people will donate their organs this year. Unfortunately, there are more than 70,000 patients currently on the national transplant waiting list. Last year a similar disparity resulted in the deaths of 6,448 patients as they waited for organs to become available. Such statistics would certainly be emotionally crushing if it were not for two sacred "truths" transplant patients and their families cling to: (1) An organ will become available in time, and (2) When an organ does become available, it will be allocated fairly. Of course these "truths" become a bit problematic when we take a critical look at not only the annual organ procurement statistics published by UNOS, but also the current organ allocation policies and regulations. With this in mind, my goal for this section is to provide an understanding of ethical and social issues that come about as a result of new strategies to increase procurement and the use of social criteria in allocation decisions. Gaining such an understanding is particularly important for ethics committees and physicians as the Joint Commission on Accreditation of Healthcare Organizations (JCAHO) requires their active participation in the development of their institution's policies and procedures with regard to procuring organs and tissues.[1]

Ever since organ transplants moved beyond experimentation there has been a significant shortfall in the number of Americans who have been willing to donate their tissues and organs. This state of affairs continues even after numerous attempts to increase the pool of donors through such policies and programs as opt-out (presumed consent), required request, financial incentives, public education, and redefining death. This last effort to increase the number of available organs is the focus of this section's first reading, by Robert Arnold and Stuart Youngner, titled "The Dead Donor Rule: Should We Stretch It, Bend It, or Abandon It?"

The authors begin their discussion by laying out the moral tenets of organ procurement: We do not take organs from people unless they are dead. We do not kill patients for their organs. Consent is obtained prior to procurement from either the patient or their family. From there, they question the sanctity of the first tenet, known as the *dead donor rule*. In 1993, when the authors wrote this article, the University of Pittsburgh Medical Center had a policy in place that allowed organs to be harvested within two minutes of a patient's cardiac arrest. Some considered this a bit too quick and felt it to be a violation of the dead donor rule. One concern repeatedly voiced in response to this policy was that this would cause people to not donate their organs for fear of being given up on too soon in order to get their organs. Taking this into account, Arnold and Youngner propose a policy that goes beyond the "Pittsburgh protocol," while at the same time addressing the aforementioned concern. They suggest doing away with the dead donor rule altogether and instead relying on the autonomous consent of the patient or their family. In this way, the number of recoverable organs would be increased as a result of not having to wait for "death" to occur, and patients would be protected from overzealous transplant teams who—according to urban legend—roam the hallways looking for organs.

Shifting to the problematic nature of the second "truth," organ allocation decisions seem to be grounded more in arbitrariness then fairness; place of residence, financial status, and character are all taken into account, sometimes significantly. For example, until this year patients who were in close proximity to an available organ were given preference over similarly situated patients who were on the other side of some random geographic line. Patients who are wealthy can travel to different transplant regions in order to be placed on the waiting lists of those transplant programs that have shorter wait times. The last example of such arbitrariness concerns the use of psychosocial screening in order to determine a patient's responsibility for her disease, so that those who "brought it upon themselves" may be given lower priority then those who are seen as "innocent victims."

This kind of moral (or social) responsibility criteria is the foundation for the next reading, "Responsibility, Alcoholism, and Liver Transplantation," by Walter Glannon. Although Glannon grounds his discussion on the fairness of giving alcoholics lower priority for liver transplants, he could have just as easily used drug abuse, smoking, obesity, or a sedentary lifestyle as justification for giving a lower priority to a patient needing a heart, kidney, or lung transplant. Glannon goes to great lengths to make clear his justification for such an allocation decision is not founded on some idea of vice, but rather it is a determination of personal responsibility that provides his justification.

Importantly, the use of this kind of character assessment in resource allocation decisions is anything but new. In 1963 Shana Alexander published an article in *Life* magazine[2] describing the world's first kidney dialysis program at the Swedish Hospital in Seattle. The program directors formed a special committee with two objectives: first, create a resource allocation protocol; and second, use their protocol to allocate ten "artificial" kidneys among some 100,000 patients. The committee's criteria weighed the patients' state of residence, church activities, marital status, occupation, net worth, income, and age.

REFERENCES

1. Joint Commission on Accreditation of Healthcare Organizations. *2000 Hospital Accreditation Standards.* Oakbrook, IL: JCAHO; 2000:81.

2. Alexander S. "They Decide Who Lives, Who Dies" *Life.* November 8, 1963:102–125.

26

THE DEAD DONOR RULE

Should We Stretch It, Bend It, or Abandon It?

Robert M. Arnold, M.D., and Stuart J. Youngner, M.D.

꧁꧂

Three important principles provide the moral framework for organ procurement in America.[1] First, the dead donor rule: Persons must be dead before their organs are taken. Second, the prohibition against active euthanasia: Although patients may be allowed to die under certain circumstances, they must never be actively killed. Third, the primacy of consent: Patient or family consent must precede organ retrieval. These rules serve to reassure people that when they enter hospitals they will not be killed or mistreated so that their organs can be taken.

By professing adherence to these principles, the Pittsburgh protocol denies that it breaks with existing policy.[2] The scholars who write in this volume seem to accept these principles as well. For the most part, their judgments about non-heart-beating cadaver donor (NHBCD) protocols rest on whether they would increase the number of transplantable organs *without violating existing ethical norms.*

We ask a more radical question—is it time to reassess the moral framework itself? By taking advantage of ambiguities in the definition and criteria of death, the Pittsburgh protocol pushes the dead donor rule to the limit. Would it be better, in our quest to fulfill the ever-greater promise of organ transplantation, to abandon rather than tamper with the dead donor rule, relying entirely on informed consent as a safe-

R. Arnold, S. Youngner. "The Dead Donor Rule: Should We Stretch It, Bend It, or Abandon It?" *Kennedy Institute of Ethics Journal.* 1993;3(2):263–278. © The Johns Hopkins University Press.

guard against abuse?[3] Or, instead, as Renée Fox[4] suggests, is it simply time to reaffirm our commitment to basic values and stop pushing for more organs? These questions become more pressing as the prohibition against active euthanasia seems to be fading.

THE DEAD DONOR RULE

Origins

Although the term *dead donor rule* was first coined by John Robertson in 1988, it aptly describes an unwritten, uncodified standard that has guided organ procurement in the United States since the late 1960s.[5] As DeVita et al.[6] have noted, because of its informal nature, the reasons for it can only be inferred. There was undoubtedly discomfort with the isolated practice of taking kidneys from patients before they died following failed bypass surgery[7] because this appeared to violate health-care professionals' admonition to "do no harm." More influential, perhaps, was the growing interest in severely brain-damaged (but heart beating) patients as a promising donor source.[7] By introducing "brain death," our society designated a subgroup of severely brain-damaged patients, those with loss of all brain functions, as an acceptable organ source. By simultaneously embracing the prohibitions of the dead donor rule, our society seemed to reassure itself that other severely compromised patients would be protected from harm; namely, they would not be killed or used as organ sources prior to their death.

Meanings of the Rule

The prohibition that persons must be dead before their organs are taken has two distinct connotations.

1. *Patients must not be killed by organ retrieval.* The first connotation is that patients must not be killed by the process of removing their organs. For example, taking an unpaired vital organ such as the heart would kill a living donor. A slightly broader interpretation prohibits killing patients so that their organs can be taken, even if organs are removed after death occurs. Both meanings are consistent with homicide laws and the strong prohibition against "mercy" killing that has characterized our society.

2. *Organs must not be taken from patients until they die.* The second connotation of the dead donor rule is that organs should not be taken from patients before they are dead, even if taking the organs does not kill them. The reasons for this prohibition are less obvious and less well articulated than those against killing, but include: a wish to prevent harm to or exploitation of the weak and vulnerable; mistrust of doctors; and concern that critically ill patients would be treated merely as a means to an end—as repositories of organs that could help others.

Unlike the prohibition against killing, the second connotation is not absolute. For example, in the case of living related donors or partial transplants, we do allow organs to be taken from living persons. The organs either are paired (kidneys) or we take only part of them (liver or pancreas). While the practice of taking one of an organ pair or parts of organs from living related donors does not violate the first connotation of the dead donor rule—i.e., the patient is not killed by organ retrieval—it does seem to violate the second connotation.

Sentiment about this issue, however, is far from unanimous. Some people argue that even consenting living donors should not be exposed to the "unnecessary" risk of organ removal since cadaver organs are nearly as successful.[7] Others point out that living related donors—especially parents of dying children—are put in a coerced position simply by giving them the choice of either donating or letting their child die.[8] Opposition to living donation grows when living donors are altruistic strangers,[9] or the surgical risk is great, and becomes downright bellicose when consideration is given to buying organs from living strangers.[8,10,11]

In summary, the dead donor rule has ensured that patients will not be killed by or for organ removal.[12] It also limits nonlethal removal of organs from living persons to a narrow category—usually healthy relatives of the potential recipient.

LIVING WITH THE DEAD DONOR RULE: DONATING ORGANS PRIOR TO DECLARING DEATH

The public has a real fear that medical treatment will be compromised in order to increase organ procurement. Surveys reveal that concern about premature declaration of death and undertreatment are the leading reasons people give for not filling out organ donor cards.[13] These fears appear in the public literature in books like *Coma*,[14] and in a storyline in *Dick Tracy*,[15] where weak and defenseless persons are murdered for their organs. To allay these fears, the dead donor rule has become central to organ procurement; strategies for increasing the donor pool have tried to operate within its confines.

One way to increase the organ supply without breaking the dead donor rule is simply to redraw the line between life and death so that it includes patients as dead who were previously considered alive. One could argue that the formulation of "brain death" was, all along, a well-intentioned effort to gerrymander the line between life and death in order to increase the donor pool without inflaming public opinion.[16] In fact, the Harvard Ad Hoc Committee that first endorsed irreversible loss of all brain function as a new criterion for determining death was quite direct in acknowledging its motivation to quell the "controversy in obtaining organs for transplantation."[17(p337)]

The whole-brain criterion for determining death was quickly and widely accepted for two reasons, neither of which had much to do with whether "brain death" was equivalent to death. First, irreversible loss of all brain function was easy to diagnose in adults, and thus seemed to offer, like the cardiopulmonary criterion, clear means for separating the living from the dead.[18] Second, once the diagnosis was evident, so too was the prognosis, which is as certain as anything in clinical medicine—patients did not regain consciousness and could not sustain a beating heart (on a respirator) for more than hours, days, or, in a few instances, weeks—despite the most aggressive treatment.[19] However as technology has advanced, making it possible to sustain the heartbeat longer—in rare cases even for months[20]—this reason may become less influential. It is these factors, plus the irresistible utilitarian appeal of organ transplantation, that greatly contributed to the acceptance of irreversible loss of all brain function as a justification for behaving as if patients were dead.[21]

While the whole-brain criterion for death did facilitate an increase in transplantable organs, it has not been without problems. First, it has become clear that it lacks a widely accepted conceptual justification. Nearly a decade passed before any concept emerged to justify exactly why persons who have lost all brain function, but whose hearts continue to beat, are dead. This concept, offered by James Bernat et al.,[22] holds that such persons are dead because they have lost the ability to function as a whole—i.e., "the spontaneous and innate activities carried out by the integration of all or most subsystems." Bernat's view has received little support in the philosophic and bioethics communities, where a higher-brain concept—loss of consciousness and cognition—finds greater acceptance.[23-26]

Moreover, there is evidence of conceptual confusion in clinical practice. A study by Youngner and his colleagues found that one-third of physicians and nurses involved in the management of "brain-dead" patients considered them to be dead because they had irreversibly lost consciousness and cognition. Youngner's study also found that another third of physicians and nurses did not perceive them as dead at all but accepted treating them as dead because they were irreparably damaged or death was imminent.[27,28] Confusion over the "real" time of death has been reported in surveys of families who donate their loved one's organs.[29] These findings, and the observation that many health professionals (and most journalists) describe "brain-dead" patients as having "died" only after either life-support machines or organs are removed, suggest that many persons disagree with or are, at a minimum, ambivalent about the conceptual status of persons whose brains have ceased functioning but whose hearts continue to beat.

The whole-brain formulation thus seems less the result of intellectual "discovery"—i.e., we figured out that some people we said were alive are really dead — and more the product of conceptual gerrymandering to solve a social problem. Unfortunately, such utilitarian justification for defining death is inherently unstable and will result in attempts at redefinition whenever utility requires it.[30] The recent attempt to redefine death to include anencephalic infants is a good example. Summarizing the argument, Fost says, "If resolution of a controversy that stands in the way of procuring organs for transplantation was a valid reason for redefining death in 1968, why would it not be a sufficient reason for another redefinition in 1988?"[31(p7),32]

Instead of grossly moving the line between life and death, the Pittsburgh protocol takes advantage of ambiguities in the way it has already been drawn. By declaring patients dead after two minutes of ventricular fibrillation, for example, the protocol makes organ retrieval possible at a time when: (1) the heart could almost certainly be restarted by medical intervention; (2) the medical evidence that it will not start up by itself (autoresuscitate) is incomplete;[33] and (3) the functional status of the brain is unknown.[33] Although "irreversible'" has been part of the definition and criterion of death, as Cole[34] and Lynn[33] point out, its theoretical meaning and practical significance have never been adequately resolved. This leaves the distinction between almost dead, maybe dead, probably dead, or dead for sure, and the effect of the possibility of treatment on these states, indeterminate. The Pittsburgh protocol merely provides answers that improve the chances for obtaining organs.[35]

The question for public policy is whether the continued readjustment of the definition of death and the criteria for determining it (which the Pittsburgh protocol exemplifies), will yield more organs or will foment suspicion and fear and turn the public against organ donation? Efforts to extend the line of death to include anencephalic infants failed after stirring considerable public controversy. How the public will react to the Pittsburgh protocol's interpretation of irreversible is unknown, but several of the scholars writing in this volume have expressed concern that it might backfire.

LIVING WITH THE DEAD DONOR RULE: THE PROHIBITION AGAINST ACTIVE KILLING

As our society has accepted that, under the right circumstances, each and every life-sustaining intervention may be withheld or withdrawn, the timing of human death has become more and more a matter of deliberate human decision. At the same time, the prohibition against active killing has provided a "bright line" that must not be crossed.[36(p250)] Indeed, as our earlier discussion suggests, society may have redrawn one line (between life and death) precisely to avoid crossing another (between killing and allowing to die).

The Pittsburgh protocol superficially respects the bright line. Under its aegis, patients who are alive are "*allowed to die*," not *killed*, when they are removed from life support. The protocol even prohibits the use of fatal doses of morphine, leaving open the possibility that patients will experience discomfort as they are withdrawn from ventilatory support before they receive analgesia.

CONCEPTUALLY DIM

For better or for worse, the bright line is growing dimmer. Brock, for example, argues that, when it comes to turning off a ventilator, the distinction between killing and allowing to die is conceptually "confused and mistaken."[37(p12)] He gives the example of a terminally ill ALS patient who is mentally competent and completely respirator dependent. When the patient's physician removes the ventilator at the patient's request, "the common understanding is that the physician thereby allows the patient to die."

Brock then changes the case so that, instead of the physician, a greedy and hostile son removes the patient from the ventilator. The son's claim that he didn't kill her, but merely allowed her to die from her ALS, "would rightly be dismissed as transparent sophistry." Brock points out that both the physician and son performed the same action with the same result. Both killed the patient; both acted in ways that resulted in the patient dying sooner than she otherwise would have. It is the nature of the motivation that makes killing morally acceptable in the first instance and blameworthy in the second. It simply makes us more comfortable to label the behavior we don't accept with the pejorative term killing.[38]

In other cultures, even honorably motivated removal of life-sustaining ventilator support is considered *killing* in a pejorative sense. While this view might be dismissed as morally "unsophisticated," perhaps the paradoxical root meaning of that word— i.e., without sophistry—is more in order. In our own hospital settings, health professionals[39] and families sometimes have trouble accepting the explanation that removing a ventilator is merely allowing to die; twnety-five years ago, few people would have accepted the explanation. The advice of the Harvard Ad Hoc Committee, in its seminal 1968 *JAMA* article, is interesting in this regard.

> It should be emphasized that we recommend the patient be declared dead before any effort is made to take him off a respirator, if he is then on a respirator. This declaration should not be delayed until he has been taken off the respirator and all artificially stimulated signs have ceased. The reason for this recommendation is that in our judgment it will provide a greater degree of legal protection to those involved. Otherwise, the physicians would be turning off the respirator on a person who is, under the present strict, technical application of law, still alive.[17(p339)]

Morally Dim

Even if one insists that removing a ventilator is not *killing,* undeniable forms of *killing—* e.g., physician-assisted suicide, in which the physician helps the patient kill herself, and lethal injection by the physician—are favored by 54 percent of Americans in recent opinion polls.[40] It is entirely possible, if not likely, that such *killing* will be legally sanctioned or at least tolerated in some U.S. jurisdictions over the next few years.

IMPLICATIONS FOR THE FUTURE: AUTONOMY AND ORGAN PROCUREMENT

The implications of these observations for the future of organ procurement are profound. The lines that forbid us to *kill* people for their organs or to take organs from people before they are dead may be, as Robertson suggests, important symbols of "the ethical concerns that arise around organ transplantation."[36(p249)] However, these symbols lose their meaning for many people as society accepts circumstances in which health professionals may hasten patients' deaths and as transplant policy makers constantly tinker with death's boundaries. Under these circumstances, bright lines dim, and symbols become detached from the moral and psychological roots from which they arose.

Consider a future in which we have abandoned the symbolic prohibitions of the dead donor rule. *Killing,* in and of itself, would no longer constitute a harm. Real harms would have to do with suffering, and violations of patient autonomy or interests.

What if, instead of continually gerrymandering the line between life and death, we simply ask, "Are there some patients whose quality of life is so unacceptable and whose death is so imminent (by fate or their own decision) that we may take their organs before they die?" Instead of pretending that we can continue to develop more accurate definitions of death (that coincidentally expand the donor pool), we would allow organ procurement from patients with severe head injuries who were irreparably damaged and near death but who have not lost all brain function. Anencephalic newborns represent a subcategory of such patients. After all, as Robertson says, there can be little harm to "a patient who is so near death, and so presumably without interests at that point, that no real harm to his interests could be shown."[36(p249)]

Fost[41] has argued for reformulating the central tenet of organ procurement to be "violates no interest" rather than "is dead," and this seems more consistent with current practices. After all, our society does not require that a patient be dead prior to the removal of life-sustaining technology; it requires only that the removal does not violate the patient's interest (as defined by either the patient or surrogate). From a patient's perspective, the consequences of organ procurement (death) may not be that different than those of forgoing life support, except that organ procurement may help others. It is therefore unclear why stricter rules should govern one than the other.[42]

How near death and how damaged a potential donor would have to be in order to be considered beyond harm is problematic. One might try to develop societal standards, although recent debates over rationing and the use of QALY's indicate that this will be quite difficult.[43-45] More likely, caregivers will rely on surrogates' assessments (as they do in decisions to forgo life-sustaining treatment).

We could minimize the problems of judging what constitutes a harm by insisting on clear and rigorous consent by the potential donors rather than their surrogates.[46] People could sign donor cards or living wills that designated the circumstances under which their organs could be taken—i.e., define their own threshold for being harmed. For example, a patient could state that if she becomes severely demented, one kidney should be removed and donated before artificial nutrition and hydration are discontinued and she is allowed to die.

Machine-dependent patients could give consent for organ removal before they are dead. For example, a ventilator-dependent ALS patient could request that life support be removed at 5:00 P.M., but that at 9:00 A.M. the same day he be taken to the operating room, put under general anesthesia, and his kidneys, liver, and pancreas removed. Bleeding vessels would be tied off or cauterized. The patient's heart would not be removed and would continue to beat throughout the surgery, perfusing the other organs with warm, oxygen- and nutrient-rich blood until they were removed.[47]

The heart would stop, and the patient would be pronounced dead only after the ventilator was removed at 5:00 P.M., according to plan, and long before the patient could die from renal, hepatic, or pancreatic failure.

If active euthanasia—e.g., lethal injection—and physician-assisted suicide are legally sanctioned, even more patients could couple organ donation with their planned deaths; we would not have to depend only upon persons attached to life support. This practice would yield not only more donors, but more types of organs as well, since the heart could now be removed from dying, not just dead, patients.

CONCLUSION

The irresistible utilitarian appeal of organ transplantation has us hell-bent on increasing the donor pool. Giving up the dead donor rule, however, raises the question of how far we are willing to go to procure more organs—and, some point out, save more lives. Are we headed for the utilitarian utopia espoused by Jack Kevorkian, where organ retrieval and scientific experimentation are options in every planned death, be it mercy killing or execution?[48]

If a look into such a future hurts our eyes (or turns our stomachs), is our discomfort any different from what we would have experienced 30 years ago by looking into the future that is today? How are we to understand such feelings? Are they merely emotional reactions and cultural habits that stand in the way of social progress?

Does the dead donor rule put our devotion to symbols ahead of the real interest dying patients have in transplantation? Why not drop the dead donor rule and replace it with a rigorous consent process and protocols that prevent real harms (e.g., the treatable discomfort which the Pittsburgh protocol allows during "weaning" from the ventilator) instead of symbolic ones (e.g., the intentional hastening of death in order to prevent pain, which the protocol forbids)? Do we really protect helpless and hopelessly damaged patients by calling them dead, by claiming that we merely allow them to die when we turn off their ventilators, or by being stingy with analgesics? Isn't this an example of respecting the symbol at the expense of the very values they represent?[49]

Proponents of the dead donor rule argue that this rationalistic interpretation of symbols "underestimates the cognitive and moral significance of symbols; it suggests that aesthetes alone traffic in them, while moralists enjoy a symbol free access to the real world."[50] Symbols keep us attuned to what we consider important. As such, they shape our self-conception and how we organize our communities. According to this view, our revulsion to a Kevorkian future is important to our moral character. Giving up the dead donor rule risks the weakening and eventual vanishing of these sentiments and thus should be opposed.[4,51-53]

Given the difficulties our society is likely to experience in trying to openly adjudicate these disparate views,[54] why not simply go along with the quieter strategy of policy creep? It seems to be getting us where we seem to want to go, albeit slowly. Besides, total candor is not always compatible with the moral compromises that inevitably accompany the formulation of public policy.[55]

Calling a spade a spade has at least one advantage, however. By framing our choices in stark rather than obfuscated terms, we may be able to choose our path more clearly and be less surprised where it takes us.

Our society is on the brink of a paradigm shift in which the production of body parts will increasingly link the intentional ending of some lives with the salvaging of others. From fetal tissue transplant to non-heart-beating cadaver donors and beyond, these practices will inevitably pit our insatiable longing for better health and longer life against deep-seated notions of the sacred and profane. How we attempt to resolve this conflict will reveal a great deal about who we are and what we value.

We would like to thank Norman Fost, MD, for his insightful comments and suggestions.

REFERENCES

1. The practices differ in other societies. For example, the Netherlands procures organs from non-heart-beating cadaver donors (NHBCDs). Under limited conditions, active euthanasia is also permitted there. Japan does not accept "brain death."

2. Caplan AL. The telltale heart: public policy and the utilization of non-heart-beating donors. *Kennedy Institute of Ethics Journal.* 1993;3:145–155.

3. Others have suggested getting rid of the requirement that consent be obtained prior to procurement. Some European countries, for example Belgium and Austria, have already adopted this policy option, called presumed consent. (Roels L, Venrenterghem Y, Waer M, et al. Three years of experience with a "presumed consent" legislation in Belgium: its impact on multiorgan donation in comparison with European countires. *Transplantation Proceedings.* 1991;23:903–904.)

4. Fox RC. "An ignoble form of cannibalism": reflections on the Pittsburgh protocol for procuring organs from non-heart-beating cadavers. *Kennedy Institute of Ethics Journal.* 1993;3:231–239.

5. Robertson JA. Relaxing the death standard for organ donation in pediatric situations. In: Mathieu D (ed.). *Organ Substitution Technology: Ethical, Legal, and Public Policy Issues.* Boulder, CO: Westview Press; 1988.

6. DeVita MA, Snyder JV, Grenvik A. History of organ donation by patients with cardiac death. *Kennedy Institute of Ethics Journal.* 1993;3:113–129.

7. Starzl TE. *The Puzzle People: Memoirs of a Transplant Surgeon.* Pittsburgh, PA: University of Pittsburgh Press; 1992.

8. Fox RC, Swazey JP. *The Courage to Fail: A Social View of Organ Transplants and Dialysis.* 2d ed. Chicago, IL: University of Chicago Press; 1978.

9. Fellner CH, Schwartz SH. Altruism in disrepute: medical versus public attitudes toward the living organ donor. *New England Journal of Medicine.* 1971;284:582–585.

10. Council of the Transplantation Society. Commercialization in transplantation. *Transplantation.* 1986;41:1–3.

11. It is ironic that we do not allow donation from living unrelated donors, who can autonomously weigh the benefits and risks of donation, while allowing donation from family members, who may be less able to make an autonomous decision because they are under extreme pressure. (Spital A. Living organ donation: shifting responsibility. *Archives of Internal Medicine.* 1991;151:234–235.)

12. "Killing" is an important distinction here. There are cases in which a surrogate's decision to "let a patient die" is influenced by organ donation. One example involves patients with severe head trauma. Families have declined aggressive treatment that would have resulted in the patients surviving in a vegetative state, when the alternative was "brain death" and organ donation.

13. Robbins RA. Signing an organ donor card: psychological factors. *Death Studies.* 1990;14:219–229.

14. Cook R. *Coma.* Boston, MA: Little, Brown; 1977.

15. Locher D, Collins M. *Pittsburgh Press.* August 4–September 25, 1991.

16. Fost, in an article that foresees many of the problems raised by NHBCDs, argues that it was not necessary for legislators to redefine death in order to give clinicians guidance regarding these difficult matters. (Fost, n. 41).

17. Ad Hoc Committee of the Harvard Medical School to Examine the Definition of Brain Death. A definition of irreversible coma. *JAMA.* 1968;205:337–340.

18. Truog and Fackler raise questions regarding this assertion. Reviewing empirical data collected over the last ten years, they demonstrate that many patients who fulfill current clinical standards for determining death by neurologic criteria still retain selective integrative brain functions. (Truog RD, Fackler JC. Rethinking brain death. *Critical Care Medicine.* 1992;20:1705–1712.) See also Halevy A, Brody B. Brain death: reconciling definitions and tests. Unpublished.

19. Britain's initial justification for "brain death" was that it predicted, with a high degree of certainty, that the patient would soon meet traditional cardiopulmonary criteria for death. Of course, this justification confuses the near dead with the currently dead. (Pallis C. ABC of brain stem death: the arguments about EEG. *British Medical Journal.* 1983;286:284–287.)

20. Parisi JE, Kim RC, Collins GH, Hilfinger MF. Brain death with prolonged somatic survival. *New England Journal of Medicine.* 1982;306:14–16.

21. A social history of the acceptance of neurologic criteria for death, within both the medical community and the public, is badly needed.

22. Bernat JL, Culver CM, Gert B. On the definition and criterion of death. *Annals of Internal Medicine.* 1981;94:389–394.

23. Gervais KG. *Redefining Death.* New Haven, CT: Yale University Press; 1986.

24. Green MB, Wilker D. Brain death and personal identity. *Philosophy & Public Affairs.* 1980;9:105–133.

25. Youngner SK, Bartlett ET. Human death and high technology: the failure of the whole-brain formulations. *Annals of Internal Medicine.* 1983;99:252–258.

26. Veatch RM. *Death, Dying, and the Biological Revolution.* New Haven, CT: Yale University Press; 1976.

27. Youngner SJ, Landefeld CS, Coulton CJ, et al. "Brain death" and organ retrieval. A cross-sectional survey of knowledge and concepts among health professionals. *JAMA.* 1989;261:2205–2210.

28. Tomlinson T. Misunderstanding death on a respirator. *Bioethics.* 1990;4:253–264.

29. Fulton J, Fulton R, Simmons R. The cadaver donor and the gift of life. In: Simmons RG, Marina SK, Simmons RL (eds.). *Gift of Life: The Effect of Organ Transplantation on Individual, Family and Social Dynamics.* New Brunswick, NJ: Transaction Books; 1977.

30. A deeper objection, both Cole and Fost (n. 31) suggest, is that death is "a natural event or process that occurs in nature quite independently of human activity and ken" (Cole, n. 34, p. 146). As such, definitions of death exist independently of purposes and cannot be modified to meet our social purposes.

31. Fost N. Organs from anencephalic infants: an idea whose time has not yet come. *Hastings Center Report.* 1988;18(5):5–11.

32. The debate about anencephalics is instructive for other reasons. First, it shows the lengths people were willing to go to avoid breaking the dead donor rule. In addition to redefining death, others have suggested treating anencephalics as a "special category" from whom organs can be removed without violating the dead donor rule, or subjecting them to intensive care solely to allow them to be defined as dead so that their organs can be procured. (Harrison MR. The anencephalic newborn as organ donor. *Hastings Center Report.* 1986;16[2]:21–23. Walters JW, Aswal S. Organ prolongation in anencephalic infants: ethics and medical issues. *Hastings Center Report.* 1988;18[5]:19–27.) Only rarely did commentators point out that another possible solution would be to do away with the dead donor rule. (Fost, nn. 31, 41. Caplan AL. Should foetuses or infants be utilized as organ donors? *Bioethics.* 1987;1:119–140.) Second, consistent with the utilitarian justification for defining death, some might argue that the reason that attempts to morally justify organ procurement from anencephalics failed was the paucity of organs that could actually be procured. (Shewmon DA. Anencephaly: selected medical aspects. *Hastings Center Report.* 1988;18[5]:11–19.)

33. Lynn J. Are the patients who become organ donors under the Pittsburgh rotocol for "non-heart-beating donors" really dead? *Kennedy Institute of Ethics Journal.* 1993;3:167–168.

34. Cole D. Statutory definitions of death and the management of terminally ill patients who may become organ donors after death. *Kennedy Institute of Ethics Journal.* 1993;3:145–155.

35. In this way, the changes suggested in the Pittsburgh protocol mirror the recent controversy regarding organ procurement from an anencephalic infant at Loma Linda. Like Loma Linda, the University of Pittsburgh Medical Center (UPMC) chose to act first and to use their actions as an attempt to force a societal response—either acceptance or rejection through public criticism, legislation, or litigation. Fost (n. 31) criticized Loma Linda for using this approach in the anencephaly debate, and Lynn (n. 33) criticized UPMC for the same reason. They argue that seeking societal consensus and approval prior to acting is much more likely to ensure that all relevant facts, interests, and arguments are included.

36. Robertson JA. Policy issues in a non-heart-beating donor protocol. *Kennedy Institute of Ethics Journal.* 1993;3:241–250.

37. Brock DW. Voluntary active euthanasia. *Hastings Center Report.* 1992;22(2):10–22.

38. In earlier writings, Brock and others pointed out that in the medical literature "killing" and "letting die" are moral descriptions of an act that can be described in a more neutral manner. (President's Commission for the Study of Ethical Problems in Medicine and Biomedical Treatment and Behavioral Research. *Deciding to Forego Life-Sustaining Treatment.* Washington, DC: U.S. Government Printing Office; 1983.)

39. Solomon MZ, O'Donnell L, Jennings B, Guilfoy V. Decisions near the end of life: professional views on life-sustaining treatment. *American Journal of Public Health.* 1993;83:14–23.

40. Malcolm AH. Giving death a hand: rending issue. *New York Times.* June 9, 1990: A6.

41. Fost N. The new body snatchers: on Scott's *The Body As Property. American Bar Foundation Research Journal.* 1983;3:718–732.

42. Some might argue that the stricter rules are needed for organ procurement because of the non-patient-related incentives to obtain organs—e.g., the desire to help others or the institutional prestige.

43. Hadorn DC. The problem of discrimination in health care priority setting. *JAMA.* 1992;268:1454–1459.

44. LaPuma J, Lawton EF. Quality-adjusted life years. Ethical implications for doctors and policy makers. *JAMA.* 1990;263:2917–2921.

45. Where on this continuum one falls will depend on the answers to a series of questions: What is meant by violates? Must donation be risk-free or is the requirement merely that the burdens are outweighed by the benefits? Are there limits to altruism as a virtue? Is the weighting of risks and benefits solely subjective or should society impose certain standards? If so, what are they and how can they be justified in a pluralistic society?

46. Relying solely on autonomy as a guiding principle for organ procurement would solve the problem of defining what constitutes a harm, but it would raise other problems. What would be done about those who had never expressed an opinion regarding procurement? This problem would be particularly acute for the never-competent, e.g., children. The philosophical justification for surrogate decision making is not as strong as autonomous decision making. (Buchanan AE, Brock DW. *Deciding for Others: The Ethics of Surrogate Decision Making.* Cambridge: Cambridge University Press; 1989.) One might, therefore, allow an autonomous patient to donate in some circumstances in which one would not allow a surrogate to consent to donation.

47. Of course, if one eliminated the first condition of the dead donor rule, one could also take the patient's heart.

48. Some will argue that this scenario is outlandish and inflammatory. We can give up the dead donor rule, they may argue, and yet keep from sliding too far along the slippery slope. However, once we abandon the dead donor rule and depend on autonomy to guide organ procurement, allowing less severely ill patients to donate their organs seems inevitable. Moreover, if recent history is any guide, active euthanasia may become a reality.

49. Feinberg J. The mistreatment of dead bodies. *Hastings Center Report.* 1985;15(1):31–37.

50. May W. Religious justifications for donating body parts. *Hastings Center Report.* 1985;15(1):38–42.

51. May W. Attitudes toward the nearly dead. *Hastings Center Studies.* 1971;1(1):3–13.

52. Welsbard AJ. A polemic on principles: reflections on the Pittsburgh protocol. *Kennedy Institute of Ethics Journal.* 1993;3:217–230.

53. Much more needs to be said about how and why this will occur if this argument is to be tenable. After all, our recent changes regarding the forgoing of life-sustaining treatment do not seem to have coarsened our moral character.

54. We are, for example, deeply ambivalent about whether the dead donor rule should be disregarded. On the one hand, we think that there is little theoretical justification for it, and that by forsaking it we might be able to procure more organs and thus save more lives. On the other hand, we are repulsed by where this move may lead us and have grave concerns about the effect on our moral characters of treating individuals as replaceable body parts. (Fox RC, Swazey JP. *Spare Parts.* New York, NY: Oxford University Press; 1992.)

55. Calabresi G, Bobbitt P. *Tragic Choices.* New York, NY: Norton; 1978.

27

RESPONSIBILITY, ALCOHOLISM, AND LIVER TRANSPLANTATION

Walter Glannon, Ph.D.

INTRODUCTION

Medical and moral arguments have been advanced in response to the question of whether patients with alcohol-related end-stage liver disease should be given lower priority for a liver transplant than those whose disease is not alcohol related. According to the medical argument, alcoholics should have lower priority than nonalcoholics because the survival rate of the former after transplantation is lower than that of the latter, owing to a fairly high probability of relapse into alcohol abuse. According to the moral argument, alcoholics should be given lower priority for a new liver because their moral vice of heavy drinking makes them responsible for their condition and effectively forfeit their claim to medical treatment.

Two challenges have been issued to the moral argument. First, Carl Cohen and Martin Benjamin[1] maintain that the argument is defective because there is no agreement about what constitutes moral virtue and vice. Moreover, E. Haavi Morreim argues that "it is generally wrong to deny medical care because of patients' lifestyles"[2(p7)] on similar grounds. And a task force on individual responsibility for health at the University of Minnesota Center for Biomedical Ethics concluded that

---

W. Glannon. "Responsibility, Alcoholism, and Liver Transplantation." *Journal of Medicine and Philosophy*. 1998;23(2):31–49. Copyright © by The Journal of Medicine and Philosophy, Inc. Reprinted by permission.

"the state of knowledge about what causes behavior and disease is inadequate to support the imposition of punitive measures,"[3(p11)] which includes giving alcoholics lower priority for liver transplants. Thus, it seems that moral evaluation of patients of any sort should be excluded from consideration of who should be treated for liver disease. Second, Alvin Moss and Mark Siegler[4] hold that alcoholism is a disease and, as such, legitimizes medical intervention to treat it, including receiving a new liver. However, they claim that while *retrospective* considerations involving causal factors leading to the disease of alcoholism should be excluded from consideration, *prospective* considerations with respect to whether they seek treatment once they already have the disease may serve to justify giving higher priority to nonalcoholics for liver transplantation. This would be the case if a person failed to enter or comply with a recovery program such as Alcoholics Anonymous to try to keep his alcoholism in remission. These considerations are not prospective in the usual sense concerning how a patient will do with a transplant, but in the sense concerning the period after alcoholism has developed but before a decision about treatment for it is made.

I shall focus on the moral rather than medical aspects of a patient's candidacy for liver transplantation and argue that neither of these two challenges refutes the claim that some patients may be given lower priority than others on the grounds that they have retrospective responsibility for their disease. My argument will proceed in two steps.

I will argue that even if disease often befalls people due to some factors beyond their control, it does not follow that it is entirely beyond their control to prevent. We have to examine the history of the disease and determine whether or to what extent one has control over the events that lead to it. I am therefore making a stronger claim than that of Moss and Siegler, maintaining that retrospective factors extending all the way back to the behavior that caused the condition in the first place, as well as prospective ones, must be considered to establish whether a person is responsible for his diseased condition and how this affects his claim to a new liver. Furthermore, I take issue with the claims by Cohen and Benjamin, Morreim, and Caplan et al. that it is unfair or indeed punitive to exclude alcoholics from consideration for liver transplantation because of moral vice or an irresponsible lifestyle. Whether alcoholics are vicious or nonalcoholics virtuous is not what matters, but rather whether patients who need a new liver have the capacity to exercise causal control over the events that lead to end-stage liver disease. If they do have this capacity for control, but fail to exercise it within reasonable expectations, then they may be responsible for their condition and thereby weaken their claim to a new organ. If so, then it may be fair, perhaps not to exclude alcoholics entirely from transplant consideration, but to give them lower priority than those who lack this control and whose disease afflicts them through no fault of their own.

CONTROL AND RESPONSIBILITY

The idea that some people may have higher or lower priority than others concerning claims to organs or other medical resources is motivated by the fact that these resources are scarce and by the belief that some people have more control over their bodily and mental functionings than others. Generally, the more control one has over one's health, the more responsible one is for a diseased condition, defined as a physical or mental state of impaired functioning.[5,6] Conversely, the less control one has, the more one's diseased condition befalls him through no fault of his own and the less responsible he is for it. Responsibility for health is a matter of degree, as is the strength of claims to be treated for a disease.

To the extent that a person has causal control over the events that determine his healthy or diseased condition, he is causally responsible for these events as well as for this condition. Furthermore, he is morally responsible for his condition just in case he is able but fails to exercise the control he has in accord with how he reasonably can be expected to behave. It is important to emphasize that it is not whether a person actually exercises causal control, but whether he has the capacity for this control, which grounds attributions of causal and moral responsibility for his good or bad health. In sum, moral responsibility for a healthy or diseased condition presupposes causal responsibility for the events that result in that condition. Causal responsibility, in turn, presupposes causal control over these events.[7-11]

Causal control over one's health consists of four components. First, a person's choices and actions must not be coerced by external factors or compelled by internal factors such as literally irresistible impulses. Broadly construed, a person's choices and actions may be externally coerced if social and economic conditions such as an abusive upbringing or extreme poverty rule out genuine alternative possibilities of choice over time concerning such things as lifestyle and diet. In this regard, social and political institutions have to be in place to ensure adequate conditions for the choices necessary to have control over one's health. These choices constitute what Amartya Sen has called "capabilities to function,"[12] where functionings represent the various things that a person is able to do in leading a life, and the capability of a person is the ability to choose between alternative ways of achieving functionings. That a person's choices and actions are neither coerced nor compelled is not sufficient for them to be autonomous, however. Autonomy, the second component of causal control, also requires the capacity for reflective self control regarding the desires, beliefs, and intentions that issue in choices and actions. One must be able critically to evaluate these springs of action and eliminate, modify, or reinforce them and come to identify with them as one's own. As Harry Frankfurt puts it, "to the extent that a person identifies himself with the springs of his actions, he takes responsibility for those actions and acquires moral responsibility for them."[13(p54),14] Third, a person must have the cognitive capacity to foresee his diseased condition at a later time as the likely consequence of his autonomous preferences, choices, and actions at earlier times. Fourth, the consequence that is a diseased condition must be sensitive to the choices and actions (or omissions) that a person makes over time, where sensitivity is formulated in counterfactual terms. That is, holding fixed all other events external to the individual, if the patient in question had made different choices and performed different actions, then the consequence of his diseased condition would not have obtained. Causal sensitivity is a necessary, not a sufficient, condition for having causal control over one's health.

Fairness in giving a former alcoholic lower priority to receive a liver transplant requires a fifth condition beyond the four conditions of causal control and responsibility which I have just articulated. When the person begins to drink at an earlier time, he must know not only that his behavior may cause the disease and the need for treatment at a later time, but also that his behavior may result in his having lower priority to receive treatment for his disease. It seems quite reasonable to assume that most people are capable of knowing that medical resources like livers are scarce, and that they are capable of inferring from this knowledge that such scarcity might require some system of priority based on control and responsibility. Assuming that an alcoholic has causal control over his condition, and that when he begins to drink he is capable of knowing that he may be given lower priority concerning treatment for his disease, it may be fair to give him lower priority.

One might object that when persons currently in need of liver transplants began to drink, say, fifteen to twenty years ago, the idea that drinking could cause liver failure would not have occurred to them. Nor did medicine have a priority system in place which might have been based on people's responsibility for their health-care needs. But both the link between drinking and cirrhosis and the scarcity of livers for transplantation have been common knowledge for some time, and even twenty years ago most people had the capacity to know the likely consequences of heavy drinking. If one is not persuaded by these points, then at the very least we can respond by saying that henceforth basing claims to health care on responsibility should become public policy, especially given the limited supply of medical resources.

Intuitively, entitlements to health care for a diseased condition are inversely proportional to control and responsibility. The more control one has over one's health, and thus the more responsible one is for it, the weaker is one's claim to receive treatment for one's condition from the health-care system. Conversely, the less control one has over one's health and thus the less responsible one is for it, the stronger is one's claim to treatment. This view is supported by the egalitarian ethic espoused by certain political philosophers who argue that society should indemnify people against poor outcomes that are the consequences of causes beyond their control, but not against outcomes that are the consequences of causes within their control, and therefore for which persons are responsible.[15-19] These same philosophers defend the related "social cost" argument, which says that it is unfair and unreasonable to demand sacrifice from some who do exercise control over their health in order to treat others for diseases or disabilities that result from having but failing to exercise this control.[19]

Applied to the case at hand, if alcoholics have control over the events that lead to cirrhosis but fail to exercise it, and if nonalcoholics with cirrhosis or some other form of end-stage liver disease do exercise this control and yet it befalls them through no fault of their own, then it seems both reasonable and fair to conclude that alcoholics should be given lower priority than nonalcoholics in receiving a liver transplant. To uphold this claim, however, I will have to examine the idea that alcoholism as a disease involves causal factors beyond our control. Moreover, I will have to address the claim that giving lower priority to alcoholics for liver transplantation unfairly singles out and even punishes them for displaying the moral vice of heavy drinking, when in fact we all display other moral vices that lead to other diseases for which we are equally responsible.

ALCOHOLISM AS A DISEASE

Some believe that we are influenced to such a degree by our genetic inheritance, upbringing, and social and economic factors that we lack the control necessary to be responsible for most diseases,[2(p7),20(p49)] and alcoholism would be included among them. Although it has been surrounded by controversy, some researchers have discovered a link between the A1 allele of the dopamine D_2 receptor and alcoholism, which suggests that people with this allele are more susceptible than others to developing alcoholism.[21-23] But from the fact that one has a disease with a genetic component, it does not follow that one cannot be responsible for contracting the disease. A gene that makes one susceptible to alcoholism only indicates the likelihood of developing the disease, not that the gene itself causally determines the disease. In most diseases with a genetic component, a faulty gene is a necessary but not sufficient cause. Sometimes an environmental insult may also be needed, as for example in schizophrenia. This disease may be caused by a mother having a virus that penetrates the placenta, which in turn causes disruption in the migration of brain cells through the neural subplate during the second trimester of fetal development.[24] Polygenic diseases such as colon cancer require more than one faulty gene to bring them about. In the case of alcoholism, even if the A1 allele makes it more likely that a person will become addicted to alcohol over time, it seems implausible to claim that it compels a person to take the first drinks that eventually lead to the addiction and liver failure.

In order to ascertain whether a person who has a disease is responsible for it, we need to examine the etiology or history of that disease. To what extent did environmental factors external to the person (e.g., an abusive upbringing) play a causal role? To what extent did a mutant gene affect one's brain biochemistry to make one more likely to become addicted to alcohol? To what extent did the patient's own autonomous choices and actions causally contribute to the disease? Retrospective as well as prospective aspects of responsibility for one's state of health need to be considered.

One could take the tack of Moss and Siegler and claim that what one is responsible for is failure to get treatment that would successfully eliminate one's alcoholism. This seems plausible, given that alcohol-related end-stage liver disease typically results from something on the order of ten to twenty years of heavy drinking. And one could insist that what is at issue here is not prospective but retrospective responsibility, where we evaluate a person's candidacy for a liver transplant depending on whether they made an effort to get treatment. Yet a recent study sponsored by the National Institute on Alcohol Abuse and Alcoholism[25] concluded that of all the alcoholics who get treatment, at least half will relapse in two to four years. Among other things, this conclusion shows the importance of prevention and thus the need to trace responsibility for alcoholism back further to the events that brought it about in the first place. Some might insist that an alcoholic cannot be responsible for his inability to avoid a relapse once he has entered a treatment program. Yet as Aristotle points out in book 3 of the *Nicomachean Ethics*, a person may be responsible for an event or condition beyond his control at a later time if, at an earlier time, he freely performs an action or series of actions which he is capable of foreseeing will lead to an impaired condition.[26(p1758)]

The following transfer principle of responsibility can be invoked to support my claim: If a person is causally and morally responsible for freely and knowingly performing an action or series of actions at an earlier time which he ought not to have performed, and if he is responsible for the fact that these actions entail certain harmful health consequences at a later time, then he is also causally and morally responsible for these consequences. In the case at hand, the responsibility transfers from the earlier presumed free acts of drinking to the later consequences, which include both the disease and the liver disease that results from it. If this reasoning is plausible, then it is equally plausible to say that a person's alcoholism and cirrhosis need not be conditions that are beyond his control. The history of how his alcoholism developed may include enough autonomy and control for him to be at least partly responsible for both the alcoholism and the end-stage liver disease. And if, when he drinks at the earlier time, he is capable of knowing that he may be given lower priority for a liver transplant at a later time on the basis of his responsibility, then it would be fair to give him lower priority.

Except for diseases caused solely by a mutation of a single gene, like Huntington's or Tay-Sachs, or where a mutation implies an extremely high risk of disease, as in the 5 to 10 percent of breast cancer cases caused by the BRCA1 or BRCA2 gene, most diseases result from the combination of genetic and environmental factors, as well as from people's autonomous choices and actions. So most diseases are not entirely beyond one's control, and one can be at least partly responsible for them. For example, while people with Type-II (adult-onset) diabetes mellitus may be genetically susceptible to the disease, usually they develop it by combining a high-fat diet with lack of exercise. Unless they live in extreme poverty and have little or no choice concerning diet and mobility, they seem to have some control over whether or not they develop diabetes and therefore may be at least partly responsible for it. Similarly, those who are more susceptible than others to become alcoholics because they have the A1 allele of the dopamine D_2 receptor gene, but are not effectively coerced into drinking by adverse environmental factors, may have enough control over their desires, choices, and actions to refrain from drinking and thus avoid the type of behavior that leads to the disease. If so, then they may be responsible for acquiring the disease. However, if the combination of genetic and environmental factors coerces or compels a person repeatedly to act in a way that leads to the disease, then he cannot be responsible for it at all because he lacks control over the sequence of events which results in alcoholism.

It may seem unfair to give lower priority for a liver transplant to a person whose alcoholism has a genetic component, when another person who also took the risk of beginning to drink did not become an alcoholic and did not later need treatment *only* because he lacked the gene which would have led to alcoholism. Are we not punishing the first individual for having the gene? Punishment is not really the issue here. Rather, the issue is whether having the gene merely disposes one to drink or compels one to drink. If the latter is true, then the person should not be given lower priority for needed health care because his condition is caused by factors completely beyond his control and thus he is not causally or morally responsible for it. If the former is true, however, then he may be given lower priority because whether he drinks or not arguably is at least partly within his control. Crucially, the D_2 gene by itself is not sufficient to cause alcoholism, but is one causal factor among others. Thus it is misleading to say that the person who has the gene and develops cirrhosis through alcoholism is treated unfairly if he is given lower priority for a new liver simply because of the gene. Responsibility for alcoholism and cirrhosis is a matter of degree, depending on the degree of control one has over the events leading to these conditions. Consequently, the strength of one's claim to treatment or a transplant may also be a matter of degree, depending on the degree of one's control and responsibility.

As Ferdinand Schoeman[27] has pointed out, determining when these factors do or do not undermine control is a notoriously difficult task. In some cases, a person does seem to have enough control over his drinking to be held responsible for his alcoholism. In others, internal or external causes may undermine his control over his drinking and thereby excuse him from responsibility for his condition.

The United States Supreme Court ruling in the case of *Traynor and McKelvey* v. *Turnage*[28] illustrates this conflict of intuitions about responsibility for alcoholism. In this case, Traynor and McKelvey sought extended benefits from the Veterans Administration on the grounds that their earlier problems with alcohol constituted a handicap for which they were not responsible. Their claim relied on a law stating that veterans are entitled to an extension of the period during which benefits can be provided if a handicap for which they are not responsible prevented them from utilizing their benefits within ten years of being discharged. Citing Herbert Fingarette's work,[29-31] Justice Byron White, writing for the majority, reasoned that alcoholism that is not the result of an underlying psychiatric disorder is not entirely beyond the agent's control as to undermine the willfulness of the drinking and thus the condition. White concluded that Traynor's and McKelvey's alcoholism should be considered a willfully incurred disability and ruled in favor of the Veterans Administration. In his dissenting opinion, Justice Harry Blackmun pointed out that both Traynor and McKelvey began drinking at an early age, and that alcohol dependence was widespread in McKelvey's family. In the light of these factors, Blackmun concluded that, even if alcoholism is not strictly speaking a disease, there are cases in which it would not be right to hold an alcohol-dependent person responsible for his condition.

What these contrasting opinions illustrate is not so much the difficulty of establishing that alcoholism is a disease, but instead the difficulty of establishing whether a person is responsible for acquiring alcoholism. Blackmun's observations about beginning to drink at an early age and a family history of alcohol dependence in McKelvey's family underscore two conditions that can excuse a person from responsibility for the disease: (1) ignorance of the likely consequences of drinking which comes with being under the age of reason; and (2) social or environmental factors that constitute forms of coercion. On the other hand, White's opinion suggests that at least some people act freely and knowingly enough willfully to acquire this condition and be responsible for it. My aim is not to take sides, but only to emphasize the difficulty in determining whether, or to what extent, one can have control over and be responsible for alcoholism. Ultimately, it depends on the desires, choices, and actions that cause the disease, specifically whether they are autonomous or else made in ignorance or under compulsion or coercion. And because some of these conditions may hold but not others, responsibility for the disease may be a matter of degree, falling somewhere between complete excuse and complete accountability.

The idea that one may be compelled to drink by certain desires raises the important issue of addiction. Many claims have been made recently about the addictive nature of alcohol, given certain features of a person's genes and brain biochemistry. If alcohol is addictive, the argument goes, then alcoholics really are compelled to have certain desires and act on them. Accordingly, they cannot appropriately be held responsible for cirrhosis because they do not have sufficient control over the events leading to this disease. There are two responses to this argument.

First, it is important to distinguish willing from unwilling addicts, only the latter of which may be excused from responsibility from behavior presumably caused by the addiction.[13(pp11-25,47-57)] A person is an unwilling addict and thus does not act freely only if the desire associated with the addiction compels him to act in a way that defeats a contrary desire to refrain from drinking. Insofar as the addiction makes him act on a desire that he does not want to have or act on, it undermines his autonomy and, correspondingly, his responsibility for his actions and their consequences. However, if the desire to drink associated with the addiction is unopposed by a competing desire to refrain from drinking, then the addict acts freely and can be held responsible for his behavior. The upshot is that addictions per se do not necessarily undermine one's autonomy or one's responsibility for alcoholism.

Second, we must examine the *history* of the addiction and how it affects brain biochemistry. An addiction usually develops only after a person repeatedly takes in a particular substance over time. Addictive drugs like cocaine, nicotine, and alcohol affect the neurotransmitter dopamine by causing heightened metabolic activity in the mesolimbic dopamine system.[32] This system connects structures high in the brain, especially the orbitofrontal cortex, the amygdala, and the nucleus accumbens. Taking these drugs repeatedly over time perturbs the dopamine system, which adapts by making dopamine less effective. Once the relevant cells adopt this defensive maneuver and become less responsive, the cells are left without normal levels of the neurotransmitter if a person stops taking a substance that floods the mesolimbic system with dopamine. These changes in turn cause a person to crave more of the drug, and the shift to addiction occurs as dopamine dependence produces chronic unpleasant feelings, depression, and the loss of motivation, which causes the need to take the drug in order to feel better.

Significantly, the dopamine system becomes altered only when nicotine, cocaine, or alcohol is taken repeatedly over time. The addiction does not explain or causally determine why the person first takes the drug which subsequently leads to the addiction. If a person is not compelled or coerced into drinking by social factors beyond his control, and is not so young or cognitively disabled as not to be capable of knowing the likely addictive consequences of drinking repeatedly over time, then he can be responsible for acquiring the addiction, as well as for its deleterious effects on his health. Even if a person becomes addicted to alcohol, the history of how this condition came about may include enough autonomy and control for him to be deemed responsible both for the addiction and the end-stage liver disease.

It is worth emphasizing that the strength of one's claim to scarce medical resources like livers is inversely proportional to the control one has over one's health. Someone who fits the description I gave above will have a weaker claim to receive a liver than someone whose end-stage liver failure is beyond his control and thus contracted through no fault of his own. A person whose liver fails because of a Hepatitis B infection contracted through a medically necessary blood transfusion would be an example of someone whose disease befalls him through no fault of his own. Yet if he knows that he may become infected with the virus by freely engaging in high-risk behavior like sharing hypodermic needles or having multiple sex partners, but negligently or recklessly does it anyway, then he may have enough control to be responsible for his condition and correspondingly have a weaker claim to receive treatment. The point here is not that developing alcoholism entails more responsibility than acquiring Hepatitis B, but whether the person with end-stage liver disease has control over the events that lead to it. If one has this control but fails to exercise it, then one is responsible for it and may be given lower priority than someone who lacks control and gets the disease through no fault of his own. Precisely because livers are scarce, it seems both reasonable and fair to employ the notions of control and responsibility in setting this order of priority.

It may well be the case that an alcoholic with end-stage liver disease does have as strong a claim to receive a liver as a nonalcoholic with the same disease. Yet this would be so only if the combination of genetic and environmental causes beyond his control actually coerced or compelled him to drink as he gradually acquired the disease, or if he was incapable of knowing the likely consequences of his drinking.

MORAL VICE AND PUNITIVE MEASURES

The second objection to using control and responsibility as moral grounds for giving some with end-stage liver disease lower priority than others is that alcoholics are unfairly and punitively singled out for the moral vice of heavy drinking. It is unfair because all of us display different vices to varying degrees (overeating, failure to exercise, etc.) which have deleterious effects on our health. It is punitive in the sense that by giving the alcoholic lower priority for, or categorically denying him from, liver transplantation, we are in effect punishing him for a morally vicious form of behavior which is more repugnant and blameworthy than others.

Cohen and Benjamin maintain that "we could rightly preclude alcoholics from transplants only if we assume that qualification for a new organ requires some level of moral virtue, or is canceled by some level of moral vice. But there is absolutely no agreement—and there is likely to be none—about what constitutes moral virtue and vice and what rewards and penalties they deserve."[1(p1299)] This view is supported by Caplan et al., who, as I noted earlier, claim that we lack sufficient knowledge of the causes of disease to justify the imposition of punitive measures. On this basis, they conclude that moral evaluation should be excluded altogether from consideration of people's need for medical treatment.

This argument is flawed because it wrongly assumes that moral evaluation of a person's candidacy for a scarce organ is understood solely in terms of virtue and vice. Surely we can discuss causal control over and moral responsibility for the actions that lead to a disease without invoking virtue and vice. To say that a person is virtuous or vicious is to make a judgment of that person's character, which consists in a general disposition to act in a certain way.[26(pp1743ff),33] But not every type of action which a person autonomously performs repeatedly over time is reflective of his character, and therefore our actions are underdetermined by our characters. In Michael Moore's words:

> Characters, to be characters, can only typically cause some class of actions, but not others. Character in this sense is inherently general, requiring typical causal connections to classes of actions; will and the choices that issue from it are in this sense particular, being equally capable of causing any particular act and not being tied to any general class of actions.[34,35(p48)]

Generally vicious people with bad characters may at times perform a praiseworthy action or series of actions. A noteworthy example of this is Oskar Schindler, the self-serving German industrialist who saved more than a thousand Jews from the Holocaust.[36] By contrast, generally virtuous people with good characters sometimes freely perform a blameworthy action or series of actions out of weakness of will or negligence. For instance, someone who is otherwise concerned about his health may continue to smoke, even though he knows that it is bad for him. But this irrational behavior does not mean that the person who engages in it is himself vicious. Autonomous choices and actions that display a failure to exercise control and which adversely affect one's health when performed over time need not and indeed should not be construed as vicious or reflective of a vicious character. Reframing the issue in terms of control and responsibility instead of virtue and vice more adequately reflects the rationale behind the shift in emphasis in health care from treatment of disease by health-care professionals to prevention by people whose own choices and actions can determine whether they are diseased or healthy.

If alcoholics have but fail to exercise the physical and cognitive control that would have enabled them to prevent getting the disease, then they can be responsible for their disease and may have a weaker claim to treatment than nonalcoholics who do exercise this control. It is important to note that this same reasoning applies to people whose liver failure is caused by the Hepatitis B virus, if they contract the virus by freely engaging in the sorts of high-risk behavior which I mentioned above. Similarly, if a person with a genetic predisposition to malignant melanoma freely spends many hours in the sun, then he, too, may be given lower priority concerning treatment than one who avoids the sun and whose melanoma afflicts him through no fault of his own (for example, if he has mutations of both the Mt S1, or multiple tumor suppressor gene, and the CDK4 gene, which binds to the regulatory protein p16 controlling the normal rate of cell division.[37] What all of these examples have in common is that they involve a moral judgment of lower or higher priority for claims to medical treatment not on grounds of virtue and vice, but on grounds of the control of their behavior which they reasonably can be expected to exercise. This control makes them either more or less responsible for their condition and in turn determines the strength of their claims to receive treatment.

Earlier, I noted the problem of social cost, which says that it is unreasonable to expect some people to bear the social costs of others' conditions that are at least partly within their control to prevent. In risky activities like alpine skiing or mountain climbing, we can distribute these costs more equally and fairly by taxing people for engaging in that behavior. Or with respect to people who ride motorcycles without helmets, the costs of head injuries can be dealt with by increasing the insurance premiums of motorcycle riders. In the case of a scarce, nonrenewable organ like a liver, though, the measures that I have just mentioned are ineffectual because liver transplantation involves not *economic* but rather *physical* scarcity of a resource. Assigning priority to receive the organ on the basis of the control the person reasonably can be expected to exercise over the preferences, choices, and actions that lead to his diseased condition, is perhaps the only fair way of resolving the problem of balancing physical scarcity of medical resources with entitlements to these resources.

The policy I have proposed should not be understood as implying that the alcoholic did something wrong and is denied a liver transplantation as punishment for this wrong. Instead, it should be understood in the following way: If a person acts on autonomously formed preferences and choices, and if he is capable of knowing what the probable consequences of his behavior will be, then he weakens his entitlement to receive treatment for a diseased condition he has brought upon himself. The weakening of the entitlement is not a form of punishment imposed on him externally, but something that he brings upon himself as the consequence of his own preferences, choices, and actions over time.

This idea is captured in what the political philosopher Thomas Scanlon[38] calls (but does not explicitly endorse) the "Forfeiture View," which is not an idea of desert, nor, conversely, of punishment. More precisely: "It is not an idea according to which certain choices, because they are foolish, immature, or otherwise mistaken, positively merit certain outcomes or consequences. The idea is rather that a person to whom a certain outcome was available, but who knowingly passed it up, cannot complain about not having it: *volenti non fit iniuria*"(p. 81). As Scanlon points out, however, this view is defensible only insofar as social and political institutions are in place to ensure the conditions necessary to make autonomous choices concerning, for example, which type of diet one should have and to what extent one should engage in physical exercise to maintain one's health. Provided that these institutions and conditions for choice are in place, if a person takes a risk by freely engaging in behavior that is harmful to his health, such as drinking, then we may conclude that he has but fails to exercise control and therefore may be responsible for his disease. And if he is responsible for it, then his entitlement to a liver transplant may be diminished.

If we do not employ the criteria of control and responsibility in assessing whether some people should be given higher priority over others in their claims to a scarce medical resource, then we risk undermining what may very well be the fairest policy available. Perhaps more importantly, we would debase rather than affirm the value of autonomy. Autonomy and responsibility are mutually entailing notions. Freedom to make choices and act on these choices entails the capacity to take responsibility for them and their consequences. By the same token, responsibility for choices, actions, and consequences presupposes that a person makes, performs, and brings them about autonomously. To say that alcoholics cannot be responsible for end-stage liver failure because alcoholism is a disease, or that it unfairly singles them out for a moral vice when nonalcoholics display other vices, threatens to divorce autonomy from responsibility. It is as if we were saying that, even if the choices that lead to the disease are not compelled or coerced, it is unfair to hold the person making those choices responsible for their consequences because we are all "sinners" capable of making bad choices that can adversely affect our health (as Caplan et al. claim). Yet autonomy and responsibility are essential features of our personhood. And the responsibility we are capable of taking for our autonomous choices and actions as well as their consequences is what makes each of us unique as a person.

So to dismiss moral responsibility from assessment of our claims to scarce medical resources in general, and to liver transplantation in particular, is to debase our autonomy and personhood. Provided that they are capable of being responsible for their choices and actions as well as for the healthy or diseased consequences of these choices and actions, giving lower priority to alcoholics than nonalcoholics is not punitive but an affirmation of people's ability to take responsibility for their own health.

It is instructive to evaluate my claims and arguments in the light of the recent shift in the rules governing priority in liver transplantation by the United Network for Organ Sharing.[39] The network has revised the long-standing policy of putting the sickest patients at the top of the list for new livers, regardless of their chances of survival. The new policy gives priority to people who face imminent death because of acute liver failure (for example, from mushroom poisoning) over those who are just as ill but whose liver failure is due to a chronic disease like cirrhosis of the liver caused by alcoholism or by a Hepatitis B or C infection. The rationale for this shift is that patients in the acute category are the sickest and have the most urgent need in that they may die within hours or days without a transplant. Not surprisingly, they also have better survival rates than patients in the chronic category. Ostensibly, this policy shift is motivated by medical reasons alone. Yet it raises the moral question of how to balance fairness and utility when there are not enough livers for all who need them. And fairness does involve responsibility insofar as it presupposes that the diseased condition that moves people to make claims to receive health care befalls them through no fault of their own. Insofar as a person knows that freely eating certain mushrooms has a high probability of causing liver failure but eats them anyway, he may be responsible for his acute condition. On the other hand, people may contract Hepatitis B or C through no fault of their own and thus not be responsible for their chronic condition. If fairness is a factor in deciding who should receive priority for a new liver, then, given the connection between fairness and responsibility, responsibility should also be a factor in addition to imminent death and survival in setting this priority.

CONCLUSION

I have argued that moral considerations may be invoked in assigning priority to some people over others concerning liver transplantation, especially in the light of the fact that livers are scarce organs. Contrary to what Cohen and Benjamin maintain, these moral considerations are not grounded in virtue or vice, nor are they punitive, as Caplan et al. suggest. Instead, they are grounded in control and responsibility. Insofar as a person's choices and actions are not compelled or coerced by addictions or adverse social circumstances like extreme poverty, and insofar as he is capable of foreseeing that his choices and actions likely will lead to cirrhosis of the liver, he has sufficient control over these events and their consequences to be responsible for this disease. In addition, if he is capable of foreseeing that his control over and responsibility for liver failure will give him lower priority for needed medical treatment, then it is fair to given him lower priority for that treatment. Furthermore, I made a stronger claim than that of Moss and Siegler, holding that retrospective as well as prospective factors must be considered when deciding whether to treat a person for a disease. That is, we must examine how the person contracted the disease in the first place and whether he had sufficient control over antecedent events to prevent it from obtaining. It may be fair to give lower priority to alcoholics *if* they have but fail to exercise control over the events that lead to their disease and liver failure, and if non-alcoholics with liver failure do exercise this control.

The view that earlier behavior under one's control can be at least a partial cause of the later need for health care has broad implications for the way we evaluate people's claims of need for medical treatment. Roughly, around forty or fifty percent of total health care measured in dollar costs involves behaviorally caused needs. Admittedly, ascertaining whether one is causally and morally responsible for one's need for treatment may result in some loss of privacy. This would represent a fundamental change in medicine's currently accepted norm that it should be need and not other factors which should determine whether one has a claim to be treated. Obviously, this issue needs further discussion that goes beyond the scope of this paper. Nevertheless, it is worth pointing out that, however difficult it may be to implement this idea in practice, in principle the economic and especially physical scarcity of medical resources may very well require differentiations to be made on the basis of causal and moral responsibility. Indeed, scarcity is the main reason why responsibility should be a factor in shaping public policy concerning health care.

In an era of scarce medical resources, there has been a necessary shift in emphasis from treatment to prevention of disease. This shift presupposes that people are able to make autonomous choices and actions and to take responsibility for their health. If we are to make good on this claim, and to affirm the value of autonomy and responsibility so essential to our personhood, then we have to hold people responsible for diseases they contract when they are able but fail to exercise control over the events that cause these diseases. This may mean giving lower priority to some versus others concerning claims to medical treatment. But provided that these decisions are based on control and responsibility, it may be fair to discriminate on these grounds.

I am grateful to two anonymous referees for very helpful comments on earlier drafts of this paper. Work on the paper was supported by a Killam Postdoctoral Fellowship.

REFERENCES

1. Cohen C, Benjamin M. Alcoholics and liver transplantation. *JAMA.* 1991;265:1999–1301.

2. Morreim EH. Lifestyles of the risky and infamous. *Hastings Center Report.* 1995;25(November/December):5–13.

3. Caplan A et al. *Sinners, Saints & Health Care: Individual Responsibility for Health—Ethical, Legal and Economic Questions.* Minneapolis, MN: University of Minnesota Center for Biomedical Ethics; 1994.

4. Moss A, Siegler M. Should alcoholics compete equally for liver transplantation? *JAMA.* 1991;265:1295–1298.

5. Boorse C. On the distinction between disease and illness. In: Cohen M, Nagel T, Scanlon T (eds.). *Medicine and Moral Philosophy.* Princeton, NJ: Princeton University Press; 1981:3–22.

6. Brock D. Quality of life measures in health care and medical studies. In: Nussbaum MC, Sen A (eds.). *The Quality of Life.* Oxford: Clarendon Press; 1993:95–132.

7. Fischer JM. Responsibility and control. *Journal of Philosophy.* 1982;79:24–40.

8. Fischer JM. *The Metaphysics of Free Will.* Cambridge: Blackwell; 1994.

9. Glannon W. Responsibility and the principle of possible action. *Journal of Philosophy.* 1995;92(May):261–274.

10. Glannon W. Sensitivity and responsibility for consequences. *Philosophical Studies.* 1997;87(September):223–233.

11. Fischer JM, Ravizza M. *Responsibility and Control: A Theory of Moral Responsibility.* New York, NY: Cambridge University Press; 1997.

12. Sen A. Capability and well-being. In: Nussbaum M, Sen A (eds.). *The Quality of Life.* Oxford: Clarendon Press; 1993:30–53.

13. Frankfurt H. *The Importance of What We Care About.* New York, NY: Cambridge University Press; 1988.

14. Taylor C. Responsibility for self. In: Rorty AO (ed.). *The Identities of Persons.* Berkeley, CA: University of California Press; 1976:281–299.

15. Rawls J. *A Theory of Justice.* Cambridge, MA: Harvard Belknap Press; 1971.

16. Rawls J. Social unity and primary goods. In: Sen A, Williams D (eds.). *Utilitarianism and Beyond.* Cambridge: Cambridge University Press; 1982:159–185.

17. Dworkin R. What is equality? Part II: equality of resources. *Philosophy and Public Affairs.* 1981;10(fall):283–345.

18. Arneson R. Equality and equal opportunity for welfare. *Philosophical Studies.* 1989;56:77–93.

19. Roemer J. A pragmatic theory of responsibility for the egalitarian planner. *Philosophy and Public Affairs.* 1993;22(spring):146–166.

20. Lockwood M. Quality of life and resource allocation. In: Bell JM, Mendus S (eds.). *Philosophy and Medical Welfare.* Cambridge: Cambridge University Press; 1988:33–55.

21. Blum K et al. Allelle association of human dopamine D2 receptor gene in alcoholism. *JAMA.* 1990;263:2055–2060.

22. Bolos A et al. Population and pedigree studies reveal a lack of association between the dopamine D2 receptor gene and alcoholism. *JAMA.* 1990;264:3156–3160.

23. Cloninger CR. D2 dopamine receptor gene is associated but not linked with alcoholism. *JAMA.* 1991;266:1833–1834.

24. Potkin S et al. Catching up on schizophrenia. *Archives of General Psychiatry.* 1996;53:456–462.

25. Babor T et al. Matching alcoholism treatments to client heterogeneity: Project MATCH posttreatment drinking outcomes. *Journal of Studies on Alcohol.* 1997;58(January):7–29.

26. Aristotle, *Nicomachean Ethics.* In: Barnes J (ed.). *The Complete Works of Aristotle.* Princeton, NJ: Princeton University Press; 1984.

27. Schoeman F. Alcohol addiction and responsibility attributions. In: Graham G, Stephens GL. *Philosophical Psychopathology.* Cambridge, MA: MIT Press; 1994:183–204.

28. *Traynor and McKelvey* v. *Turnage,* 108 S. Ct. 1372 (1988).

29. Fingarette H. The perils of Powell: in search of a factual formulation for the disease concept of alcoholism. *Harvard Law Review.* 1971;83:793–812.

30. Fingarette H. Legal aspects of alcoholism and other addictions: some basic conceptual issues. *British Journal of Addiction.* 1981;76:125–132.

31. Fingarette H. *Heavy Drinking: The Myth of Alcoholism As a Disease.* Berkeley, CA: University of California Press; 1988.

32. Koob G. Drug addiction: the yin and yang of hedonic homeostasis. *Neuron.* 1996:893–896.

33. Kupperman J. *Character.* New York, NY: Oxford University Press; 1991.

34. Moore M. *Law and Psychiatry: Rethinking the Relationship.* Cambridge: Cambridge University Press; 1984.

35. Moore M. Choice, character, and excuse. In: Paul EF, Miller F, Paul J (eds.). *Crime, Culpability, and Remedy.* Cambridge: Cambridge University Press; 1990;29–58.

36. Kenneally T. *Schindler's List.* London: Penguin; 1982.

37. Dracopoli N et al. Mutations associated with familial melanoma impair p16INK4 function. *Nature Genetics.* 1995;10(May):114–116.

38. Scanlon T. The significance of choice. In: Darwall S (ed.). *Equal Freedom.* Ann Arbor, MI: University of Michigan Press; 1995:39–104.

39. Kolata G. In shift, prospects for survival will decide liver transplants. *New York Times.* November 15, 1996:1, 15.

Part 11

ISSUES IN
MANAGED CARE

❦

When it is our turn to be that "someone else" who is critically ill or injured, we expect to be provided with whatever tests, procedures, surgeries, and medications are necessary to bring about the quickest and most effective recovery, as we see it. The cost of our ICU bed, physical therapy, IVs, and reconstructive surgery never enters our awareness—that is, until our health insurer (HMO, PPO, and the like) denies coverage. In recent years our newspapers have become quite efficient in demonstrating that this does not always happen to someone else. This awareness has ingrained into our collective consciousness that modern medicine is as much a business as it is an art and a science.

Using financial incentives, drug formularies, gag clauses, gatekeeping, utilization review, and precertification, health insurers struggle to balance our desire for patient care that is high quality, cost effective, and accessible. Obviously, something has to give, as we are spending almost 15 percent of our GDP on health care, almost 7 percent more than all other industrialized nations. The Joint Commission on Accreditation of Healthcare Organizations (JCAHO) considers these efforts morally significant enough to require that all healthcare institutions address the effects of such cost containment schemes in their code of ethics. In particular, JCAHO's "Organizational Ethics" standard requires the code of ethics to ensure the integrity of clinical decision making is protected.[1] To that end, this following readings discuss two important issues regarding the formation of a code of organizational ethics: (1) the meaning of and process for determining what is and is not medically necessary, and (2) the effect of cost-containment policies on the patient–health-care provider relationship.

In "Who Should Determine When Health Care Is Medically Necessary?" Sara Rosenbaum, David Frankford, and Brad Moore discuss how "medical necessity" assessments have become the newest cost-containment technique. Using various sources of data, health insurers have tried to determine what tests, procedures, medications, and rehab programs are "beneficial" for populations of patients, and then apply their findings to cases of specific patients. In this short reading, the authors raise several important issues such as appropriate sources of data, problems with generalized data, and the need for national reform concerning the definition of medical necessity. One of the key ethical issues they raise concerns exceptions to medical necessity; for example, if a watchmaker (or pianist, tennis star, surgeon, etc.) severely injures her wrist, she will receive the same treatment options as the random person off the street. Yet these particular patients need a top hand surgeon whereas the random person off the street needs only a "standard" hand surgeon. Without taking account of what constitutes "normal" for both individuals and populations, a health insurer's definition of medical necessity will be unjust, as it will approve treatment that is appropriate for some and substandard for others.

In "The Impact of Managed Care on Patients' Trust in Medical Care and Their Physicians," David Mechanic and Mark Schlesinger carefully lay out the ways in which various cost-saving schemes used by health insurers can harm the patient–health-care provider relationship. In particular, the authors address financial incentives (e.g., capitation), utilization review, and the process of treatment and referral. In a capitated environment health insurers contract with physicians and physician groups to provide care by paying them a set amount of money per enrollee (aka subscriber). At the end of each year, whatever is left over from the capitated fee is kept by the physician or physician group. The primary concern this business relationship raises is that every test, procedure, and/or hospital admission translates into less money kept by the physician at the end of the year. As the authors make clear, this corporatization of medicine has placed the financial interests of the physician in direct conflict with the health interests of the patient, as physicians obviously have a strong incentive to do less.

On the other hand, when physicians do provide a particular intervention, utilization review comes in. Simply, utilization review retrospectively determines whether a test or procedure was needed, with "need" being defined soley by the insurer. If it is determined the treatment was not needed then it will not be covered; in other words, the patient is stuck with the bill. A variation of this scheme is called "precertification," which requires physicians to submit the proposed treatment to the health insurer for review prior to its provision. Needless to say, insurers do not pay for treatment they determine to be unnecessary. Some precertification clauses stipulate that even if the insurer would have determined the treatment was necessary, if it is not submitted for prior review the claim will be denied. A particularly morally dubious cost-containment technique that is also addressed is confidentiality (or gag) clauses. These are contractual clauses in which physicians agree: (1) to not discuss the financial incentive program with their patients; (2) to not disparage the health insurer or its policies; (3) to not recommend test or treatment options that are not covered by a patient's plan; and (4) to not give a patient information about tests or treatment options that are not covered by the patient's plan. The ethical issues raised by such clauses clearly go to the very core of what it means to make an informed decision. When information is withheld from a patient regarding treatment options, his ability to make an informed decision has all but been removed.

NOTE

1. Joint Commission on Accreditation of Healthcare Organizations. *2000 Hospital Accreditation Standards.* Oakbrook, IL: JCAHO; 2000:83.

28

WHO SHOULD DETERMINE WHEN HEALTH CARE IS MEDICALLY NECESSARY?

Sara Rosenbaum, J.D., David M. Frankford, J.D.,
Brad Moore, M.D., M.P.H., and Phyllis Borzi, J.D., M.A.

I n the United States there has been a radical shift in the power to determine when health care is medically necessary and therefore covered by insurance. From the 1950s through the late 1970s, physicians' medical opinions largely dictated coverage and were rarely challenged by insurers. Physicians no longer have this extraordinary level of autonomy. Insurers now routinely make treatment decisions by determining what goods and services they will pay for. The line between clinical decisions about necessary medical care and decisions about insurance coverage is particularly blurred in managed-care plans. The power of insurers to determine coverage potentially gives them the power to dictate professional standards of care for all but the wealthiest patients.

At present, the power of insurers is constrained by law in two ways. First, insurance contracts typically use clinically derived professional standards of care as the basis for determinations of medical necessity and coverage. The courts frequently reverse insurers' attempts to deviate from these standards, particularly where the insurer has ignored the patient's medical record, the opinion of the treating physician, experts' opinions, and pertinent data from government-sponsored or peer-reviewed studies.[1-4] Second, in cases in which patients have appealed insurers' decisions under the Employee Retirement Income Security Act (ERISA), the courts have consistently overturned decisions that were arbitrary and capricious and that represented an abuse of the trust between the insurer and the insured.[1,2,4] The courts are particularly sensitive to the fact that insurers have a conflict of interest because they stand to gain financially from denying coverage.[3]

ERISA regulates health and welfare benefits for more than 140 million workers and their families; thus, many determinations of medical necessity are now held to a minimal standard of fairness. Even this minimal level of protection is threatened, however. Insurers are learning how to write contracts so that standards of medical necessity are not only separated from standards of good clinical practice but also essentially not subject to review.[5,6] Insurers are also pushing for legislation to change ERISA. Legislation passed by the House[7] and introduced in the Senate[8] would have granted insurers the explicit power to define medical necessity apart from current standards of medical practice by allowing them to classify as medically unnecessary any procedure not specifically found to be necessary by the insurer's own technical-review panel. The Senate proposal would also have granted insurers the power to determine what evidence would be relevant in evaluating a claim for coverage and would have permitted insurers to classify some coverage decisions as exempt from administrative review. An alternative bipartisan bill introduced in the Senate would have required that insurers' standards of medical necessity reflect "generally accepted principles of professional medical practice"; prohibited insurers from "arbitrarily interfer[ing] with or alter[ing] the decision of the treating physician"; required insurers to provide an external administrative review of any coverage decision; and required that the external reviewer consider, among other evidence, the patient's health and medical information, the opinion of the treating physician, valid and replicable studies in the peer-reviewed literature, the results of professional consensus conferences, practice guidelines based on government-funded studies, and guidelines prepared by insurers that have been determined to be "free of any conflict of interest."[9] None of these proposals became law, but similar bills are likely to be introduced in the next session of Congress.

Groups such as the Advisory Commission on Consumer Protection and Quality in the Health Care Industry have recommended only procedural protection for patients, such as the right to a timely review of an adverse decision about coverage.[10] Although procedural reforms are important, no amount of procedural protection can help patients if insurers are given broad power to determine what standards will be used to make decisions about coverage. Such "protection" would be an instance of winning a battle but losing the war.

In our view, an insurer should be able to set aside the recommendations of a treating physician only in restricted circumstances. Decisions about coverage should continue to be weighed against clinically accepted standards of medical practice. An insurer's decision should be lawful only if the insurer can prove that the decision rests on valid and reliable evidence that is relevant to a patient's individual circumstances. We advocate neither a return to total autonomy for treating physicians in determining insurance coverage nor a system in which insurers decide on coverage according to criteria that are totally independent of professional standards of clinical practice. Rather, we propose maintaining the middle position represented by current law. This middle position requires insurers to act reasonably and weighs the reasonableness of their conduct against professional standards of practice as reflected by valid and reliable evidence.

BACKGROUND

Deciding whether proposed medical care is covered by insurance involves the interpretation of legal terms found in a health-plan contract. A contract typically defines covered services as those that are "medically reasonable and necessary." Usually, coverage hinges on the answers to two questions. First, is the proposed service a type that is covered? For example, radiography is covered as a type of diagnostic service. Second, even if the contemplated care is a type generally covered, is its use medically reasonable and necessary in this particular case and thus warranted? To answer the second question, the decision-making process should be individualized and factual. Three general issues are made explicit in the case law governing decision making by private insurers. First, who has the power to decide what is medically necessary? Second, what evidence can and must be used to justify that decision? Third, who bears the burden of proof: must the insurer demonstrate with acceptable evidence that a recommended treatment is unnecessary, or does the patient bear the burden of demonstrating that the treatment in question is necessary?

Traditionally, insurers considered care and services medically necessary whenever treating physicians said they were necessary. However, as the cost of health insurance escalated, commercial insurers, Medicare, and Medicaid began to review the medical necessity of physicians' treatment recommendations as the basis for determining which procedures and services would be covered.[11] Even so, for more than two hundred years, the courts in malpractice cases have turned to clinical practices for evidence of when and under what circumstances medical care should be considered medically necessary,[12] and insurers therefore have relied on the prevailing clinical standards of care.

Recently, however, it has been suggested that the definition of medical necessity should be separated from clinical practices. Eddy proposed that coverage of medical care should be determined largely on the basis of studies showing its benefit in a population.[13] Havighurst championed the inclusion of provisions in health-plan contracts that explicitly delineate covered and uncovered services and that generally separate coverage from what he termed "professional control."[14] Implicit in such recommendations is the belief that insurers should have the power to make a conclusive and nonreviewable decision that a particular service is unnecessary and therefore excluded from coverage. Thus, for example, in applying a contract provision that excluded high-dose chemotherapy for certain forms of "advanced cancer," an insurer would be allowed to decide unilaterally that a patient's cancer was sufficiently advanced to trigger the exclusion.

In response to the pressures of cost, insurers may add provisions to contracts that exclude coverage of care for specific diseases and that link medical necessity to broad standards based on evidence involving large groups of patients rather than to clinically derived professional standards applied to particular patients. Such provisions would be unfortunate, for three reasons. First, a sole reliance on broad standards derived from generalized evidence is at odds with good medical practice. Second, there are practical limits to designing studies that can answer all clinical questions. Even if such studies could be conducted, it would be impractical to incorporate all the results into contract provisions. Third, much of the existing evidence that might be used to justify wholesale, nonreviewable exclusions of coverage is of insufficient scientific quality to displace clinical judgment.

PROBLEMS WITH THE USE OF GENERALIZED EVIDENCE OF MEDICAL NECESSITY

The practice of medicine has a core ethical dimension and requires that the physician use his or her knowledge of the particular patient in deciding on the course of treatment along with the patient. Thus, even when there are good data on the effectiveness of an intervention, it is bad medical policy to apply general rules arbitrarily to all cases. A recent case involving a child with severe cerebral palsy illustrates this point. The child's pediatrician and pediatric neurologist prescribed physical therapy to prevent muscular atrophy and possibly allow the child to walk. On the basis of a single article in a medical journal, however, the insurer's medical director decided that intensive physical therapy can never speed the development of such children. A federal appeals court found the decision to be without any rational basis and required that the insurer cover the physical therapy.[2]

All standards of care, including those based on rigorous scientific evidence, implicitly or explicitly use outcomes as the benchmark, and the choice of an outcome is inherently value laden. Take the example of a patient with a broken wrist. For most patients who perform ordinary activities with their hands, simply setting the bone might suffice to restore a reasonable range of motion. For a concert pianist, however, who requires a wider range of motion, more aggressive surgery might be essential. Which outcome should be the basis for the decision about insurance coverage: the functional level necessary for playing the piano or the functional level required for ordinary activities? Even in such a simple case, much less a more complicated one, this question cannot be answered without taking into account the value of the surgery, which in turn depends on the identity, goals, and values of the individual patient. Accounting for individual variation is part and parcel of clinical practice and is largely what medical practice is all about. Insurance provisions regarding medical necessity must be flexible enough to take into account the needs and circumstances of each patient.

Decisions about insurance coverage that rely solely on broad standards derived from generalized evidence diminish the ability of clinicians to perform their roles, because they lock in certain outcomes and effectively impose "one size fits all" values. Such decisions also formalize the generalizations based on large-scale evidence and incorporate them into the insurance contract as a hidden limitation of coverage. At the extreme, physicians and patients are left with no discretion. The clinician's knowledge of the individual patient is rendered irrelevant.

PRACTICAL LIMITATIONS OF GENERALIZED EVIDENCE

There are also practical limitations to basing decisions about medical necessity on generalized evidence. Much of medical practice is the result of tradition and collective experience. Many basic medical interventions have not been studied rigorously. Researchers often examine intermediate results or report process measures rather than ultimate outcomes. Furthermore, aside from a handful of procedures that are explicitly identified as covered or not covered, most medical care is not specifically described in a health-plan contract, and for good reason: the number of procedures and the circumstances of their application are limitless. No amount of effort could produce a contract that specified all of them. If coverage depended on generalized evidence concerning large classes of patients, then most care would not be covered.

Many evidence-based studies of medical interventions examine their efficacy in a controlled clinical setting rather than in actual practice.[15] Interventions are often studied in isolation, yet physicians need to know the benefits of one over another. Moreover, randomized clinical trials are expensive to conduct, particularly if attempts are made to account for variations in the characteristics of patients, coexisting conditions, and other such factors. Given the enormous number of procedures and the individual circumstances of patients, limiting insurance coverage to a host of separately validated and specifically described procedures is impractical.

THE RIGORS OF SCIENCE

In addition, we must consider the actual circumstances in which insurance companies apply evidence of medical necessity. Carefully developed criteria for coverage are of relatively limited consequence if the decision maker is allowed to disregard critical evidence or use flawed, biased, or otherwise unreliable evidence in deciding whether a particular patient's situation meets the criteria.

Decision making by insurers about medical care is not well understood. In one study of the evidence considered by insurers in making decisions about coverage, researchers collected data on the process and information used by 231 physicians at health plans representing 66 percent and 72 percent of the U.S. population covered by health maintenance organizations and indemnity plans, respectively.[16] Medical directors were asked to rank the sources of information they used to make decisions. They were offered many choices, including medical journals, opinions of local or national experts, documents of the Food and Drug Administration, practice guidelines, Medicare policies, National Institutes of Health (NIH) consensus conferences, and the practices of other, larger plans. Even the most highly ranked source of information—medical journals—was used or considered optimal by less than 60 percent of the respondents. Most sources of information were used or considered optimal by 40 percent or less of the respondents, and information generated by the trade associations representing the health plans and undefined practice guidelines was ranked ahead of information from national experts, government documents, and NIH consensus conferences. In another study, insurers consistently denied coverage for growth hormone therapy for children, even in the case of diagnoses for which there was a 96 percent treatment-approval rate (virtual consensus) among surveyed pediatric endocrinologists.[17] These findings are consistent with the fact that materials such as the practice guidelines prepared by Milliman and Robertson,[18] a well-known actuarial firm, often rely on insurers' own decisions rather than on well-designed scientific research.

The need to control costs and generate profits also brings into question the reliability and soundness of decision making by insurers. The sine qua non of scientific research is the production of objective results, and objectivity is ensured through a process of open and vigorous debate among persons who have no financial stake in the outcome. Yet much of the decision making about insurance coverage is based on unpublished, proprietary, and unreviewed data. Furthermore, methods are undisclosed and unexamined unless litigation ensues. An endeavor that operates in this fashion and is subject to the conflict of interest inherent in the insurance industry cannot justifiably be called scientific.

THE NEED FOR NATIONAL REFORM

National legislation is needed to ensure continued linkage between decisions about the medical necessity of care for individual patients and clinical practice, for three reasons. First, the states have little or no power in this regard, because ERISA shields many or most decisions about medical necessity from the reach of state laws that govern insurance contracts.[19] Second, although patients may sue under ERISA to reverse an adverse determination of medical necessity, they can recover only the value of the benefits denied, not damages for injuries sustained as a result of the denial. Thus, even though a federal court ultimately reinstated coverage of physical therapy for the child with cerebral palsy, the family could not sue the insurer to recover damages for harm suffered by the child while they awaited the ruling. Third, even ERISA's limited remedy will be precluded, as insurance contracts are rewritten to give insurers the authority to base decisions about medical necessity on generalized, questionable evidence that is separate from clinical practice and that does not take into account the circumstances of particular patients.[5,6] National action is needed, not only to ensure a rapid and fair process for review of coverage decisions, but also to guard against arbitrary exclusion of services from coverage.

Congress should enact legislation that maintains the link between medical necessity and professional practice standards. An insurer should be able to set aside the decision of the treating physician only if the insurer can show that the proposed treatment conflicts with clinical standards of care or that there is substantial scientific evidence, regardless of clinical practices, that the proposed care would be unsafe or ineffective or that an alternative course would lead to an equally good outcome. By substantial evidence, we mean a sizable number of studies published in peer-reviewed journals that meet professionally recognized standards of validity and replicability and that are free of conflicts of interest. These are the requirements currently written into most contracts and enforced by the courts, which require insurers to act reasonably and not arbitrarily.[1,2] There is obviously room for interpretation of what is meant by substantial scientific evidence and for debate about the validity and replicability of various methods of evaluation, such as randomized clinical trials, consensus-based standards of appropriate care, and meta-analyses. Similarly, there is room for debate about how generalized evidence might affect an individual patient. Such debate is necessary and healthy. Finally, Congress should ensure that patients have access to a speedy, external administrative review of all coverage decisions, not merely those that insurers decide are subject to review. Congress should also stipulate that external reviewers may consider a broad array of evidence.

REFERENCES

1. *Adams* v. *Blue Cross/Blue Shield of Maryland*, 757 F. Supp. 661 (D. Md. 1991).

2. *Bedrick* v. *Travelers Insurance Co.*, 93 F.3d 149 (4th Cir. 1996).

3. *Firestone Tire and Rubber* v. *Bruch*, 489 U.S. 101 (1989).

4. *McGraw* v. *Prudential Insurance Company of America*, 137 F.3d 1253 (10th Cir. 1998).

5. *Fuja* v. *Benefit Trust Life Insurance Co.*, 18 F.3d 1405 (7th Cir. 1994).

6. *Harris* v. *Mutual of Omaha Co.*, 992 F.2d 706 (7th Cir. 1993).

7. H.R. 4250, Title I, Subtitle B, §111(b) and (e) of ERISA, as added by §1101(b)(2)(4); §503(b), as added by §1201(a) (105th Cong., 2d Sess.).

8. S. 2330, Title I, Subtitle C, §503(e)(1) and (4) of ERISA, as added by §121(a) (105th Cong., 2d Sess.).

9. S. 2416, §102(b)(1) and (4); §106(b)(3) (105th Cong., 2d Sess.).

10. President's Advisory Commission on Consumer Protection and Quality in the Health Care Industry. *Quality First: Better Health Care for All Americans*. Washington, DC: US Government Printing Office; 1998.

11. Bergthold LA. Medical necessity: do we need it? *Health Affairs*. 1995;14(4):180–190.

12. *Slater* v. *Baker and Stapleton*, 95 Eng. Rep. 860, 862 (King's Bench 1767), holding that in determining the liability of a surgeon for malpractice the proper standard of review was "the usage and the law of surgeons ... the rule of the profession ..." and the proper evidence was the testimony of other surgeons.

13. Eddy DM. Rationing resources while improving quality: how to get more for less. *JAMA*. 1994;272:817–824.

14. Havighurst CC. Prospective self-denial: can consumers contract today to accept health care rationing tomorrow? *University of Pennsylvania Law Review*. 1992;140:1755–1808.

15. Franklin C. Basic concepts and fundamental issues in technology assessment. *Intensive Care Medicine.* 1993;19:117–121.

16. Steiner CA, Powe NR, Anderson GF, Das A. The review process used by US health care plans to evaluate new medical technology for coverage. *Journal of General Internal Medicine.* 1996;11:294–302.

17. Finkelstein BS, Silvers JB, Marrero U, Neuhauser D, Cuttler L. Insurance coverage, physician recommendations, and access to emerging treatments. *JAMA.* 1998;279:663–638.

18. *Healthcare Management Guidelines.* New York: Milliman and Robertson; 1996–1998.

19. *Corcoran* v. *United HealthCare,* 965 F.2d 1321 (5th Cir.), cert. den. 506 U.S. 1033 (1992).

29

THE IMPACT OF MANAGED CARE ON PATIENTS' TRUST IN MEDICAL CARE AND THEIR PHYSICIANS

David Mechanic, Ph.D., and Mark Schlesinger, Ph.D.

T rust always has been central to relationships between physicians and patients. Throughout this century, the medical community made extraordinary efforts to build confidence in physicians' competence and ethics through rigorous standards for education and accreditation and through active public relations. However, in recent decades there have been many challenges to the public's trust in U.S. medicine, a consequence of changing organizational and financial arrangements, well-publicized disputes about treatment and training practices, and a greater consumer orientation by many patients. As a result, confidence in medicine collectively has plummeted.[1] Nevertheless, Americans remain confident in their personal physicians.[2] In this context, the growth of managed care potentially challenges the ability of individual physicians to sustain trust. It also raises important questions about the forms of trust appropriate for medical care, questions that the American Medical Association (AMA) code of ethics, current physician training, and prevailing public policies are ill-equipped to address.

Mechanic D, Schlesinger M. "The Impact of Managed Care on Patients' Trust in Medical Care and Their Physicians." *Journal of the American Medical Association.* 1996;275(21): 1693–1697. ©American Medical Association. Reprinted by permission.

THE MEANING AND IMPORTANCE OF TRUST

Trust refers to the expectations of the public that those who serve them will perform their responsibilities in a technically proficient way (competence), that they will assume responsibility and not inappropriately defer to others (control), and that they will make patients' welfare their highest priority (agency). Implicit in these criteria are the further expectations that responses will be sensitive and caring, that they will encourage honest and open communication, and that rules of privacy and confidentiality will be respected. People may place their trust in other individuals (interpersonal trust) or in collective institutions (social trust). The two forms of trust are to some extent functional substitutes for each other. Patients who trust their physicians may worry less about the trustworthiness of the hospitals or health maintenance organizations (HMOs) through which they get their services, since they count on their physicians to make appropriate referrals or to monitor the quality of services. Similarly, trust in one's physicians and nurses can flow from confidence in the competence and commitment of the institutions with which they are affiliated. It is usually assumed that trusted institutions maintain recruitment, selection, and performance standards, that they have in place appropriate supervisory structures, and, most important, that their clinicians are among the best.

But interpersonal trust and social trust are also different in important ways. Interpersonal trust has deep roots in socialization, personality development, and primary relations, it is often closely associated with strong affect, and it develops gradually in the course of repeated interactions through which expectations about a person's trustworthy behavior can be tested over time.[3] Social trust, in contrast, is more remote, influenced by media exposure and general reputation more than by firsthand knowledge. It is also likely connected with broader forms of confidence in social institutions generally.

Both forms of trust have potentially important roles in medical care. Interpersonal trust is a prerequisite for many aspects of effective care, including patients' willingness to reveal potential stigmatizing information about health-related behaviors (e.g., sexual practices and substance use), their description of personal feelings and thoughts that are necessary to differentiate mental from physical disorders, and their acceptance of treatment practices or prescribed changes in personal behavior that are difficult or risky. The most fundamental "caring" aspects of medicine depend on the sort of personal bonding that is only possible with those one trusts. Conversely, patient-physician relationships that are characterized by suspicion and distrust are more likely to foster litigation and the costly practices of defensive medicine.[4]

Social trust plays a different but important role. Trust is associated with patient loyalty, essential for maintaining stable patient populations. The absence of trust creates substantial social costs as patients or purchasers seek information about physician performance and second and third opinions or otherwise guard themselves against possible adverse outcomes.[5,6] A 1991 study[7] estimated that utilization management and review alone cost $2.3 billion. Collectively, distrust in the medical-care system fosters external controls by public and private agencies desiring to maintain accountability for the health care that they are purchasing. In short, a health-care system without social trust diverts a large share of the medical-care dollar away from treatment to self-protection, regulatory enforcement, and physician compliance

MANAGED CARE AND TRUST

In its broadest sense, managed care refers to organizational arrangements that seek to alter treatment practices so that care of acceptable quality can be provided at lower cost. More specific to current concerns, managed care refers to organizational structures and strategies designed to constrain expenditures. This is accomplished through capitation, selective financial incentives for physicians and patients such as bonuses and withholds, gatekeeper arrangements or other factors constraining treatment or referral practices, and utilization review, including the use of protocols and practice standards. Each of these features has potentially important implications for how patients perceive competence, control, and agency. With different combinations of managed care arrangements, there are many different permutations and an equally wide range of effects on both interpersonal and social trust. In the limited space available, we focus only on three aspects of managed care: financial incentives for physicians, utilization review, and factors governing the process of treatment and referral.

TRUST AND FINANCIAL INCENTIVES

Managed care plans use a variety of financial incentives. They use them because they work.[8,9] Varied in form, virtually all of these mechanisms rely on withholding a portion of the physicians' incomes until the end of the year, basing year-end payments on costs of treatment for a group of patients, ranging from the physician's own patients to all the plan's enrollees. The smaller the risk pool, the stronger the financial incentives to conserve on treatment.

Strong financial incentives raise questions about the quality of treatment provided under managed care. But our concern here is less with the actual quality of care than with the trust it engenders. We know very little about the ways in which patients might interpret different payment arrangements. However, the limited evidence available suggests that many are uncomfortable with incentives that require physicians to balance the benefits of their medical care against the costs that it engenders for the plan.[10] Thus, payment arrangements could significantly undermine patients' beliefs that their physicians are acting as their agents.

Currently, there is neither government regulation of compensation arrangements in managed care nor any effective mechanisms for informing enrollees about the ways in which physicians are paid. The AMA's code of ethics requires that physicians discuss with new patients how they are paid by the plan. For a variety of reasons, disclosure requirements of this sort are unlikely to reduce distrust. In the absence of any effective enforcement mechanism, it seems unlikely that many physicians actually convey this information. Even if they did, patients would be placed in a difficult position of trying to interpret what they were told, trying to understand the implications; of different risk pools, and/or trying to assess the consequences of financial risk. Even if they do understand, many patients face restricted options because of lack of choice or few significant differences among the plans available to them.

Most important, disclosure of this information, however it is conveyed or interpreted, seems more likely to elicit distrust than trust. The disclosure comes early in the patient's interactions with the physician, but interpersonal trust is created largely through ongoing interactions. This creates initial reasons for doubt, without any offsetting reasons to trust. If an unfortunate medical outcome subsequently occurs, initial doubts may blossom into stronger suspicions. Studies of blame attribution suggest that if people doubt motives and then an undesirable outcome occurs and the key actor is seen as responsible (that is, in control), the key actor tends to be blamed for the outcome.[11–13]

TRUST AND UTILIZATION REVIEW

Various forms of utilization review or management (including precertification, concurrent review, second opinions, and case management for high-cost patients) have become common. In traditional notions of patient-physician relationships, the physician was assumed to do everything reasonably helpful for the patient, explaining the costs and benefits of varying options, including economic considerations where they were relevant. When patients observe that the care their physicians consider best is not the care that their insurance companies will pay for—and, unless they are well-to-do, the care that they will actually receive—patients can no longer have faith that their physicians, however well-intentioned, can actually get them the treatment that they need. This is most likely to occur when it is the patient's responsibility to contact the plan to obtain prior authorization and when the managed-care firm informs them directly when treatment has not been authorized.

Patients could, of course, interpret this sequence of events as suggesting that their physician was not competent to begin with. Their interpretation depends on whether they have more faith in the decisions made by their personal physician or by the utilization review process. Where patients have well-established relationships with physicians, they would almost certainly place greater faith in them. When the patient has recently switched physicians or been recently referred to a specialist, doubts about which party is more trustworthy may be more common.

These consequences are mitigated in the short run if the patient never becomes aware that utilization review has altered his or her treatment. Recognizing this, some managed-care plans have attempted to discourage physicians from discussing utilization review with their patients. For example, a recent directive to physicians in an Ohio Kaiser Permanente HMO prohibited them from discussing proposed treatments with patients prior to authorization or even describing to them the authorization procedure.[14]

While such gag rules reduce some short-term threats to trust, they raise long-term threats that are more disturbing. Efforts to restrict physician communication with patients are objectionable not only because they limit the autonomy of both physicians and patients, but also because they undermine physicians' responsibilities to their patients. At the heart of an effective and caring relationship between physicians and patients is honest and open communication from both parties. Limits on openly discussing options, suggesting alternatives, and advising on the constraints that limit access to care in a given plan undermine two important components of the trust relationship, those relating to agency and control.

The spread of utilization review also raises additional questions about physicians' capabilities to advocate effectively for their patients. All utilization review incorporates several stages of appeals after an initial denial. Given the difficulty of determining whether treatment is warranted on initial review, effective appeals processes are essential for utilization review to function appropriately. In 1993, about 20 percent of all treatment requests that were initially denied were reversed on appeal.[15] But appeals, as with all stages of utilization review, require considerable physician time and effort.[5] This is not a role for which physicians have been trained. Many physicians will view their advocacy role with discomfort or distaste because it takes time and attention away from treatment. If this discourages them from appealing for needed treatment, they have failed their patients. While there are many anecdotes, we know virtually nothing systematic about physicians' willingness and ability to deal with utilization review.

TRUST AND CARE STRUCTURES

While utilization review affects primarily what physicians decide in terms of treatment, other managed-care practices have their impact on how treatment decisions are made. Perhaps the most widely recognized are limitations on choice of physician or plan. Studies suggest that enrollees who are not given a choice of managed-care plans are significantly less satisfied with their treatment.[16] Although trust has not been measured directly, it is plausible that individuals who can choose their plans and are, therefore, more satisfied with them will be more trusting than those who have arrangements imposed on them. Choice is important to interpersonal trust because patients have more confidence in physicians they select for themselves than those that are assigned to them. Conversely, when patients know that they may be required to switch physicians whenever their employer changes health plans or when physicians leave a plan or network, they may invest less in their relationship with physicians. Given free choice of physicians, patients will change physicians when trust breaks down. If this safety valve is restricted, trust between physicians and patients is likely to erode.

The role of physician gatekeepers may have even more pronounced consequences for trust. When primary care physicians are given gatekeeping authority, they must diagnose a broader range of conditions to determine if a referral is warranted. Many HMOs also provide primary care physicians with a financial incentive to limit referrals. This encourages them to treat more conditions themselves. The literature suggests that for some conditions, treatment by primary care physicians is less expensive and of comparable quality to treatment by specialists.[17] But there are also conditions (e.g., cancer[18] or depression[19,20]) where recognition, diagnosis, and treatment are less effective. Although debate continues about the relative efficiency and effectiveness with which primary care physicians and specialists provide care for varying conditions is likely that many patients will have strong views on these issues and will resent limited access to specialty referral. Patients with the acquired immunodeficiency syndrome (AIDS), for example, have been critical of their access to appropriate specialized care in HMOs.[21]

Compounding issues of competence are those of agency. Although the ideal primary care relationship is based on trust and open communication, it is widely understood that many physicians are uncomfortable dealing with family difficulties, sexual practices, domestic violence, or substance use among their patients. In an unmanaged system, patients who recognize this discomfort can simply seek care for these services elsewhere. With primary care gatekeepers, this is no longer possible. Aware that their physicians are uncomfortable with some issues, patients must either directly broach the issue, which may undermine their close relationship, or keep their problem to themselves and thus forgo treatment that would be covered by their insurance. Either way, trust in the physician is strained.

Gatekeeper requirements reflect a broader process through which the roles and images of physicians and insurance plans are becoming enmeshed. This is clearly in the interests of insurers because social trust in insurance is so much lower than interpersonal trust in physicians.[1,2] Enmeshment is fostered by various contractual requirements. As managed-care plans increasingly encourage or require physicians to establish exclusive contracts, patients will tend to see physicians as surrogates for a particular plan, replete with its paperwork, coverage limitations, and utilization review. This connection would be further strengthened if patients believed their physicians were more loyal to the plan than to them.[22] One contractual arrangement is almost guaranteed to foster these doubts: confidentiality clauses that prohibit physicians from providing patients with any information that might damage the reputation of the plan.[23] Choice Care in Cincinnati, Ohio, for example, requires physicians to agree that they will "take no action or make any communication which undermines or could undermine the confidence of enrollees, potential enrollees, their employers, plan sponsors, or the public in Choice Care, or in the quality of care which Choice Care enrollees receive."[14] Although there are no comprehensive data on the prevalence of these gag rule clauses, anecdotal reports from lawyers and benefit consultants familiar with managed care suggest that they are becoming the norm.

HOW MUCH AND WHAT KIND OF TRUST IN MEDICAL CARE?

We have identified a variety of ways in which managed care may affect trust in medicine. Given its importance, loss of trust in any form has real costs. But these may be costs worth bearing if there are other benefits that offset them. Primary care gatekeepers may be the most effective means of coordinating medical services, even if this increases discomfort for some patients. Similarly, patients can be too trusting if their trust makes them less sensitive to real risks they face in choosing among physicians, plans, or treatments.[24] The complexities of this balancing act, coupled with the ways in which increasing some forms of trust may serve to undermine others, make it difficult to identify responses to all the issues that we have raised in this article. Nonetheless, several strategies appear promising and feasible.

The ubiquity of utilization review symbolically challenges the competence of the medical profession. Since utilization review is likely to remain a feature of U.S. medicine in the foreseeable future, it is imperative that physicians develop the skills and motivation to be effective advocates for their patients, who must be able to trust that their interests are being effectively represented. To some extent, states can more effectively regulate the appeals process to ensure its accessibility to all clinicians. But given the myriad ways in which the review and appeals processes can be structured, public regulation is likely to be too crude to ensure effective advocacy. Therefore, the medical community must commit to making physicians effective and reliable advocates by encouraging an advocacy orientation and developing and teaching advocacy models in the curricula of medical schools and continuing medical education programs. This is but a small step, but an important one in defining physician responsibility. Physicians must also work cooperatively with regulatory agencies facilitating disclosure and review of the utilization review process and in guaranteeing an objective and fair appeals process.

A more complicated issue involves the relationship between information and trust. Trust can be maintained in the short run by suppressing information, but only at the cost of long-term erosion of the bedrock of trust on which the profession of medicine rests. Private managed-care plans, driven by market pressures, may pursue a short-term perspective, as evidenced by the spread of confidentiality clauses and gag rules. Even if plans do not act often on these rules, their presence alone deters communication. We believe that interpersonal trust can be preserved only in an atmosphere of complete and honest communication.

To date, the profession has been concerned with disclosure of financial arrangements.[25] Expecting physicians to explain financial arrangements that they are ill-equipped to assess creates disclosure requirements that are ill-timed for building patient trust. It would be more useful to shift obligations for financial disclosure to plans, which would be required annually to report their financial arrangements with physicians to state health agencies, purchasers, and enrollees in a standard form. The requirements for reporting might differ depending on the audience. Routine disclosure by plans is preferable to disclosure by physicians early in patient relationships because it is less likely to undermine the initial development of interpersonal trust crucial to patient-physician relationships. Plans should further be prohibited from using incentives to put too high a proportion (perhaps more than a fifth) of physicians' incomes at risk.

Determination of appropriate bounds depends on how income incentives are combined with quality assurance mechanisms and requires careful consideration by the profession and appropriate regulatory agencies. The Health Care Financing Administration recently issued final rules for comment affecting incentive payments in the Medicaid and Medicare programs. Health plans that exceed a 25 percent threshold would be required to meet a variety of conditions, including the provision of stop-loss protection, detailed disclosure, and specified enrollment surveys.[26] These new Health Care Financing Administration rules represent a sensible step, but they seem too limited in several senses. They apply only to managed-care plans that contract with Medicare or Medicaid, and they require disclosure only if incentives exceed the 25 percent threshold and only if enrollees explicitly request this information. Although quality of medical care may not be at risk, trust may be undermined by a wide variety of financial arrangements. We believe that all patients should be informed about the way in which their physicians are paid to provide their medical care.

Putting requirements on plans rather than physicians would relieve physicians of reporting their financial arrangements. But we would correspondingly increase expectations that they fully communicate with patients about options for treatment as well as report outcomes of negotiations with utilization reviewers. Open disclosure of these negotiations would increase physicians' inclinations to negotiate aggressively. To facilitate such communication, contractual obligations with insurance plans requiring confidentiality should be declared unambiguously a violation of codes of ethics and prohibited as a matter of law. But this in itself is insufficient. The profession must adopt and encourage a norm of open communication, which does not at this point exist.[27]

We recognize the difficulty of "putting teeth" in professional codes and view this as an evolutionary process. Public discussion and external rules as in state regulations can help establish an enabling climate. But the profession must use its various points of leverage to eliminate restraints on physician behavior that undermine trust and to encourage physicians to have full and open communication with their patients. Physicians working together and with others have had success in changing some managed-care practices such as early discharge following childbirth and the use of gag rules by US Healthcare. Similar actions are required to protect physicians from being "deselected" by plans if they speak frankly with patients. Protections against termination without cause could be modeled on existing protections available to employees in the workplace. Patients' trust depends on their perceptions that physicians are free to act in their best interests.

As managed care comes to dominate the medical marketplace, the public increasingly will identify individual physicians with managed-care plans (and vice versa). This may be an asset to managed care in building social trust, but it erodes interpersonal trust in physicians. Managed care may need greater social trust, but a close association may be a bad trade for physicians as well as society as a whole. It is necessary and inevitable that physicians participate and cooperate with the managed-care process. But it is also important that they retain as much independence as they can to remain strong patient advocates when they believe that quality of care is being compromised. For example, the insistence of general practitioners in England to remain contractors rather than employees of the National Health Service may seem largely symbolic, but this nuance probably contributed to maintaining an independent voice.

The current focus of organized medicine is to seek legislation that allows physician-sponsored plans. The logic is that physicians themselves can garner the resources that increasingly go to managers and stockholders while protecting their autonomy from managerial intrusions. The drawback of such ventures is that they further combine and confuse the sometimes conflicting interests of plans and physicians. This argues for professional norms and public policies that encourage clear separation of the interests of physicians and plan financing and organization. We need measures to ensure trustworthy forms of managed care either by encouraging particular organizational forms (nonprofit vs. profit, for example) or through explicit incentives for them to market themselves accurately and then function in a trustworthy way. But in the final analysis, trust will depend more on the quality of the patient-physician relationship than all else. Protecting this relationship from conflicts of interest and suspicion will ultimately best preserve those aspects of trust that are most important to the public and vital to ensuring the quality of their future health care.

This work was supported in part by Robert Wood Johnson Foundation Investigator Awards in Health Policy Research to the authors.

REFERENCES

1. Blendon RJ, Hyams TS, Benson JM. Bridging the gap between expert and public views on health care reform. *JAMA.* 1993;269:2573–2578.

2. Blendon RJ, Taylor, H. Views on health care: public opinion in three nations. *Health Affairs.* 1989;8:149–157.

3. Mechanic D. Changing medical organization and the erosion of trust. *Milbank Quarterly.* 1996;74:171–189.

4. Ryan KJ. The threat of litigation. *Journal of the Royal Society of Medicine.* 1994;87(supp. 22):17–18.

5. Emmons D, Chawla A. Physician perceptions of the intrusiveness of utilization review. In: Marder W (ed.). *Socioeconomic Characteristics of Medical Practice.* Chicago, IL: American Medical Association; 1991.

6. Luhman N. *Trust and Power.* New York, NY: John Wiley & Sons Inc.; 1989.

7. Sheils JF, Young GJ, Rabin RJ. O Canada: do we expect too much from its health system? *Health Affairs.* 1992;11:7–20.

8. Hillman A, Welch WP, Pauly M. Contractual arrangements between HMOs and primary care physicians: three-tiered HMOs and risk pools. *Medical Care.* 1992;30:136–148.

9. Hillman A, Pauly M, Kerstein JJ. Do financial incentives affect physicians, clinical decisions and the financial performance of health maintenance organization? *New England Journal of Medicine.* 1989;321:86–95.

10. Mechanic D, Ettel T, Davis D. Choosing among health care options. *Inquiry.* 1990; 27:14–23.

11. Shaver KG. *The Attribution of Blame: Causality, Responsibility, and Blameworthiness.* New York, NY: Springer-Verlag; 1985.

12. McGraw KM. Avoiding blame: an experimental investigation of political excuses and justifications. *British Journal of Political Science.* 1989;20:119–142.

13. Hibbard J, Weeks E. Consumerism in health care: prevalence and predictions. *Medical Care.* 1987;25:1019–1032.

14. Pear R. Doctors say HMO's limit what they can tell patients. *New York Times.* December 21, 1995: A1.

15. Schlesinger M, Gray B, Perreira K. Deprofessionalization or reprofessionalization: the impact of utilization review on American medicine. *Health Affairs.* In press.

16. Davis K, Collins KS, Schoen C, Morris C. Choice matters: enrollee views of their health care plans. *Health Affairs.* 1995;14:99–112.

17. Greenfield S, Rogers W, Mangotich M, Carney MF, Tarlov AR. Outcomes of patients with hypertension and non-insulin-dependent diabetes mellitus treated by different systems and specialties: results from the Medical Outcomes Study. *JAMA* 1995;274:1436–1444.

18. Gillis CR, Hole DJ. Survival outcome of care by specialist surgeons in breast cancer: a study of 3786 patients in the west of Scotland. *BMJ.* 1996; 312: 145–148.

19. Wells KB, Hays RD, Burnam MA, Rogers W, Greenfield S, Ware JE Jr. Detection of depressive disorders for patients receiving prepaid or fee for service care—results from the Medical Outcomes Study. *JAMA.* 1989;262:3298–3302.

20. Hays RD, Wells KB, Sherbourne D, Rogers W, Spritzer K. Functioning and well-being of patients with depression compared with chronic medical conditions. *Archives of General Psychiatry.* 1995;52:11–19.

21. Rosenthal E. Managed care has trouble treating AIDS, patients say. *New York Times.* January 15, 1996: 1.

22. Macklin R. *Enemies of Patients.* New York, NY: Oxford University Press; 1993.

23. Kassirer JP. Managed care and the morality of the marketplace. *New England Journal of Medicine.* 1995;333:50–52.

24. Lupton D, Donaldson C, Lloyd P. Caveat emptor or blissful ignorance? patients and the consumerist ethos. *Social Science and Medicine.* 1991;33:559–568.

25. Rodwin M. *Medicine, Money, and Morals: Physicians' Conflicts of Interest.* New York, NY: Oxford University Press; 1993.

26. Health Care Financing Administration. Medicare and Medicaid Programs; Requirements for Physician Incentive Plans in Prepaid Health Care Organizations. 42 CFR §417 and 434; April 12, 1996.

27. Emanuel E, Dubler N. Preserving the physician-patient relationship in the era of managed care. *JAMA.* 1995;273:323–329.

Part 12

ISSUES IN RESOURCE ALLOCATION

❦

The ongoing escalation of health-care costs, along with the scarcity of livers, hearts, and ICU beds, has long provided the media with fodder for exposés on health-care rationing. While these exposés usually involve high-tech tests or procedures, rationing decisions take place in almost every patient encounter and often go unrecognized as such. Physicians make rationing decisions every time they decide how many minutes they will allocate to a specific patient's office visit. Nurses make rationing decisions when they "decide" how much compassion they will allocate to a particular family. Paramedics make rationing decisions when they decide how far they are willing to go when a patient's needs are more social than medical. And hospital CEOs make rationing decisions when they decide how many nurses will work the day shift. It is the recognition of these morally subtle rationing decisions that is the goal of this section. With this recognition in hand, health-care providers will be better prepared to appreciate when they are in fact making rationing decisions—the obvious corollary being that health-care providers will make more reflective and just decisions. Even though the next two readings address the more obvious examples of rationing, the theoretical foundation the authors set out is certainly germane to the more frequent mundane rationing decisions.

As health-care providers and ethics committees develop "rationing" policies (e.g., drug formulary additions, allocation of pediatric ICU beds, etc.) they must explicitly balance the financial realities of our current health-care system with the Joint Commission on Accreditation of Healthcare Organizations's organizational ethics standards. In particular, *Patient Rights and Organizational Ethics* standard RI.4.4 requires a "hospital's code of ethical business and professional behavior . . . to . . . protect the integrity of clinical decision making, regardless of how the hospital compensates or shares financial risk with its leaders, managers, clinical staff and licensed independent practitioners."[1]

In this section's first reading, "Rationing By Any Other Name," David Asch and Peter Ubel help us to appreciate how subtle and removed some rationing decisions can be. Using five vignettes they discuss the ethical issues that come about when a physician decides to recommend a less efficacious treatment in order to save money. Of course, this justification presupposes the money saved will actually be redistributed to those with a greater need, as opposed to the institution's shareholders. Grounding this article is the premise that due to our current financial crisis in health care, there is no way to avoid compromises between quality and access. From this premise the authors focus their discussion on what counts as a valid justification for specific instances of rationing.

Concluding this section is "Recognizing Bedside Rationing: Clear Cases and Tough Calls," by Peter Ubel and Susan Goold. As the authors define it, bedside rationing occurs when a physician has control over a resource (e.g., medication, surgery, etc), he withholds or withdraws that resource from a patient, and he does so in order to benefit someone other than his patient. At the core of this reading is the question of obligation: Specifically, is a physician obligated to further the interests of only his patients, or is he obligated to balance his patients' interests against the interests of the community, insurer, medical profession, or even himself? Using six vignettes, the authors provide an understanding of rationing that will help guide health-care providers as they try to provide good patient care in a time of scarce resources.

REFERENCE

1. Joint Commission on Accreditation of Healthcare Organizations, *2000 Hospital Accreditation Standards.* Oakbrook, IL: JCAHO; 2000:73–74.

30

RATIONING BY ANY OTHER NAME

David A. Asch, M.D., and Peter A. Ubel, M.D.

Although many clinicians and health policy makers are comfortable with the notion that some beneficial health-care services are simply too expensive to provide, fewer are comfortable using the word "rationing" to describe these compromises. The word is so loaded that some cannot use or hear it without thinking of policies that discriminate against vulnerable population groups. Some policy makers carefully avoid the word, substituting euphemistic phrases such as "emphasizing truly beneficial services." When the word is used in medical contexts, it is usually to discredit an insurance program or a suggested health policy that cuts too close to a favored program.

Besides having negative connotations, the word "rationing" also suffers from inconsistent definitions.[1] To most economists, rationing is simply the process of allocating goods in the face of scarcity. In health-care settings, however, the word is frequently invoked to describe distributions based on cost and, in particular, decisions to limit some clinical services because they are thought to be too expensive for society. On the other hand, some argue that rationing includes only explicit decisions taken at a systemwide level to limit services to some categories of people.[2] This definition would exclude less explicit mechanisms, such as market pressures based on price. Others believe that rationing properly refers only to cost-based limitations on "nec-

D. Asch, P. Ubel. "Rationing by Any Other Name." *New England Journal of Medicine.* 1997;336:1668–1671. Copyright ©1997 Massachusetts Medical Society. All rights reserved.

essary services" rather than limitations on beneficial services that, although effective and desired, are beyond what would be considered basic needs.[3]

Whatever words one uses and whatever definitions one gives to those words, the reality is that clinical services believed to be beneficial are limited because those services are seen as too costly to provide. All around us are examples of practices and policies that promote such compromises. At the same time, since clinicians, managers, and policy makers rarely say that they are engaged in rationing, what is it that they say they are doing?

In this paper, we describe several alternative characterizations of rationing. Each alternative is introduced with a case. These cases are based on our own experience or on situations we have been told about. In each case, a physician decides in favor of a treatment choice that he or she believes to be both less effective (from the perspective of the patient) and less expensive (from the perspective of society, the healthcare plan, or the clinical practice, but not the patient). Our purpose in presenting these scenarios is to illustrate that compromises in clinical care are pervasive, varied, and often disguised. If there is to be a resolution to the debate about compromise in clinical care, it must come from discussion of what actually happens rather than of the language used to describe it.

THINKING BEYOND THE INDIVIDUAL PATIENT

Dr. Smith is about to perform coronary arteriography on Mr. Stevens and is deciding whether to use ionic or nonionic radiocontrast dye during the procedure. He decides on the less expensive ionic contrast dye, even though he believes the nonionic dye is less likely to cause complications. Dr. Smith reasons, "If everybody used nonionic contrast dye, some patients would be better off, but not enough to justify the large increase in cost to society."

Here the clinician opts for a less costly clinical strategy by considering the effects of a more expensive strategy on overall social welfare. In this case, the tension between the cost of the alternative and its benefit is overt but is displaced from the patient at hand to a wider field. Dr. Smith could have assumed an individual perspective and considered only the welfare of this particular patient. Had he assumed an individual perspective, he might have been uncomfortable choosing the less effective agent. Instead, he considers the effect among many other patients and clinicians. Although this switch from an individual to a group perspective may seem transparent, there is evidence that physicians make different decisions for individual patients and for groups of similar patients.[4,5]

APPEALING TO THE "STANDARD OF CARE"

Mr. Green complains to his physician, Dr. Brown, of a new, persistent headache. Dr. Brown orders a computed tomographic (CT) scan to evaluate the possibility of a brain tumor, even though she believes magnetic resonance imaging (MRI) would be more sensitive. In discussing the issue with Mr. Green, Dr. Brown mentions that, in general, ordering a CT scan in this situation is the "standard of care."

In this instance, the physician opts against the more effective and more expensive MRI, arguing to the patient or to herself that the less expensive CT scan is the standard of care. Nevertheless, the standard of care is itself often influenced by considerations of the cost to society. One reason it is not the standard of care to obtain MRIs for patients such as Mr. Green is that the resulting costs would be too high. If MRIs were less costly, the standard of care for patients with headaches might be different.

It is possible to view Dr. Brown's actions in many ways. Is Dr. Brown playing with words in order to reduce social costs? Is she making peace with herself in resolving a potentially difficult conflict? Is she following a long-standing professional norm that just happens to have incorporated the consideration of costs to society? Whatever the view, in many situations physicians appeal implicitly or explicitly to the "standard of care." In many cases the standard of care reflects some consideration of cost, yet most physicians in these situations probably do not feel that they are trading off their patients' welfare against social cost.

DISPLACING RESPONSIBILITY

Ms. Johnson sees her general internist, Dr. Edwards, about her gastroesophageal reflux disease. She is surprised when Dr. Edwards prescribes cimetidine rather than omeprazole, which she has heard is the best treatment. Dr. Edwards explains that although he believes omeprazole would probably be somewhat better for relieving Ms. Johnson's symptoms, the health-care company's formulary policy restricts the prescription of omeprazole to patients whose need for the drug has been determined by a gastroenterologist.

In this situation, Dr. Edwards justifies or explains his less costly choice by appealing to an external rule. Dr. Edwards apparently believes that one drug would be better than another but shifts the responsibility for choosing the less effective, less expensive agent onto the health-care company. The way one views this situation depends not only on clinical factors (for example, how much difference one perceives there really is between the two drugs), but also on professional and institutional factors (how much independence Dr. Edwards really has in making a choice). Some of these decisions may actually be out of the individual physician's control, but others may not. For example, perhaps the responsibility in fact rests with the formulary committee. On the other hand, if Dr. Edwards truly believes that omeprazole is better, he could refer the patient to a gastroenterologist.

Responsibility can be displaced, appropriately or not, in many different directions. The justification that "in general, we don't consider omeprazole to be first-line therapy for gastroesophageal reflux disease" in effect shifts the decision from an individual physician to a professional norm. In doing so, it resembles the "standard of care" argument presented earlier. Justifications such as, "Your policy doesn't cover a glucometer unless you require insulin," may reveal a firmer rule, although sometimes even these can be bent. Physicians might blame the medical marketplace: "If I were to order an MRI for every patient with a headache, I would be identified as a high-cost clinician and managed-care organizations would drop me from their panels." Or clinicians might shift responsibility to the patient: "Doxycycline is as effective as azithromycin; you just have to take it for a week." These justifications are all intended to transfer responsibility for perceived cost-quality trade-offs away from the physician. And in general, external rules are both limiting and liberating: A formulary that restricts access to expensive drugs can simultaneously tie physicians' hands and allow them to avoid decisions they do not want to make.

Suppose Ms. Johnson did not mention omeprazole to Dr. Edwards, but instead asked for cimetidine. In this case, Dr. Edwards would be spared the need to explain his choice. It would certainly be convenient for him that Ms. Johnson asked for the less expensive medicine, which he would have prescribed, rather than the more expensive medicine, which he thought was clinically superior.

One way to view this situation is to recognize that patients' preferences should always be considered when making medical choices. Preferences for medical rather than surgical approaches to certain conditions, for example, may reflect deeper attitudes about risk or aggressive therapy that ought to be considered in making decisions. But incorporating the expressed preferences of patients into medical decision making may not be enough if patients do not adequately understand the available alternatives. Ms. Johnson may not have heard of omeprazole. Although Dr. Edwards would have done exactly what Ms. Johnson requested in the second instance, he would have taken a passive stance in serving as her advocate.

MAKING DO WITH LESS THAN THE BEST

Mrs. Glenn sees her family practitioner, Dr. Shepard, for a referral to an orthopedist for a total knee replacement. There are two orthopedists in the community. Dr. Aldrin is considered a national expert in the procedure, but the plan under which Dr. Shepard sees Mrs. Glenn has an arrangement with Dr. Grissom, a general orthopedist. Dr. Shepard anticipates Mrs. Glenn's concern: "I know that you would like a referral to Dr. Aldrin, because she is considered the expert in knee replacements, but Dr. Grissom is an able orthopedist."

One can imagine many different financial or organizational reasons why Dr. Shepard would refer Mrs. Glenn to Dr. Grissom, and these differences might affect how one views the situation. Common to any of these unstated arrangements is the question of whether Dr. Shepard's responsibility is to arrange the best possible care for Mrs. Glenn or simply to arrange good care. Even if Dr. Aldrin really is the better orthopedist, perhaps she is not able to operate on all the patients in the community who need her help. Immutable constraints such as these increase our tolerance for making do and might make Dr. Shepard more comfortable with his actions, even if he would have referred his own mother to Dr. Aldrin.

USING THE "BEST TREATMENT" ONLY AFTER OTHERS FAIL

Ms. Cooper sees her general internist, Dr. Kelley, about her seasonal allergies. Dr. Kelley explains that although he believes a nonsedating antihistamine is likely to be better tolerated, he thinks it is reasonable to try a less expensive conventional antihistamine first and to use the more expensive kind only if Ms. Cooper is troubled by sedation.

It takes a broad definition of "compromise" to argue that Dr. Kelley is compromising Ms. Cooper's care in order to save money. After all, Dr. Kelley intends to prescribe the more expensive agent that he believes is more effective, but only if the less expensive agent fails. There are many situations in which physicians start with an inexpensive approach and move to a more costly and generally more effective one only if it is necessary.

We might think differently if Dr. Kelley used to prescribe the more expensive agent as first-line therapy in similar cases but developed this new strategy only after his health-care company introduced financial incentives favoring the less expensive approach. Still, some might argue that Dr. Kelley should have been following a strategy like this all along. Nevertheless, if Dr. Kelley really believes that one drug is more likely to succeed than the other, he has made a compromise, albeit a small one, in the care of Ms. Cooper.

DISCUSSION

We suspect that many physicians will recognize elements of their own practices in these cases. Does this mean that they are rationing care? Perhaps not, if rationing refers only to practices that are in some way unethical or unprofessional. Perhaps so, if rationing refers to any decrease in the quality of care intended to save money. Or perhaps it does not matter at all what we call these cases, because whatever words we use, all the cases still involve decisions that favor a less expensive option even though it is perceived to be less effective. Each case reflects a compromise. As physicians, patients, insurers, and others face trade-offs between cost and quality, the debate should not be about some global notion of rationing or compromise, but about which justifications are valid and which compromises are appropriate.

For example, in many situations the practice of thinking beyond the individual patient may be an effective way to link individual decisions to broader issues. Clinicians practicing in public or nonprofit settings, in which savings in one area can support costs in another, are justified in making compromises within this wider perspective. The same reasoning is less persuasive when savings in one area leave the system in the form of profits for owners.

Compromises embedded in the standard of care make sense as long as the standard of care itself makes sense, but not otherwise. In some cases, an appeal to the standard of care is just a shorthand way of describing good medical practice—when good medical practice reflects a wider social perspective. But an appeal to the standard of care should not justify or legitimize a choice unless that choice makes sense for other reasons.

Efforts to displace responsibility are hard to evaluate in the abstract. One should look at the effects of the compromise, at the underlying motivations of those imposing the constraints, and at the extent to which the physician's traditional fiduciary posture is weakened. Although physicians have strong and historic obligations to individual patients, clearly they cannot fight every battle relentlessly. Nor should they abdicate their professionalism in favor of some wider institutional or social mission. Although these extremes are well defined, drawing the correct line between them is likely to remain a matter of specific circumstances and personal judgment.

Cost containment that occurs passively, because the patient is not aware of the alternatives, is not justified by this fact alone. Although physicians interested in cost containment may find it convenient when patients request a less expensive but less effective treatment or test, physicians should not rely on these expressed preferences. There may be legitimate reasons for making such a choice, but the expressed preference of an uninformed patient is not one of them. Taking advantage of one patient's less expensive preferences makes no more sense than giving in to a request for an inappropriately expensive test or treatment from another.

Finally, using the "best" but most expensive treatment only after others fail will be seen by many physicians as a timeless and essential part of practicing medicine. The compromise embodied in this approach is that sometimes symptoms are not relieved as fast as they might be or conditions are prolonged or exacerbated while one waits to see whether the first treatment will succeed. In practice, however, any ill effects of compromises such as these are usually small.

Indeed, the best measure of all compromises is their magnitude. Using the "best" treatment first makes more sense when the second-best one is much less likely to work, or when the clinical stakes are higher. Thinking beyond the individual patient is easier and more tolerable when the individual patient is not likely to lose much. Because there is no uniform way of dealing with these trade-offs, they always require personal judgment and they will always involve gray areas when those judgments vary. Our goal is not to eliminate the gray areas when choices are hard and when judgments vary, because we believe gray areas are unavoidable. Rather, in making these different rationales explicit and demonstrating that many of the practices in our scenarios are pervasive, we hope to help move discussion beyond the loaded question of whether rationing is acceptable to the more constructive question of what kinds of compromise are justified. The goal, in the end, is to help physicians learn to practice medicine more effectively when compromise is inevitable.

REFERENCES

1. Ubel PA, Goold S. Recognizing bedside rationing: clear cases and tough calls. *Annals of Internal Medicine.* 1997;126:74–80.

2. Reiman AS. Is rationing inevitable? *New England Journal of Medicine.* 1990;322:1809–1810.

3. Hadorn DC, Brook RH. The health care resource allocation debate: defining our terms. *JAMA.* 1991;266:3328–3331.

4. Redelmeir DA, Tversky A. Discrepancy between medical decisions for individual patients and for groups. *New England Journal of Medicine.* 1990;322:1162–1164.

5. Asch DA, Hershey JC. Why some health policies don't make sense at the bedside. *Annals of Internal Medicine.* 1995;122:846–850.

31

RECOGNIZING BEDSIDE RATIONING

Clear Cases and Tough Calls

Peter A. Ubel, M.D.,
and Susan Goold, M.D., M.H.S.A., M.A.

❦

Physicians are under great pressure to contain medical costs. They are being asked to consider not only the clinical implications of their decisions but also whether particular services are "worth" the cost of providing them. When should physicians order low-yield screening tests, prescribe expensive new antibiotic agents, or request consults from highly paid specialists? Whether physicians should be engaged in this "bedside rationing," whether they should be making judgments about the costworthiness of medical services, is debated. Some argue that physicians should serve only as advocates for their patients, as "perfect agents," and that they should never put economic interests ahead of patients' interests.[1-5] According to these arguments, bedside rationing is wrong because it harms the physician-patient relationship, creates possibilities for injustice, and leaves moral decisions in the hands of physicians who are not trained to make them. Others argue that, at times, physicians' rationing decisions are morally justified.[6-8] According to these arguments, some amount of bedside rationing is acceptable because this rationing is the most effective and clinically flexible way to ration care. Still others claim that it is inevitable that rationing decisions will be made by physicians and that many of the decisions physicians now make, such as how much time to spend with a patient or whether to transfer a patient to a distant care center, are rationing decisions that have gone unrecognized.

P. Ubel, S. Goold. "Recognizing Bedside Rationing: Clear Cases and Tough Calls." *Annals of Internal Medicine.* 1997;126:74–80.

Thus, the threshold for recommending a service may change, but the difference is one of degree, not of kind.[9,10]

Whatever position one holds about the inevitability or morality of bedside rationing, it is clearly important to clarify what counts as "bedside rationing." If one argues that bedside rationing is morally impermissible, then it is necessary to identify exactly what sorts of activity are proscribed. Alternatively, even persons who consider bedside rationing morally permissible agree that it raises moral problems and must be done cautiously.[7] Politicians and the media label health-care policy proposals as attempts at "rationing" when they want to denigrate or discredit those proposals, and they present alternative proposals that, in turn, receive the "*R*-word" label from opponents. The moral and political debate about rationing in general and bedside rationing in particular cannot proceed without a clear and consistent understanding of the concept. Physicians need guidelines for making rationing decisions, if indeed they are or will be making them. When are these decisions justified? When are they not? When should physicians play a key role, and when should other agents take primary responsibility? When do instances of bedside rationing need to be disclosed to individual patients? Without a fuller understanding of what qualifies as bedside rationing, these questions cannot be addressed.

We propose to clarify what does and does not count as bedside rationing. We describe three conditions that, in our view, must be met if physicians' actions are to qualify as bedside rationing. These conditions are illustrated with examples of actions that do and do not qualify as bedside rationing. Our effort may have an important and advantageous side effect: Once we have clarified what qualifies as bedside rationing, persons who are opposed to any form of it and those who consider it inevitable or justifiable may find that what appeared to be an irresolvable disagreement rests on different interpretations of the behavior in question rather than on a deep or abiding incompatibility of worldviews.

WHAT IS BEDSIDE RATIONING?

Bedside rationing is the withholding by a physician of a medically beneficial service because of that service's cost to someone other than the patient. Three conditions must be met, in our view, before a physician's action qualifies as bedside rationing. The physician must (1) withhold, withdraw, or fail to recommend a service that, in the physician's best clinical judgment, is in the patient's best medical interests; (2) act primarily to promote the financial interests of someone other than the patient (including an organization, society at large, and the physician himself or herself); and (3) have control over the use of the medically beneficial service.

An example helps show what types of actions qualify as bedside rationing.

A patient arrives at his local emergency department with the classic signs and symptoms of acute myocardial infarction. The emergency department physician decides to administer thrombolysis with streptokinase rather than tissue plasminogen activator even though the latter is slightly better for this type of heart attack. Tissue plasminogen activator costs ten times as much as streptokinase, and the physician thinks that the benefits of this therapy are not worth the additional cost.

This is an example of bedside rationing because the physician withheld a service that would have been in the patient's best medical interests; tissue plasminogen activator would have been a better treatment for this patient than streptokinase.[11] In addition, the physician had control over the resource and withheld it because of a desire to save money for society as a whole. This is a relatively clear example of bedside rationing, but other cases are less clear. Thus, we elaborate on these three conditions through a series of additional examples. In some cases, we provide examples that fail to meet one or more of the conditions to emphasize the importance of each condition. In these cases, we propose changes that would make the cases qualify as examples of bedside rationing.

CONDITION 1: THE PHYSICIAN WITHHOLDS A SERVICE THAT IS IN THE PATIENT'S BEST MEDICAL INTERESTS

For a physician's action to qualify as bedside rationing, it must first and foremost be an example of health-care rationing. Although there is no single accepted definition of health-care rationing,[8] for our purposes, we consider health-care rationing to be the withholding of a service that is in the patient's best medical interests. Defining the first condition in these terms helps physicians decide whether withholding a service is an example of health-care rationing of any kind. (The other two conditions help the physician decide whether the rationing in question is bedside rationing or some other form of rationing.) The case of thrombolysis used to treat myocardial infarction, described above, is an example of health-care rationing because the physician withheld a service, the administration of tissue plasminogen activator, that was in the patient's best medical interests. If streptokinase had been better than tissue plasminogen activator, then the case would not be an example of health-care rationing.

Treatment of Mild Hypertension

An otherwise healthy forty-two-year-old man presents to his physician with mild hypertension. He has been dieting and exercising for 6 months, but his blood pressure is still elevated. His physician institutes therapy with generic hydrochlorothiazide. The physician is chided by her colleagues for using this old, inexpensive medicine when newer antihypertensive agents are available. The physician feels uncomfortable because she knows that she prefers this older agent partly because it is less expensive than the newer ones.

At first glance, this case appears to be an example of bedside rationing: A physician prescribed hydrochlorothiazide rather than a new antihypertensive agent because hydrochlorothiazide was less expensive. However, although this physician considered costs, she did not ration at the bedside, because the more expensive alternatives were no better than the less expensive one. Newer, more expensive antihypertensive agents have not been shown to be better than hydrochlorothiazide at controlling mild hypertension,[12,13] nor have they been shown to have better side-effect profiles. Thus, the physician should not have felt uncomfortable about considering the costs of treatment. Instead, she should have recognized that she eliminated waste by offering an equally beneficial and less expensive medicine.

Many persons argue that physicians do not need to ration health care but merely need to eliminate waste in the medical system.[2] This assertion may or may not hold up under close scrutiny, but physicians should certainly eliminate waste whenever possible. Considering costs when services are of equal benefit is morally praiseworthy because it can provide other needed services in the context of limited resources without producing additional burdens. Considering costs is not necessarily bedside rationing.

One can easily imagine a change in this case that would make it meet the first condition of bedside rationing. Suppose that the patient had been diabetic. In this case, there would have been good reason to think that angiotensin-converting enzyme inhibitors, a more expensive class of antihypertensive medicine, would be better for this patient than hydrochlorothiazide because of their beneficial effects on kidney function[14] and their lower potential for aggravating glucose intolerance.

Although providing an equally beneficial but cheaper service is clearly praiseworthy, it is not always easy to know which medical options are in a patient's best medical interests. Many health-care services have not been proven to be better or worse than others. When such services are involved, it is up to physicians to do their best to evaluate the available evidence. If evidence is lacking or if a service is of disputed benefit, it is often morally justifiable to use cost as a reason to choose one treatment over another. One needs to recognize, however, that even judgments about the strength and quality of evidence are value judgments and are influenced by culture and context, including cost constraints.[15] These judgments may be a particularly well-hidden form of rationing because they are disguised as "medical" or "objective" determinations. What counts as justification for a particular alternative may also depend on the nature of the choice that is confronted. Forced, high-stakes choices, such as promising but unproven treatments for the acquired immunodeficiency syndrome, may be made on the basis of weak evidence if strong evidence is lacking.[16]

Physicians themselves may differ in their skepticism about new treatments, their judgments about evidence, and their assessments of the importance of the patient's medical interests that are at stake. Thus, judgments about benefit are likely to vary among physicians. A caution, however, is in order and is illustrated in the next case.

Prostate-Specific Antigen Testing

A sixty-year-old asymptomatic man visits his primary care physician and asks whether he should have the "blood test for prostate cancer." The physician describes the risks and benefits of prostate-

specific antigen testing and the controversy surrounding its use. The patient says, "Doctor, I'd still like to get the test. My closest friend just got diagnosed with prostate cancer and has it all over his body. I'd rather go through anything than have that happen to me." Although the physician thinks that, in general, the risks of this testing outweigh its benefits, he knows several urologists and primary care physicians who routinely use it for screening.

Where reasonable physicians would disagree, the patient's preference may influence the physician's judgment about whether the service would be medically beneficial in a given case.[17,18] Physicians (and other health-care providers) are in an ideal position to account for such strongly felt preferences, and they should consider these preferences relevant to judgments about risk versus benefit and cost versus benefit. The medical benefit of a service needs to be evaluated from the patient's perspective in individual physician-patient decision making.[19,20] Refusing to authorize a test, even if the patient would pay for it, abuses the power discrepancy in the physician-patient relationship and fails to respect the patient's values and goals. To prevent these considerations from overwhelming all judgments of clinical effectiveness, however, the request should fit within the range of reasonable medical opinion. Where consensus exists about the potential benefits of a service, requests for particular services should be given less weight. Similarly, cases in which the potential harms of a withheld intervention clearly and uncontroversially outweigh the intervention's benefits (as with exercise stress tests for young, asymptomatic women) are not examples of bedside rationing because the decision to withhold the intervention is based on the balance between risks and benefits and not on cost considerations.

Considering costs is thus a necessary but not a sufficient condition for bedside rationing. For rationing to occur, a medical benefit that is valued by the patient must be withheld. Despite the difficulty of always knowing what the best alternative is for a given patient, the moral point should remain straightforward. Bedside rationing does not occur unless there is good reason to think—taking into account the physician's best clinical judgment and the patient's preferences and values—that the patient has not received a service that would have been medically beneficial. One way to address this question in the clinical setting is to ask oneself, "Would I be willing to provide or authorize this service if it were free or if the patient were paying for it himself or herself?" In this way, one can at least separate cases in which the harms outweigh the benefits from cases in which the benefits do not seem to be worth the costs. In addition, however, one must be open to patients' preferences and must recognize that one's own medical opinion is open to challenge where controversy or disagreement exists among physicians.

CONDITION 2: THE PHYSICIAN ACTS PRIMARILY TO PROMOTE THE FINANCIAL INTERESTS OF SOMEONE OTHER THAN THE PATIENT

According to the first condition, health-care rationing occurs when a service that is in the patient's best medical interests is withheld. In such cases, consideration of the second and third conditions helps to determine whether the rationing is bedside rationing or another form of health-care rationing.

Antibiotic Treatment of a Urinary Tract infection

A thirty-six-year-old woman presents to her physician with urinary frequency and urgency. Urinalysis shows leukocytes and many bacteria. The patient has no known allergies but has never taken sulfa drugs. The physician prescribes a 3-day course of trimethoprim-sulfamethoxazole, even though ciprofloxacin, an expensive broad-spectrum antibiotic, would have a better chance of curing the patient and a smaller risk for side effects.[21] She chooses this treatment primarily because of concern about increasing antibiotic resistance.

This case meets the first condition of bedside rationing: A service that was in the patient's best medical interests was withheld. It does not, however, meet the second condition. Ciprofloxacin was withheld not for financial reasons but to prevent the development of resistance to an important broad-spectrum antibiotic agent.[22] To maintain the effectiveness of broad-spectrum antibiotics in patients with severe illnesses, it is necessary to use less potent antibiotics for common conditions, such as the one afflicting this patient. Thus, as this case shows, the second condition of bedside rationing is important because many of the decisions that physicians make are intended to promote public health or other important objectives rather than the financial interests of someone other than the patient. These decisions do not qualify as examples of bedside rationing because they balance the nonmonetary benefits and harms accruing to others against the medical benefit to the patient. Instead, these decisions qualify as other forms of health-care rationing.

In this case, the choice of trimethoprim-sulfamethoxazole is an example of noneconomic rationing. In noneconomic rationing, the patient does not receive the best medical treatment for a nonfinancial reason. In this case, the reason was the promotion of public health. Another example of noneconomic rationing is the decision to withhold scarce transplant organs from some patients because those patients are less likely than others to benefit from transplantation.[23] The next case is an example of an economic form of health-care rationing that does not qualify as bedside rationing.

Out-of-Pocket Costs of Antihistamines

A twenty-year-old college student presents to her physician with seasonal allergic rhinitis. The physician discusses treatment options with the patient and recommends a trial of antihistamines.

He mentions that inexpensive, over-the-counter antihistamines are often effective for allergy symptoms but can cause drowsiness. More expensive antihistamines that do not cause drowsiness are available. Because the student has no prescription coverage, she asks to try the less expensive antihistamine first.

Although cost was a factor in this physician's decision about treatment, the decision was clearly made primarily to promote the patient's interests by reducing her out-of-pocket expenses. Physicians need to remember that patients' interests are not purely medical. In addition, this decision was made primarily by the patient: The physician explained the relative merits and drawbacks of the treatment alternatives, and the patient was able to weigh the costworthiness of the more expensive medication using her own valuation of costs and benefits. Thus, this is an example of rationing, but the decision was not made by the physician and was not made with interests other than the patient's in mind.

Imagine that the physician had prescribed the less expensive medicine without discussing the more expensive alternative. If that had occurred, the physician may have been motivated by the patient's financial interests, but it would be unclear whether those interests had been served, because some patients might be willing to spend more money to avoid possible sedation. The only way to know what a patient wants is to discuss the alternatives with the patient. Similarly, patients often make their own rationing decisions about services that are available only at a great geographic distance. Here, the "cost" of travel and inconvenience may tip the balance against an otherwise medically beneficial service. Discussions about cost when patients care about cost are an integral and important part of informed consent.[24]

If this patient had not had out-of-pocket expenses or had had a copayment that did not vary with the cost of the medication and if the physician had offered only the less expensive medication without discussing the alternative treatment, this case would be a clear example of bedside rationing. The physician would have judged that the additional benefit of the more expensive drug was not worth the extra cost. This decision may be justifiable if, for instance, the patient had known that physicians make such judgments as part of a health-care plan or had known that physicians are expected to follow established guidelines for the use of expensive medications. It may also be justifiable if the physician had told the patient, "There is a more expensive medication that causes less drowsiness, but it is much more expensive and, in our managed-care plan, we reserve it for truck drivers and others whose need for it is more pressing." The patient could choose to pay for the medication herself or could explain that she, too, has a special or pressing need. Physicians in these situations need to be sensitive to the power discrepancy inherent in the physician-patient relationship. Physicians, because of their knowledge and power, can influence patients' decisions and even the way that patients express their values. It is important to recognize that when the patient makes the value judgment, bedside rationing does not occur; in bedside rationing, the physician makes the value judgment that a service is not worth its cost.

CONDITION 3: THE PHYSICIAN HAS CONTROL OVER THE USE OF THE MEDICALLY BENEFICIAL SERVICE

Hospital Control of Contrast Agents

A physician orders intravenous pyelography for a patient with no known allergies. The patient is injected with a high-osmolar contrast agent and has moderate nausea. Later, the patient learns that low-osmolar contrast agents are less likely to cause this uncomfortable side effect.[25] The physician is sorry that the patient had the side effect, but hospital policy had precluded her from ordering low-osmolar contrast agents for a patient without a high risk for a serious adverse reaction.

This case meets the first condition: A service that was in the patient's best interest was withheld. It meets the second condition because, in general, policies such as the one maintained by this hospital are in place to conserve societal resources.[26] However, it does not meet the third condition. This physician did not have control over use of the low-osmolar contrast agent. Instead, it was the hospital that limited the use of the better, but more expensive, contrast agent.

Rationing often occurs outside of individual physician-patient encounters. Formulary committees, utilization reviewers, and third-party payers can all limit physicians' actions.[7] Physicians may even play crucial roles as sources of information or expertise in these organizational rationing decisions. For example, many physicians work on hospital formulary committees. Although formulary committees must think about the moral implications of their decisions,[27] physicians working on formulary committees are not bound by the same moral duties that apply when they work directly with patients. Similarly, physicians may work in government-designed rationing plans, such as Oregon's Medicaid experiment.[28] Physicians who limit the use of expensive medicines through formulary committees are not involved in bedside rationing but are making population-based, organizational-level rationing decisions that may later influence what is available for their individual patients. Similarly, physicians who follow policies established by governments or organizations are not rationing at the bedside.

Use of Scarce Magnetic Resonance Imaging Slots

A neurologist works at a county hospital that does not have a magnetic resonance image (MRI) scanner. The hospital puts money aside each year so that six patients can receive an MRI at a nearby hospital. A physician evaluates a patient who has a "soft indication" for an MRI. The physician could order an MRI for the patient. However, he knows that if he requests an MRI for this patient, he denies an MRI to another patient, who may need it more. Thus, he tells the patient that an MRI is unnecessary.

At first glance, this case does not appear to be an example of bedside rationing. It is not, one might argue, the price of the service that prevented this physician from ordering an MRI but rather the scarcity of time slots, the "absolute scarcity" of this service. In addition, this physician does not appear to have control over the service, because the hospital limits the number of MRIs that can be ordered in a year. However, these appearances are deceptive. In fact, it is the physician who decides when and whether to order the MRI; thus, he has control over the decision. The decision, indirectly, conserves services (scarce MRI "slots") in the interests of other, presumably needier patients. Although it is not dollars per se that are being saved, restrictions on numbers of services—or intensive care beds, or staff members—are ultimately made for financial reasons. Money is, after all, merely the medium of exchange for all health-care (and other) resources.

One could argue that these MRI slots, like intensive care beds or solid organs, are an absolutely scarce resource, whereas money is a relatively scarce resource. This distinction, however, is false. Resources are always limited. They may be stringently limited, as in this case, or more gently limited (as they would have been if this hospital had had its own MRI equipment and could have scanned hundreds of patients per year).

Thus, withholding and not recommending a potentially beneficial MRI counts as bedside rationing. It may be morally justified but should not be dismissed as a noneconomic decision. This example illustrates the importance of "economic honesty." Only openness about these kinds of choices will allow discussion of their merits and morality to proceed.

CLEAR CASES AND TOUGH CALLS

As the above cases show, tough and often subtle calls need to be made when one tries to decide whether a clinical decision qualifies as an instance of bedside rationing. It is not always easy to know what is in a patient's best medical interests. Medical data about the risks and benefits of many health-care services are frequently unclear, and assessment of evidence is itself a value-laden process. Nor is it easy to know what is in a patient's best financial interests when patients may not know their copayment responsibilities. Moreover, physicians frequently make decisions that have implications for public health.

There will always be tough cases, but it is helpful for physicians to be able to recognize when their actions definitely qualify or do not qualify as instances of bedside rationing. The figure summarizes how physicians can recognize when the withholding of a service might qualify as an example of bedside rationing. Physicians should ask themselves the following three questions.

Is the service that is being withheld in the patient's best medical interests? If a withheld service is not in the patient's best medical interests, no rationing of any type has occurred. If the service is clearly in the patient's best medical interests, then the case involves some form of health-care rationing. If the patient's best medical interests are

Ask yourself the following three questions about the service being withheld:

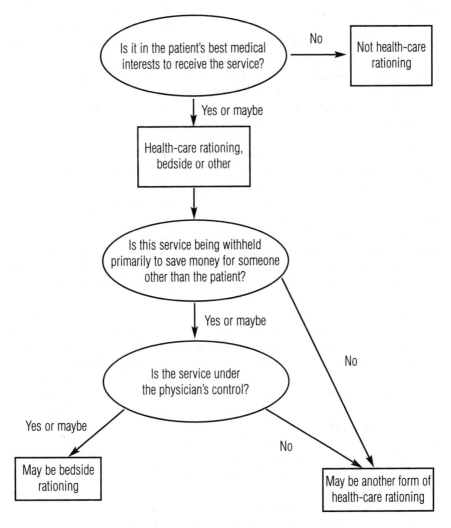

**Figure. How to Recognize When the Withholding
of a Service Qualifies As Bedside Rationing.**

unclear, the question of whether the case involved rationing is also unclear. In such cases, physicians should ask themselves the next two questions to avoid missing any cases that qualify as instances of bedside rationing. It is better to err on the side of overidentification so that physicians can try to decide whether their actions in particular cases are justified.

Is the service being withheld primarily to save money for someone other than the patient? If physicians withhold a service to promote public health or to pursue other nonmonetary goals, they are not engaged in bedside rationing. Similarly, if a patient chooses a less expensive option because of its cost, the rationing is being done not by the physician but by the patient. Physicians may want to pay attention to this "self-imposed" rationing. For example, physicians may choose to take a more active role in influencing health-care or organizational policies that cause patients to have high out-of-pocket costs.

Is the service in question under the physician's control? If a physician's use of a service is limited by, for example, administrative mechanisms, then the withholding of that service is not an example of bedside rationing but an example of rationing through administrative mechanisms. If the physician has complete control over use of the service, then the decision to withhold the service is an example of bedside rationing. In many cases, how much control the physician has is unclear. A physician may need to spend time to get approval for a service, and sometimes such an inordinate amount of time is necessary that it becomes nearly impossible for the physician to obtain the service. At that point, the physician needs to decide whether to spend that time.

In cases in which the answer to all three questions is "yes," physicians have rationed at the bedside. In these cases, physicians need to seriously consider whether their rationing decisions are justified. The medical profession has yet to decide whether bedside rationing is ever morally justified, and, if so, under what circumstances. Physicians may indeed have an important role to play in limiting the use of marginally beneficial services because they are able to consider patients' individual characteristics and preferences (clinical guidelines, for example, cannot do this).

In cases in which the answer to one or more of the questions is "no," physicians do not need to worry that they have participated in bedside rationing. In cases in which the answers to one or more of the questions are unclear—for example, if the best medical interests of the patient are unclear—then whether the physician has participated in bedside rationing is not obvious. Physicians should take cases in this gray area as seriously as if they definitely involved bedside rationing, and they should carefully consider whether their decisions are morally justified.

Only by recognizing what counts as bedside rationing can the next, more controversial step be taken: discussion among physicians, ethicists, patients, and society about the circumstances of, constraints on, and justifications for bedside rationing.

The authors thank Cynthia McNamara, MD, Jane McCort, MD, and David Asch, MD, MBA, for comments on an earlier draft of the manuscript.

REFERENCES

1. Abrams FR. Patient advocate or secret agent? *JAMA.* 1986;256:1784–1785.

2. Angell M. Cost containment and the physician. *JAMA.* 1985;254:1203–1207.

3. Cassell EJ. Do justice, love mercy: the inappropriateness of the concept of justice applied to bedside decisions. In: Shelp EE (ed.). *Justice and Health Care.* New York, NY: D. Reidel; 1981:75–82.

4. Hiatt HH. Protecting the medical commons: who is responsible? *New England Journal of Medicine.* 1975;293:235–241.

5. Sulmasy DP. Physicians, cost control, and ethics. *Annals of Internal Medicine.* 1992;116:920–926.

6. Welch HG. Should the health care forest be selectively thinned by physicians or clear cut by payers? *Annals of Internal Medicine.* 1991;115:223–226.

7. Ubel PA, Arnold RM. The unbearable rightness of bedside rationing. Physician duties in a climate of cost containment. *Archives of Internal Medicine.* 1995;155:1837–1842.

8. Hall M. Rationing health care at the bedside. *New York University Law Review.* 1994;69:693–780.

9. Goold SD, Brody H. Rationing decisions in managed care settings: an ethical analysis. In: Misbin RI, Jennings B, Orentlicher D, Dewar M (eds.). *Health Care Crisis? The Search for Answers.* Frederick, MD: University Publishing Group; 1995.

10. Morreim EH. Fiscal scarcity and the inevitability of bedside budget balancing. *Archives of Internal Medicine.* 1989;149:1012–1015.

11. An international randomized trial comparing four thrombolytic strategies for acute myocardial infarction. The GUSTO investigators. *New England Journal of Medicine.* 1993;329:673–682.

12. Alderman MH. Which antihypertensive drugs first—and why? *JAMA.* 1992;267:2786–2787.

13. Moser M. Current hypertension management: separating fact from fiction. *Cleveland Clinical Journal of Medicine.* 1993;60:27–37.

14. Viberti G, Mogensen CE, Groop LC, Pauls JF. Effect of captopril on progression to clinical proteinuria in patients with insulin-dependent diabetes mellitus and microalbuminuria. European Microalbuminuria Captopril Study Group. *JAMA.* 1994;271:275–279.

15. Anspach RR. *Deciding Who Lives: Fateful Choices in the Intensive-Care Nursery.* Berkeley, CA: University of California Press; 1993.

16. James W. *The Will To Believe and Other Essays in Popular Philosophy.* Cambridge, MA: Harvard University Press; 1979.

17. Wolf AM, Nasser JF, Wolf AM, Schorling JB. The impact of informed consent on patient interest in prostate-specific antigen screening. *Archives of Internal Medicine.* 1996;156:1333–1336.

18. Ubel PA. Informed consent. From bodily invasion to the seemingly mundane [editorial]. *Archives of Internal Medicine.* 1996;156:1262–1263.

19. Barry MJ, Mulley AG Jr, Fowler FJ, Wennberg JW. Watchful waiting vs immediate transurethral resection for symptomatic prosta tism. The importance of patients' preferences. *JAMA.* 1988;259:3010–3017.

20. Pauker SG, McNeil BJ. Impact of patient preferences on the selection of therapy. *Journal of Chronic Diseases.* 1981;34:77–86.

21. Grubbs NC, Schultz HJ, Henry NK, Ilstrup DM, Muller SM, Wilson WR.

Ciprofloxacin versus trimethoprim-sulfamethoxazole: treatment of community-acquired urinary tract infections in a prospective, controlled, double-blind comparison. *Mayo Clinic Proceedings.* 1992;67:1163–1168.

22. Lipsitch M. Fears growing over bacteria resistant to antibiotics. *New York Times.* September 12, 1995: C1.

23. Ubel PA, Arnold RM, Caplan AL. Rationing failure. The ethical lessons of the retransplantation of scarce vital organs. *JAMA.* 1993;270:2469–2474.

24. Ubel P, Loewenstein G. The role of decision analysis in informed consent: choosing between intuition and systematicity. *Social Science and Medicine.* 1997;44(5):647–656.

25. Steinberg EP, Moore RD, Powe NR, et al. Safety and cost effectiveness of high-osmolality as compared with low-osmolality contrast material in patients undergoing cardiac angiography. *New England Journal of Medicine.* 1992;326:425–430.

26. Eddy DM. Clinical decision making: from theory to practice. Applying cost-effectiveness analysis. The inside story. *JAMA.* 1992;268:2575–2582.

27. Hochla PK, Tuason VB. Pharmacy and Therapeutics Committee: cost-containment considerations. *Archives of Internal Medicine.* 1992;152:1773–1775.

28. Garland MJ. Rationing in public: Oregon's priority-setting methodology. In: Strosberg MA, Wiener JM, Baker R, Fein IA (eds.). *Rationing America's Medical Care: The Oregon Plan and Beyond.* Washington, DC: Brookings Institution; 1992.

Part 13

ORGANIZATIONAL ETHICS

꧁꧂

W ithout the encouragement and support of their administrations, health-care providers have little reason to consider, address, and develop solutions to the ethical and social issues they face when caring for patients and families. Even with encouragement and support, for health-care providers to continue such endeavors their recommendations must be taken seriously such that when appropriate, institutional policies and procedures change in response to their recommendations. When health-care organizations do not give staff suggestions appropriate attention, they are implicitly showing a lack of respect for their employees and making it clear that the staff are not considered valuable resources for bringing about institutional improvement. Conversely, when their insights and recommendations are taken seriously and acted upon, the staff's sense of professional ethics is not only fulfilled but, as made clear in part 6, patient and family care will also be improved. The correlation between outcomes and the administration's corporate culture is well recognized by the Joint Commission on Accreditation of Healthcare Organizations (JCAHO), which requires a code of ethics that addresses marketing, admission, transfer, discharge, billing, and professional relationships.[1] Following JCAHO's lead, this section seeks to help ethics committees broaden their focus from the duties and obligations of individual health-care providers to the duties and obligations of institutions, including hospitals, hospice, and long-term care facilities.

In the first reading, "Patient Rights and Organization Ethics: The Joint Commission Perspective," Paul Schyve begins by setting out a health-care institution's obligations and the foundation for those obligations. With this framework in hand, he considers the challenges posed to these obligations by the various health-care financing schemes, particularly managed care. As a senior vice president of JCAHO, his perspective on the business ethics of health care is certainly one to be given serious consideration. In essence, Schyve claims there are two sources of an institution's obligations: the patient–health-care provider relationship and the customer-supplier relationship that exists among patients and institutions. He goes on to make it clear that JCAHO holds these obligations as going well beyond simple "medical treatment" to include respect, nondiscrimination, privacy, confidentiality, and consent.

Although the moral issues raised by managed care are the primary focus of his article, Schyve emphasizes that all health-care financing schemes have their own "ethical challenges." In order to resolve these various challenges, he suggests a five-step process: (1) acknowledge the problem; (2) talk about it openly; (3) work to find a solution built on consensus; (4) establish a proactive program to prevent its recurrence; and (5) take responsibility for ensuring that the solution is carried out. From there he looks at the issues raised by the (non)disclosure of financial incentives, drug formularies, risk sharing, and the underutilization services, all of which are endemic to managed care.

The second reading, by Kevin Wildes, is titled "Institutional Identity, Integrity and Conscience." Wildes takes a more intimate look at what it means for an inanimate object—such as a hospital, hospice, or nursing home—to have a conscience. Importantly, even though he situates his discussion within the context of a Catholic health system, his insights are certainly relevant to nonreligious health-care institutions.

A health-care institution's integrity arises from an amalgam of individual acts and endeavors, beginning with an administration's earnest support of its institutional ethics committee. Providing secretarial support, a budget, and a place to meet are certainly necessary forms of support but are by no means sufficient for an ethics committee to flourish. A committee needs the active and open support of its board, CEO, department heads, managers, and assistant managers. No matter what else an administration does it must begin by openly suggesting that its ethics committee consider the various ethical issues identified in department, unit, and/or board meetings. The administration clearly and loudly demonstrates its support to the entire institution by simply asking the ethics committee to look into those issues raised in such meetings and report back with an assessment and recommendations. Wildes goes on to identify and discuss several prime indicators of a health-care institution's integrity, such as its mission statement, strategic plan, budget, and the staff's right of conscience.

REFERENCE

1. Joint Commission on Accreditation of Healthcare Organizations. *2000 Hospital Accreditation Standards.* Oakbrook, IL: JCAHO; 2000:RI.4., 4.1, 4.2, 4.3, 4.4: 73–74.

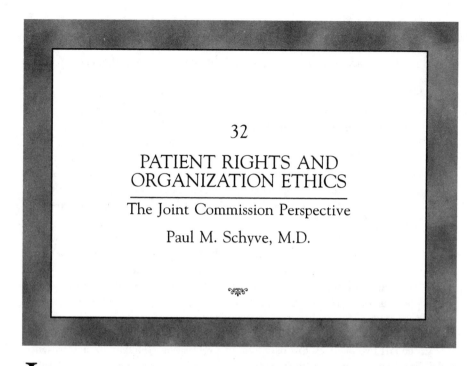

32

PATIENT RIGHTS AND
ORGANIZATION ETHICS

The Joint Commission Perspective

Paul M. Schyve, M.D.

In 1995, the Joint Commission on Accreditation of Healthcare Organizations changed the name of its standards chapters on "Patient Rights" to "Patient Rights and Organization Ethics," to reflect the addition of standards on ethical business behavior. What lies behind this change? This paper will address the relationship of a health-care organization's ethics to patient rights, key themes in an organization's business ethics that are addressed in Joint Commission standards, and special ethical challenges raised by the growth of managed care. Consideration of these issues leads to suggestions concerning the future role of ethics services in health-care organizations.

AN EXPANDING PARADIGM

The paradigm for health-care ethics has been gradually expanding. The earliest paradigm focused on the *practitioner's* obligation to the patient. The third-century B.C.E. Oath of Hippocrates states

> Whatever house I may visit, I will come for the benefit of the sick, remaining free of all intentional injustice.

P. Schyve. "Patient Rights and Organization Ethics: The Joint Commission Perspective." *Bioethics Forum.* 1996;12(2):13–20. Reprinted by permission of the Midwest Bioethics Center.

In 1859, Florence Nightingale echoed this theme of "do the sick no harm" in her *Notes on Hospitals*.

But in the latter half of the twentieth century, the paradigm's focus expanded from the professional's obligation to include a source of that obligation—the rights of *patients*. This expansion arose from three sources:

1. The idea that a person does not forfeit his or her universal human rights by virtue of having become a patient; every patient has the right to be treated with respect as an individual. Both the atrocious experiments on patients in World War II and sociological studies on the inevitable loss of dignity that accompanies routine medical care emphasized the need for respect of persons in health care;

2. The realization that a patient who participates in his or her own health care—from decision making to therapeutic activity—is more likely to have a desirable outcome than is the person who does not participate; and

3. The advent of consumerism in health care, in which key elements of a supplier-customer relationship have been recognized as part of the clinician-patient relationship (i.e., the choosing and using of a service, irrespective of paying for it).

In the last two decades, this paradigm of professionals' obligations and patients' rights has further expanded to include the health-care organization's obligation to respect patients' rights. The first national emphasis on this organizational obligation was reflected in the "Statement on Rights of Patients" published in 1970 in the Joint Commission's 1971 *Accreditation Manual for Hospitals*. This statement said:

> The patient's perception of and response to his environment [of care] are important factors in his progress and recovery. Environmental considerations are reflected in the standards in certain general principles which may be said to represent a set of rights accruing to the patient. . . .

The 1972 "Patient's Bill of Rights" published by the American Hospital Association echoed this idea with the clear statement that the "institution itself has a responsibility to the patient."

Themes of the joint Commission's 1970 statement included that the patient has the right to:

- Ethical and humane treatment
- Respect for his or her individuality and dignity
- No discrimination based on race, color, creed, national origin, or source of payment
- Physical privacy
- Confidentiality of communication
- Information about his or her problem, planned treatment and procedures, prognosis, and how to care for himself or herself.

An important expansion of this list of rights occurred in the 1978 *Accreditation Manual for Hospitals*, with the addition of the patient's right to informed participation in decisions involving his or her care. To enable the patient to give voluntary informed consent, the patient has the right to clear, concise, understandable information about his or her condition and proposed procedures, which includes the probability of success, the possibilities of any risk or problems that might arise, and significant alternatives to the proposed treatment. Should there be any lingering question, the right to refuse treatment (to the extent permitted by law) was explicit. The 1978 statement had another significant addition. It introduced the idea that the patient has rights as a customer or consumer, i.e., the patient is entitled to an itemized, detailed explanation of his or her bill.

This brief, historical summary suggests that a health-care *organization's* obligation to patients derives from two relationships:

1. The patient-provider relationship that is built on the patient's acceptance and trust in the provider's commitment to do no harm, to treat the patient with respect and dignity, and to make the patient a full participant in decisions about his or her care.
2. The customer-supplier relationship that is built on the trust derived from the organization's business practices.

The former relationship is governed by "clinical" ethics, and the latter relationship is governed by "business" ethics. But these two relationships and their ethical dimensions are not independent. For example, bad customer-supplier relationships can lead to avoidance by patients of needed care, provision of unneeded care (with its attendant risks) to patients, and failure of patients to participate effectively in their treatment, i.e., to "comply" with treatment recommendations. Any of these are likely to lead to less-than-optimum health outcomes. That is, there may be clinical "harm" to the patients that arises through acts of commission or omission in business behavior.

CHALLENGES IN BUSINESS ETHICS

Challenges in health-care business ethics have been attributed to the financing mechanisms and organizational structures in the health-care system. Consequently, some observers have proposed that the solution is one or another mechanism or structure. But each mechanism and structure brings its own ethical challenges, such as the following:

- Fee-for-service incentives that favor overutilization of services, with the subsequent unnecessary risks and costs that accompany some diagnostic tests and treatment;
- Risk-sharing (e.g., DRGs and capitation) incentives that reward underutilization of services and not informing the patient about alternative, perhaps more effective, treatments;
- Independent services provided by multiple organizations with incentives involving fee splitting for referrals, or, less overtly, mutually beneficial reciprocal referrals that do not reflect the patient's best interests; and

- Integration of services within one organization, which promotes self-referral for unneeded but separately reimbursed services (e.g., outpatient consultants acting as "recruiters" for nursing homes that are part of their system).

Clearly, ethical challenges are unavoidable. In some cases, the challenge derives from a conflict between the interest of the patient and the success, at least for the short term, of the organization. In other cases, the conflict is between two ethical principles, such as the good of the individual versus the good of the community. What should be the organization's response? It could try to resolve the challenge by telling the patient caveat emptor, but most providers and patients would find this not only unsatisfactory but unethical in itself. The organization could rely on the personal ethics of each practitioner and administrator in the health-care system to withstand all temptation and to do the right thing. This, however, doesn't account for the fact that some individuals do not live by high ethical principles, that most of us have occasional ethical lapses, and that knowing the "right thing" can be difficult when ethical principles conflict. Or, organizations can face the ethical challenges and meet them.

How are these ethical challenges managed? There are five steps:

- *Recognizing* and *acknowledging* the challenge;
- *Discussing* the challenge openly with stakeholders and decision makers, gathering pertinent information, listening to the various viewpoints, identifying pertinent ethical values, and identifying relevant ethical principles;
- *Resolving* the challenge, through consensus whenever possible;
- Building in *protections* against behaviors and outcomes that the resolution desires to avoid; and
- Being *accountable* to the public—patients and other health-care consumers—for the resolution and its implementation.

THE JOINT COMMISSION RESPONSE

Within this context, the Joint Commission introduced new standards on organizational ethics in all its 1995 and 1996 accreditation standards manuals (i.e., for ambulatory care, behavioral health care, health-care networks, home care, hospitals, long-term care, and pathology and laboratory services). These new standards arose out of well-publicized concerns about abuses in which patients were admitted to hospitals unnecessarily and were discharged or transferred only after their insurance expired. Patient advocates and health-care professionals proposed that the Joint Commission address these abuses because unnecessary admissions and inappropriate discharges can affect patient care quality. Some health-care professionals also believed that a response by a professionally sponsored standard-setting body would convey to the public that most professionals were opposed to such unethical behavior.

The standards (in the language of the 1996 *Accreditation Manual for Hospitals*) are as follows:

- The hospital [or other health-care organization] operates according to a code of ethical behavior;

- The code addresses marketing, admission, transfer and discharge, and billing practices; and
- The code addresses the relationship of the [organization] and its staff to other health-care providers, educational institutions, and payers.

The intent of these standards is as follows:

An [organization] has an ethical responsibility to the patients and community it serves. Guiding documents such as the [organization's] mission statement and strategic plan provide a consistent, ethical framework for its patient care and business practices. But a framework alone is not sufficient. To support ethical operations and fair treatment of patients, an [organization] has and operates according to a code of ethical behavior. The code addresses ethical practices regarding: marketing; admission transfer; discharge; and billing and resolution of conflicts associated with patient billing. The code ensures that the [organization] conducts its business and patient care practices in an honest, decent, and proper manner.

To meet the intent of these standards, the organization must recognize and acknowledge the ethical challenges it faces in these areas and must discuss and resolve them in order to generate its own code of ethical business behavior. What mechanisms can be used for discussion and resolution?

Since 1992, standards in the "Patient Rights" chapter of the accreditation manuals have required every organization accredited by JCAHO to have a mechanism for consideration of ethical issues that arise in the care of patients, and to provide education to staff and patients about ethical issues in health care. The standards do not specify the mechanism to be used, but give examples that include ethics committees, ethics consultation services, and formal ethics forums. This deliberate reticence acknowledges that different mechanisms may best meet the needs of different organizations and that innovation in developing more effective mechanisms is to be encouraged. The common mechanisms currently in use—ethics committees and consultation services—have generally focused on issues in clinical ethics, often involving the care of an individual patient. While not required by Joint Commission standards, it is suggested that existing mechanisms, such as ethics committees and consultation services, be expanded to provide services to those facing challenges in the area of business ethics. This suggestion is based on the following two considerations:

1. The boundary between "clinical" ethics and "business" ethics is not clear and in many cases is nonexistent. While marketing and admission practices are seen as issues related to "business" ethics, they can lead to unneeded admissions or demand for unneeded services, both of which can unnecessarily expose the patient to the risk of side effects or complications. Likewise, underutilization of needed services is likely to lead to less-than-optimal health outcomes.

2. The knowledge and expertise of the individuals in existing mechanisms, such as ethics committees and consultation services, have much to contribute to the resolution of challenges in business ethics. For example, effective members of ethics committees and consultation services have: knowledge of ethical prin-

ciples; knowledge of how to reason about ethical questions; skills in communicating and educating about these ethical principles and methods of reasoning; and skills in facilitating ethical dialogue and decision making.

Each of these bodies of knowledge and skills is necessary to resolve ethical challenges in business decisions and practice, and their expansion to that realm will help prevent artificial separations between "clinical" and "business" ethical issues. But this suggested expansion in the scope of the ethics mechanism may require an expansion in the expertise of participants (usually through augmenting membership of existing committees and consultation services to include administrators and other nonclinicians) and will require that the mechanisms be accessible to the organization's nonclinical administration and staff.

If an organization recognizes and acknowledges the challenges and discusses and resolves the issues, it must also protect and be accountable to the public for its actions. Ultimately, accountability means telling health-care consumers what risks they face from the ethical challenges, how they are being protected from those risks, and how successful the organization is at protecting them. Effective ways to protect the patient and other health-care consumers are to make public the organization's code of business ethics and its criteria for admission, transfer, and discharge, and to encourage patients to review their bills. Public disclosure not only is an incentive to the organization and its staff to make good ethical decisions and to live by them, but also enlists the patient as a participant in his or her own care, including protecting himself or herself from harm.

Just as there has been advice to patients to ask the doctors and nurses about the medication they receive, likewise, they should be encouraged to ask questions about their admission, discharge, and treatments and to inquire about alternatives. This encouragement should go beyond the requirements set forth in current Joint Commission standards, which stipulate that the organization have a publicized mechanism to review and expeditiously resolve complaints from patients and their families and to inform the complainant of the outcome.

ISSUES IN MANAGED CARE

As noted above, a health-care organization such as a managed-care organization that is at financial risk in providing care to a defined population faces a potential ethical challenge that culminates in risk of underutilization of necessary services. Because of financial risk borne by the organization, there can be a temptation to provide fewer services and the least expensive services to an enrollee. This temptation could influence the ordering of diagnostic tests, referrals to specialty care, admission to a more intensive setting (e.g., the hospital), the use of specialty services (e.g., rehabilitation), the list of medications included in the approved formulary, the organization's policy on off-formulary prescribing, and recommendations for therapeutic and rehabilitative procedures.

The need for the organization to contain costs within a fixed income can place pressures on clinicians and administrators to act in ways that are not in a patient's best interest. Certain methods of risk sharing with clinicians and /or administrators can transfer this pressure from the organization as a whole to the individual. For example, if a portion of a physician's income is based on how much money is not spent on patient care, the physician may be tempted to avoid services needed by the patient. Associated with these pressures is another risk: some managed-care organizations have, by written or unwritten policy or through incentives, restricted the physician's freedom in informing the patient about alternative treatments that are either costly or not offered within the organization's benefit package.

These pressures tend to exacerbate certain ethical challenges including those that involve:

- The interest of the patient versus the interest of the organization, including employees and their families;
- The interest of the one—the individual patient—versus the interest of the many—the population served by the organization; and
- The interest in constraining choice so that it involves using the most cost-effective intervention versus the patient's right to be informed about alternative treatments (some of which may have merits other than cost-effectiveness, or which may not yet have received adequate study regarding cost-effectiveness) and to participate in decision making.

To address these challenges and risks, in 1994 the Joint Commission expanded the scope of the organizational ethics standards for managed care organizations accredited under its Health Care Network Accreditation Program. The following new standard was added (in the language of the 1996 *Accreditation Manual for Health Care Networks*):

> The network's code of ethical business and professional behavior protects the integrity of clinical decision making, regardless of how the network compensates or shares financial risk with its leaders, managers, clinical staff, and licensed independent practitioners.

The intent of this standard is

> to avoid compromising the quality of care, clinical decisions, including tests, treatments, and other interventions that are based solely on member health care needs. The network's code of ethical business and professional behavior specifies that the network implements policies and procedures that address this issue. Policies and procedures and information about the relationship between the use of services and financial incentives are available on request to all members, clinical staff, licensed independent practitioners, and network personnel.

This intent statement makes clear that the standard requires that the organization recognize and acknowledge the ethical challenges that arise in connection with financial incentives or sharing of financial risk, and requires that the organization discuss and resolve the ethical challenges in order to create its own code of ethical business and professional behavior. The organization must then protect the public—patients and enrollees—from these risks by establishing policies and procedures that reflect and implement the resolutions embodied in the code, and it must be accountable to the patients and enrollees by publicly disclosing the source of the risk ("the relationship between the use of services and financial incentives") and its method of protection from this risk ("policies and procedures").

The pressure to reduce costs could also tempt a managed-care organization to base the composition of its practitioner panel predominantly on financial consideration. While managed-care organizations or fee-for-service settings, including hospitals, may use economic, including utilization, criteria in appointment and reappointment, these decisions can affect the quality of care. Not only could they be disruptive of a patient's long-standing doctor-patient relationship, but they could also be unintentionally biased toward practitioners who succumb to the incentives for underutilization of needed services. To address this risk, the Joint Commission introduced the following standard in its 1996 *Accreditation Manual for Hospitals* and *Accreditation Manual for Health Care Networks* (in the language of the Network manual):

> Decisions on appointments or reappointments [and clinical privileges in hospitals] consider criteria directly related to the quality of care.

Thus, when a contemplated decision is based on financial aspects or considerations other than quality of care, the potential impact of the decision on the quality of care must be considered before it is implemented. That is, the organization must *recognize* and *acknowledge* the potential risk, and must *discuss* and *resolve* it, making its own record of its decision and rationale.

CONCLUSION

In today's turbulent environment, health-care organizations face ethical challenges on a daily basis. Some challenges seem directly related to decisions about an individual's care, and have been traditionally thought of as issues in *clinical* ethics. Other challenges seem more related to business decisions, and have been thought of as issues in *business* ethics. In both realms, the health-care organization, as an organization, plays a role, whether in establishing procedures for obtaining informed consent—a focus of clinical ethics—or in establishing guidelines for truth in marketing—a focus of business ethics. Hence, in a health-care organization, clinical ethics and business ethics together comprise its *organization* ethics.

However, the boundaries between clinical ethics and business ethics may turn out to be ephemeral or illusory. For example, business decisions and practices in marketing, admissions, discharges, transfers, and reimbursement mechanisms can all affect patient care and, ultimately, patient health outcomes and patient satisfaction.

Patient health outcomes are as close to *clinical* as one can get. Separating business ethics from clinical ethics in practice, therefore, is unlikely to serve the best interests of either the patient or health-care organization or those who are trying to resolve the ethical challenges in health care. Regardless of the issues from which the challenge arises, a sound approach to resolving the challenge has the same elements: *recognition* and *acknowledgment* of the challenge, *discussion* and *resolution* of the challenge, *protection* against failure to act in accordance with the resolution, and *accountability* to those at risk—the public, including individual patients and plan members—for the organization's decisions and actions.

The basic knowledge and skills needed to successfully use this approach in resolving ethical challenges often can be found in existing organizational structures and mechanisms used to resolve ethical issues that arise in the care of patients, such as clinical ethics committees and ethics consultation services. An expansion in the scope and business ethics expertise of these mechanisms, and in their accessibility, would build on the mechanisms' strengths, and would help avoid an often artificial and unproductive compartmentalization of ethical issues.

While the Joint Commission, through its standards, has called upon health-care organizations to act ethically in their business practices, it is the organizations themselves that must struggle with the ethical challenges they face and resolve them in the contexts of their own ethical values. Ultimately, the public will hold them accountable for those values and decisions.

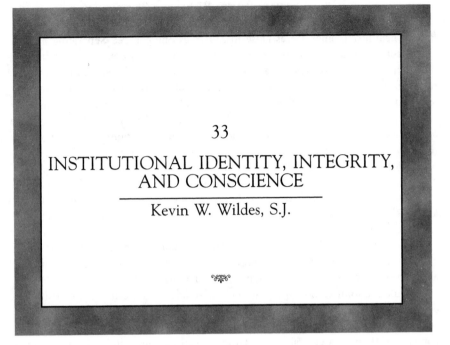

33
INSTITUTIONAL IDENTITY, INTEGRITY, AND CONSCIENCE

Kevin W. Wildes, S.J.

Conscience is almost always discussed in reference to individuals. The essays by James Childress, for example, continue his important work on individual conscience.[1-3] I will argue, however, that conscience can apply, analogously, to institutions and corporations. I will further argue that, given changes in contemporary health care, bioethics will be inadequate if we in the field only look at individuals and fail to look at institutional practices and questions. Indeed, several years ago Ezekiel Emanuel[4] challenged the bioethics community to turn its attention from particular cases and principles to institutional arrangements and structures.

I hope to argue successfully that an important area of development for ethics and bioethics, especially in the context of managed care, is to conceive of ethical issues as issues not only for individual persons, but for systems and social structures as well. This is a shift that must be made for both ethics and health care. The institutional and social structures that support and surround health care will not allow us to ask ethical questions as if they existed only at the level of individual choice. Too many of the ethical issues of the clinic are well beyond the control of the individuals involved. The issues of bioethics have moved beyond the bedside, the clinic,

K. Wildes. "Institutional Identity, Integrity, and Conscience." *Kennedy Institute of Ethics Journal.* 1997;7(4):413–419. © The Johns Hopkins University Press.

and the stand-alone hospital. These changes call for an important shift in the moral imagination to situate ethical questions in the web of institutional patterns and relationships. Institutional conscience can be an important tool in this development.

It may be helpful for my argument to begin by placing the present American health-care situation in a broader historical context. Medicine has been both a product of and resistant to the forces of modernity, until now. The shifts to models of managed care, corporate medicine, have moved important parts of health care from the guild model of the late Renaissance to the corporate model of modernity. Managed care completes the move of medicine into modernity. This context and change create new questions of ethics. It is in this context that one can and should think about institutional identity and institutional conscience.

MEDICINE AND MODERNITY

There are many ways to talk about modernity. The different debates about "postmodernity" serve to illustrate just how difficult it can be to define modernism and the modern age. One way to characterize modernity is to examine the dominant model of knowledge in the modern age: science. In the modern age, science has replaced theology, the model of the Middle Ages, as the central method of human knowing. In the modern age, even theology aspires to be "scientific." In modernity scientific knowledge is characterized as universal and objective. True knowledge is not based on the particular or the subjective. The particular is treated as a part of a universal—e.g., the class of patients with a particular disease. What cannot be universally understood or measured is treated as subjective and private.

Modernity can also be characterized by important economic shifts. There has been a move away from an agrarian society to an industrialized society. Industrialization has given rise to the scientific welfare state. In this way modernity has supported the evolution of the centralized state and the rise of bureaucratic structures to address basic human needs (welfare systems). Changes in the economic order—e.g., industrialization/technology and capital markets—have led to more bureaucratic structures in social life and the development of centralized bureaucracy and government. Systems of education and health care arose not only in response to the explosion of knowledge but also to replace and support what families used to do but can no longer do in the urbanized economic order.

Until recently, medicine in the United States has had a peculiar relationship to modernity. On the one hand, medicine has benefited enormously from the rise of the scientific model. Scientific knowledge has redefined the purpose of medicine as "cure." Hospitals, as centers of technology, reflect the modern, bureaucratic structures to deliver health care. At the same time, however, physicians in the United States have retained a guild or artisan model of operation.[5] The model for physicians has been solo practitioners. Even hospitals have been largely standalone operations.

The development of managed care in the United States can be understood as the continuation of the pattern of modernization for American medicine. While the surge in managed care has been driven by the cost of fee-for-service medicine, the models of managed care are tied to the patterns of modern, bureaucratic, corporate life. Managed care represents the completion of the shift from the guild model to the model of corporate and bureaucratic health care. It represents the completion of the movement of medicine into the modern age. The change in economic structure completes a transition for medicine into the modern age.

The change to the model of managed care moves the practice of medicine to focus on the care of populations and not only the patient who is before the physician. To view medicine as addressing the needs of particular patients is an incomplete reading of the modern context. Managed care forces physicians to see themselves as part of larger teams. Furthermore, managed care brings to medical practice many of the fruits of scientific study and knowledge—e.g., evidence-based medicine, outcome studies, patient assessment, and the like. Through the use of statistical knowledge, practice guidelines, outcome studies, and utilization reviews, managed care has emphasized the "science" of medicine over the "art" of medicine.

A NEW CONTEXT FOR ETHICS

The traditional context for questions of ethics in health care has been a focus on particular patients, that is, individuals. The traditional focus has been physician ethics. What should I do? How should the patient be treated? What is my role as a health-care professional in this situation? However, the shift toward managed care puts the questions that must be faced by individual physicians and patients into a different context and adds a new dimension to ethical discourse. The physician is no longer the solo practitioner. The hospital is no longer a stand-alone facility. Patients are no longer seen in the singular but are now seen as part of a patient population, and treatment is guided by statistical analysis. Institutions and professionals are set in a maze of relationships and obligations.

Some are skeptical about any talk of institutional conscience or institutional moral integrity.[6] However, there is at least one history of institutional experience that points to the possibility of institutional moral integrity and conscience. In the last century, Roman Catholic health-care facilities have struggled with the question of institutional identity and agency. This is not a history or experience to be copied by others. It is, however, a history from which we can learn.

This experience provides two important elements for thinking about institutional conscience. The first element is from Roman Catholic social thought and social ethics. A crucial insight of the social justice tradition has been that justice involves concerns not only about how goods are distributed, but also with how a society is ordered and structured, a topic that raises the fundamental questions of *social justice*. This line of thought reminds us that an institution's structures, processes, and corporate culture reflect the fundamental moral commitments of the institution. In a discussion of institutional moral identity and conscience such structures become important tools for analysis.

A second element from Roman Catholic experience involves the idea of institutional identity and cooperation. As Catholic institutions have been in the world and part of the fabric of different societies and cultures, the Roman Catholic community has been concerned with how institutional identity can be maintained.[7,8] This concern has lead to a series of guidelines and directives for Roman Catholic institutions in the United States. These guidelines are an example of a group of institutions struggling to articulate and maintain a moral identity.

In light of these two elements from the experience of Catholic health-care institutions, I would argue that an institution can have a moral identity and conscience. A necessary condition for talking about institutional conscience is the moral identity of an institution. One way to explore this moral identity is to look at the mission of an institution. How does an institution understand itself? How does it present itself?[9] A mission will not be comprised exclusively in terms of moral values and commitments. But if there are common moral commitments for the institution, the mission should be articulated in such a way that the moral commitments can be identified.

In writing about conscience, James Childress has noted that appeals to conscience involve appeals to moral standards, but conscience itself is not a moral standard. Like "integrity" or "wholeness," conscience needs content.[10] For an institutional conscience the articulation of a mission is central. Within the broad institutional parameters of mission one can begin to think about moral integrity. That is, does the institution live out its moral commitments? Such a living-out need not be thought of as simply unimaginative consistency. Circumstances, contexts, and problems change and develop. So too integrity will involve creativity and fidelity.

Developing an understanding of mission should give an institution the criteria to develop the tools to evaluate mission effectiveness and shape and implement institutional conscience. For example, one might look at the Ethical and Religious Directives (ERD) for Roman Catholic health-care institutions in the United States[7] as setting out a broad framework in which Roman Catholic institutions can articulate their mission. The ERD are best known, perhaps, for the prohibitions they contain—e.g., against abortion, euthanasia, and sterilization. However, an equally important part of the ERD is the positive vision they articulate for Catholic health-care institutions.

TOOLS FOR LIVING OUT THE IDENTITY

Assuming that an institution or system can articulate a mission, how does that mission get implemented? How can a vision become real? It is essential to the development of institutional conscience that, whatever form a mission takes, the mission has a common ownership within an institution. The mission supplies the vision against which institutional structures and procedures can be evaluated.

A critical tool for the integrity and conscience of an institution is the *budget*. A budget should be understood as a planning document. It is an articulation of an institution's mission. For example, if an institution says in its mission statement that it is committed to care of the poor, but makes no line-item commitment to care of the poor, one can say that the institution either is in deep self-deception or is lying.

Along with a budget, an institution's *strategic plan* and *planning process* are important to its mission, identity, and conscience. Just as individuals plan according to life goals and objectives, so, too, health-care institutions and systems need to deploy a planning process. A measure for the conscience of an institution is the degree to which the moral commitments of the institution are part of its strategic planning. They ought to shape the long-term goals and the means that are used to achieve them.

The process of planning involves a process of self-study and evaluation. One could well imagine a hospital *ethics committee* or some analogous structure that reviews the practices and policies of an institution. The focus would be not only on patients and particular issues of clinical care but also on the whole moral culture of the institution, including, for example, advertisement.

In this whole process, the role of the institution's *trustees/directors* is crucial. They have a special role in the articulation of institutional mission and identity and a special responsibility to call and lead the institution in fidelity to that mission. While others may be more concerned with the day-to-day details of patient care and institutional management, the duty of trustees is to ask for accountability for broader questions of institutional identity and life.

If there is to be development of an institutional moral identity and conscience, then there needs to be an ongoing process of *education* to shape the culture of the institution. Education is important for ongoing renewal and adaptation. It is also important for consent. That is, the members of the institution, patients, workers, and professionals, need to consent to the mission. They need to be aware of the culture of the institution they are joining. Of course, there is rarely a "perfect fit" of individuals and institutions. Another crucial tool, therefore, will be the provisions made for the *protection of individual conscience*.

CONCLUSION

The changing character of health care raises a new area of investigation and discourse for bioethics: institutional ethics. I have argued that there can be an institutional moral identity and an institutional conscience. Institutional conscience is shaped by the mission of the institution, and it is implemented by the structures of the institution such as budgeting and planning. Internal practices provide a way to measure what an institution really is, and institutional structures provide a way to evaluate how well an institution lives out the mission it announces.

REFERENCES

1. Childress JF. Conscience and conscientious actions in the context of MCOs. *Kennedy Institute of Ethics Journal.* 1997;7:403–411.

2. Childress JF. Appeals to conscience. *Ethics.* 1979;89:315–355.

3. Childress JF. Civil disobedience, conscientious objection, and evasive noncompliance: a framework for the analysis and assessment of illegal actions in health care. *Journal of Medicine and Philosophy.* 1985;10:63–83.

4. Emanuel E. Medical ethics in the era of managed care: the need for institutional structures instead of principles for individual cases. *Journal of Clinical Ethics.* 1995;6:335–338.

5. Madison D. Preserving individualism in the organizational society: "cooperation" and American medical practice, 1900–1920. *Bulletin of the History of Medicine.* 1997;70:442–483.

6. Rie M. Defining the limits of institutional agency in health care: a response to Kevin Wildes. *Journal of Medicine and Philosophy.* 1991;16:221–224.

7. United States Catholic Conference. Ethical and religious directives for Catholic health care services. *Origins.* 1994;24:449, 451–461.

8. Wildes KW. A memo from the central office: the "ethical and religious directives for Catholic health care services." *Kennedy Institute of Ethics Journal.* 1995;5:133–139.

9. Collins JC, Porras JI. Building your company's vision. *Harvard Business Review.* 1996(September/October):65–77.

10. Wildes KW. Institutional integrity: approval, toleration and holy war, or "always true to you in my fashion." *Journal of Medicine and Philosophy.* 1991;16:211–220.

Part 14

ISSUES IN
GENETIC TESTING

❦

T he number of patients who have elected to undergo genetic testing has become astonishing, as is their ability to choose from over 550 different tests. This interest in genotyping is not new, as ten years ago the interest was widespread enough that *Consumer Reports* actually rated genetic tests in their July 1990 issue. Genetic testing has gone from being a widespread phenomenon to medicine's new magic bullet, thanks in particular to the completion of a working draft to the human genome in June of 2000. With this achievement in hand there will soon be an unprecedented upsurge in not only the number of traits that can be tested for, but also in the number of patients, employers, and health insurers who will want them. This conclusion requires little in the way of predictive powers as by mid-2000, the U.S. Patent and Trademark Office had already awarded some two thousand gene patents, with twenty-five thousand or so applications still pending.

For many in health care all this hoopla about genetic testing is far removed from their everyday work, but that will change. Fortunately, this lag time presents health-care providers and ethics committees with a unique opportunity in medical ethics: the ability to proactively address the ethical and social issues brought about by a new technology. To that end, the following readings discuss the scientific basis of genetic testing, when genetic tests might be used, and what the potential benefits and burdens of these tests might be for patients and their families. The goal of this section is to help health-care providers address their patients' concerns regarding whether they should be tested, what a positive test could mean, and how a positive test could affect their insurability or employment. This section also seeks to help ethics committees reformulate their policies on privacy and confidentiality in light of genetic testing, as well as establish a new policy on genetic testing itself.

As was put forth in part 3, before doing anything else we must "collect the facts and understand the medical reality." This has unfortunately been made rather difficult by the news media, which have continually failed to give an accurate account of both genetic testing and disease causation.

Contrary to popular belief, genetic testing does not definitively identify who will actually "get" a disease, and most of them leave wide open the question of how someone will be affected by a disease, presuming they do get it. The BRCA1 test for breast cancer provides a good example of the limits to genetic testing. A positive test for a BRCA1 gene mutation is believed to indicate a 55 to 65 percent lifetime chance of developing breast cancer if the person being tested is in an "at risk" population. The problem with patients, insurers, and employers relying on this as a basis for action is threefold: First, testing positive for the BRCA1 mutation does not mean the patient will actually get breast cancer, it simply means she is at an increased risk. Second, testing negative for the BRCA1 mutation (meaning the patient has a normal BRCA1 gene) does not mean the patient will not get breast cancer; it means she has the same 1-in-9 chance of getting breast cancer as the rest of the population. And third, patients, insurers, and employers are applying the test results of those in an "at risk" population to the test results of those not in an "at risk" population. Hence, a patient's decision to have a prophylactic mastectomy, a health insurer's decision to deny coverage, and an employer's decision to deny employment are all based on test results that do not mean what they think they mean.

With regard to disease causation it would be instructive to briefly consider the problematic nature of classifying a disease as being either wholly "genetic" or wholly "environmental" (epigenetic). Cystic fibrosis (CF) has traditionally been thought of as a paradigm of a recessive[1] genetic disease, as it was seen as having 100 percent penetrance.[2] Once the gene was sequenced, however, the situation became much more complicated as it was discovered that there are multiple alleles[3] at the CF locus[4] that can produce the truncated[5] protean, the most common of which is the ΔF508 mutation, that can cause the signs and symptoms of CF. In other words, the problems inherent in testing for breast cancer via the BRCA1 mutation apply to testing for CF via the sweat chloride test, which looks for the ΔF508 mutation. The problem with relying on genetic tests for CF became apparent when researchers found patients who had all the signs and symptoms of CF, but did not have the ΔF508 mutation. There are also individuals who have the ΔF508 mutation but are completely asymptomatic, when it is this mutation that is correlated with the more sever symptoms of CF. Strangely enough, researchers have even found patients with severe symptoms but only minor mutations, while at the same time finding patients with significant mutations but only mild symptoms. Although the full meaning of these observations is still unknown, they certainly make it problematic to continue classifying CF as a paradigm of genetic disease.

The goal of the preceding example was to illustrate the complexity of disease causation, as there are myriad genetic and epigenetic factors that must be present for someone to actually "have" a disease. By appreciating this complexity we are in a better position to understand the issues raised in the following two articles on genetic testing. We begin with "Genetic Tests: Evolving Policy Questions" by Drs. David Asch and Michael Mennuti. This article looks at the benefits and burdens of patient-initiated testing (through the physician), testing by an employer, and testing by a health insurer.

Patient-initiated genetic testing can be beneficial but only so long as the patient is mindful of the test's limitations. One such benefit can come about when a patient learns he has a certain genotype that is a known contributing factor to a disease. The authors cite a positive test for Ataxia-telangiectasia, an autosomal[6] recessive disease, as an example. Those with this gene have an increased risk for cancer as a result of being particularly sensitive to radiation. This knowledge allows patients to avoid common sources of radiation such as diagnostic X-rays and mammograms. In contrast, genetic tests can also do harm both physically and emotionally. If a genetic test is used to determine the "cause" of an unknown illness, a positive result could actually be harmful because potentially beneficial treatment options may be ruled out, or not even considered, because they are outside the official treatment "box." In another vein, a positive result could cause significant emotional harm while offering no benefit in the balance. The authors use the test for Huntington's to raise this issue by asking how patients' interests are served by knowing their genotype is a major contributing factor to a deadly disease when nothing can be done.

The remainder of their discussion focuses on the usefulness of genetic tests to health insurers and employers. Taking into account the ever-present quest to reduce health-care expenditures, Asch and Mennuti raise the specter of a genetic underclass that would be uninsurable and unemployable. These fears are certainly well grounded, as surveys have begun to reveal that companies are actively gathering genetic information on prospective and current employees, through interviews and required genetic testing. For now it is a small percentage, but some employers are using genetic information to decide who to hire and who to promote, as there are currently no federal laws preventing genetic discrimination in the workplace. Health insurers, on the other hand, do not have this luxury, as federal law currently prevents them from discriminating on the basis of genetic information. However, this law only protects those enrolled in group health plans, leaving some thirteen to fifteen million self-insured Americans vulnerable to such discrimination.

The next reading in this section opens with two cases, the first of which explores the emotions and conflicts that are brought about when a family must decide whether to have a prenatal genetic test for Huntington's. In "Ethical Implications of Genetic Testing," Deborah Raines provides us with a fundamental understanding of the science of genetic testing so that we are able to gain greater insight into the ethical and social issues raised by disease, carrier, and prenatal genetic testing, particularly the latter.

Raines's first case evolves as Mary, who is pregnant, begins to suspect that her husband's family has a long history of Huntington's disease. Through this case it quickly becomes apparent that there is something very unique about genetic testing: connectedness. If a patient has a genetic test, in a manner of speaking his family is also having a genetic test, without their consent or knowledge. To return to the case at hand, if Mary tests her fetus, then she is also having her husband, Jim, tested; a positive test for the fetus is a positive test for Jim. Even when she simply turns to her family and friends for support, Mary is preempting Jim's right to decide who, if anyone, knows about his "condition." Through Jim's predicament, Raines goes on to make clear the need for ethics committees to reformulate their policies on privacy and confidentiality to include considerations for the families of those who undergo genetic testing. This technology also necessitates the formation of a new section within the genetic testing consent forms. In particular, patients must appreciate that not only can they harm their families by violating their privacy, they can also harm them by "forcing" them to know potentially unwanted and emotionally harmful information. Therefore, by including this issue in consent forms, patients are encouraged to consider ways they can share their health issues with their families without forcing unwanted information on them. Although such a balancing act may not always be possible, at least patients will be aware that this is something else to take into account.

REFERENCES

1. A minimal or no phenotypic effect when occurring in a heterozygous condition that has a contrasting allele.

2. The proportion of individuals with a particular genotype that expresses its phenotypic effect in a given environment.

3. An alternative form of a gene that occurs at a particular locus.

4. The position of a particular gene or allele in a chromosome.

5. A protean that is lacking an expected or normal element.

6. A non-sex-linked chromosome.

34

GENETIC TESTS

Evolving Policy Questions

David A. Asch, M.D., and Michael T. Mennuti, M.D.

❦

Rapid advances in molecular biology are changing the world and the way we think of ourselves. As the Human Genome Project moves forward, we will identify more and more of the estimated 100,000 genes that make up our genome. This information will help us understand, identify, and eventually treat many genetic disorders and other diseases in which genetic predisposition plays an important role.[1]

A central challenge posed by these advances is that the technology to diagnose genetic conditions and predispositions inevitably precedes the ability to intervene with specific treatments. During this window, genetic information has little therapeutic outlet and may find social outlets with desirable but also undesirable consequences. For example, the gene for cystic fibrosis was identified in 1989, making it possible in many cases to identify heterozygous carriers of this mutation who, though unaffected themselves, may bear children with cystic fibrosis. This discovery was an important medical advance, but it posed a challenge because there is no definitive treatment for this disorder. In such cases, genetic information may have undesirable social consequences.[2-7]

Current or soon-to-be-available genetic tests such as these raise the issue of potential uses and misuses of information. This is an issue of which both clinicians and the public need to be aware.

D. Asch, M. Mennuti. "Genetic Tests: Evolving Policy Questions." *IEEE Technology and Society.* Winter 1996/1997. ©1996 IEEE. Reprinted with permission.

SCREENING AND STAKEHOLDERS

As the genes for more diseases are identified, our concept of screening for genetic diseases is changing. The entire population is becoming the potential audience for genetic tests. Screening is no longer performed only in specialized medical settings by those experienced with interpreting and delivering genetic information, but in the offices of other health professionals, and in employment and insurance settings where safeguards for counseling and confidentiality cannot be assumed. This promises to make potentially valuable information available to more patients, but raises concerns about how this information will be transmitted and used. A report from the House Committee on Government Operations states that the complex problems that will result from our expanding knowledge of the human genome must be addressed "before inappropriate uses of genetic information become institutionalized."[2]

Different stakeholders will use genetic information differently. Patients, the most obvious and most legitimate stakeholders, have the most to benefit or lose from genetic information. They benefit from a genetic test when they learn they are not at risk for a familial condition or, if at risk, that they can minimize or eliminate that risk. They may lose if the information causes uncompensated anxiety or distress, or leads to social stigma or discrimination. Similar potential benefits and losses are provided by other medical tests that do not have a genetic basis, but there are important differences as well.

Genetic tests have special meaning because of their implications for the health prospects of relatives and future generations. Knowledge that an individual carries genetic mutations may be at once valuable and troublesome for relatives. Tests to detect infection with the human immunodeficiency virus raise similar issues: sexual contacts and children of a tested individual have a stake in the test results and may benefit or lose.

Physicians, genetic counselors, and other health professionals are stakeholders as well. Increasingly they will be asked to educate patients about the tests. and to help them make decisions about their use. Employers and insurers may also feel they have a stake in genetic information because it may help in their hiring practices or risk ratings.

Finally, advances in testing impact on social and religious values. Genetic testing often takes place in the prenatal setting and is linked with decisions regarding reproduction. Also, the ability to identify certain conditions and predispositions as genetically based will change the way these conditions are viewed. If we identify a partial genetic basis for phenomena that we previously thought had only a social basis—like criminal behavior—our views toward responsibility and punishment may change.

Some uses of genetic tests achieve legitimate social and personal goals. But often the distinction between desirable and undesirable uses of genetic tests depends on one's perspective and values.

GENETIC TESTING FOR INDIVIDUAL DIAGNOSIS

The use of genetic tests for diagnosis of symptomatic patients is the most direct benefit of our expanding ability to probe the genome. Detection of two cystic fibrosis mutations in a child may establish the diagnosis even though the clinical findings are equivocal. Genetic tests are also beneficial when they identify predispositions that can be mitigated. Ataxia-telangiectasia, an autosomal recessive disorder, is associated with an increased sensitivity to ionizing radiation. The cancer rate for homozygotes for this trait is about 100 times greater than in the general population. Recent evidence suggests that heterozygotes also are more sensitive to radiation and have approximately a fourfold increased risk of certain cancers. The individual and public health implications of this finding are profound. Although the homozygous condition is rare, approximately 1.4 percent of the population is heterozygous for the gene. Such carriers, identified by DNA testing, will have a strong reason to minimize their exposure to diagnostic radiation. For heterozygous women the risk of mammography-induced breast cancers may exceed the benefits of early detection.

Individuals may also benefit from presymptomatic testing, although the benefits of such testing are not always clear. Huntington's disease, an autosomal dominant disorder, causes severe neurologic symptoms that do not develop until middle age. Individuals with an affected parent face a 50 percent chance of eventually manifesting the disease. There is a predictive test for Huntington's disease, but the disease is incurable. The test is a mixed blessing: learning that one has inherited the gene is disturbing and the information cannot be used in managing one's health, but it may be important in reproductive planning.[3] Moreover, the information has implications for children already born. For these reasons, many at risk do not want to be tested, and the mere availability of the test can cause anguish.

The recent discovery of the BRCA1 gene,[4,5] associated with breast and ovarian cancer, raises similar troublingissues for an even more common disease. About 1 in 200 to 400 women are believed to carry this gene. These women may have an 85 percent lifetime risk of developing breast cancer. Screening for this gene can identify these women, but the clinical value of this information is unclear. Preventive management, for example with tamoxifen[6] or prophylactic bilateral mastectomy[7,8,9] is of uncertain benefit. There is no evidence that prophylactic mastectomy reduces breast cancer risk, but much of the public and the medical profession seems eager to accept its promise. In a recent survey, 90 of 700 Maryland surgeons reported performing at least one preventive mastectomy.[10] Moreover, most women who will eventually develop breast cancer do not carry a detectable mutation in this gene. Negative screening for BRCA1 mutations may create a false sense of security, leading women to forego conventional periodic breast examination or mammography.[11] Confusion is likely to increase among patients and clinicians as other genes related to breast cancer are uncovered.

Even for less significant disorders, genetic information may be more stressful than other types of medical information, and the communication of screening results and interpretation presents special challenges. Genetic traits are more likely to be a source of stigma and discrimination, perhaps because people often define personal identity in terms of one's genes. Genetic traits cluster along ethnic or racial lines, which also can be sources of discrimination, and they can create intense feelings of guilt and responsibility among relatives. Whatever the explanation, genetic testing often has more profound emotional consequences than other medical tests. At the same time, the test results can be difficult to contain, both because they have implications for family members and because family members, for some tests, must also provide DNA samples to complete testing for the proband and may inadvertently receive information they wish to avoid.[12]

Many social concerns of genetic testing resemble those of testing for infection with the human immunodeficiency virus. Both raise issues of privacy, stigma, discrimination, and voluntarism. Genetic disorders are not communicable, but they are transmitted vertically to future generations, and relatives in many ways resemble contacts. Individuals learning they carry a gene for Tay Sachs disease, for example, simultaneously learn that their siblings have a 50 percent chance of carrying that gene as well. Because this knowledge may be valuable to them, it may create obligations to disclose.[13] This conflict between the right of privacy and the duty to disclose is a perennial problem in public health that has no clear solution. Genetic testing provides another setting for this dilemma.

Another challenge is how to convey and interpret the results of genetic tests, which are genetic often probabilistic in nature. One quarter of a sample of middle class pregnant women in one study equated chances of 1 in 1000 and 10 percent, showing the widespread difficulty that many people have in interpreting probabilistic information.[14] Many genetic tests have the potential for false positive and false negative results, which further complicates their interpretation.

Thus genetic testing creates problems for informed consent and the need for more genetics education for the general public and health professionals. More testing will increase the need for genetic counseling. Counseling for cystic fibrosis carrier screening alone might require approximately one-third of the currently board-certified genetic counselors.[15]

REPRODUCTIVE PLANNING

Genetic testing can provide couples with information useful in reproductive planning. Despite its obvious benefits, prenatal testing has been controversial because it is often linked with the option of abortion. Also, it may target certain genotypes as undesirable and promote the implicit goal of reducing their prevalence.

Opportunities for genetic testing in the reproductive setting are increasing rapidly. Approximately one in 25 Caucasians in the United States carries a cystic fibrosis mutation; in approximately one in 625 couples both partners are carriers. For these couples, each pregnancy faces a one in four chance of being affected with cystic fibrosis. Carrier screening, now available, can help identify couples at risk, and prenatal diagnosis can help identify affected fetuses.[16] Prenatal diagnosis can help couples decide whether to continue a pregnancy, and if the pregnancy is not terminated, it can be valuable in planning the delivery and arranging future care.

Alternatively, couples can undergo carrier screening before a pregnancy and decide whether or not to conceive on the basis of test results, or whether to conceive with different partners through the donation of eggs or sperm from noncarriers.

For many, however, the important issue is not abortion, but whether genetic testing in a reproductive setting is a form of eugenics. The issue is what, if any, genetic characteristics are legitimate targets for screening. Nobody knows how many pregnancies are terminated for sex selection, although the practice certainly occurs. As we increase our ability to perform prenatal diagnostic tests earlier in pregnancy less invasively, and for many new indications, more pregnancies will be terminated as a result of genetic tests. In vitro fertilization has further expanded prospects for prenatal diagnosis. A single cell can be removed from an embryo fertilized in vitro and new molecular techniques used to amplify and determine some of its genetic characteristics. From this information, one can decide whether to select that embryo, among the others similarly tested, for implantation.[17-19] The availability of such tests will lead to demand for using them, because couples may see the tests as answering personal needs, and because of external pressures to use them.[20]

Physicians may be a source of such pressures. Obstetricians may fuel the demand for carrier screening and prenatal diagnosis if they fear future malpractice suits if a child is born with a condition that could have been identified in advance. Physicians may yield also to marketing pressures. Both of these factors have been cited in the rapid diffusion of alpha-fetoprotein screening for neural tube defects. Future genetic tests are likely to follow the same pattern.

Public opinion is a source of pressure as well. A recent survey found that 39 percent of Americans believe every pregnancy should be tested to determine if the fetus has any serious genetic defects; 22 percent believe that a pregnant woman should have an abortion if the fetus has a serious genetic defect; and 10 percent believe an indigent woman should be required by law to have an abortion rather than have the government help pay for the care of a child with a genetically based condition.[21] These public attitudes add to the stigma faced by parents of children with genetic conditions, and may increase demand for genetic tests. Women are particularly likely to be targets of such pressures, because they are often viewed as responsible for adverse outcomes of pregnancy, are more commonly the recipients of reproductive health care, and are more likely to become the subjects of screening programs.

Past experience with carrier screening has raised other concerns. Sickle cell carrier screening programs, begun in the 1970s, have been fraught with difficulties. In many states mandatory sickle cell screening raised concerns about racist and eugenic motivations. Patients and the public often equated carrier status with sickle cell disease, believed sickle cell disease to be communicable or sexually transmitted, believed that carriers should not have children, or believed that childbirth could be hazardous.[22] These misconceptions increased the stigma and discrimination faced by carriers and those affected with the disease.

These problems underscore the need for widespread efforts to educate medical professionals, the public, and screened individuals about the meaning of test results. Despite the obvious difficulties, it seems possible to design carrier screening programs that are sensitive to these concerns. Carrier screening for Tay-Sachs disease began at about the same time as screening for sickle cell trait, and has generally been regarded as a success.[23] Screening programs were designed with heavy participation from the Jewish communities at risk for the disease. Screening has been voluntary, although some have suggested that the community provides some coercive pressure.[24] One orthodox community in New York, where marriages are arranged, originated the program of Chevra Dor Yeshorim. In this program, young adults are screened for Tay Sachs disease and results are kept secret in a central registry. To minimize the chances of stigma and discrimination, no one is informed of his or her result until a marriage is proposed. Only if both prospective partners are carriers are they told their carrier status; they are then referred for counseling, and new matches may be sought.[25] These efforts suggest that screening programs can be designed to address cultural needs and concerns.

Screening programs like Chevra Dor Yeshorim illustrate the use of genetic screening tests by individuals in the selection of partners. Another example is from Cyprus, where the high prevalence of beta-thalassernia led to a national effort in the early 1970s to screen potential carriers and provide counseling and prenatal diagnosis to couples at risk. In 1983, the Greek Orthodox Church, which opposes abortion to prevent affected births, began requiring couples to show evidence of screening and counseling before blessing a marriage. This led to a 97 percent decrease in the number of children born with beta-thalassemia. Since 1985 there has been a 20 percent reduction in the number of couples in which both partners screen positive, suggesting that carriers are now less likely to marry other carriers.[26]

GENETIC TESTING BY EMPLOYERS

Questions arise about the legitimacy of genetic screening in the employment setting for several reasons. First, employers might avoid hiring individuals with a genetic predisposition to medical illnesses that might increase their absenteeism, reduce their productivity, or increase the costs of recruitment and training new workers. A company might use a test to detect and exclude prospective workers who are likely to die of premature coronary artery disease, for example. Less likely, prospective employees might use genetic tests to choose career paths.

Second, employers might use genetic screening tests to avoid hiring individuals who are likely (or who have family members likely) to incur high health-care or disability costs. Screening prospective employees for the purposes of identifying those likely to have high future health costs is prohibited under the Americans with Disabilities Act. Nevertheless, self-insured employers are permitted to limit coverage for specific conditions after employees are hired: The ADA provides only limited protections.

Third, employers might use genetic screening tests to avoid hiring workers who have genetic predispositions that might endanger public safety. Tremendous pressures might develop to use a test that could screen prospective airline pilots or bus drivers for a gene linked to alcoholism, for example, even if its predictive ability was limited.[27]

Finally, employers might use genetic screening tests to identify workers especially vulnerable to workplace exposures. About fifty genetic conditions are known that enhance susceptibility to workplace exposures.[28(p83)] Tests for sickle cell trait, glucose-6-phosphate dehydrogenase deficiency, and alpha 1-antitrypsin deficiency have been used at one time or another to exclude certain workers from jobs felt to present them with special risk,[29] and some companies prohibit fertile women from working in settings that are potentially hazardous to fetal development.[28(p148)]

Efforts to identify susceptible workers might benefit them, especially if they are offered alternative positions, but it is not clear that such screening has uncovered real risks that may be mitigated.[30] Testing in the workplace is less voluntary than testing in the physician's office, and the same safeguards for confidentiality and counseling do not exist. Patients can ignore the advice of their physicians, but employees, especially prospective employees, cannot similarly ignore the "advice" of employers.

Some critics suggest that screening workers for susceptibility to occupational hazards shifts the blame for occupational hazards from environmental exposures to genetic predisposition. Screening may substitute for efforts to clean up the workplace that might benefit others who are not hypersusceptible.[27] In a recent case involving the potential risk of lead exposure to fetuses carried by women involved in the production of batteries, the Supreme Court ruled that company fetal protection policies are unlawful if they ban fertile women from sites because of possible fetal injury.[31]

With many of these concerns in mind, the American Medical Association (AMA) recently issued an opinion that identified no role for the screening of workers for nonoccupationally related health risks, and only a very limited role for the screening of employees for susceptibility to workplace exposures. The AMA considered the latter to be appropriate only when the workplace hazard is so serious and develops so rapidly that monitoring the exposure would be ineffective in preventing the injury; when the test is highly predictive of a significantly increased susceptibility; when alternative means of lowering the exposure are extraordinarily expensive; and when the worker provides informed consent for the screening.[27]

Despite the many ways employers *might* use genetic screening, it is unclear how prevalent the practice really is. A 1982 survey commissioned by the Office of Technology Assessment suggested that fewer than 2 percent of Fortune 500 companies engage in any form of genetic screening or monitoring. Another 1989 survey found that 5 percent of Fortune 500 companies engage in genetic screening or monitoring.[28] This suggests that the practice is neither widespread nor increasing rapidly. The potential savings of employee-screening programs might not offset their costs. Nevertheless, the social hazards of workplace screening are real, and one reason for the expanded scope of the ADA is that clear motivations exist for engaging in more testing. Whether or not genetic testing by employers offers some benefits in limited settings, it clearly provides an opportunity for unfair employment discrimination. It is not yet clear how well the ADA or the opinions of organized medicine can steer the use of genetic tests by employers away from these discriminatory uses.

GENETIC TESTING BY INSURERS

Genetic testing by life and health insurers raises other concerns. Insurers rate individuals according to their perceived health risks and determine their insurability and the premium to charge. Genetic tests expand the ability of insurance companies to determine individual risks, and might change the practice of insurance risk rating.

Only about a third of health insurance policies and about half of life insurance policies in this country are individual policies. The rest are group insurance, typically obtained through empowers and not subject to individual risk rating. Because employers have parallel incentives to reduce their financial exposure. as discussed above, genetic information might he equally relevant to those covered by both group and individual policies.

Individuals might hesitate to use genetic tests if the results might later be used to deny insurance coverage. This is similar to "job lock," in which employees receiving employment-based health insurance are unable to change jobs because recently diagnosed conditions would represent "preexisting conditions" that would not be covered if health insurance policies are changed. Genetic tests are different from other medical tests in this setting because they change the very nature of what might be considered preexisting. Most health insurers that responded to a 1991 Office of Technology Assessment (OTA) survey considered genetic conditions, such as cystic fibrosis or Huntington's disease, to be "preexisting" conditions.[32(p195)] Predictive genetic tests blur the distinction between an increased risk of disease and a preexisting condition.

An example illustrates a related concern. A couple with a child affected with cystic fibrosis learned through prenatal diagnosis that another pregnancy was affected. When the couple decided to continue the pregnancy, their insurance company argued that it should not have to pay for health care of the child related to cystic fibrosis, since it had paid for the prenatal diagnosis ostensibly to avoid the birth of the affected child. Under pressure, the insurance company later reversed its position.[33] Other similar cases show that this was not an isolated instance.[34] This anecdotal evidence shows that insurance companies can use genetic information irresponsibly.

A related question is whether insurers would use genetic testing before issuing individual policies. OTA's 1991 survey of insurers found that most health insurers believe it is "fair for insurers to use genetic tests to identify individuals with increased risk of disease" and that they "should have the option of determining how to use genetic information in determining risks." Few insurers, however, predicted they would in fact be using genetic tests in this way in five or ten years.[32(p33)] This might change if accurate tests to predict breast cancer or low back pain, for example, became available.

Genetic screening will probably be more expensive than other methods of obtaining actuarially relevant medical information, such as questions about family medical history. Why, then, might insurers use such tests?

One reason is that individuals can undergo genetic testing on their own. and if they discover that they are at greater medical risk they might purchase more insurance. This phenomenon, known as adverse selection, puts insurance companies at a disadvantage if they lack access to the same information. To level the playing field, insurance companies might have a legitimate interest in the results of genetic tests already performed, and might have an incentive to initiate testing for selected conditions. When one insurer begins to use genetic information in its risk rating, others must follow or they will disproportionately attract individuals who are denied coverage elsewhere.

This suggests that insurance companies will inevitably begin to use genetic information in risk rating, despite the expense and complexities involved. Some analysts have argued that this inexorable trend contradicts the rationale for insurance in the first place. As genetic tests increase our ability to refine risk so that individuals are placed in ever smaller risk pools, administrative costs for insurance will soar as the ability to distribute financial risks vanishes.[35] These trends may constitute an independent argument for new systems of health-care financing that eliminate individual insurance policies and risk rating.

FUTURE POLICY OPTIONS

Advances in molecular biology offer tremendous promise for diagnosing disease. But the lack of effective therapies following genetic diagnosis creates dilemmas. Genetic information that cannot be used for treatment might be used for undesirable social purposes. We need to gain the most good from our expanding knowledge and avoid the pitfalls. Clinicians, the public, and policy makers share this challenge.

Experience with past and present genetic testing programs provide some direction. Past problems with sickle cell screening programs vividly demonstrate the need to educate the public and health-care professionals alike about the meaning and implications of genetic tests. We need to strengthen our genetic curriculum at all educational levels, and also train more health-care providers who can counsel patients about the benefits and risks of these tests. The experience with sickle cell screening also illustrates the need for strict protection of confidentiality to avoid the stigma and discrimination that may occur in social, employment, and insurance settings. This may require the strengthening of the ADA and similar legistlation.

We must identify the best balance in our *overall* approach to genetic disorders. Should we screen to avoid diseases, or devote those resources to helping those who are or will be affected?

Genetic testing raises broader health policy issues as well. These include: whether to foster the development of new diagnostic information when treatment is not immediately available, how to control the diffusion of new medical technologies in commercial environments or the role of social pressures and defensive medicine in the adoption of these technologies, and the role of health insurance in providing equitable access to care. These policy concerns, most of which are not unique to genetic testing, need to be addressed as the technology expands.

Perhaps most importantly, we need to match our increasing understanding of genetic diagnosis with efforts to increase our acceptance of those affected. As we learn to detect, prevent, and alter previously immutable characteristics, we risk reducing our tolerance for genetic variation. We must continue to view genetic diversity as both a biological and a social good. The American values of diversity and individual rights will undoubtedly continue to inform U.S. policies, but we should recognize that other countries and other cultures may develop substantialy different policies. Health policy for genetic testing must be formed through the exploration of human values.

REFERENCES

1. National Center for Human Genome Research. *Understanding Our Genetic Inheritance: The U.S. Genome Project.* NIH Publication 90-1590. Springfield, VA: National Technical Information Service; 1990.

2. House of Representatives Committee on Government Operations. Designing genetic information policy: the need for an independent policy review of the ethical, legal, and social implications of the human genome project. *House of Representatives Rep. 102-478.* April 1, 1992: 25.

3. Meissen GJ, Myers RH, Mastromauro CA, et al. Predictive testing for Hundington's disease with use of a linked DNA marker. *New England Journal of Medicine.* 1988;318:535–542.

4. Hall JM, Lee MK, Newman B, et al. Linkage of early onset breast cancer to chromosome 17q21. *Science.* 1990;250:1684–1689.

5. Miki Y, Swensen J, Shattuck-Eidens S, et al. A strong candidate gene for the breast and ovarian cancer susceptibility gene BRCA 1. *Science.* 1994;266:66–71.

6. Nayfield SG, Karp JE, Ford LG, Dorr PA, Kramer BS. Potential role of tamoxifen in prevention of breast cancer. *Journal of the National Cancer Institute.* 1991;83:1450–1459.

7. Zeigler LD, Kroll SS. Primary breast cancer after prophylactic mastectomy. *American Journal of Clinical Oncology.* 1991;14:451–454.

8. Nelson H, Miller SH, Buck D, Demuth RJ, Fletcher WS, Buehler P. Effectiveness of prophylactic mastectomy in the prevention of breast tumors in C3H mice. *Plastic and Reconstructive Surgery.* 1989;83:662–669.

9. Goodnight JE, Quagliana JM, Morton L. Failure of subcutaneous mastectomy to prevent the development of breast cancer. *Journal of Surgical Oncology.* 1984;26:198–201.

10. Cowley G. Family matters. *Newsweek.* December 6, 1993: 46–52.

11. Biesecker BB, Boehnke M, Calzone K, et al. Genetic counseling for families with inherited susceptibility to breast and ovarian cancer. *Journal of the American Medical Association.* 1993;269:1970–1974.

12. Milan FA, Curtis A, Mennie M, et al. Prenatal exclusion testing for Huntington's disease: a problem of too much information. *Journal of Medical Genetics.* 1989;26:83–85.

13. Pelias MZ. Duty to disclose in medical genetics: a legal perspective. *American Journal of Medical Genetics.* 1991;39:347–354.

14. Chase GA, Faden RR, Holtzman NA, et al. The assessment of genetic risk by pregnant women: implications for genetic counseling. *Social Biology.* 1986;33:57–64.

15. Wilford BA, Fost N. The cystic fibrosis gene: medical and social implications for heterozygote detection. *Journal of the American Medical Association.* 1990;263:2777–2783.

16. Asch DA, Patton JP, Hershey JC, Mennuti MT. Reporting the results of cystic fibrosis screening. *American Journal of Obstetrics and Gynecology.* 1993;168:1–6.

17. Verlinsky Y, Pergament E, Strom C. The preimplantation genetic diagnosis of genetic diseases. *Journal of In Vitro Fertilization and Embryo Transfer.* 1990;7:1-5.

18. Handyside AH, Lesko JG, Tar'n JJ, Winston ML, Hughes MR. Birth of a normal girl after in vitro fertilization and preimplantation diagnostic testing for cystic fibrosis. *New England Journal of Medicine.* 1993;327:905–909.

19. Simpson JL, Carson SA. Preimplantation genetic diagnosis. *New England Journal of Medicine.* 1992;327:951–953.

20. Clarke A. Is non-directive genetic counseling possible? *Lancet.* 1991;338:998–1002.

21. Singer E. Public attitudes toward genetic testing. *Population Research and Policy Review.* 1991;10:235–255.

22. Reilly P. *Genetics, Law, and Social Policy.* Cambridge, MA: Harvard University Press; 1977.

23. Roberts L. One worked: the other didn't. *Science.* 1990;247:18.

24. Holtzman NA. *Proceed with Caution: Predicting Genetic Risks in the Recombinant DNA Era.* Baltimore, MD: Johns Hopkins University Press; 1989: 217–218.

25. Metz B. Matchmaking scheme solves Tay-Sachs problem. *Journal of the American Medical Association.* 1987;258:2636–2639.

26. Angastiniotis M. Cyprus: Thalassaemia program. *Lancet.* 1990; 119–129.

27. American Medical Association Council on Ethical and Judicial Affairs. Use of genetic testing by employers. *Journal of the American Medical Association.* 1991;266:1827–1830.

28. U.S. Congress. Office of Technology Assessment. *Genetic Monitoring and Screening in the Workplace, OTA-BA-455.* Washington, DC: U.S. Government Printing Office; 1990.

29. Reinhardt CF. Genetic hypersusceptibility. *Journal of Occupational Medicine.* 1978;20:319–322.

30. Draper E. *Risky Business: Genetic Testing and Exclusionary Practices in the Hazardous Workplace.* Cambridge, MA: Cambridge University Press; 1991.

31. *United Automobile Workers* v. *Johnson Controls, Inc.* 111 SC 1196. 1991.

32. U.S. Congress. Office of Technology Assessment. *Cystic Fibrosis and DNA Tests: Implications for Carrier Screening, OTA-BA-532.* Washington, DC: U.S. Government Printing Office; 1992.

33. Caskey CT. New technology brings new ethical consideration. *Legal and Ethical Issues Raised by the Human Genome Project.* Conference materials. Houston, TX; March 7–9, 1991.

34. Billings PR, Kohn MA, de Cuevas M, Beckwith J, Alper JS, Natowicz MR. Discrimination as a consequence of genetic testings. *American Journal of Human Genetics.* 1992;50:476–482.

35. Light DW. The practice and ethics of risk-related health insurance. *Journal of the American Medical Association.* 1992;267:2503–2508.

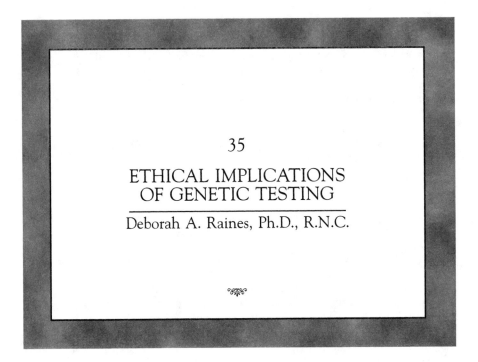

35

ETHICAL IMPLICATIONS OF GENETIC TESTING

Deborah A. Raines, Ph.D., R.N.C.

Advances in biotechnology have created previously unforseen possibilities to determine the genetic makeup of individuals and to predict the health of future societies. Advances in recombinant technology mean that for several of the single-gene disorders, the risk of being a carrier or the risk of an affected pregnancy can be ascertained with a high degree of accuracy. The biomedical model views genetic testing as neutral and proposes that expanded testing capabilities and increased knowledge will open new horizons for reproductive health.[1] Most of the literature related to the emerging genetic knowledge and technologies have focused on the safety, accuracy, and financial costs of genetic testing but not on the broader implications of the use of that knowledge within the context of society. The ability to influence the type of individual produced through a pregnancy and the identification of genetic traits of individuals raise complex questions about what is normal and abnormal and what is desirable and undesirable, and it regenerates fears of eugenics and the goal of creating a society of perfect individuals. Within a societal culture that has valued autonomous choice, individuality, and diversity, the concept of predefined biogenetic definitions appears contradictory.

Consider the following situations that illustrate the potential ethical dilemmas inherent in the widespread use of recombinant molecular genetic technology.

D. Raines. "Ethical Implications of Genetic Testing." *Nursing Clinics of North America.* 1998;33(2):275–286. Reprinted by permission of W. B. Saunders Company.

Mary and Jim meet at college. After a brief romance, they choose to marry. Not long after their marriage, Mary discovers that she is pregnant. Although the pregnancy was not planned, Mary and Jim are both happy about the pregnancy and impending parenthood. Jim and Mary plan a trip for her to meet his family and to share the news of their pregnancy. Mary knows little about Jim's family.

He has told her only that they are close, treasure their privacy, and do not accept outsiders readily. Mary's observations of Jim's family cause her to become concerned. She begins to suspect that she had married into a family with the presence of a genetic disease. Mary arrives at this conclusion after meeting the family and learning that numerous family members experienced early death after what was described as "not being themselves for an extended period of time." Mary begins to suspect that these individuals died of Huntington's disease. Huntington's disease is an autosomal dominant disorder characterized by a variety of jerky, complex movements and progressive mental deterioration, dementia, and eventually death. The typical onset is during the early forties, with death occurring within ten to fifteen years after onset. Mary shares her observations and concerns with Jim. Jim denies any knowledge of this problem within his family but admits he really does not know much about the early deaths of his ancestors or the behavioral changes, including loss of short-term memory, currently being exhibited by his father and some of his father's siblings. Jim does remind Mary that this family does not like others looking into their private matters and advises her to stop pursuing this issue.

Upon returning home, Mary shares her observations and suspicions with her obstetrician. She asks if it is possible to test the fetus she is carrying for the presence of the gene for Huntington's disease. Mary is approximately twelve weeks pregnant and is anxious to have the option of abortion available if the fetus is affected. Mary shares her desire to have the fetus tested with Jim and even urges Jim to have himself tested. Jim becomes angry and tells Mary to stop looking for problems. Jim refuses to have himself tested and emphatically states that he does not want his future child tested.

The dilemma inherent in this situation is Jim's right not to know his genetic status (if the fetus tests positive for the gene, then Jim also must be positive for the gene), which conflicts with Mary's right to know about the health of the fetus she is carrying, as well as issues related to the benefits and burden, for the future child, of the knowledge of a condition that does not have any clinical signs or symptoms for approximately forty years.

Consider the case of Sarah, a forty-two-year-old woman with a significant family history of heart disease. Sarah presents with a severe lipid problem and is diagnosed with hyperlipidemia. Sarah agrees to undergo genetic testing to confirm her genetic predisposition to familial heart disease and the genetic contribution to her current health status. The identification of the presence of a genetic component is useful information in the development and implementation of a treatment plan for Sarah. However, when the test results are received, the physician discovers that Sarah not only has the genetic alteration consistent with familial heart disease and explanatory of her hyperlipidemia but also has a double dose of this genetic alteration, a condition found in only a small percentage of the population. The significance of this finding is that a double dose of this particular gene is strongly associated with the onset of Alzheimer's disease.

The dilemma in this case is what the health-care provider does with this additional information, which was not part of the intended testing and diagnostic procedure but may have a significant impact on the client's future. Principles of informed consent, information disclosure, and truth telling are integral to this type of situation.

These technologic advances and the ethical questions inherent in this advanced scientific ability are a direct result of the Human Genome Project. The Human Genome Project is a fifteen-year endeavor based on the premise that advanced biologic research and medical advances ultimately will benefit human kind. In other words, the underlying assumption is that the more health-care providers and scientists know about the genetic map of healthy, normal human beings, the better they can predict and correct deviations in the genetic map and the resulting health-related sequelae. However, these research advances and scientific achievements are paralleled by the debate over the promises and threats that this new knowledge holds for individuals and society. As stated by Carol Tauer, "the human genome project carries a dramatic metaphor: the notion that our genes are the program that determines who we are and that when we know all the genes we will know the human being, both genetically and individually."[2] However, if human existence is viewed by the highly mechanistic model that a person is determined solely by the composition of his or her genes, the issue of accountability and motivation for personal actions and behaviors, choices, and acts becomes nonexistent. Further genetic composition has the potential to become the measuring stick to determine status, importance, nature, and the values of human life.

The Human Genome Project has increased the ability to identify genes linked to diseases. As more genes are discovered, it is becoming possible to test individuals for an expanding list of genetic diseases, disorders, and traits. However, the relationship between a genetic abnormality and the individual's functional abilities and health status is not based on a simple cause-and-effect model. The individual's values, lifestyles, health practices, and other intrinsic and extrinsic influences impact whether the information learned through genetic testing is beneficial or burdensome to the individual, the family, and society as a whole. Consequently, the ethical dilemmas related to genetic testing are not limited to unraveling the human genome per se but also apply to the application of the resulting technology that goes beyond pattern detection and forces individuals and society to question the fundamental nature of the technology itself and the application of the technology to human beings.

THE SCIENTIFIC BASES OF GENETICS

The genome is the total genetic material of an organism.[3] Genes are composed of DNA, a large molecule composed of a five-carbon sugar (deoxyribose) with a phosphate attached and four different nucleotides (nitrogen bases): adenine, thymine, guanine, and cytosine. These nucleotides are the fundamental building blocks of the genes. Genes function by determining the ordering of the nucleotides that is the structure of the peptide chain or string of amino acids that form proteins. At the cellular level, these proteins create structures and act as enzymes to carry out cellular processes. If the genetic blueprint contains an error or a minute alteration in the genetic material, the protein that is created does not function in the usual manner and the resulting abnormalities culminate in the signs or symptoms of a genetically inherited disease or trait.

The human genome is found on the forty-six chromosomes (twenty-two pairs of autosomes and one pair of sex chromosomes) unique to the human species. Each chromosome is a linear strand of DNA that contains many genes or combinations of nucleoticles. Each cell in an individual contains a complete copy of the individual's genome. Estimates state that approximately three billion nucleotides of DNA comprise the genes in the human genome.[1]

GENETIC TESTING

Genetic testing broadly describes diagnostic techniques that identify the presence of a genetic mutation or a gene protein product that may result in abnormal function. The most widely recognized types of genetic testing are prenatal testing, traditionally used to identify a developing fetus' genetic complement or number of chromosomes, and the mandatory neonatal screening programs legislated by state governments to provide a population-wide approach for testing newborns for a variety of genetic disorders. However, newer techniques have expanded the number and the types of conditions that can be identified through prenatal testing and have introduced the option of obtaining knowledge of one's genetic makeup throughout the life span. Genetic techniques for identification of abnormal genes fall into three categories: disease testing, carrier testing, and prenatal testing. Gene tests generally are performed on a sample of living tissue, usually a blood sample, but in some procedures a cheek swab or skin sample may be needed. A gene test is performed on the tissue's DNA, which is a stable chemical that can be extracted from the tissue and analyzed for the sequence of the component nucleotides.

Disease Testing

Disease testing identifies the presence of a genetic alteration or a specific gene mutation in an individual. Diagnostic testing can be confirmatory, presymptomatic, or predispositionary. Confirmatory testing is implemented to confirm the genetic basis of a disorder consistent with the clinical presentation of the individual. For example, the young child who presents to the pediatric health-care setting with a history of recurrent respiratory infections, chronic cough, and respiratory congestion and alteration in sodium homeostasis may be tested to confirm the presence of the genetic alteration consistent with a diagnosis of cystic fibrosis. In this situation, the genetic testing confirms a diagnosis that is formulated based on the individual's clinical presentation. Thus, confirmatory testing helps to determine what is wrong with the individual. Consequently, disease testing results provide objective scientific information that can be used in implementing a treatment strategy for that individual and in making prognostic evaluations.

However, some genetic diseases have no early signs or symptoms or only manifest later in life. A classic example of a late-onset genetic disease is Huntington's disease, an autosomal dominant disorder that typically presents during the fourth decade of life. Presymptomatic testing enables healthy individuals to learn with certainty whether they will develop this genetic condition. Presymptomatic testing is most useful in identifying conditions caused by a single gene mutation that is fully penetrate, that is, the gene is always expressed regardless of other external influences. Presymptomatic testing is most commonly used in families with a documented history of diseases such as Huntington's disease. Presymptomatic testing answers the question regarding what the future holds for the individual's health status specific to the disorder in question. However, until preventive measures or treatment interventions are available to prolong or prevent the onset of the disorder itself, some individuals ask whether knowledge of future health status is a benefit or a burden.

Predisposition testing entails identifying individuals who possess some genetic characteristic that places them at greater risk than the general population for a disease. In other words, the individual has a better-than-average chance of developing the disorder at some time, but the individual also has a chance of never being affected with the disorder. One of the areas of ambiguity in the understanding of predisposition testing is how much the actual onset of the disease associated with the genetic alteration is influenced by genetics and how much is related to external factors such as environmental exposures, lifestyle, and health-care practices. Currently, predisposition testing is being applied on a limited base to individuals with a strong family history of diseases such as particular types of heart disease, breast cancer, ovarian cancer, colon cancer, and Alzheimer's disease.[4] It could be argued that predisposition testing is a benefit because the knowledge of increased risk status motivates the individual to implement behavioral and environmental changes to minimize the external factors that influence disease development. However, it is evident from years of data and public education about the risk of lung cancer associated with smoking and the minimal relationship between knowledge of risk and behavioral change that scientific data alone may not be a primary motivator of individual behavior.[5] However, unlike the smoking risk data that are population based, the consequence of a positive genetic disease test finding indicates a definite personal risk; thus, compliance and behavioral change may be greater.

In the future, disease testing—confirmatory, presymptomatic, and predispositionary—may be the prelude to gene therapy or the ability to manipulate or alter the abnormal gene to decrease the severity or eliminate the presence of the disease-causing gene. Currently, however, knowledge and ability to identify genetic alteration have outpaced the knowledge and ability to intervene to treat or cure these genetic alterations. Consequently, a positive test result may leave the individual with no options for interventions related to the identified disease or disorder. In addition, it is unclear whether prophylactic measures such as elective mastectomy or oopherectomy are beneficial to individuals who test positive for genetic disposition to diseases such as breast or ovarian cancer or if the risk of complications and sequella from the prophylaxis are a greater burden than the genetic risk. Thus, the question of whether knowledge of the presence of a genetic disease or disease predisposition is a benefit or burden to the individual must be considered and will become more complicated as knowledge and identification of the components of the human genome continue to outpace clinical interventions.

Another possible outgrowth of the acceptance of disease testing is individual accountability and allocation of health-care resources. Based on the results of genetic testing, are individuals accountable for behavioral change, health screening, and preventive measures to facilitate a delayed onset of symptoms, early diagnosis, and treatment, and less severe disease course where possible? For example, would the individual who is identified with the genetic predisposition to various types of cancers or familial heart disease be held accountable for adhering to dietary, exercise, and environmental modifications known to decrease the severity and incidence of a disorder or disease? Would this be an individual or societal responsibility? In addition, the knowledge of an individual's genome may refine the use of clinical assessments and diagnostic procedures and the most efficient use of scarce health-care resources. On the other hand, genetic test findings may lead some individuals to additional risk-taking behaviors and the lack of health-promoting practices based on their perception that their destiny is predetermined and individual actions have minimal consequences. The lack of a genetic marker for a particular disease also may be used erroneously as a proxy for the standard accepted norm for monitoring or early detection of a disease; for example, an individual who does not have the gene for breast cancer who believes that breast self-examination and mammography are unnecessary. However, in other cases, such as the genetic predisposition for Alzheimer's disease or presymptomatic testing for Huntington's disease, there are no known preventive measures. Yet one may argue that even if no scientific-based medical interventions exist, the interval between genetic diagnosis and clinical presentation may be beneficial to the individual in terms of planning for personal concerns and life choices, thereby decreasing the burden on the family when the individual is no longer able to participate in the decision-making process. On the other hand, it could be argued that knowledge without an available action plan simply places an unreasonable burden, that is, dreaded anticipation of premature loss of self-determination, on the individual.

The issue of opportunity within society is another issue integral to the use of genetic testing. Would individuals who test positive for the predisposition or presymptomatic state of a disease or disorder be denied the same options and opportunities within the greater society? The issue of insurance coverage, which is based on risk assignment, is debated frequently. An individual with the genetic trait for

Huntington's disease uses more of the insurer's resources for medical and long-term care; therefore, should this individual be required to pay more into the pool or be denied coverage because of the known additional risk and needs?

With knowledge comes a responsibility for reasonable use of the information available and for implementation of individual action. As the use of society's resources continues to be scrutinized, the question of individual accountability for acting responsibly to promote individual well-being could become linked to one's genome. The danger is that no clear boundary exists between genetic and nongenetic contributing factors to disease development and the disease's progression and its ultimate impact may vary among individuals.

Carrier Testing

The objective of carrier testing is to identify individuals whose genome includes the presence of a disease-related recessive gene. Carrier testing usually is performed in adults who are healthy and exhibit no symptoms of the genetic disease. However, these individuals may carry the genetic material that places them at risk for passing a genetic condition onto their offspring. With a recessive gene disorder, there is a 25 percent chance of the offspring inheriting the genetic material and actually exhibiting signs and symptoms of the condition. For an individual to be affected with a recessively inherited disorder, the individual must inherit two abnormal genes or one gene from each carrier parent. In other words, both parents must be carriers of the genetic alteration in order to produce an affected offspring. Consequently, knowledge of one's carrier status can influence procreation practices through actions such as selecting a sex partner who is not a carrier, refraining from having children, or seeking help from sperm or ovum donations in order to produce healthy children.[6] If pregnancy is chosen, the individual knows that there is a 25 percent chance the pregnancy will be affected and has the option of pursuing prenatal diagnosis of the developing fetus' genome. Based on that information the individual can make an informed choice about the disposition of the pregnancy.

Many of the common genetic diseases such as cystic fibrosis, sickle cell anemia, B-thalassemia, and Tay-Sachs disease are recessive disorders. Theoretically, the use of carrier testing and prudent procreative choices could eliminate the mutant gene from the gene pool over time. There has been limited evidence of this in the cases of Tay-Sachs disease and B-thalassemia, in which carrier testing, reproductive counseling, and informed decision making have been used effectively to decrease the incidence of these disorders.[7] However, who has the ultimate choice in reproductive decisions and who is responsible for the outcomes of that choice? The goal of genome identification must be clarified as providing information and not direction.

Carrier testing is accomplished by testing for a gene protein product; however, variants of a gene can make carrier testing potentially misleading. For example, more than two hundred variants of the cystic fibrosis gene have been discovered, yet 90 percent of the cystic fibrosis cases are accounted for by approximately six of these variants.[8] Consequently, the current mode of carrier testing for cystic fibrosis is a compromise that tests only for the most common variants of the gene protein product, which results in the possibility of false-negative results or individuals who are not carriers of the variant being tested for. However, a carrier of another variant of the gene may still have the potential to pass the genetic alteration to offspring.[8]

Prenatal Testing

Prenatal testing is most commonly performed on a fetus during pregnancy to provide predictive information about the health status of the developing baby. However, newer techniques in conjunction with in vitro fertilization advances have been developed to facilitate genetic testing of the developing embryo or blastomere before implantation of the potential pregnancy into the uterus. Methods using a maternal blood sample and fetal cell separation during early pregnancy to perform fetal genetic analysis also have been developed. Identification of affected pregnancies is believed to be beneficial because in the pediatric population, genetic diseases are expensive to treat and chronic in nature. It has been estimated that in the United States, 50 percent of pediatric hospital admissions are gene related and that 20 percent of infant deaths are due to genetic disorders.[9]

In the early years of prenatal testing, the diseases looked for were considered grave ones, counseling efforts were nondirective, and the decision about continuing or terminating the pregnancy belonged to the couple. These early prenatal testing modalities primarily examined the fetus' chromosome complement or number of chromosomes and identified trisomic conditions such as Down syndrome, trisomy 18, and Klinefelter's syndrome and monosonic conditions such as Turner's syndrome. These conditions have fairly well-defined clinical presentations and known consequences for fetal well-being and childhood morbidity and mortality. Prenatal testing also offers individuals known to be carriers of a genetic trait the option of contributing to the genetic endowment of their offspring but not bringing an affected child into the world by providing the option of abortion after diagnosis of an affected pregnancy.

However, advances in recombinant technology mean that many single gene disorders can be ascertained with a high degree of accuracy during a pregnancy.[10] In addition, the new technology and findings of the Human Genome Project have added to the list of choices in prenatal screening available to prospective parents. For example, as the genes for hair color, height, weight, or athletic ability are identified, should potential parents be offered the opportunity to undertake genetic testing for these attributes of their fetus and make decisions about continuing or terminating the pregnancy based on these traits? Another possible outcome of increased prenatal testing potential is seeking prenatal testing with the desire for a genetic alteration and nonacceptance of a pregnancy without the genetic alteration. For example, two individuals with congenital deafness seek prenatal testing to determine if the fetus is also deaf and state that they refuse to give birth to and raise a hearing child.[8] A similar scenario can occur with achondroplasia dwarfism, an autosomal dominant disorder. If these individuals procreate with other dwarfed individuals, they have a 25 percent chance of conceiving a non-dwarf child. For some couples the prospect of giving birth to and parenting a "normal"-sized child is unacceptable. These situations raise the difficult question of parental choice conflicting with the biomedical model of neutrality and the goal of the Human Genome Project, which is identification of genetic traits to promote the elimination of disease. When the disorders identified by genetic testing had grave sequelae for the child, the problems faced by health care professionals and parents were less complex. The use of genetic testing as a guise for gender determination, with subsequent pregnancy termination based solely on the parents' preference for one gender over another, is an acknowledged but disturbing practice among many practitioners.[8] It is logical to hypothesize that decisions about the disposition of a pregnancy based on other genetic attributes that are not related to disease will be equally troubling. The new technological advances in recombinant genetics and techniques in prenatal diagnosis are forcing a reexamination of the ideologic concept of neutrality and its application to genetic counseling standards.

Prenatal testing not only is becoming increasingly available but also is being increasingly recommended during pregnancy. Technological and scientific advances have increased the ability to examine the fetus and to identify genetic traits at progressively earlier gestational ages. These abilities have transformed the pregnancy itself and the developing fetus from a mysterious event to an entity to be tested and the recipient of health care. Another issue to consider in the widespread use of prenatal genetic testing is that some of the traits identified may not manifest clinical signs or symptoms until many years after birth. Thus, does the choice about the impact of the condition belong with the parent or the child? In addition, it must be recognized that conditions detected currently that are considered untreatable and undesirable may become treatable or even curable within the lifetime of the affected child.[11] Another difficult dilemma is related to the child's rights. If the genetic testing is positive for a presymptomatic or predispositionary condition, should the child be told of the genome? When is the appropriate time for sharing of this information? Unlike other forms of genetic testing, the parents, not the fetus or child, make the choice to pursue testing. What if the parents choose to withhold information from the child, especially in the situations in which lifestyle or behavioral changes may influence expression of the genetic trait? What is the impact of the child knowing at an early age that he or she is predestined to develop a life-threatening and life-shortening disease at some time? Consequently, issues of autonomy and disclosure of information are integral to the use of prenatal genetic testing. Although beyond the scope of this article, prenatal genetic diagnosis also has implications for the essence of the pregnancy experience and the rights of pregnant women as autonomous decision makers and active participants in their health care as opposed to containers for the production of desirable offspring.[11]

MEANING OF GENETIC INFORMATION

What is the purpose of genetic testing and what is the meaning of the information known about an individual's genome? The stated purpose of the Human Genome Project is to identify all the components of the human genome with the ultimate goal of increased understanding of the causes and treatments of human disease. From a pure bench science perspective, this is an admirable pursuit. However, when this outcome is applied to human beings in the context of real-life situations, the potential ethical dilemmas become evident. The potential dilemmas are based in the definition of normal or desirable traits, the implication of having or not having a particular genetic attribute, and the individual's right to autonomous choice for making decisions about self balanced with the needs of the greater good of the family or society.

If an accepted long-term goal of continued advancement in recombinant technologies is the elimination or correction of abnormal genes, then society is embracing the concept that anything else is of lesser value. However, as additional genes are identified and the genetic influence of physical, emotional, and cognitive attributes is identified and open to manipulation, the question of which attributes are desirable, normal, and healthy must be addressed. Inherent in these definitions of desirable, normal, and healthy is the issue of whose values, perspectives, and beliefs are dominant and whether one standard is applied to all individuals or might there be variation by group affiliation or individual choice? How does having a societally determined undesirable trait, such as a physical attribute (e.g., hair color, height, or weight), impact society's response to the individual and thus the individual's opportunities within the larger societal context?

As the list of attributes that are identifiable through genetic testing but are unrelated to disease states continues to grow, the ideology of nondirectiveness in counseling and diagnostic pathways, combined with the increased number of choices available to the clients and the application of genetic technologies to real-life situations, becomes more complex. A parent's choice not to give birth to a child with a particular genetic attribute may be a sound and defensible position based on the factual and contextual nature of that parent's perspective yet may be morally disturbing to the provider and the larger community. The example cited earlier in this article, in which parents desired offspring like themselves (e.g., with a congenital hearing loss or dwarfism) is an exemplar of the use of technology to meet individual values and needs but to achieve and outcome that is contrary to the prevailing thought of the traditional biomedical model of technology's application to reproductive choices. Consequently, the implication of identifying individual genes goes beyond labeling and must address questions related to quality of life, productivity and contribution to society, resource use, and the value of individuality.

Genetic testing raises a number of ethical issues because of attributes that make it different from most other testing methods in health care. With the exception of confirmatory disease testing, genetic testing is predictive in nature. In other words, healthy people learn of their future risk of pathologic conditions without an equal quantity of information about the severity, duration, or impact of the condition. Because of the predictive nature of genetic testing and the numerous ambiguities associated with the applied meaning of the test finding, the risk/benefit analysis of knowing one's genome can be debated. The traditional medical model of informed consent supports full disclosure or telling a client everything that is known or knowable. However, health-care ethics also support the client's autonomous decision making. Therefore, as illustrated in the scenario at the beginning of this article, people may choose not to know their genetic composition and the implications of their individual genetic code.

The issue of informed knowing is additionally complex as applied to genetics because genetic testing involves families, not just individuals. Based on the laws of inheritance, one person who tests positive for a predictive or predispositive trait immediately reveals information about the possible risk that first-degree relatives are also affected. Consequently, whether intended or not, genetic testing is often a family affair by necessity.

CONCLUSION

The possible uses of genetic technology require scientists, health-care professionals, and society at large to reexamine the benefits of technologic advances moved from the scientist's laboratory to the practitioner's laboratory or the real world. Are increased knowledge, choice, and the possibility of improving one's genome a benefit or a burden to humanity? One of the greatest dangers of the emerging genetic technologies and associated value-based choices is the risk that some may view humanity as nothing more than a college of nucleotides in the form of genes. Identifying and understanding the technological bases of the human genome are part of human evolution, yet some people fear the impact of this advancing technology in future societies. However, as Samuels[12] points out, "technology is an extension of our hands and minds, whatever there is to fear is a fear of ourselves. We create, select and shape technologies and deal with their aftermath through the creation of still another technology." As health-care providers with a holistic perspective, nurses can play an integral role in challenging the ethical and social issues posed by genetic technologies in the clinical setting.

REFERENCES

1. Holtzman NA. Discovery, transfer and diffusion of technology for the detection of genetic disorders. *International Journal of Technology Assessment in Health Care.* 1994;10:562–572.

2. Tauer C. The human significance of the genome project. *Midwest Medical Ethics.* 1992;81:3–12.

3. Munro CL, Pickler RH. The basis of heredity: a genetic primer. *Neonatal Network.* 1996;15:710.

4. Murray TH. Assessing genetic technologies. *International Journal of Technology Assessment in Health Care.* 1994;10:573–582.

5. Rosenau PV. Reflections on the cost consequences of the new gene technology for health policy. *International Journal of Technology Assessment in Health Care.* 1994;10:545–561.

6. Holtzman NA. *Proceed with Caution: Predicting Genetic Risk in the Recombinant DNA Era.* Baltimore, MD: Johns Hopkins University; 1989.

7. Kaback M. Perspectives in genetic screening. *International Journal of Technology Assessment in Health Care.* 1994;10:592–603.

8. Murray TH, Livny E. The human genome project: ethical and social implications. *Bulletin of the Medical Library Association.* 1995;83:14–21.

9. Hall J. Impact of genetic diseases on pediatric health care. In: Kaback M, Shapiro L (eds.). *Frontiers in Genetic Medicine.* Report of the 92nd Ross Pediatric Research Conference. Columbus, OH; 1987: 1–3.

10. Rona RJ, Beech R, Mandalia S, et al: The influence of genetic counseling in the era of DNA testing on knowledge, reproductive intentions and psychological well-being. *Clinical Genetics.* 1994;46:198–204.

11. Raines DA. Fetal surveillance issues and implication. *Journal of Obstetric, Gynecologic, and Neonatal Nursing.* 1996;25:559.

12. Samuels SW. Ethical and metaethical criteria for an emerging technology: risk assessment. *Occupational Medicine.* 1997;47:241–246.

Part 15

ISSUES IN CLINICAL INTEGRITY

❧

M ore than two thousand years ago Plato wrote a story called "The Ring of Gyges." Simply, the main character acquired a ring that rendered him invisible. Imagine the power such a ring would bring its user. That power is similar to the power health-care providers have over patients. As patients, we allow complete strangers to probe us, poke us, look at us naked, and ask deeply personal questions. We do so even though we have no idea whether our health-care provider is knowledgeable, technically proficient, or even nice. This kind of relationship can only exist when a health-care profession itself is trusted. When the profession is trusted, individual members are trusted. It is this trust by association that gives a patient reason to believe it is safe, physically and emotionally, to put herself in the hands of a health-care provider she has just met.

Now, consider what our health-care system would be like if patients no longer trusted the health-care professions. Patients would avoid seeking health care for fear of being harmed. Personal (or embarrassing) information would not be openly shared. Diagnoses and recommendations would be seen as "untrustworthy." And suggested procedures and tests would be viewed as just as likely to be harmful as beneficial. With the consequences of this "world without trust" scenario in mind, consider the repercussions from the Tuskegee syphilis study, the U.S. government's human radiation experiments, gene therapy trials, and "emergency" research. Physicians, prestigious universities, medical researchers, public-health workers, nurses, pharmacists, and paramedics have actually carried out experiments (some of which were classified "top secret") without consent in any form. Even though the fiftieth anniversary of the Nuremberg trial—after which the Nuremberg code set out basic moral principles for conducting human research, including the basic tenet requiring voluntary consent of all research subjects—has just passed, we are still deeply entrenched in scandals regarding the lack of basic protections for human research subjects.

The goal of this section is to provide ethics committees and health-care providers with a foundation in the ethical issues of human research. The Joint Commission on Accreditation on Healthcare Organizations (JCAHO) sets out seven standards regarding research ethics that must be addressed in a health-care institutions' policies and procedures.[1] To that end, this section begins with the consent requirements for human research as set out by the federal government.

The consent requirements for human research have been set forth by the U.S. Food and Drug Administration and the U.S. Department of Health and Human Services in the U.S. Code of Federal Regulations, last revised on April 1, 1999. These regulations require all potential research subjects to be informed as to the research protocol's purpose; its duration; what exactly will be done to the subject; what the "foreseeable" risks and benefits are; who will have access to the subject's personal information; and what, if any, compensation will be provided. Researchers are also required to ensure that the subject's decision is voluntary and that he has had "sufficient opportunity to consider whether or not to participate."

The second reading in this section is "The Study of Untreated Syphilis in the Negro Male," by Otis Brawley. His article provides us with an account of the Tuskegee syphilis study that was conducted in Macon County, Alabama, from 1931 to 1972. Some 399 men with syphilis were enrolled for the sole purpose of documenting the disease's natural progression. At no time during the study were the men told they had syphilis; they were simply told they had "bad blood." As a result of this omission the subjects continued to have sexual relations with their wives and girlfriends, thus furthering the number of infected individuals. The circumstances that made this research study so egregious was twofold. First, numerous articles were published during the course of the experiment in many of the most prestigious medical journals. Even though the study was well-known within the medical community, nothing was said, no protests were made—and the study went on for forty-one years. Second, at the same time that the Allied "judicial system" was condemning Nazi physicians at Nuremberg, American physicians were violating almost every moral tenet that was so passionately being used against the accused in Germany.

The final reading is written by Henry Beecher, a famed professor of anesthesiology at Harvard University. In "Ethics and Clinical Research," Beecher describes twenty-two studies, published in prominent medical journals, in which consent of the human subjects was not obtained. As with the syphilis study, the medical community was well aware of the morally problematic nature of these studies, but nothing was ever said or done. Beecher begins his discussion by providing a sense of where these problems begin: funding. In 1945 the National Institute of Health gave out $701,800 in grants for medical research; in 1965 that amount had increased to $436,600,000.

During this past decade human research has become an even greater industrial complex as the Human Genome Project alone was awarded a $3-billion federal grant.

REFERENCE

1. Joint Commission on Accreditation of Healthcare Organizations. *2000 Hospital Accreditation Standards.* Oakbrook, IL: JCAHO; 2000:72–73.

36

INFORMED CONSENT
OF HUMAN SUBJECTS

Title 21 Food and Drugs
Chapter 1 Food and Drug Administration, Department
of Health and Human Services
Part 50 Protection of Human Subjects
50.20, 50.23.,50.24, 50.25, 50.27
[Revised as of April 1, 1999]

SEC. 50.20: GENERAL REQUIREMENTS
FOR INFORMED CONSENT

Except as provided in Secs. 50.23 and 50.24, no investigator may involve a human being as a subject in research covered by these regulations unless the investigator has obtained the legally effective informed consent of the subject or the subject's legally authorized representative. An investigator shall seek such consent only under circumstances that provide the prospective subject or the representative sufficient opportunity to consider whether or not to participate and that minimize the possibility of coercion or undue influence. The information that is given to the subject or the representative shall be in language understandable to the subject or the representative. No informed consent, whether oral or written, may include any exculpatory language through which the subject or the representative is made to waive or appear to waive any of the subject's legal rights, or releases or appears to release the investigator, the sponsor, the institution, or its agents from liability for negligence.

SEC. 50.23: EXCEPTION FROM
GENERAL REQUIREMENTS

(a) The obtaining of informed consent shall be deemed feasible unless, before use of the test article (except as provided in paragraph [b] of this section), both the investigator and a physician who is not otherwise participating in the clinical investigation certify in writing all of the following:

(1) The human subject is confronted by a life-threatening situation necessitating the use of the test article.

(2) Informed consent cannot be obtained from the subject because of an inability to communicate with, or obtain legally effective consent from, the subject.

(3) Time is not sufficient to obtain consent from the subject's legal representative.

(4) There is available no alternative method of approved or generally recognized therapy that provides an equal or greater likelihood of saving the life of the subject.

(b) If immediate use of the test article is, in the investigator's opinion, required to preserve the life of the subject, and time is not sufficient to obtain the independent determination required in paragraph (a) of this section in advance of using the test article, the determinations of the clinical investigator shall be made and, within five working days after the use of the article, be reviewed and evaluated in writing by a physician who is not participating in the clinical investigation.

(c) The documentation required in paragraph (a) or (b) of this section shall be submitted to the IRB within five working days after the use of the test article.

(d) (1) The Commissioner may also determine that obtaining informed consent is not feasible when the Assistant Secretary of Defense (Health Affairs) requests such a determination in connection with the use of an investigational drug (including a biological product) in a specific protocol under an investigational new drug application (IND) sponsored by the Department of Defense (DOD). DOD's request for a determination that obtaining informed consent from military personnel is not feasible must be limited to a specific military operation involving combat or the immediate threat of combat. The request must also include a written justification supporting the conclusions of the physician(s) responsible for the medical care of the military personnel involved and the investigator(s) identified in the IND that a military combat exigency exists because of special military combat (actual or threatened) circumstances in which, in order to facilitate the accomplishment of the military mission, preservation of the health of the individual and the safety of other personnel require that a particular treatment be provided to a specified group of military personnel, without regard to what might be any individual's personal preference for no treatment or for some alternative treatment. The written request must also include a statement that a duly constituted institutional review board has reviewed and approved the use of the investigational drug without informed consent. The Commissioner may find that informed consent is not feasible only when withholding treatment would be contrary to the best interests of military personnel and there is no available satisfactory alternative therapy.

(2) In reaching a determination under paragraph (d)(1) of this section that

obtaining informed consent is not feasible and withholding treatment would be contrary to the best interests of military personnel, the Commissioner will review the request submitted under paragraph (d)(1) of this section and take into account all pertinent factors, including, but not limited to:

(i) The extent and strength of the evidence of the safety and effectiveness of the investigational drug for the intended use;

(ii) The context in which the drug will be administered, e.g., whether it is intended for use in a battlefield or hospital setting or whether it will be self-administered or will be administered by a health professional;

(iii) The nature of the disease or condition for which the preventive or therapeutic treatment is intended; and

(iv) The nature of the information to be provided to the recipients of the drug concerning the potential benefits and risks of taking or not taking the drug.

(3) The Commissioner may request a recommendation from appropriate experts before reaching a determination on a request submitted under paragraph (d)(1) of this section.

(4) A determination by the Commissioner that obtaining informed consent is not feasible and withholding treatment would be contrary to the best interests of military personnel will expire at the end of one year, unless renewed at DOD's request, or when DOD informs the Commissioner that the specific military operation creating the need for the use of the investigational drug has ended, whichever is earlier. The Commissioner may also revoke this determination based on changed circumstances.

SEC. 50.24: EXCEPTION FROM INFORMED CONSENT REQUIREMENTS FOR EMERGENCY RESEARCH

(a) The IRB responsible for the review, approval, and continuing review of the clinical investigation described in this section may approve that investigation without requiring that informed consent of all research subjects be obtained if the IRB (with the concurrence of a licensed physician who is a member of or consultant to the IRB and who is not otherwise participating in the clinical investigation) finds and documents each of the following:

(1) The human subjects are in a life-threatening situation, available treatments are unproven or unsatisfactory, and the collection of valid scientific evidence, which may include evidence obtained through randomized placebo-controlled investigations, is necessary to determine the safety and effectiveness of particular interventions.

(2) Obtaining informed consent is not feasible because:

(i) The subjects will not be able to give their informed consent as a result of their medical condition;

    (ii) The intervention under investigation must be administered before consent from the subjects' legally authorized representatives is feasible; and

    (iii) There is no reasonable way to identify prospectively the individuals likely to become eligible for participation in the clinical investigation.

(3) Participation in the research holds out the prospect of direct benefit to the subjects because:

    (i) Subjects are facing a life-threatening situation that necessitates intervention;

    (ii) Appropriate animal and other preclinical studies have been conducted, and the information derived from those studies and related evidence support the potential for the intervention to provide a direct benefit to the individual subjects; and

    (iii) Risks associated with the investigation are reasonable in relation to what is known about the medical condition of the potential class of subjects, the risks and benefits of standard therapy, if any, and what is known about the risks and benefits of the proposed intervention or activity.

(4) The clinical investigation could not practicably be carried out without the waiver.

(5) The proposed investigational plan defines the length of the potential therapeutic window based on scientific evidence, and the investigator has committed to attempting to contact a legally authorized representative for each subject within that window of time and, if feasible, to asking the legally authorized representative contacted for consent within that window rather than proceeding without consent. The investigator will summarize efforts made to contact legally authorized representatives and make this information available to the IRB at the time of continuing review.

(6) The IRB has reviewed and approved informed consent procedures and an informed consent document consistent with Sec. 50.25. These procedures and the informed consent document are to be used with subjects or their legally authorized representatives in situations where use of such procedures and documents is feasible. The IRB has reviewed and approved procedures and information to be used when providing an opportunity for a family member to object to a subject's participation in the clinical investigation consistent with paragraph (a)(7)(v) of this section.

(7) Additional protections of the rights and welfare of the subjects will be provided, including, at least:

    (i) Consultation (including, where appropriate, consultation carried out by the IRB) with representatives of the communities in which the clinical investigation will be conducted and from which the subjects will be drawn;

    (ii) Public disclosure to the communities in which the clinical investigation will be conducted and from which the subjects will be drawn, prior to initiation of the clinical investigation, of plans for the investigation and its risks and expected benefits;

(iii) Public disclosure of sufficient information following completion of the clinical investigation to apprise the community and researchers of the study, including the demographic characteristics of the research population, and its results;

(iv) Establishment of an independent data monitoring committee to exercise oversight of the clinical investigation; and

(v) If obtaining informed consent is not feasible and a legally authorized representative is not reasonably available, the investigator has committed, if feasible, to attempting to contact within the therapeutic window the subject's family member who is not a legally authorized representative, and asking whether he or she objects to the subject's participation in the clinical investigation. The investigator will summarize efforts made to contact family members and make this information available to the IRB at the time of continuing review.

(b) The IRB is responsible for ensuring that procedures are in place to inform, at the earliest feasible opportunity, each subject, or if the subject remains incapacitated, a legally authorized representative of the subject, or if such a representative is not reasonably available, a family member, of the subject's inclusion in the clinical investigation, the details of the investigation and other information contained in the informed consent document. The IRB shall also ensure that there is a procedure to inform the subject, or if the subject remains incapacitated, a legally authorized representative of the subject, or if such a representative is not reasonably available, a family member, that he or she may discontinue the subject's participation at any time without penalty or loss of benefits to which the subject is otherwise entitled. If a legally authorized representative or family member is told about the clinical investigation and the subject's condition improves, the subject is also to be informed as soon as feasible. If a subject is entered into a clinical investigation with waived consent and the subject dies before a legally authorized representative or family member can be contacted, information about the clinical investigation is to be provided to the subject's legally authorized representative or family member, if feasible.

(c) The IRB determinations required by paragraph (a) of this section and the documentation required by paragraph (e) of this section are to be retained by the IRB for at least three years after completion of the clinical investigation, and the records shall be accessible for inspection and copying by FDA in accordance with Sec. 56.115(b) of this chapter.

(d) Protocols involving an exception to the informed-consent requirement under this section must be performed under a separate investigational new drug application (IND) or investigational device exemption (IDE) that clearly identifies such protocols as protocols that may include subjects who are unable to consent. The submission of those protocols in a separate IND/IDE is required even if an IND for the same drug product or an IDE for the same device already exists.

Applications for investigations under this section may not be submitted as amendments under Secs. 312.30 or 812.35 of this chapter.

(e) If an IRB determines that it cannot approve a clinical investigation because the investigation does not meet the criteria in the exception provided under paragraph (a) of this section or because of other relevant ethical concerns, the IRB must document its findings and provide these findings promptly in writing to the clinical investigator and to the sponsor of the clinical investigation. The sponsor of the clinical investigation must promptly disclose this information to FDA and to the sponsor's clinical investigators who are participating or are asked to participate in this or a substantially equivalent clinical investigation of the sponsor, and to other IRB's that have been, or are, asked to review this or a substantially equivalent investigation by that sponsor.

SEC. 50.25: ELEMENTS OF INFORMED CONSENT

(a) Basic elements of informed consent. In seeking informed consent, the following information shall be provided to each subject:

(1) A statement that the study involves research, an explanation of the purposes of the research and the expected duration of the subject's participation, a description of the procedures to be followed, and identification of any procedures which are experimental.

(2) A description of any reasonably foreseeable risks or discomforts to the subject.

(3) A description of any benefits to the subject or to others which may reasonably be expected from the research.

(4) A disclosure of appropriate alternative procedures or courses of treatment, if any, that might be advantageous to the subject.

(5) A statement describing the extent, if any, to which confidentiality of records identifying the subject will be maintained and that notes the possibility that the Food and Drug Administration may inspect the records.

(6) For research involving more than minimal risk, an explanation as to whether any compensation and an explanation as to whether any medical treatments are available if injury occurs and, if so, what they consist of, or where further information may be obtained.

(7) An explanation of whom to contact for answers to pertinent questions about the research and research subjects' rights, and whom to contact in the event of a research-related injury to the subject.

(8) A statement that participation is voluntary, that refusal to participate will involve no penalty or loss of benefits to which the subject is otherwise entitled, and that the subject may discontinue participation at any time without penalty or loss of benefits to which the subject is otherwise entitled.

(b) Additional elements of informed consent. When appropriate, one or more of the following elements of information shall also be provided to each subject:

(1) A statement that the particular treatment or procedure may involve risks to

the subject (or to the embryo or fetus, if the subject is or may become pregnant) which are currently unforeseeable.

(2) Anticipated circumstances under which the subject's participation may be terminated by the investigator without regard to the subject's consent.

(3) Any additional costs to the subject that may result from participation in the research.

(4) The consequences of a subject's decision to withdraw from the research and procedures for orderly termination of participation by the subject.

(5) A statement that significant new findings developed during the course of the research which may relate to the subject's willingness to continue participation will be provided to the subject.

(6) The approximate number of subjects involved in the study.

(c) The informed consent requirements in these regulations are not intended to preempt any applicable Federal, State, or local laws which require additional information to be disclosed for informed consent to be legally effective.

(d) Nothing in these regulations is intended to limit the authority of a physician to provide emergency medical care to the extent the physician is permitted to do so under applicable Federal, State, or local law.

SEC. 50.27: DOCUMENTATION OF INFORMED CONSENT

(a) Except as provided in Sec. 56.109(c), informed consent shall be documented by the use of a written consent form approved by the IRB and signed and dated by the subject or the subject's legally authorized representative at the time of consent. A copy shall be given to the person signing the form.

(b) Except as provided in Sec. 56.109(c), the consent form may be either of the following:

(1) A written consent document that embodies the elements of informed consent required by Sec. 50.25. This form may be read to the subject or the subject's legally authorized representative, but, in any event, the investigator shall give either the subject or the representative adequate opportunity to read it before it is signed.

(2) A short form written consent document stating that the elements of informed consent required by Sec. 50.25 have been presented orally to the subject or the subject's legally authorized representative. When this method is used, there shall be a witness to the oral presentation. Also, the IRB shall approve a written summary of what is to be said to the subject or the representative. Only the short form itself is to be signed by the subject or the representative. However, the witness shall sign both the short form and a copy of the summary, and the person actually obtaining the consent shall sign a copy of the summary. A copy of the summary shall be given to the subject or the representative in addition to a copy of the short form.

37

THE STUDY OF UNTREATED SYPHILIS IN THE NEGRO MALE

Otis W. Brawley, M.D.

❦

INTRODUCTION

When we think of the Tuskegee Institute, the first thing we should think of is its rich history—Booker T. Washington, George Washington Carver, and the Tuskegee Airmen. The first thing we think of should not be the Tuskegee Syphilis Study. Indeed, the study, officially titled "The Tuskegee Study of Untreated Syphilis in the Negro Male," should really be referred to as the "U.S. Public Health Service (PHS) Study of Untreated Syphilis in the Negro Male."

My purpose here is to recount the facts of the study and its historical context. Unfortunately, the facts of what truly happened from 1931 to 1972 are widely misunderstood. Rumor and prejudice have replaced fact, a situation that has been made worse by the recent Home Box Office film entitled "Miss Ever's Boys." This television movie, which was billed as "fiction based on a factual event," certainly deviated from the truth. Despite this deviation, it is largely viewed as fact and not the fiction that it is. Finally, incomplete and inaccurate news coverage has obscured what really happened.

The history recounted here is taken from a review of documents gathered during the U.S. Senate hearings and investigation in 1972, original papers located in

O. Brawley. "The Study of Untreated Syphilis in the Negro Male." *International Journal of Radiation, Oncology, Biology, Physics.* 1998;40(1);5–8. Reprinted with permission from Elsevier Science.

the National Library of Medicine, and the book *Bad Blood* by James Jones.[1] This history is conveyed through the eyes of an African American physician who has designed and conducted clinical trials. As I recount the history, I will attempt to discern established fact from interpretation.

It is my belief that the lessons of the PHS syphilis study are numerous. These lessons apply not only to those of us who conduct clinical trials, but to literally everyone involved in any aspect of medicine. These lessons apply to the counseling of and the informing of the lay public by medical professionals and lay advocates. Many of the individuals who supported or helped conduct this tragic study likely deceived themselves into believing that they were doing the right thing. The first lesson involves the obligation of those of us who take a leadership role in the delivery of health care to learn and understand medicine ourselves. The second lesson involves the obligation of health-care providers and advocates to go beyond merely informing to teaching. Patients must understand the ramifications of a decision and freely choose to participate in a study or accept health care.

THE AMERICAN SOUTH IN THE 1920s

The context of the times is important to the history of the study. In the late 1920s, a number of survey studies suggested that over 35 percent of black men in the rural South were infected with syphilis. These surveys suffered from selection biases that likely magnified the estimates. The conclusions of these studies were widely publicized by concerned parties and organizations in an effort to force public health officials to do something. The limits of and potential selection biases of the studies were not widely disclosed.

At this time "race medicine" was still widely accepted in the United States. Central to "race medicine" was the belief that blacks were different from whites and that a disease could have differing effects on blacks versus whites. There was considerable belief that syphilis was a more indolent disease in blacks than in whites. It was noted that many blacks had syphilis and few were dying of it. This argument and the fiscal limitations of the depression made it even easier for federal, state, and local public health officials to ignore the problem of syphilis in blacks.

The common therapies for syphilis at that time were difficult to administer, expensive, painful, and dangerous. The efficacy of the these therapies (arsphenamine, bismuth, and mercurial compounds) were, and still are, debated within the medical community. Importantly, these were the accepted treatments of the time. Few American blacks were treated for syphilis because medical care was expensive. Indeed, most southern Negroes, being poor, had never seen a physician for any reason.

In the 1920s and 1930s, the discipline called "public health" was relatively new. The Division of Venereal Diseases of the U.S. Public Health Service was comprised of a group of committed young public health physicians. The PHS teamed with representatives of several charitable foundations, and began treating blacks for syphilis in several sites in the southern United States. These activities were to demonstrate that both logistically and medically difficult antisyphilis treatments could be administered to rural blacks.

One of the demonstration projects was in Macon County, Alabama, home of the Tuskegee Institute. Macon County was rural and more than 80 percent black. The poor living conditions of Macon County were startling to the PHS officers; chronic malnutrition and other diet-related illnesses, such as pellagra, were common. One PHS officer, Thomas Parran, who later would become U.S. Surgeon General, wrote about the poverty of Macon County in his book *Shadow on the Land.*[2] The demonstration project started in 1930 and was terminated in just over a year due to insufficient funds, with many people having received an incomplete course of therapy.

The Initial Study

In 1933, the PHS returned to Macon County. There was such a high incidence of unusual syphilitic pathology that it was felt that a study of persons with a long history of syphilis could be done. PHS physician Dr. Taliafero Clark devised a study that would provide data on how syphilis differed in the "Negro vs. the White." The initial plan was to identify people who had syphilis for a long time, examine them, and record physical and laboratory findings. The original project, as planned, would last less than a year and would treat those diagnosed with syphilis. There was some concern that the persons involved would not get the standard eighteen months of treatment, but it was felt that some treatment would be better than no treatment. Some speculated that, at least, these people would be rendered uninfectious to others.

The PHS officers went to the all-black Andrew Hospital at the Tuskegee Institute to enlist support. The principal of the institute and the director of the hospital (both black men) enthusiastically agreed to support the project. Tuskegee and Andrew Hospital would be paid to provide clinical space, as well as laboratory and radiological support to the study. This would also be a beneficial learning experience for the young black medical interns at Andrew Hospital. Tuskegee would provide hospitalization, when necessary, and be the site of autopsies. Tuskegee agreed to hire one of its nurse graduates interested in public health, Eunice Rivers, R.N., to serve as data manager for the study.

This was to be a study of tertiary syphilis. Late in the design phase, the study was changed to a survey of men because women, having internal genitalia, frequently did not know when they were infected. This study enrolled 399 men with syphilis and 201 uninfected men to serve as controls. All men enrolled were at least twenty-five years old at enrollment.

The Second Study

The initial survey was completed, as planned, in about a year. It was at this point that all therapy was terminated. Some men received as little as a month of antisyphilitic therapy, and others received therapy for several months. It was decided that the pathology seen was so impressive that PHS physicians would return annually to follow the course of these patients, and they did so for three decades to assess men at so-called round-ups. Rivers, whose employment was eventually transferred to the U.S. Public Health Service, was entrusted to keep track of the study subjects to assure that as few as possible were "lost to follow-up."

The men in this trial participated voluntarily and most continued coming to round-ups believing there was value in the annual physical examinations; however, there is no evidence that any diagnosed illnesses were treated. Vitamins, tonic, and aspirin may have been given to some men who complained of minor pains and ailments.

Some men submitted to lumbar punctures, believing that the procedure was a therapeutic "spinal shot"; however, it was purely for research purposes. The morbidity associated with these spinal shots should not be underemphasized; indeed, it was a most terrible experience. Men who received these shots experienced severe back pain, headache, and even temporary paralysis. Some men suffered from the results of these "spinal shots" for years.

In the late 1930s, several men died and were not autopsied. The Milbank fund was convinced to provide funds to the Tuskegee Institute for fifty-dollar burial stipends. This was a successful effort to encourage families to notify Nurse Rivers immediately upon death of a study subject, so that an autopsy could be arranged. Participation of the Tuskegee Institute and its hospital decreased significantly after 1945, although the burial stipends, some laboratory tests, X-rays, and autopsies continued to be performed by Andrew Hospital physicians into the 1960s. The Tuskegee Veterans Administration Hospital, another predominantly black institution, also provided some support of the trial into the late 1960s.

Many of the strategies we discuss today as necessary for overcoming barriers to clinical trials recruitment were pioneered in this study. Nurse Rivers would recruit patients to the trial by going to their places of work, going to barber shops, going to churches, and providing transportation. She was the educated and respected friend who guided these men through the study. Other things done to preserve the trial were quite unusual and extreme. In 1941, more than 250 of the men were less than forty-five years old and draftable. The PHS, however, was able to convince the local draft board not to conscript any of these men, therefore preventing the men from being moved out of the area, diagnosed, and treated.

Several beliefs about this study, commonly held by the public, are clearly false. Many think that men in the study were infected by those running the study. The trial actually enrolled men who could identify a syphilitic skin lesion more than five years before entry. Controls who developed infection were continued in the study and, clearly, some men in the study infected others during the trial. Today, many erroneously believe that these men were unaware that they were in a study. Many men bragged that they were taking part in "Nurse River's Study." Indeed, in Macon County, it was a social honor to be in her study. Although they were informed, it is obvious that those who had syphilis did not understand that they had a sexually transmittable disease, and many in the control group did not know or believe they were healthy. However, the men were aware that they had "bad blood," but did not know what that meant.

In 1943, penicillin was introduced in the PHS national antisyphilis campaign. Unlike previous therapies, it was clearly effective, inexpensive, and easy to administer. It is unknown who made the decision to continue the study and not treat these men. The PHS did convince the local draft board to support the study by excluding participants from the draft. If drafted, a participant would be diagnosed and treated. Penicillin was used in Macon County by the PHS, but care was taken not to treat the men in the Study. Local physicians, some of them black, supported the study by agreeing not to treat men on the trial. There is no evidence that these men were informed that a cure for syphilis existed and that decision had been made not to cure them. There is some evidence that, in the mid 1940s, some PHS officers discussed treatment and felt that penicillin might be harmful to men with a long history of syphilis.

It is unclear why the study continued for three decades after the development and widespread availability of penicillin. Some involved with the trial actually claimed that it was a unique opportunity to learn the natural history of syphilis and that the trial was more important than ever, given that there was an effective treatment. Even if the physicians really believed this, they were forgetting that many men in the trial had been partially treated prior to the advent of penicillin. It is obvious that they felt no obligation to the men in the trial, and did not learn from the Nuremberg trials of the late 1940s that led to the Nuremberg Code of Principles of Human Experimentation or the many changes in how clinical research was conducted.

Contrary to common belief, the study was not a secret. From 1933 to 1965, more than a dozen peer-reviewed papers with results from the study were published in respected journals such as *Public Health Reports, Archives of Internal Medicine,* and the *Journal of Chronic Diseases.* These articles explained that the data came from a study in which a large number of black men with syphilis were being observed and not treated. The title of one paper was "Untreated Syphilis in the Male Negro: A Prospective Study of the Effect on Life Expectancy."[3] Ironically, some of these papers have become classics and are still cited in the literature today. Nurse Rivers was the first black to be coauthor in several prestigious medical journals.

Few in the American medical community really questioned the study until the middle 1960s. In 1965, one physician did write to the PHS and ask how this study could be performed, but his letter was not answered. In 1968, the PHS even convinced a group of predominantly black physicians in Macon County to endorse the study and agree not to treat participants. It was not until a PHS officer named Peter Buxton, who read a paper about the trial, raised questions about the trial, that questions led to the trial's end.

THE END OF THE TRIAL

After several years of questioning by Mr. Buxton, several news articles were published, leading to a Senate investigation headed by Senator Edward Kennedy. The investigation forced the trial's closure in 1972. The reaction to the trial would lead to enactment of legislation establishing the Office for Protection from Research Risks within what is now the Department of Health and Human Services, and the requirement for Institutional Review Boards. Institutional Review Boards are designed to assure that trials are ethical and participants in clinical studies give informed consent.

A lawsuit was filed by the famed civil rights attorney Fred Gray against the Centers for Disease Control, of which the PHS Division of Venereal Disease had become part in the 1940s. A suit of the Federal government was complicated, and it was finally settled out of court for $10 million. Syphilitic men or their estates (in the case of men who had died) received up to $37,500 apiece. Controls received up to $16,000. Survivors of the trial and some wives and children affected by syphilis also received free medical care for the remainder of their lives. Mr. Gray received a $1-million fee for his legal work. No individual associated with the trial was ever sued, prosecuted, or even formally reprimanded. In May 1997, the president of the United States formally apologized to the trial participants and their families. It was the federal government's first official admission of responsibility, and that inappropriate things occurred in the conduct of the study. Seven survivors of the trial were alive at the time of the apology.

LESSONS TO LEARN

Alfred North Whitehead once said that "those who do not understand history are doomed to repeat it." The lessons of the U.S. Public Health Study of Untreated Syphilis in the Negro male include the dangers of paternalism, arrogance, blind loyalty, and misuse of science.

Many have judged the PHS officers who ran the trial as evil racists. Those who initially started the trial actually had reputations as committed public health physicians with commitment and concern regarding the health of Negroes. They argued in scientific papers that the high prevalence rates of syphilis among blacks were not due to inherent racial susceptibility, but to their poor social and economic status. They also helped many of the black Andrew Hospital interns receive postgraduate training at elite, traditionally all-white institutions. Indeed, several were critics of the poverty and circumstance of blacks in the South. It is conceivable that these physicians somehow fooled themselves into believing they were doing a service to blacks as a whole by running this study.

The concept of "race medicine" remains with us. Unfortunately, it can still lead us to scientific tragedies and social injustice. It is interesting that some current literature (medical and lay) and legislation assume the old "race medicine" premise that blacks are biologically different from whites, who are biologically different from Asians, and so on. In fact, scientists frequently publish rates by race or ethnicity, encouraging many to quickly conclude that if a disease occurs more frequently in or appears to be more deadly in a particular race or ethnic group, it must be because of inherent biological or genetic differences. Furthermore, outcomes are often attributed to race when modifiable factors, such as culture or socioeconomic status, might be the major underlying cause.

The tragedy of the study can be attributed in large part to the arrogance and paternalism of the people running the study. Arrogance prevented complete peer review, which might have prevented the study from being started, and even intermittent peer review by persons concerned with the safety of the men in the trial certainly would have stopped it with the advent of penicillin.

Furthermore, there were a number of black physicians and laboratory technicians assisting in the conduct of this trial, especially in the early years but even into the 1960s. Some may even have been guilty of believing that they were better than the uneducated poor blacks entering this trial. Classism among blacks did and, unfortunately, still does exist. Some blacks and some whites were likely guilty of failing to understand and learn all about the trial on which they were working.

Much has been made of Rivers's participation. She retired from the study in 1965, but came back as a consultant every year until its termination. From interviews and depositions given by Rivers after the trial was stopped, it appears that she was a sincere woman who cared about the men and the study and just did not understand.

PHS officials in the 1950s and 1960s were guilty of not rigorously assessing the value of the trial and, clearly, did not consider its ethics. They allowed the trial to become entrenched in the PHS bureaucracy and felt no sense of personal responsibility. Furthermore, government personnel may not have questioned the trial because it was historically associated with several distinguished PHS officers: Thomas Parran, who had gone on to become Surgeon General, and John R. Heller, who became head of what would become the National Cancer Institute.

One person with a profound respect for the truth could have, and eventually did, stop this tragedy. Additionally, going beyond merely informing participants to instructing participants about the study and receiving truly informed consent might also have prevented this tragedy. This lesson is still valid today for those of us involved in routine clinical practice and trials. It is our obligation not just to inform our participants, but to go beyond and assure that our patients fully understand the study. There is also the obligation that we ourselves must fully comprehend any subject matter before we teach or advocate it.

As more sophisticated screening, diagnostic, and treatment technologies are developed, it must be realized that the errors of this study can and do occur today. Those of us who counsel patients, whether lay health advocates, nurses, or physicians, have a personal responsibility to be fully informed and an obligation to fully inform. We must have a commitment to tell our patients the truth. The urge to oversimplify a complicated concept and deny individuals information that will allow them to make informed decisions affecting their lives is still frequent.

REFERENCES

1. Jones J. *Bad Blood: The Tuskegee Syphilis Experiment.* New York, NY: Free Press; 1981.

2. Parran T. *Shadow on the Land: Syphilis.* New York, NY: Putnam; 1937.

3. Shafer JK. Untreated syphilis in the male Negro: A prospective study of the effect on life expectancy. *Public Health Reports.* 1954;69:688–692.

38

ETHICS AND CLINICAL RESEARCH

Henry K. Beecher, M.D.

Human experimentation since World War II has created some difficult problems with the increasing employment of patients as experimental subjects when it must be apparent that they would not have been available if they had been truly aware of the uses that would be made of them. Evidence is at hand that many of the patients in the examples to follow never had the risk satisfactorily explained to them, and it seems obvious that further hundreds have not known that they were the subjects of an experiment although grave consequences have been suffered as a direct result of experiments described here. There is a belief prevalent in some sophisticated circles that attention to these matters would "block progress." But, according to Pope Pius XII,[1] " . . . science is not the highest value to which all other orders' of values . . . should be subordinated."

I am aware that these are troubling charges. They have grown out of troubling practices. They can be documented, as I propose to do, by examples from leading medical schools, university hospitals, private hospitals, governmental military departments (the Army, the Navy, and the Air Force), governmental institutes (the National Institutes of Health), Veterans Administration hospitals and industry. The basis for the charges is broad.*

I should like to affirm that American medicine is sound, and most progress in it soundly attained. There is, however, a reason for concern in certain areas, and I

H. K. Beecher. "Ethics and Clinical Research." *New England Journal of Medicine.* 1966;274:1354–1360. Copyright ©1966 Massachusetts Medical Society. All rights reserved.

believe the type of activities to be mentioned will do great harm to medicine unless soon corrected. It will certainly he charged that any mention of these matters does it disservice to medicine, but not one so great, I believe, as a continuation of the practices to he cited.

Experimentation in man takes place in several areas: in self-experimentation; in patient volunteers and normal subjects; in therapy; and in the different areas of *experimentation on a patient not for his benefit but for that, at least in theory, of patients in general*. The present study is limited to this last category.

REASONS FOR URGENCY OF STUDY

Ethical errors are increasing not only in numbers but in variety—for example, in the recently added problems arising in transplantation of organs.

There are a number of reasons why serious attention to the general problem is urgent.

Of transcendent importance is the enormous and continuing increase in available funds, as shown below.

Money Available for Research Each Year

Massachusetts General Hospital	National Institutes of Health[a]
1945	$ 500,000[b]	$ 701,800
1955	2,222,816	36,063,200
1965	8,384,342	436,600,000

[a]National Institutes of Health figures based upon decade averages, excluding funds for construction, kindly supplied by Dr. John Sherman, of National Institutes of Health.

[b]Approximation, supplied by Mr. David C. Crockett, of Massachusetts General Hospital

---

Since World War II the annual expenditure for research (in large part in man) in the Massachusetts General Hospital has increased a remarkable 17-fold. At the National Institutes of Health, the increase has been a gigantic 624-fold. This "national" rate of increase is over 36 times that of the Massachusetts General Hospital. These data, rough as they are, illustrate vast opportunities and concomitantly expanded responsibilities.

Taking into account the sound and increasing emphasis of recent years that

---

*At the Brook Lodge Conference on Problems and Complexities of Clinical Research, I commented that "what seem to be breaches of ethical conduct in experimentation are by no means rare, but are almost, one fears, universal." I thought it was obvious that I was by "universal" referring to the fact that examples could easily be found in all categories where research in man takes place to any significant extent. Judging by press comments, that was not obvious; hence, this note.

experimentation in man must precede general application of new procedures in therapy, plus the great sums of money available, there is reason to fear that these requirements and these resources may be greater than the supply of responsible investigators. All this heightens the problems under discussion.

Medical schools and university hospitals are increasingly dominated by investigators. Every young man knows that he will never be promoted to a tenure post, to a professorship in a major medical school, unless he has proved himself as an investigator. If the ready availability of money for conducting research is added to this fact, one can see how great the pressures are on ambitious young physicians.

Implementation of the recommendations of the President's Commission on Heart Disease, Cancer, and Stroke means that further astronomical sums of money will become available for research in man.

In addition to the foregoing three practical points there are others that Sir Robert Platt[2] has pointed out: a general awakening of social conscience; greater power for good or harm in new remedies, new operations, and new investigative procedures than was formerly the case; new methods of preventive treatment with their advantages and dangers that are now applied to communities as a whole as well as to individuals, with multiplication of the possibilities for injury; medical science has shown how valuable human experimentation can be in solving problems of disease and its treatment; one can therefore anticipate an increase in experimentation; and the newly developed concept of clinical research as a profession (for example, clinical pharmacology)—and this, of course, can lead to unfortunate separation between the interests of science and the interests of the patient.

FREQUENCY OF UNETHICAL OR QUESTIONABLY ETHICAL PROCEDURES

Nearly everyone agrees that ethical violations do occur. The practical question is, how often? A preliminary examination of the matter was based on 17 examples, which were easily increased to 50. These 50 studies contained references to 186 further likely examples, on the average 3.7 leads per study; they at times overlapped from paper to paper, but this figure indicates how conveniently one can proceed in a search for such material. The data are suggestive of widespread problems, but there is need for another kind of information, which was obtained by examination of 100 consecutive human studies published in 1964, in an excellent journal; 12 of these seemed to be unethical. If only one quarter of them is truly unethical, this still indicates the existence of a serious situation. Pappworth[3] in England, has collected, he says, more than 500 papers based upon unethical experimentation. It is evident from such observations that unethical or questionably ethical procedures are not uncommon.

THE PROBLEM OF CONSENT

All so-called codes are based on the bland assumption that meaningful or informed consent is readily available for the asking. As pointed out elsewhere,[4] this is very often not the case. Consent in any fully informed sense may not be obtainable. Nevertheless, except, possibly, in the most trivial situations, it remains a goal toward which one must strive for sociologic, ethical, and clear-cut legal reasons. There is no choice in the matter.

If suitably approached, patients will accede, on the basis of trust, to about any request their physician may make. At the same time, every experienced clinician investigator knows that patients will often submit to inconvenience and some discomfort, if they do not last very long, but the usual patient will never agree to jeopardize seriously his health or his life for the sake of "science."

In only 2 of the 50* examples originally compiled for this study was consent mentioned. Actually, it should be emphasized in all cases for obvious moral and legal reasons, but it would be unrealistic to place much dependence on it. In any precise sense statements regarding consent are meaningless unless one knows how fully the patient was informed of all risks, and if these are not known, that fact should also be made clear. A far more dependable safeguard than consent is the presence of a truly *responsible* investigator.

EXAMPLES OF UNETHICAL OR QUESTIONABLY ETHICAL STUDIES

These examples are not cited for the condemnation of individuals; they are recorded to call attention to a variety of ethical problems found in experimental medicine, for it is hoped that calling attention to them will help to correct abuses present. During ten years of study of these matters it has become apparent that thoughtlessness and carelessness, not a willful disregard of the patient's rights, account for most of the cases encountered. Nonetheless, it is evident that in many of the examples presented, the investigators have risked the health or the life of their subjects. No attempt has been made to present the "worst" possible examples; rather, the aim has been to show the variety of problems encountered.

References to the examples presented are not given, for there is no intention of pointing to individuals, but rather, a wish to call attention to widespread practices. All, however, are documented to the satisfaction of the editors of the *Journal*.

---

*Reduced here to 22 for reasons of space.

Known Effective Treatment Withheld

Example 1. It is known that rheumatic fever can usually be prevented by adequate treatment of streptococcal respiratory infections by the parenteral administration of penicillin. Nevertheless, definitive treatment was withheld, and placebos were given to a group of 109 men in service, while benzathine penicillin G was given to others.

The therapy that each patient received was determined automatically by his military serial number arranged so that more men received penicillin than received placebo. In the small group of patients studied, two cases of acute rheumatic fever and one of acute nephritis developed in the control patients, whereas these complications did not occur among those who received the benzathine penicillin G.

Example 2. The sulfonamides were for many years the only antibacterial drugs effective in shortening the duration of acute streptococcal pharyngitis and in reducing its suppurative complications. The investigators in this study undertook to determine if the occurrence of the serious nonsuppurative complications, rheumatic fever and acute glomerulonephritis, would be reduced by this treatment. This study was made despite the general experience that certain antibiotics, including penicillin, will prevent the development of rheumatic fever.

The subjects were a large group of hospital patients; a control group of approximately the same size, also with exudative Group A streptococcus, was included. The latter group received only nonspecific therapy (no sulfadiazine). The total group denied the effective penicillin comprised over 500 men.

Rheumatic fever was diagnosed in 5.4 percent of those treated with sulfadiazine. In the control group rheumatic fever developed in 4.2 percent.

In reference to this study a medical officer stated in writing that the subjects were not informed, did not consent, and were not aware that they had been involved in an experiment, and yet admittedly 25 acquired rheumatic fever. According to this same medical officer *more than 70* who had had known definitive treatment withheld were on the wards with rheumatic fever when he was there.

Example 3. This involved a study of the relapse rate in typhoid fever treated in two ways. In an earlier study by the present investigators, chloramphenicol had been recognized as an effective treatment for typhoid fever, being attended by half the mortality that was experienced when this agent was not used. Others had made the same observations, indicating that to withhold this effective remedy can be a life-or-death decision. The present study was carried out to determine the relapse rate under the two methods of treatment; of 408 charity patients, 251 were treated with chloramphenicol, of whom 20, or 7.97 percent, died. Symptomatic treatment was given, but chloramphenicol was withheld in 157, of whom 36, or 22.9 percent, died. According to the data presented, 23 patients died in the course of this study who would not have been expected to succumb if they had received specific therapy.

Study of Therapy

Example 4. TriA (triacetyloleandomycin) was originally introduced for the treatment of infection with gram-positive organisms. Spotty evidence of hepatic dysfunction emerged, especially in children, and so the present study was undertaken on 50 patients, including mental defectives or juvenile delinquents who were inmates of a children's center. No disease other than acne was present; the drug was given for treatment of this. The ages of the subjects ranged from thirteen to thirty-nine years. "By the time half the patients had received the drug for four weeks, the high incidence of significant hepatic dysfunction . . . led to the discontinuation of administration to the remainder of the group at three weeks." (However, only two weeks after the start of the administration of the drug, 54 percent of the patients showed abnormal excretion of bromsulfalein.) Eight patients with marked hepatic dysfunction were transferred to the hospital "for more intensive study." Liver biopsy was carried out in these 8 patients and repeated in 4 of them. Liver damage was evident. Four of these hospitalized patients, after their liver-function tests returned to normal limits, received a "challenge" dose of the drug. Within two days hepatic dysfunction was evident in 3 of the 4 patients. In one patient a second challenge dose was given after the first challenge and again led to evidence of abnormal liver function. Flocculation tests remained abnormal in some patients as long as five weeks after discontinuance of the drug.

Physiologic Studies

Example 5. In this controlled, double-blind study of the hematologic toxicity of chloramphenicol, it was recognized that chloramphenicol is "well known as a cause of aplastic anemia" and that there is a "prolonged morbidity and high mortality of aplastic anemia" and that " . . . chloramphenicol-induced aplastic anemia can be related to dose. . . ." The aim of the study was "further definition of the toxicology of the drug.

Forty-one randomly chosen patients were given either 2 or 6 g of chloramphenicol per day; 12 control patients were used. "Toxic bone-marrow depression, predominantly affecting erythropoiesis, developed in 2 of 20 patients given 2 g and in 18 of 21 given 6 g of chloramphenicol daily." The smaller dose is recommended for routine use.

Example 6. In a study of the effect of thymectomy on the survival of skin homografts 18 children, three and a half months to eighteen years of age, about to undergo surgery for congenital heart disease, were selected. Eleven were to have total thymectomy as part of the operation, and 7 were to serve as controls. As part of the experiment, full-thickness skin homografts from an unrelated adult donor were sutured to the chest wall in each case. (Total thymectomy is occasionally, although not usually, part of the primary cardiovascular surgery involved, and whereas it may not greatly add to the hazards of the necessary operation, its eventual effects in children are not known.) This work was proposed as part of it long-range study of "the growth and development of these children over the years." No difference in the survival of the skin homograft was observed in the 2 groups.

Example 7. This study of cyclopropane anesthesia and cardiac arrhythmias consisted of 31 patients. The average duration of the study was three hours, ranging from two to four and a half hours. "Minor surgical procedures" were carried out in all but one subject. Moderate to deep anesthesia, with endotracheal intubation and controlled respiration, was used. Carbon dioxide was injected into the closed respiratory system until cardiac arrhythmias appeared. Toxic levels of carbon dioxide were achieved and maintained for considerable periods. During the cyclopropane anesthesia a variety of pathologic cardiac arrhythmias occurred. When the carbon dioxide tension was elevated above normal, ventricular extrasystoles were more numerous than when the carbon dioxide tension was normal, ventricular arrhythmias being continuous in one subject for ninety minutes. (This can lead to fatal fibrillation.)

Example 8. Since the minimum blood-flow requirements of the cerebral circulation are not accurately known, this study was carried out to determine "cerebral hemodynamic and metabolic changes . . . before and during acute reductions in arterial pressure induced by drug administration and/or postural adjustments." Forty-four patients whose ages varied from the second to the tenth decade were involved. They included normotensive subjects, those with essential hypertension, and finally a group with malignant hypertension. Fifteen had abnormal electrocardiograms. Few details about the reasons for hospitalization are given.

Signs of cerebral circulatory insufficiency, which were easily recognized, included confusion and in some cases a nonresponsive state. By alteration in the tilt of the patient "the clinical state of the subject could be changed in a matter of seconds from one of alertness to confusion and for the remainder of the flow, the subject was maintained in the latter state." The femoral arteries were cannulated in all subjects, and the internal jugular veins in 14.

The mean arterial pressure fell in 37 subjects from 109 to 48 mm of mercury, with signs of cerebral ischemia. "With the onset of collapse, cardiac output and right ventricular pressures decreased sharply.

Since signs of cerebral insufficiency developed without evidence of coronary insufficiency the authors concluded that "the brain may be more sensitive to acute hypotension than is the heart."

Example 9. This is a study of the adverse circulatory responses elicited by intraabdominal maneuvers:

> When the peritoneal cavity was entered, a deliberate series of maneuvers was carried out [in 68 patients] to ascertain the effective stimuli and the areas responsible for development of the expected circulatory changes. Accordingly, the surgeon rubbed localized areas of the parietal and visceral peritoneum with a small ball sponge as discretely as possible. Traction on the mesenteries, pressure in the area of the celiac plexus, traction on the gall bladder and stomach, and occlusion of the portal and caval veins were the other stimuli applied.

Thirty-four of the patients were sixty years of age or older; 11 were seventy or older. In 44 patients the hypotension produced by the deliberate stimulation was "moderate to marked." The maximum fall produced by manipulation was from 200/105 to 42/20; the average fall in mean pressure in 26 patients was 53 mm of mercury.

Of the 50 patients studied, 17 showed either atrioventricular dissociation with nodal rhythm or nodal rhythm alone. A decrease in the amplitude of the T wave and elevation or depression of the ST segment were noted in 25 cases in association with manipulation and hypotension or, at other times, in the course of anesthesia and operation. In only one case was the change pronounced enough to suggest myocardial ischemia. No case of myocardial infarction was noted in the group studied although routine electrocardiograms were not taken after operation to detect silent infarcts. Two cases in which electrocardiograms were taken after operation showed T-wave and ST-segment changes that had not been present before.

These authors refer to a similar study in which more alarming electrocardiographic changes were observed. Four patients in the series sustained silent myocardial infarctions; most of their patients were undergoing gall bladder surgery because of associated heart disease. It can be added further that in the 34 patients referred to above as being sixty years of age or older, some doubtless had heart disease that could have made risky the maneuvers carried out. In any event, this possibility might have been a deterrent.

Example 10. Starling's law—"that the heart output per beat is directly proportional to the diastolic filling"—was studied in 30 adult patients with atrial fibrillation and mitral stenosis sufficiently severe to require valvulotomy. "Continuous alterations of the length of a segment of left ventricular muscle were recorded simultaneously in 13 of these patients by means of a mercury-filled resistance gauge sutured to the surface of the left ventricle." Pressures in the left ventricle were determined by direct puncture simultaneously with the segment length in 13 patients and without the segment length in all additional 13 patients. Four similar unanesthetized patients were studied through catheterization of the left side of the heart transeptally. In all 30 patients arterial pressure was measured through the catheterized brachial artery.

Example 11. To study the sequence of ventricular contraction in human bundle-branch block, simultaneous catheterization of both ventricles was performed in 22 subjects; catheterization of the right side of the heart was carried out in the usual manner; the left side was catheterized transbronchially. Extrasystoles were produced by tapping on the epicardium in subjects with normal myocardium while they were undergoing thoracotomy. Simultaneous pressures were measured in both ventricles through needle puncture in this group.

The purpose of this study was to gain increased insight into the physiology involved.

Example 12. This investigation was carried out to examine the possible effect of vagal stimulation on cardiac arrest. The authors had in recent years transected the homolateral vagus nerve immediately below the origin of the recurrent laryngeal nerve as palliation against cough and pain in bronchogenic carcinoma. Having been impressed with the number of reports of cardiac arrest that seemed to follow vagal stimulation, they tested the effects of intrathoracic vagal stimulation during 30 of their surgical procedures, concluding, from these observations in patients under satisfactory anesthesia, that cardiac irregularities and cardiac arrest due to vagovagal reflex were less common than had previously been supposed.

Example 13. This study presented a technique for determining portal circulation time and hepatic blood flow. It involved the transcutaneous injection of the spleen and catheterization of the hepatic vein. This was carried out in 43 subjects, of whom 14 were normal; 16 had cirrhosis (varying degrees), 9 acute hepatitis, and 4 hemolytic anemia.

No mention is made of what information was divulged to the subjects, some of whom were seriously ill. This study consisted in the development of a technique, not of therapy, in the 14 normal subjects.

Studies to Improve the Understanding of Disease

Example 14. In this study of the syndrome of impending hepatic coma in patients with cirrhosis of the liver certain nitrogenous substances were administered to 9 patients with chronic alcoholism and advanced cirrhosis: ammonium chloride, diammonium citrate, urea, or dietary protein. In all patients a reaction that included mental disturbances, a "flapping tremor," and electroencephalographic changes developed. Similar signs had occurred in only one of the patients before these substances were administered:

> The first sign noted was usually clouding of the consciousness. Three patients had a second or a third course of administration of a nitrogenous substance with the same results. It was concluded that marked resemblance between this reaction and impending hepatic coma, implied that the administration of these [nitrogenous] substances to patients with cirrhosis may be hazardous.

Example 15. The relation of the effects of ingested ammonia to liver disease was investigated in 11 normal subjects, 6 with acute virus hepatitis, 26 with cirrhosis, and 8 miscellaneous patients. Ten of these patients had neurologic changes associated with either hepatitis or cirrhosis.

The hepatic and renal veins were cannulated. Ammonium chloride was administered by mouth. After this, a tremor that lasted for three days developed in one patient. When ammonium chloride was ingested by 4 cirrhotic patients with tremor and mental confusion the symptoms were exaggerated during the test. The same thing was true of a fifth patient in another group.

Example 16. This study was directed toward determining the period of infectivity of infectious hepatitis. Artificial induction of hepatitis was carried out in an institution for mentally defective children in which a mild form of hepatitis was endemic. The parents gave consent for the intramuscular injection or oral administration of the virus, but nothing is said regarding what was told them concerning the appreciable hazards involved.

A resolution adopted by the World Medical Association states explicitly: "Under no circumstances is a doctor permitted to do anything which would weaken the physical or mental resistance of a human being except from strictly therapeutic or prophylactic indications imposed in the interest of the patient." There is no right to risk an injury to one person for the benefit of others.

Example 17. Live cancer cells were injected into 22 human subjects its part of a study of immunity to cancer. According to a recent review, the subjects (hospitalized patients) were "merely told they would be receiving 'some cells'"—"the word cancer was entirely omitted. . . . "

Example 18. Melanoma was transplanted from a daughter to her volunteering and informed mother, "in the hope of gaining a little better understanding of cancer immunity and in the hope that the production of tumor antibodies might be helpful in the treatment of the cancer patient." Since the daughter died on the day after the transplantation of the tumor into her mother, the hope expressed seems to have been more theoretical than practical, and the daughter's condition was described as "terminal" at the time the mother volunteered to be a recipient. The primary implant was widely excised on the twenty-fourth day after it had been placed in the mother. She died from metastatic melanoma on the four hundred fifty-first day after transplantation. The evidence that this patient died of diffuse melanoma that metastasized from a small piece of transplanted tumor was considered conclusive.

Technical Study of Disease

Example 19. During bronchoscopy a special needle was inserted through a bronchus into the left atrium of the heart. This was done in an unspecified number of subjects, both with cardiac disease and with normal hearts.

The technique was a new approach whose hazards were at the beginning quite unknown. The subjects with normal hearts were used not for their possible benefit, but for that of patients in general.

Example 20. The percutaneous method of catheterization of the left side of the heart has, it is reported, led to 8 deaths (1.09 percent death rate) and other serious accidents in 732 cases. There was, therefore, need for another method, the transbronchial approach, which was carried out in the present study in more than 500 cases, with no deaths.

Granted that a delicate problem arises regarding how much should be discussed with the patients involved in the use of a new method, nevertheless where the method is employed in a given patient for his benefit, the ethical problems are far less than when this potentially extremely dangerous method is used "in 15 patients with normal hearts, undergoing bronechoscopy for other reasons." Nothing was said about what was told any of the subjects, and nothing was said about the granting of permission, which was certainly indicated in the 15 normal subjects used.

Example 21. This was a study of the effect of exercise on cardiac output and pulmonary-artery pressure in 8 "normal" persons (that is, patients whose diseases were not related to the cardiovascular system), in 8 with congestive heart failure severe enough to have recently required complete bed rest, in 6 with hypertension, in 2 with aortic insufficiency, in 7 with mitral stenosis, and in 5 with pulmonary emphysema.

Intracardiac catheterization was carried out, and the catheter then inserted into the right or left main branch of the pulmonary artery. The brachial artery was usually catheterized; sometimes, the radial or femoral arteries were catheterized. The subjects exercised in a supine position by pushing their feet against weighted pedals. "The ability of these patients to carry on sustained work was severely limited by weakness and dyspnea." Several were in severe failure. This was not a therapeutic attempt but rather a physiologic study.

Bizarre Study

Example 22. There is a question whether ureteral reflux can occur in the normal bladder. With this in mind, vesicourethrography was carried out on 26 normal babies less than forty-eight hours old. The infants were exposed to X-rays while the bladder was filling and during voiding. Multiple spot films were made to record the presence or absence of ureteral reflux. None was found in this group, and fortunately no infection followed the catheterization. What the results of the extensive X-ray exposure may be, no one can yet say.

COMMENT ON DEATH RATES

In the foregoing examples a number of procedures, some with their own demonstrated death rates, were carried out. The following data were provided by three distinguished investigators in the field and represent widely held views.

Cardiac catheterization. Right side of the heart, about 1 death per 1000 cases; left side, 5 deaths per 1000 cases. "Probably considerably higher in some places, depending on the portal of entry." (One investigator had 15 deaths in his first 150 cases.) It is possible that catheterization of a hepatic vein or the renal vein would have a lower death rate than that of catheterization of the right side of the heart, for if it is properly carried out, only the atrium is entered en route to the liver or the kidney, not the right ventricle, which can lead to serious cardiac irregularities. There is always the possibility, however, that the ventricle will be entered inadvertently. This occurs in at least half the cases, according to one expert—"but if properly done is too transient to be of importance."

Liver biopsy. the death rate here is estimated at 2 to 3 per 1000, depending in considerable part on the condition of the subject.

Anesthesia. The anesthesia death rate can be placed in general at about 1 death per 2000 cases. The hazard is doubtless higher when certain practices such as deliberate evocation of ventricular extrasystoles under cyclopropane are involved.

PUBLICATION

In the view of the British Medical Research Council[5] it is not enough to ensure that all investigation is carried out in an ethical manner: It must be made unmistakably clear in the publications that the proprieties have been observed. This implies editorial responsibility in addition to the investigator's. The question rises, then, about valuable data that have been improperly obtained.* It is my view that such material should not be published.[5] There is a practical aspect to the matter: Failure to obtain publication would discourage unethical experimentation. How many would carry out such experimentation if they *knew* its results would never be published? Even though suppression of such data (by not publishing it) would constitute a loss to medicine, in a specific localized sense, this loss, it seems, would be less important than the far-reaching moral loss to medicine if the data thus obtained were to be published. Admittedly, there is room for debate. Others believe that such data, because of their intrinsic value, obtained at a cost of great risk or damage to the subjects, should not be wasted but should be published with stern editorial comment. This would have to be done with exceptional skill, to avoid an odor of hypocrisy.

SUMMARY AND CONCLUSIONS

The ethical approach to experimentation in man has several components; two are more important than the others, the first being informed consent. The difficulty of obtaining this is discussed in detail. But it is absolutely essential to *strive* for it for moral, sociologic, and legal reasons. The statement that consent has been obtained has little meaning unless the subject or his guardian is capable of understanding what is to be undertaken and unless all hazards are made clear. If these are not known this, too, should be stated. In such a situation the subject at least knows that he is to be a participant in an experiment. Secondly, there is the more reliable safeguard provided by the presence of an intelligent, informed, conscientious, compassionate, responsible investigator.

Ordinary patients will not knowingly risk their health or their life for the sake of "science." Every experienced clinician investigator knows this. When such risks are taken and a considerable number of patients are involved, it may be assumed that informed consent has not been obtained in all cases.

The gain anticipated from an experiment must be commensurate with the risk involved.

An experiment is ethical or not at its inception; it does not become ethical *post hoc*—ends do not justify means. There is no ethical distinction between ends and means.

---

*As far as principle goes, a parallel can be seen in the recent *Mapp* decision by the United States States Supreme Court. It was stated there that evidence unconstitutionally obtained cannot be used in any judicial decision, no matter how important the evidence is to the ends of justice.

In the publication of experimental results it must be made unmistakably clear that the proprieties have been observed. It is debatable whether data obtained unethically should be published even with stern editorial comment.

REFERENCES

1. Pope Pius XII. Address. Presented at First International Congress on Histopathology of Nervous System. Rome, Italy, September 14, 1952.

2. Platt R, 1st bart. *Doctor and Patient: Ethics, Morals, Government.* London: Nuffield Provincial Hospitals Trust; 1963:62–63.

3. Pappworth MH. Personal communication.

4. Beecher HK. Consent in clinical experimentation: myth and reality. *JAMA.* 1966;195:34.

5. Great Britain Medical Research Council. Memorandum, 1953.

Part 16

ISSUES IN PROFESSIONALISM

❦

While in a restaurant, repair shop, or airport, it is not uncommon for a customer to complain, for a variety of reasons, that an employee acted "unprofessionally." At the same time, we have all said to ourselves, for a variety of reasons, that someone acted "like a professional." When we use these labels we are expressing how a particular individual compares with what we conceive to be the ideal plumber, mechanic, insurance agent, and so forth. Although we may get angry when we are treated unprofessionally, we certainly do not expect the plumber's association to place an unprofessional plumber on probation or require him to take a class on professionalism (or ethics!). Yet when patients use these labels to describe a physician, nurse, psychologist, or paramedic, this is exactly what they expect to happen. As a society we expect health-care providers who commit unprofessional acts to be held strictly accountable for their conduct. Such accountability can be cashed out in terms of a fine, a requirement to undergo therapy, a remedial education requirement, probation, suspension, or even the permanent loss of a health-care provider's right to practice.

The goal of this section is twofold: first, to provide a foundation for appreciating the distinction between acting like a professional and being a professional; and second, to explicate the special boundaries and duties that are fundamental to the health-care professions. This section will be particularly helpful for physicians who serve on peer review committees and state medical boards, as well as ethics committees that develop policies on professionalism.

To be a professional, at the most rudimentary level, is to posses a body of esoteric knowledge that is applied within a fiduciary relationship. As an esoteric knowledge base, only those within the profession are able to determine what it takes to obtain that knowledge (e.g., premed requirements, medical school curriculum, etc.), as well as what constitutes the appropriate application of that knowledge (e.g., standards of care, treatment protocols, etc.). Professionals are also self-regulatory as they alone have the right to decide who shall be admitted to the profession and who shall be expelled. A code of ethics is another fundamental requirement of a profession. Such codes are not ideals, as is the case for many trades; they are standards by which members of the profession will be judged and held accountable by their peers and the courts.

In this section's first reading, "Professional Boundaries in the Physician-Patient Relationship," Glen Gabbard and Carol Nadelson address the kinds of interpersonal boundaries that are necessary for a therapeutic relationship to exist. The primary focus of their discussion concerns the most common boundary violation: sexual contact. Importantly, they also address other forms of boundary violations that tend to be less media-worthy, such as gift giving, inappropriate language, special attention, self-disclosure, nonsexual physical contact, and dual relationships. The latter can come about when health-care providers and patients become social friends, business partners, or even mutual confidantes. "Love, Boundaries and the Patient-Physician Relationship," by Neil Farber, Dennis Novack, and Mary O'Brien, deals with similar issues but pays particular attention to the issues that are raised when it is the patient who violates a boundary. Although both readings were explicitly written about the physician-patient relationship, the issues they raise and the strategies they develop for preventing such violations are certainly relevant to the rest of the health-care professions.

In this section's last reading, titled "Am I My Brother's Warden?" E. Haavi Morreim looks at the moral, practical, and political difficulties that permeate the medical professions' attempts to police their own. As with the first two readings, the issues raised and recommendations given are relevant to all health-care providers. Morreim begins by setting out a detailed grounding from which the duty to police one's colleagues arises. The remainder of her article deals with how physicians ought to assess their colleagues' performance and moral conduct, and how they ought to respond when their assessment reveals a colleague who is either incompetent or unethical.

39

PROFESSIONAL BOUNDARIES IN THE PHYSICIAN-PATIENT RELATIONSHIP

Glen O. Gabbard, M.D., and Carol Nadelson, M.D.

T he subject of professional boundaries (and boundary violations) has received a great deal of recent attention in the psychiatric literature.[1-5] The emphasis on defining guidelines for professional conduct has expanded beyond the confines of ethics committees and has worked its way into licensing boards charged with disciplining physicians whose behavior jeopardizes the well-being of patients. The Massachusetts Board of Registration in Medicine,[6] for example, has recently issued detailed guidelines on such matters as self-disclosure, dual relationships, sexual relationships with patients, and other professional boundaries to help define for the public and for the profession the parameters of professional conduct in the practice of psychotherapy by physicians. While specialists in psychiatry have been debating the pros and cons of issuing such guidelines, nonpsychiatric physicians have yet to involve themselves so extensively in similar discussions. In this article, we will provide a conceptual framework for discussion of professional boundaries in the physician-patient relationship and offer our view of measures the profession can take to prevent serious violations of these boundaries. We will use instances from our own clinical experiences or those of our trainees to illustrate the relevant issues.

Gabbard GO, Nadelson C. "Professional Boundaries in the Physician-Patient Relationship." *Journal of the American Medical Association.* 1995;273(18):1445–1449.©American Medical Association. Reprinted by permission.

WHAT ARE BOUNDARIES?

Professional boundaries in medical practice are not well defined. In general, they are the parameters that describe the limits of a fiduciary relationship in which one person (a patient) entrusts his or her welfare to another (a physician), to whom a fee is paid for the provision of a service. Boundaries imply professional distance and respect, which, of course, includes refraining from sexual involvement with patients. While sexual contact is perhaps the most extreme form of boundary violation, many other physician behaviors may exploit the dependency of the patient on the physician and the inherent power differential. These include dual relationships, business transactions, certain gifts and services, some forms of language use, some types of physical contact, time and duration of appointments, location of appointments, mishandling of fees, and misuses of the physical examination. The transgressions of some of these boundaries may at times be necessary and helpful. For example, it would certainly be appropriate to hold the hand of a patient who reaches out to a physician after losing a family member. One can differentiate minor boundary crossings from devastating boundary violations that ruin professional careers and seriously damage patients.[3] Similarly, some problems arise from corrupt and unethical physician behavior, while others arise from honest misunderstandings.

Much of the medical profession's increased interest in boundaries has derived from the awareness of the damaging effects of sexual misconduct. Examination of instances of physician-patient sexual relationships has revealed that sexual exploitation is usually preceded by a progressive series of nonsexual boundary violations, a phenomenon generally described as the "slippery slope."[2,3,7] In this regard, what appear to be trivial violations may in reality be considerably more serious when viewed in the context of a continuum. Attention to nonsexual boundary issues may therefore be an effective way to prevent sexual boundary transgressions. This approach is especially salient because it has become clear that many of the nonsexual boundary violations may in and of themselves cause harm to patients irrespective of the possibility that they also may lead to sexual involvement.[1,3-5]

As a result of the intense concern that has been generated by sexual exploitation in the physician-patient relationship, much more research has accumulated on sexual boundary violations than on nonsexual boundary violations. Hence, our discussion of professional boundaries will begin with a consideration of sexual misconduct and progress from there to an examination of other forms of professional boundary transgressions.

Sexual Boundary Violations

Six studies[8-13] have sought to determine the prevalence of sexual misconduct in the physician-patient relationship (see Table).

A comparison of the U.S. studies with the survey from the Netherlands and with the studies from Canada suggest that the problem is one that is not unique to

Self-Report Surveys of Sexual Contacts between Physicians and Patients

Source, y	Sample Size	Specialties	Return Rate, %	Men Acknowledging Contact, %	Women Acknowledging Contact, %
Kardener et al.,[8] 1973	1000 male physicians	Gynecology. psychiatry, internal medicine, surgery, general practice	46	12	Not applicable
Gartrell et al.,[9] 1986	5574	Psychiatry	26	7.1	3.1
Gartrell et al.,[10] 1992	10000	Family practice, internal medicine, gynecology, surgery	19	10	4
College of Physicians and Surgeons of British Columbia,[11] 1992	2082	All specialties	69.5	3.8 (8.1*)	0.3(4.3*)
Wilbers et al.,[12] 1992	975	Gynecology, ENT	74	4	4†
Lamont and Woodward,[13] 1994	792	Gynecology	78	3	1

*Percentage of sexual contacts with former patients.
†This figure is for gynecologists. Only five female ear, nose, and throat (ENT) specialists were in the study.

U.S. physicians and that it occurs with roughly the same frequency in the United States as in other countries where sexual misconduct has been studied. The problem is not unique to medicine. Other professions are also vulnerable, including other health care professionals, the clergy, and the law. Research aimed at psychologists, social workers, and teachers reveals that sexual exploitation is a pervasive problem in fiduciary relationships. [2,14-16]

The studies listed in the table must be viewed as less than definitive because of the fundamental methodological problems inherent in questionnaire surveys. These include low return rates, raising the possibility that the sample is by no means representative. Other problems include the possibility that some practitioners might not answer the questions honestly because they question the anonymity of the method. Also, some who have engaged in sexual misconduct may not return the questionnaire. On the other hand, other professionals who have transgressed sexual boundaries might feel the need to anonymously confess. In essence, we do not know the true prevalence of sexual misconduct.

While the data suggest that sex between a male physician and a female patient is the most common, all gender configurations also are seen with some regularity. In a series of more than two thousand cases of therapist-patient sex, Schoener et al.[17] noted that approximately 20 percent of cases involved a same-sex dyad, and 20 percent of the therapists were women (some overlap was present in these two groups).

Concern about sexual exploitation by physicians in Canada has resulted in major task force reports in British Columbia,[11] Alberta,[18] and Ontario.[19] In the United States, the American Medical Association (AMA) Council on Ethical and Judicial Affairs considered the problem extensively and issued a 1991 statement: "Sexual contact or romantic relationships concurrent with the physician-patient relationship may be unethical."[20(p2741)]

The ethics standard proposed by the council subsumes a wide range of situations encountered in medical practice. These would include, but would not be limited to, the following categories:

(1) Predatory physicians with serious personality disorders who systematically attempt to seduce patients.

(2) Those who claim to use sex for therapeutic purposes.

(3) Cases involving abuse of the physical examination procedure (e.g., a physician who does a breast or pelvic examination when not indicated, or a physician who does an appropriate examination in an inappropriate, erotized manner).

(4) Situations in which a physician asks a patient on a date during the initial visit to his or her office or to an emergency department.

(5) Cases in which a long-standing physician-patient relationship evolves into an intense lovesickness or infatuation.

(6) Situations in which a rural general practitioner who is the only physician in town dates a patient because virtually anyone who is a potential romantic partner is also a patient.

(7) Cases in which patients are raped or fondled (while awake or under anesthesia) in the operating room or office.

(8) Cases related to sexual harassment in which the physician makes erotic or suggestive comments to the patient.

The Medical Council of New Zealand[21] has recognized the spectrum of sexual misconduct by dividing the behaviors into three categories: (1) sexual impropriety, (2) sexual transgression, and (3) sexual violation.

Sexual impropriety refers to expressions or gestures that are disrespectful to the patient's privacy and sexually demeaning to the patient. This category would include such behaviors as inappropriate draping practices, sexualized comments made by a physician to a patient, or sexually demeaning remarks about a patient's body or undergarments.

Sexual impropriety as defined by the Medical Council of New Zealand would also include instances of sexual harassment. According to the U.S. Equal Employment Opportunity Commission,[22] any unwanted and repeated verbal or physical advances, derogatory statements or sexually explicit remarks, or sexually discriminatory comments made by someone in the workplace is sexual harassment if the recipient is offended or humiliated and job performance suffers as a result. Although these guidelines do not apply legally outside the employment context, the situation of the physician-patient relationship involves a person in a less powerful position at risk for being subjected to harassing behavior by someone who is more powerful, the classic paradigm of sexual harassment. It is important to note that there are gender differences in the perception of sexual harassment.[23] While many male physicians may view sexual comments as humorous, a female patient or health professional observing such remarks is not as likely to view them in the same way.

The second category in the New Zealand set of definitions, sexual transgression, refers to inappropriate and sexualized touching of a patient that stops short of overt sexual relations. This category would include such items as sexualized kissing, touching of breasts or genitals when not appropriate for the physical examination, or performing a pelvic examination without gloves.

The third category, sexual violation, involves physician-patient sexual relations, regardless of who initiated the relationship, and would include genital intercourse, oral sexual relations, anal intercourse, and mutual masturbation.

Regarding sexual relationships between former patients and physicians, the AMA Council on Ethical and Judicial Affairs[20] is less absolute, implying that individualized case review is necessary to ascertain whether exploitation of a still emotionally dependent patient is involved. A one-time contact with a specialist or an emergency department physician may be quite different from an ongoing physician-patient relationship of many years' duration. However, a focus on the length of the relationship alone misses other dimensions of equal importance. For example, a patient may only see a surgeon for one procedure, but if that procedure is life saving, the patient may retain a persistently idealized and dependent attitude toward that surgeon, which would compromise the capacity for mutual consent. Likewise, an obstetrician may have a single contact with a patient during a difficult delivery and capture the patient's fantasy as a hero or rescuer.

These considerations lead us directly into an examination of why physician-patient sex is considered unethical. Several reasons have emerged from case law, from the deliberations of ethics committees and licensing boards, and from clinical work with patients who have been exploited by their physicians. First, it is a breach of the trust that is fundamental in a fiduciary relationship. Second, it calls into question the physician's capacity for objective professional judgment. A third reason derives from the psychological state of the patient induced by the clinical situation. Patients rapidly develop feelings toward their physicians that have been called "transference." This involves the displacement of feelings derived from past relationships onto the current physician-patient relationship. The physician can thus be viewed as an all-knowing parent, and a great deal of power is turned over to the physician by the patient.

Brody[24] has pointed out that the physician may have greater power because of greater knowledge and skills regarding diagnosis and treatment, because of higher socioeconomic and educational status, and because of an inherent social or charismatic power. The patient, on the other hand, "gains power only by virtue of being surrounded by boundaries that the physician cannot cross without egregiously violating moral rules."[24 (p62)]

The combination of transference and the power imbalance between the physician and the patient makes mutual consent, in the usual sense, highly questionable. As Johnson[25(p1559)] has stressed, those who argue that mutual consent is possible between physician and patient stand "in sharp contrast to the implied presumption of disproportionate professional control underlying the AMA's opinion on sexual misconduct." Finally, studies find that there is the potential for considerable harm to the patient as a result of such sexual relationships.[26-28]

Dual Relationships

An essential element of the physician's role is the notion that what is best for. the patient must be the physician's first priority. Physicians must set aside their own needs in the service of addressing the patient's needs. Other kinds of relationships that coexist simultaneously with the physician-patient relationship have the potential to contaminate the physician's ability to focus exclusively on the patient's well-being and can impair the physician's judgment. As noted herein, patients can transfer residual longings from other relationships onto the person of the physician; and they can view the physician as parent, spouse, lover, adversary, or friend. If the physician tries to maintain both roles with the patient, objective decision making may be jeopardized. For example, financial relationships or business transactions may lead to resentment or dependency that interferes with the physician's ability to be empathic, sensitive, and selfless in the physician-patient relationship. Similarly, romantic ties or intimate friendships with patients may make it difficult for the physician to confront noncompliance with treatment or to bring up unpleasant medical information. The long-standing practice of referring family members to another physician grows out of similar considerations regarding compliance and compromised objectivity.[29] Even in the case of a rural family practitioner who treats everyone in the community, a romantic relationship that begins to develop with a patient should result in referring the patient, if possible, to another physician in a neighboring town for care.

Gifts and Services

Grateful patients often wish to show their appreciation by bringing gifts to their physician. In other instances, a patient may offer to perform services for the physician in lieu of payment or in addition to payment. A range of services, such as filing, typing, babysitting, and cleaning, have been offered and accepted by physicians. In some places, barter is a common form of payment when patients without insurance coverage or financial means wish to pay the physician in goods or services. An example is a farmer who gives a chicken to the physician for delivering a baby.

Different forms of barter involve different boundary issues. While the provision of poultry may not violate any significant boundaries, services that involve contact with confidential records or with the physician's family may present problems. For example, if a physician's baby is injured while a patient is baby-sitting, the physician-patient relationship maybe permanently damaged. If a patient paints the physician's house, but the physician is dissatisfied with the quality of the work, the ensuing tension may also adversely affect the alliance between physician and patient.

While small gifts may represent benign boundary crossings rather than serious violations, services and more significant and expensive gifts may be problematic from two standpoints. First, gift giving may be a conscious or unconscious bribe designed to keep aggression, negative feelings, or unpleasant subjects out of the physician-patient relationship. Second, there is often a secret quid pro quo involved in performing services or bestowing a gift. As implied by the saying, "There is no free lunch," expectations arise from gifts. The same can apply to the physician who gives patients gifts or refrains from charging a fee for a particular patient. Although done with the best of intentions, the patient may feel burdened by a sense of obligation that can never be openly discussed with the physician. Similarly, physicians who receive expensive gifts may feel an obligation that influences their clinical judgment in much the same way the gifts from drug companies may.[30]

Time and Duration of Appointments

Maintaining an orderly schedule of patient appointments is an aspect of professional conduct that is often neglected. While all physicians must cancel or delay appointments periodically because of an emergency or other extenuating circumstances, some practitioners keep patients waiting while extending their time with others, perhaps those they find fascinating, charming, or attractive. The special patient may be flattered by the extra time but also may wonder which of the physician's own needs are being gratified by extending the appointment. Those patients who are kept waiting may feel their physician has utter disregard for their needs and concerns, as well as their schedules.

Related problems may occur around the time of day at which appointments are scheduled. A female patient scheduled to see her male internist at 9 P.M., after the office staff have gone home, may wonder why she is being seen so late without anyone else around. She may feel sufficiently uncomfortable that she will not return to see that particular physician. It is noteworthy, in this regard, that attorneys have discovered that some cases of sexual misconduct occur with patients who are scheduled during the last appointment of the day when no one else is around. As a result, they view such scheduling as reflective of the possibility of other boundary violations.[3] In general, unless an emergency occurs, physicians are wise to see patients only during office hours with someone else in the office.

Language

An essential component of professional conduct is respect for the patient's dignity. Within this framework, the physician's language is a boundary that should not be overlooked. In general, patients feel some loss of dignity merely by being in the patient role, by having to disrobe and wear a gown, and by depending on the physician's knowledge to explain what is going on with them. Addressing patients by pet names or by first name when they are not well known to the physician may be experienced as a further loss of dignity.[31] Similarly, avoiding slang names that may be offensive also maintains a sense of professionalism and respect in the relationship.

One variant of this boundary is the use of language in a seductive or erotic way designed to make the patient uncomfortable or to sexually excite the patient. One male pediatrician told a sixteen-year-old female patient, "You're developing a very nice set of breasts!" The patient felt embarrassed and humiliated, and she reported the comment to her mother. When the mother called the pediatrician to complain, he defended himself by insisting that he was complimenting her. This vignette is typical of some sexual harassment scenarios mentioned previously in which a man in a position of power may think he is being humorous or flattering, while the woman on the receiving end of the comment may feel intensely uncomfortable.

Self-Disclosure

While physicians commonly chat with their patients about matters of mutual interest in an effort to build rapport and put the patient at ease, excessive self disclosure may create difficulties for the patient and strain the rapport. A common starting point on the slippery slope to sexual involvement with a patient is a role reversal in which the physician starts disclosing personal problems to the patient. Even if revealing personal issues to a patient does not lead progressively to more extreme boundary violations, self-disclosure is itself a boundary problem because it is a misuse of the patient to satisfy one's own needs for comfort or sympathy. It is also inappropriate to try to extract care for oneself when a patient is paying for the physician's time. Moreover, the patient may find sharing health concerns extremely difficult if the physician is perceived as needy and vulnerable.

The Physical Examination

Patients are often anxious and uncomfortable during a physical examination but willingly go along with whatever the physician asks them to do. One female patient seeing her physician for a sore throat submitted to a breast examination even though she couldn't see the purpose of it. She later said that at the time of the examination she felt as though she were being raped but felt paralyzed to stop the examination. Another female patient described how her gynecologist asked her about her sexual history during a pelvic examination. She experienced the questioning as an indication that her physician was "nosy and intrusive."

At the very least, the physician should explain to the patient why examining the genitals, breasts, or other sensitive areas is necessary. If the patient hesitates, the physician should encourage questions or expressions of concern that can then be clarified, empathized with, and understood. Body areas that are draped should remain draped whenever possible. The relevance of sexual history questions also should be made clear to the patient.

What about situations in which the physician encounters sexual arousal on the patient's part while conducting a physical? One female medical student was examining an elderly male patient when she noticed that his penis was erect. She completed the examination without remarking on the erection but later consulted her clinical tutor about the situation. Her tutor explained to her that she had done precisely the right thing. The medical student commented that nothing on this subject had been taught in the classroom and that if she had not had a mentor with whom to consult, she would have continued to feel insecure about the appropriate response.

The presence of a chaperone during the physical examination may also be reassuring to the patient. However, guidelines on when to use a chaperone are not well established. While traditionally within medicine a female chaperone is present when a male physician is examining a female patient, this advice is too general and does not allow for problems that arise in other gender constellations. The use of chaperones is always a matter of good clinical judgment, but we would strongly recommend having a chaperone present in the following situations: (1) with a patient who has a known history of sexual abuse; (2) with a patient who has extreme anxiety or a psychiatric disorder; (3) with a litigious patient; (4) with a patient undergoing a pelvic examination; and (5) with a patient who for any reason raises concerns in the physician.

Some of these recommendations may be modified for long-standing patients when a good physician-patient alliance exists. A nurse who is in and out of the room during the course of the examination may be sufficient.

Physical Contact

Physical contact outside the context of the physical examination varies widely. Some physicians routinely shake the hands of their patients on greeting them, a practice that is well within the scope of professional conduct. Others hold the hand of a patient when delivering stressful news. When hugs and kisses enter into the picture, the situation becomes murkier. Some patients experience a hug or a kiss as a promise of a different kind of relationship. Maybe the physician will be a parent or lover who will make up for disappointments with others in those roles from the past. In these cases, the physician has raised false hopes in the patient, who will ultimately be disillusioned.

Other patients, particularly those with histories of sexual abuse, may experience a hug or a kiss as an assault, a repeat of early boundary violations that have left scars on the patient's psyche. One physician was charged with sexual misconduct by a patient who insisted that he had had "genital contact" with her. The physician adamantly denied it. When further inquiry was made, it became clear that during a hug the patient had experienced the pressure of the physician's genitals on her pelvis as "genital contact," reawakening old trauma.

There are, of course, cultural variations on the appropriateness of hugs or kisses. However, cultural differences can be used to rationalize behavior that patients perceive as offensive. Licensing boards frequently encounter physicians who claim that they are unfamiliar with American customs regarding touch. They may claim that within their culture, the kind of contact they had with the patient is entirely acceptable. A critical issue in these situations, of course, is that the patient may not be from the same culture and may feel extremely uncomfortable with the kind of contact initiated by the physician.

Beyond hugs or kisses, other forms of physical contacts may be viewed as a violation of the professional relationship. One woman reported that her gynecologist sensually rubbed her back while discussing the findings of her pelvic examination with her. Regardless of his intent, she perceived him as deriving sexual gratification from his contact with her.

PREVENTION OF BOUNDARY VIOLATIONS

The key to preventing boundary violations lies largely in education, although certain physicians whose character defects lead them to this behavior may not be deterred by such efforts. Medical students and residents should be taught the concept of professional conduct in conjunction with learning interviewing and physical diagnosis. Sensitivity to professional boundaries should be as routine as auscultating the chest. These issues should be discussed not exclusively in the context of ethics courses, but in all clinically oriented courses. They are the fabric of the physician patient relationship.

Information about the widespread prevalence of sexual abuse and its connection with subsequent revictimization also should be taught in medical school as part of this preventive education. It is well known that patients who have been sexually abused are at high risk for being sexually exploited by physicians and psychotherapists.[26,28,32] While we do not intend to blame patients for the boundary transgressions of their physicians, medical students need to be aware of the common dilemmas presented by sexually abused patients, particularly the rescue fantasies they inspire in physicians, who may gradually become overinvolved in an effort to repair the damage from the past.

Another area of education that would be productive in the prevention of boundary violations is sensitivity to gender issues and gender differences. Professional conduct should take into account differences in the gender configuration of the physician-patient dyad and how that influences the perception of the physician and the content of the physician's communication. A corollary to this principle is the need to be empathic and nonjudgmental when taking into account differences related to sexual orientation and sexual preference.[33]

A crucial component of education is sensitivity to the diversity of the population and the associated cultural and individual differences, particularly regarding the meaning of touch and other forms of physical contact. What is therapeutic touch to one patient may be experienced as assaultive by another. Because the physician cannot know how a certain patient is likely to respond to various aspects of touch inherent in the physical examination, clear communication is of paramount importance. Physicians also must develop an empathic attunement to their patients so that they can sense the impact of any aspect of the examination that might be routine from their perspective but has special meaning to the patient. This attention to careful communication about examination procedures has enormous significance in a managed-care era in which patients are routinely seeing new physicians with whom no sense of trust has developed. Similarly, following our previously mentioned guidelines for the presence of a chaperone may also be of particular value for new patients.

Role modeling cannot be overemphasized in medical education. The obverse of professional misconduct is, of course, professional conduct, which encompasses all the features of a humane physician-patient relationship as well as the sum total of professional boundaries. This overarching demeanor can best be learned by watching role models relate to their patients in the course of rounds, examinations, and other clinical settings. Teachers also must make it clear to their trainees that they are available as supervisors or consultants when students find themselves attracted to patients and are confused about how to manage such feelings.

In the midst of our enthusiasm for preventive education, we must also acknowledge that it is not a panacea. Some unscrupulous practitioners with severe personality disorders will be completely untouched by educational efforts. Their predatory behavior with patients is simply an extension of predatory behavior outside their professional lives.[2] The best we can hope for is that such individuals, who constitute a relatively small number of physicians, can be identified early in the medical school process and redirected toward other careers.

REFERENCES

1. Frick DE. Nonsexual boundary violations in psychiatric treatment. In: Oldham JM, Reba MB (eds.). *American Psychiatric Press Review of Psychiatry*. Washington, DC: American Psychiatric Press; 1994; 13:415–432.

2. Gabbard GO. Sexual misconduct. In: Oldham JM, Reba MB (eds.). *American Psychiatric Press Review of Psychiatry*. Washington, DC: American Psychiatric Press; 1994;13:433–456.

3. Gutheil TG, Gabbard GO. The concept of boundaries in clinical practice: theoretical and risk-management dimensions. *American Journal of Psychiatry*. 1993;150:188–196.

4. Epstein RS. *Keeping the Boundaries*. Washington, DC: American Psychiatric Press; 1994.

5. Epstein RS, Simon RL. The exploitation index: an early warning indicator of boundary violations in psychotherapy. *Bulletin of the Menninger Clinic*. 1990;54:450–465.

6. Massachusetts Board of Registration in Medicine. *General Guidelines Related to the Maintenance of Boundaries in the Practice of Psychotherapy by Physicians (Adult Patients)*. Boston, MA: Massachusetts Board of Registration in Medicine; 1994.

7. Strasburger LH, Jorgenson L, Sutherland P. The prevention of psychotherapist sexual misconduct: avoiding the slippery slope. *American Journal of Psychotherapy*. 1992;46:544–555.

8. Kardener SH, Fuller M, Mensh IN. A survey of physicians' attitudes and practices regarding erotic and nonerotic contact with patients. *American Journal of Psychiatry*. 1973;130:1077–1081.

9. Gartrell NK, Herman J, Olarte S, et al. Psychiatrist-patient sexual contact: results of a national survey, I: prevalence. *American Journal of Psychiatry*. 1986;143: 1126–1131.

10. Gartrell NK, Milliken N, Goodson WH, et al. Physician-patient sexual contact: prevalence and problems. *Western Journal of Medicine*. 1992;157:139–143.

11. Committee on Physician Sexual Misconduct. *Crossing the Boundaries: The Report of the Committee on Physician Sexual Misconduct*. Vancouver, BC: Prepared for the College of Physicians and Surgeons of British Columbia; November 1992.

12. Wilbers D, Veensstra G, van d Wiel HBM, et al. Sexual contact in the doctor-patient relationship in the Netherlands. *BMJ*. 1992;304:1531–1534.

13. Lamont JA, Woodward C. Patient-physician sexual involvement: a Canadian survey of obstetrician-gynecologists. *Canadian Medical Association Journal.* 1994;150:1433–1439.

14. Pope KS. Teacher-student sexual intimacy. In: Gabbard GO (ed.). *Sexual Exploitation in Professional Relationships.* Washington, DC: American Psychiatric Press; 1989:163–176.

15. Brodsky AM. Sex between patient and therapist: psychology's data and response. In: Gabbard GO (ed.). *Sexual Exploitation in Professional Relationships.* Washington, DC: American Psychiatric Press; 1989:15–26.

16. Gechtman L. Sexual contact between social workers and their clients. In: Gabbard GO (ed.). *Sexual Exploitation in Professional Relationships.* Washington, DC: American Psychiatric Press; 1989:27–38.

17. Schoener GR, Milgrom JH, Gonsisorek JC, et al. (eds.). *Psychotherapists' Sexual Involvement with Clients: Intervention and Prevention.* Minneapolis, MN: Walk-In Counseling Center; 1989.

18. College of Physicians and Surgeons of Alberta. *Doctor/Patient Sexual Involvement: Policy Paper and Future Initiatives.* Edmonton, AB: College of Physicians and Surgeons of Alberta; November 1992.

19. College of Physicians and Surgeons of Ontario. *The Final Report of the Task Force on Sexual Abuse of Patients.* Toronto, ON: College of Physicians and Surgeons of Ontario; November 25, 1991.

20. Council on Ethical and Judicial Affairs, American Medical Association. Sexual misconduct in the practice of medicine. *JAMA.* 1991;266:2741–2745.

21. Medical Council of New Zealand. Sexual abuse in the doctor-patient relationship: discussion document for the profession. *Newsletter of the Medical Council of New Zealand.* 1992;6:4–5.

22. Equal Employment Opportunities Commission. Guidelines on discrimination because of sex. *Federal Register.* 1980;45:7467–74677.

23. Goleman D. Sexual harassment: about power, not sex. *New York Times.* October 22,1991:B5–B8.

24. Brody H. *The Healer's Power.* New Haven, CT: Yale University Press; 1992.

25. Johnson SH. Judicial review of disciplinary action for sexual misconduct in the practice of medicine. *JAMA.* 1993;270:1596–1600.

26. Feidman-Summers S, Jones G. Psychological impacts of sexual contact between therapists or other health care practitioners and their clients. *Journal of Consulting and Clinical Psychology.* 1984;52:1054–1061.

27. Williams MH. Exploitation and inference: mapping the damage from therapist-patient sexual involvement. *American Psychologist.* 1992;47:412–421.

28. Kluft RP. Incest and subsequent revictimization: the case of therapist-patient sexual exploitation, with a description of the sitting-duck In: Kluft RP (ed.). *Incest-Related Syndromes of Adult Psychopathology.* Washington, DC: American Psychiatric Press; 1990:263–287.

29. La Puma J, Priest ER. Is there a doctor in the house? an analysis of the practice of physicians' treating their own families. *JAMA.* 1992;267:1810–1812.

30. Chren MM, Landefeld CS, Murray TH. Doctors, drug companies, and gifts. *JAMA.* 1989;262:3448–3451.

31. Bradshaw S, Burton P. Naming: a measure of relationship in a ward milieu. *Bulletin of the Menninger Clinic.* 1976;40:665–670.

32. Chu JA. The revictimization of adult women with histories of childhood abuse. *J Psychother Pract Res.* 1992;1:259-269.

33. Robinson TE. Treating female patients. *Canadian Medical Association Journal.* 1994;150:1427–1430.

40

LOVE, BOUNDARIES, AND THE PATIENT-PHYSICIAN RELATIONSHIP

Neil J. Farber, M.D., Dennis H. Novack, M.D.,
and Mary K. O'Brien, Ph.D.

❧

Bonds may form whenever patients and physicians interact. This bond is characterized by a particular form of love akin to the Greek *agape*, or brotherly love.[1] The love that forms is an integral part of the patient-physician relationship. This love is not characterized by romantic feelings, but rather denotes a platonic relationship and one in which intimacy is used to benefit the patient.

While medical education and the profession of medicine have been characterized throughout recent history as aspiring to objective detachment,[2] it is a profession of caring and empathy as well. Physicians are capable of the extremes of detachment or attachment with patients, as witnessed by physician involvement in the atrocities of Nazi Germany[3] or, conversely, some physicians who have sexual relations with patients.[4]

For most physicians, compassionate and empathetic care for their patients is balanced with avoidance of becoming overinvolved.[3] Gabbard and Nadelson[5] have indicated that physicians can do this by maintaining professional distance and respect in the form of boundaries, while still caring for the patient. They also cite accepted ethical guidelines in the patient-physician relationship, e.g., a strict proscription of sexual or romantic contact. Professional boundaries have been described within the context of the psychiatric encounter, in which distance must be maintained because

Farber NJ, Novack DH, O'Brien MK. "Love, Boundaries, and the Patient-Physician Relationship." *Archives of Internal Medicine.* 1997;157:2291–2294. ©American Medical Association. Reprinted by permission.

of the issue of transference and the possibilities of exploitation by psychiatrists of emotionally vulnerable patients.[6] However, there has been little discussion of the nature and origin of role boundaries in the medical literature. This understanding is key for physicians to maintain an empathetic yet objective relationship with their patients. Previous articles[4,5] in the medical literature have dealt with physician boundary transgressions, while patient transgressions and how to effectively deal with them have not been explored.

We describe role boundaries and how they are formed and explore boundary violations by patients. We discuss how these violations can be avoided through a process of physician self-awareness, an examination of family of origin issues, and communication with patients.

PROPOSING A THEORETICAL FRAMEWORK FOR BOUNDARIES IN PATIENT CARE

Boundaries in patient care are mutually understood, unspoken, physical, and emotional limits of the relationship between the trusting patient and the caring physician.[5] Boundaries are important in situations where a power differential may exist,[7] as in the patient-physician relationship. Boundary parameters include the contact time between the two individuals, the amount of information shared by the patient and the physician, the degree of shared decision making, and the shared physical and emotional space. These interpersonal boundaries are distinct from the social roles that the participants play in the interaction,[8] e.g., most notably that of the patient and physician. While social roles define how the physician and patient will individually act within the relationship, the boundaries within the relationship define how the two parties may acceptably interact with one another.

Boundaries define the relationship. For example, the boundaries in psychotherapeutic relationships prevent inappropriate forms of intimacy, such as sexual relations, while enhancing others, like connectedness.[9] Boundaries in the patient-physician relationship prevent exploitation of either of the two parties[10] by allowing the two parties to set appropriate limits during the interaction. Patients are often ill and therefore vulnerable. Trust in their physicians may cause patients to behave in ways that hinder self-protection. Mutually understood boundaries provide protection for the patients in the relationship by allowing certain limits on physical space and contact and emotional involvement. Physicians also may have a number of psychological vulnerabilities.[11] Caring for patients may foster strong emotions in physicians; boundaries protect the physician from overextending in this regard.

FACTORS THAT AFFECT PHYSICIAN AND PATIENT BOUNDARIES

Cultural and sociodemographic aspects of the physician's and patient's family and peers, such as gender, ethnicity, age, and attitudes toward illness and death, play a major role in the formation of boundaries.[4] For example, physicians who have been physically or sexually abused as children by male figures may have a difficult time in dealing with aggressive male patients. Physicians' attitudes toward their role as professionals may affect the setting of boundaries. Some physicians who view their role as an avocation may encourage telephone calls at home; others who view their professional role as a job may refuse these calls.

The physician's practice will also have an effect on the boundaries inherent in the relationship. For example, psychiatrists who have different models of office counseling have different types of boundaries.[12] The activity of the practice and the amount of time a physician has to spend with the patient on any given day will also influence the boundaries in the relationship. In many cases, physicians who have busier practices may be able to spend less time with patients (one of the interpersonal boundaries noted above). In addition, health insurance coverage may impose various parameters on the relationship, such as defining the amount of time spent with the patient in a managed care environment.

Perhaps most important in the formation of boundaries is the underlying social and psychological development of the physician and patient. Family-of-origin issues, such as birth order and family role expectations, may be key in how individuals form relationships.[13] For example, families may emphasize the role of caretaker to the oldest child. These children may then be overinvolved with patients as adult physicians. Several physicians in a number of workshops conducted by two of us (N.J.F. and D.H.N.) have described instances of giving money to patients and helping them shop for food on weekends. Boundaries define distinctions between members of the family, such as the differences in roles, rights, and expectations between one's parents and oneself.[8] These roles can be individual or complementary, such as brother-sister. The boundaries that are an inherent part of a functional family system allow one to differentiate from the other members of the family to develop one's sense of self-identity.[14]

Often in dysfunctional families, boundaries are either too diffuse (porous) or inflexible.[8] In the former case, the family becomes enmeshed so that no one within the family can differentiate as an individual, while in the latter case, individuals within the family are excessively distanced from one another. Unmet and denied needs as a child may lead to overly involved relationships by the physician, while a problem with trust during development may make feelings of dependence from a patient threatening.[15] These unmet needs may cause the development of dysfunctional beliefs on the part of the physician: limitations in knowledge is a personal failing; responsibility is to be borne alone by physicians; altruistic devotion to work and denial of self is desirable (physicians may feel the need to do and be everything for certain patients); and it is "professional" to keep one's uncertainties and emotions to oneself.[16] Instability during childhood may also cause physicians to have some of their dependency needs (e.g., love, caring) met by the patient.[11] Patients with family-of-origin issues of trust and unmet dependency needs may cause the patient to have unrealistic expectations of the physician or the patient may become aggressively independent.

Another major component in the patient-physician relationship as it relates to boundaries is that of the development of trust. Trust evolves out of past experiences and interactions between two parties, and therefore develops to some degree as the patient-physician relationship evolves.[17] Thus, as the patient-physician relationship matures, an increase in trust by both parties occurs and boundaries in the relationship will change. It is the changes in trust that cause flexibility in the boundaries of the interaction, allowing for a greater closeness and sharing between the physician and patient. These changes are often beneficial to both the patient and physician as the closeness can be used therapeutically.[18]

BOUNDARY TRANSGRESSIONS BY PATIENTS

When the limits of the patient-physician relationship are differently understood, unaccepted, or disrespected, transgressions can occur. These transgressions can be on the part of the physician or the patient. We address those transgressions committed by the patient. Recent studies[5,12,19–22] have focused on transgressions by physicians and therefore these are not addressed herein.

Why Do Patient Boundary Transgressions Occur?

In three workshops conducted by two of us (N.J.F. and D.H.N.) at the annual and mid-Atlantic regional meetings of the Society of General Internal Medicine, a total of seventy physicians pointed to a number of concerns about patient transgressions: patients who want more time than the physician has to give; patients who are overly friendly, seductive, or overly curious about the physician's personal life; and patient gift giving. These transgressions are especially prevalent in patients with borderline personality.[23] Many borderline patients are unable to separate their fantasies from the reality around them[22] and, especially when under stress, these patients tend to "fuse" with the physician.[23] Even patients without such severe psychopathological conditions can sometimes lose sight of the well-established boundaries in the patient-physician relationship. This can be especially prevalent at times of stress, when the therapeutic touch can have strong meanings for the patient.[24] Patients who may become needy and unfulfilled may find themselves attempting to validate their worth and gain acceptance through the physician.[25]

Sexual Contact by the Patient

Marjorie Connors, a fifty-two-year-old woman, was seeing one of the residents in clinic, Dr. Steven Todd. Mrs. Connors, a recent widow, wrote the number thirty on a piece of paper and showed it to Dr. Todd. When he asked about it, Mrs. Connors said that if she was thirty again she would like him very much.

Boundary transgressions involving sexual behavior are often initiated by the patient. Schulte and Kay[26] found that 71 percent of female medical students and 29 percent of male medical students indicated that they had experienced at least one instance of patient-initiated sexual behavior during the course of their medical school years. Twelve percent of the female medical students indicated that there was sexual touching or grabbing by the patient. Almost one-third of practicing psychiatrists who had some sexual contact with their patients indicated that the patient initiated the occurrence.[21] However, as in the above situation, occurrences that are not clearly sexual will need to be interpreted individually by the physician in the context of the relationship with the patient.

Gift Giving

A frequent transgression by patients is gift giving. Small gifts given in gratitude may sometimes be welcomed and not viewed as a boundary violation.[5] However, repeated attempts at gift giving or gifts accompanied by compliments and other evidence of seductive behavior may represent an attempt by the patient to consciously or unconsciously control the patient-physician interaction.[27] Larger or more expensive gifts are clear and serious boundary transgressions,[5] unless they are given as a charitable donation to a nonprofit institution, rather than as a personal gift to the physician.

Conversely, patients occasionally transgress patient-physician boundaries by requesting money from the physician. The physician may be tempted to help a needy patient, but this can lead to repeated attempts at soliciting funds that is ultimately detrimental to the relationship. Repeated requests for socializing or assisting in the patient's home are also beyond the normal scope of the patient-physician relationship and constitute a transgression of boundaries.

Language and the Relationship

Physicians may transgress boundaries by referring to patients by their first names. Sometimes a patient may call the physician by his or her first name.[28] This may occur because of a patient's wish for control of the relationship or envy of the physician. At an extreme, patients may even verbally or emotionally abuse the physician. In a study of Canadian internists, more than 75 percent indicated they had experienced such abuse at least once by patients.[29]

Other transgressions by patients may occur. Some patients may attempt to extend the visit with the physician. Time is an important issue for many physicians, especially in managed-care settings. In addition, transgressions of the limits set by the physician may occur. For example, patients may ask personal questions of the physician. The dependency needs of the patient should be explored when a role reversal is perceived by the physician.

PREVENTING AND DEALING WITH BOUNDARY TRANSGRESSIONS

The key to preventing boundary transgressions is the establishment of clear, mutually understood, and accepted boundaries within the patient-physician relationship.[9] These boundaries must be most clear in the case of sexual feelings for patients. Gabbard[30] has described occurrences of erotic transferences in psychoanalysis; these occurrences are also common in physicians of all specialties.[19] Physicians who face these feelings for patients must recognize their existence.[20] A key aspect of self-awareness is the recognition of physicians' unmet needs and how they are stimulated by patients. Thus, physicians must become aware of their own emotional and physical needs[25] to avoid the possibility of transgressing sexual boundaries with their patients by acting on sexual feelings.

Physicians must also be wary of transgressions of nonsexual touching. While touch can have significant therapeutic benefits,[18] too much touching can cause a decrease in satisfaction by the patient.[31] There may be difficulty in distinguishing nonsexual from sexual touching[19] and misinterpretations by the patient may occur because of differences in experiences and values between the patient and the physician. Thus, physicians must communicate clearly with their patients and have clear boundaries as regards nonsexual touching (for example, in addition to handshakes, touches on the arm of a patient who is emotionally wrought), since it has been shown that physicians who are freer with nonsexual contact with their patients are more likely to engage in sexual contact with them as well.[32]

Physicians must recognize their own needs for companionship, security, and physical contact—aspects of a relationship that are not appropriately found with patients. Thus, physicians should have a clear sense of self to establish appropriate boundaries and to function most effectively as a physician.[9] One important mechanism for achieving this sense of self and for understanding the dynamics of the patient-physician relationship is to examine one's family of origin.[33] Physicians can collect information about all the members in their family of origin, as well as the various relationships and interactions in the family. This information can be organized using a genogram as described in the method by Bowen.[34] Physicians may then be able to examine how their own family patterns may be reflected in the relationship with the patient. This will allow the physician to set adequate boundaries and to deal appropriately with a problematic patient. Other methods, such as support groups and Balint groups, can also help physicians.[35] When family-of-origin exploration and other methods cannot resolve the difficulties, possibilities include referring the patient, collaborating with another physician,[13] or seeking psychotherapy.

Strategies for dealing with patients who can occasionally become abusive include communicating clear expectations and setting limits with these patients.[36] In dealing with patients who attempt to engage in sexual contact with the physician, the physician should be clear about the boundaries within the relationship and the professional nature of the interaction[23] and should always ensure that a nurse is present during any examination. The physician must also acknowledge and address the patient's psychological need that initiated this attempt at a boundary transgression[26] by directly discussing the patient's motivations and feelings, toward the physician. Thus, in the above vignette Dr. Todd might indicate to Mrs. Connors that the kind of relationship she desires is not possible, but he would like to explore why Mrs. Connors feels the way she does.

Setting limits prevents other types of patient transgressions and can be used to diffuse potential transgressions. For example, one should set limits when encountering a patient who flatters the physician and continually attempts to give small gifts.[27] The patient who is trying to control the relationship in this manner will often cease the behavior when told that the physician will accept the patient even without the need for gifts and flattery.

Medical training has not provided information to physicians about role and interpersonal boundaries and potential transgressions.[37] Gartrell et al.[21] reported that 56 percent of physicians indicated that the issue of sexual contacts with patients had never been addressed in medical school or residency, and only 3 percent had ever participated in a continuing medical education course on the topic. Medical education at all levels of training and in continuing medical education is the key to physicians' understanding of boundaries and the prevention of transgressions.[5] Trainees should be allowed to experience erotic and other feelings that occur in the relationship, know that they are normal, and understand that acting on them is unacceptable.[10] Role models are extremely important in medical students and residents' development of appropriate role and interpersonal boundaries.[5]

CONCLUSIONS

An understanding of boundaries and how they are formed will allow physicians to be able to find a connection with their patients, yet prevent enmeshment from occurring. We explored the psychosocial aspects of boundaries and some aspects of their origin, along with an exploration of patient transgressions. Medical education and the processes of self awareness and exploration of family-of-origin issues will help physicians to understand their roles and the interpersonal boundaries that are inherent in the patient-physician relationship and help prevent these transgressions.

REFERENCES

1. Bignall J. Learning and loving. *Lancet* 1994;343:249–250.

2. Spiro H. What is empathy and can it be taught? *Annals of Internal Medicine.* 1992;116:843–846.

3. Friedman E. The perils of detachment. *Healthcare Forum Journal.* 1990;33:9–10.

4. Zinn WM. Doctors have feelings too. *JAMA.* 1988;259:3296–3298.

5. Gabbard GO, Nadelson C. Professional boundaries in the physician-patient relationship. *JAMA.* 1995;273:1445–1449.

6. Epstein AS, Simon RI. The Exploitation Index: an early warning indicator of boundary violations in psychotherapy. *Bulletin of the Menninger Clinic.* 1990;54:450–465.

7. Blackshaw SL, Miller JB. Boundaries in clinical psychiatry. *American Journal of Psychiatry.* 1994;151:293.

8. Wood B, Talmon M. Family boundaries in transition: a search for alternatives. *Family Practice.* 1983;22:347–357.

9. Ryder RG, Bartle S. Boundaries as distance regulators in personal relationships. *Family Practice.* 1991;30:393–406.

10. Strasburger LH, Jorgenson L, Sutherland P. The prevention of psychotherapist sexual misconduct: avoiding the slippery slope. *American Journal of Psychotherapy.* 1992;46:544–555.

11. Vaillant GE, Sobowale NC, McArthur C. Some psychologic vulnerabilities of physicians. *New England Journal of Medicine.* 1972;287:372–375.

12. Gutheil TG, Gabbard GO. The concept of boundaries in clinical practice: theoretical and risk-management dimensions. *American Journal of Psychiatry.* 1993;150:188–196.

13. McDaniel SH, Campbell TL. Seaburn D. *Family-Oriented Primary Care.* New York, NY: Springer-Verlag; 1990:361–373.

14. Mengel MB. Physician ineffectiveness due to family-of-origin issues. *Fam Systems Med.* 1987;5:176–190.

15. Christie-Seely J, Fernandez R, Paradis G, Talbot Y, Turcotte A. The physician's family. In: Chrislie-Seely J (ed.). *Working With the Family in Primary Care.* New York, NY: Praeger Publishers; 1983:524–546.

16. Martin AR. Stress in residency: a challenge to personal growth. *Journal of General Internal Medicine.* 1986;1:252–257.

17. Rempel JK, Holmes JG, Zanna MP. Trust in close relationships. *Journal of Personality and Social Psychology.* 1985;49:95–112.

18. Jensen PS. The doctor-patient relationship: headed for impasse or improvement? *Annals of Internal Medicine.* 1981;95:769–771.

19. Council an Ethical and Judicial Affairs, American Medical Association. Sexual misconduct in the practice of medicine. *JAMA.* 1991;266:2741–2745.

20. Simon RI. Sexual exploitation of patients: how itbegins before it happens. *Psychiatric Annals.* 1989;19:104–112.

21. Gartrell N, Herman J, Olarte S, Feldstein M, Localio R. Psychiatrist-patient sexual contact: results of a national survey, I: prevalence. *American Journal of Psychiatry.* 1986;143:1126–1131.

22. Gartrell NK, Milliken N, Goodson WH, Thiemann S, Lo B. Physician-patient sexual contact: prevalence and problems. *Western Journal of Medicine.* 1992;157:139–143.

23. Gutheil TG. Borderline personality disorder: boundary violations, and patient-therapist sex: medicolegal pitfalls. *American Journal of Psychiatry.* 1989;146:597–602.

24. Lehrman NS. Pleasure heals: the role of social pleasure—love in its broadest sense—in medical practice. *Archives of Internal Medicine.* 1993;153:929–934.

25. Kardener SH. Sex and the physician-patient relationship. *American Journal of Psychiatry.* 1974;131:1134–1136.

26. Schulte HM, Kay J. Medical students' perceptions of patient-initiated sexual behavior. *Academic Medicine.* 1994:69:842–846.

27. Hainer BL. Recognition and management of the overly affectionate patient. *Journal of Family Practice.* 1982;14:47–49.

28. Bradshaw S. Burton P. Naming: a measure of relationships in award milieu. *Bulletin of the Menninger Clinic.* 1976;40:665–670.

29. Cook DJ, Griffith LE, Cohen M, Guyatt GH, O'Brien B. Discrimination and abuse experienced by general internists in Canada. *Journal of General Internal Medicine.* 1995;10:565–572.

30. Gabbard GO. On love and lust in erotic transference. *Journal of the American Psychoanalytic Association.* 1992;42:385–403.

31. Larsen KM, Smith CK. Assessment of nonverbal communication in the patient-physician interview. *Journal of Family Practice.* 1981;12:481–488.

32. Kardener SH, Fuller M, Mensh IN. Characteristics of "erotic" practitioners. *American Journal of Psychiatry.* 1976;133:1324–1325.

33. Crouch M. Working with one's own family: another path for professional development. *Family Medicine.* 1986;18:93–97.

34. Bowen M. *Family Therapy in Clinical Practice.* New York, NY: Jason Aronson; 1978:337–387, 461–547.

35. Novack DH, Suchman AL, Clark W, Epstein A, Naiberg E, Kaplan C. Calibrating the physician: personal awareness and effective patient care. *JAMA.* 1997;278(6):502–509.

36. Sparr LF, Rogers JL, Beahrs JO, Mazur DJ. Disruptive medical patients: forensically informed decision making. *Western Journal of Medicine.* 1992;156:501–506.

37. Perry JA. Physicians' erotic and nonerotic physical involvement with patients. *American Journal of Psychiatry.* 1976;133:838–840.

41

AM I MY BROTHER'S WARDEN?

Responding to the Unethical
or Incompetent Colleague

E. Haavi Morreim, Ph.D.

"A physician should expose, without fear or favor, incompetent or corrupt, dishonest or unethical conduct on the part of members of the profession."[1] It is a commandment easier issued than followed. Although a rising interest in quality assessment has led to increased disciplinary actions by state boards and to treatment programs for impaired physicians,[2] strong social norms reject spying and "snitching" on colleagues in favor of respecting professional privacy and individual responsibility.

Professional self-policing is particularly challenging with respect to physicians who are incompetent or unethical, as distinct from impaired. An impaired physician is unable to practice medicine with reasonable skill and safety by reason of physical or mental illness. He or she may be hindered by waning eyesight, dementia, or substance abuse. The incompetent physician, on the other hand, is not ill, but ignorant or unskillful, while the unethical physician knowingly and willingly violates fundamental norms of conduct toward others, especially his or her own patients.

Impairment commonly elicits sympathy and a wish to help. Even a drastic intervention, such as to remove an aging surgeon from the operating room, can be done with charity toward the physician. And in the process one may help that physician. Many states have confidential programs to treat substance abusers and return them to practice, benefiting both them and their patients.[3] In contrast, one feels less charitable toward the incompetent and not at all benevolent toward the unethical physician.

E. H. Morreim. "Am I My Brother's Warden?" *Hastings Center Report.* 1993;23(3):19–27. Reproduced by permission. © The Hastings Center.

Furthermore, the standards by which we define impairment are considerably clearer than those by which we identify incompetence or poor ethics. Though there are borderline cases, usually we know what it is to be going blind or to be an addict. In contrast, it is not always clear what constitutes "standard" medical knowledge and skill. Practice parameters can suggest routine management of common problems, but cannot define competent care. Patients and their illnesses vary widely, and it can be difficult to distinguish between poor management of an ordinary situation and good management of an unusually complex situation.[4]

Ethical standards are at least as difficult. Some things, of course, are clear. It is plainly wrong to demand sexual intercourse from a fourteen-year-old girl while holding a gun to her head,[5] or to trade forty-four prescription pain pills for a pair of machine guns.[6] But elsewhere standards are not so clear. We may never agree whether euthanasia or even assisted suicide is morally acceptable.

If identifying standards is particularly difficult in the case of competence and ethics, the same is true for gathering evidence. On the one hand, indications of impairment can be relatively straightforward. Blood tests can reveal alcohol, and medical evaluation can diagnose dementia. In contrast, incompetence is seldom easy to detect, partly because the competence of care depends on the clinical context. The patient may have looked very different when he first presented to his primary care physician, for example, than he did hours later for a consulting physician. Furthermore, incompetence typically requires not just one error, even a serious one, but a pattern of them. Not often does any one colleague have the opportunity to observe such a pattern. Unethical conduct is commonly even more difficult to detect, as a devious doctor takes great care to conceal his misdeeds.

Although we must distinguish impaired, incompetent, and unethical physicians, these categories can of course overlap. The demented physician is also incompetent. A surgeon who continues to operate despite failing eyesight commits moral as well as medical wrongs. Still, the concepts are distinct. And while impairment has received considerable scholarly attention, incompetent and unethical physicians have not. In this article I will therefore focus on the latter two, and will begin the analysis by looking more closely at why professional self-policing is so difficult.

POLICING ONE'S OWN

It is difficult for physicians to monitor each other for many reasons. As noted, judgments about competence and ethics require standards and facts that are often neither clear nor readily available. The practice of medicine is permeated by uncertainty, and the best physician is bound to make errors, including some serious ones. To condemn someone else is to invite scrutiny of oneself.

Beyond this, careless or unjust allegations can harm the accused economically, professionally, and personally, as they may drive away patients, reduce collegial esteem, and leave the physician feeling betrayed by those he trusted. Patients, too, can be harmed if a good medical relationship is destroyed or if a capable physician is removed from practice. Even a raised-eyebrow innuendo about a physician's qualifications can raise troubling uncertainties that the patient is in no position to resolve. Neither is the profession as a whole enhanced by widespread mud-slinging or an accusatory, punitive atmosphere. In current times of increasing economic competition among physicians, the danger of such an atmosphere is real.

Finally, the physician who challenges a colleague may herself be harmed, even if her accusations are correct. Whistle blowers can suffer retribution[7] or be sued for slander, libel, or discrimination.[8] More recently, they can face antitrust allegations. Those who sit on peer review committees and other disciplinary bodies are sometimes sued on the ground that they are attempting not to police the profession, but merely to stifle competition.[9] Losers in such suits pay treble damages.

To sue, of course, is not necessarily to win. Peer review that satisfies the requirements set forth by the Health Care Quality Improvement Act (HCQIA) of 1986— good faith, good facts, good procedures, and good reasoning—enjoys antitrust immunity.[10] Still, even a small prospect of legal wrangling can inhibit physicians from pointing accusatory fingers at colleagues.

The individual physician has not only reasons to be cautious, but also some reassurance that the profession already monitors its own. Physicians have a number of avenues, such as weekly morbidity/mortality conferences, by which to critique and improve each other's performance. Most medical specialty boards now plan or require periodic recertification as a regular means of improving quality of care. Hospitals have assorted forums, from credentials review to tissue committees, to monitor staff physicians' performance. The HCQIA of 1986 established a National Practitioner Data Bank that requires reports ranging from malpractice awards and state licensure actions, to adverse judgments rendered by hospitals and medical societies. Hospitals are required to check this data bank before granting or biennially renewing staff physicians' credentials.[11] State medical boards can revoke or suspend licenses and impose other discipline, actions also requiring reports to the data bank.

The legal system also monitors physicians. Tort law lets injured patients seek compensation for negligent injuries and broken contracts, while criminal law prosecutes those who practice without a license or commit fraud. Administrative law enforces the standards of quality and efficiency expected of physicians caring for federally insured patients: the Health Care Financing Administration uses peer review organizations (PROs) to monitor quality and necessity of care, while the Department of Health and Human Services has its Office of Inspector General to enforce laws against kickbacks, fraud, patient abuse, and incompetence.

Economics also spurs quality. Health insurance companies review utilization to identify inappropriate care, particularly overutilization, and many malpractice insurance companies aggressively monitor their physician-subscribers' quality of service. Reviewing such factors as medical judgment, patient rapport, and record keeping, these companies educate and supervise physicians whose poor performance could cost the company too much.[12] Patients also demand quality in an increasingly competitive market for health care.[13]

Unfortunately, these measures are generally conceded to be inadequate. State medical boards are typically hampered by inadequate funding, heavy case loads, and a demanding standard of proof that permits actions in only the worst cases.[14] Hospital and medical society committees have been hindered by inadequate funding and by political pressures. PROs concentrate more on fraud and excess costs than on incompetence. And the medical community itself, perhaps feeling under siege by myriad lawsuits and a plethora of new peer review requirements, is often so reluctant to pursue errant colleagues that the public perceives an intense mutual protectionism. Let us consider, then, why each physician should personally help to pursue incompetent and unethical colleagues. The reasons include professionalism, patient autonomy, law, and economics.

Professions, by definition, are complex fields involving esoteric knowledge that serves some important human need. Only the members of a profession are qualified to establish their standards of care, and they have an obligation to police their own ranks. In medicine this duty is magnified by patients' vulnerability. Aside from the physical, emotional, and rational impairments accompanying illness, patients usually lack the knowledge to diagnose or treat their ailments, or even to judge for themselves the quality of care they are receiving. Physicians' obligations of fidelity therefore include protecting patients from substandard colleagues—by not referring the patient to a colleague whom one knows to be unethical or incompetent,[15] and by removing or reforming unsuitable colleagues.

Autonomy encompasses not only the patient's right to make medical decisions, but also to make an informed choice among providers who are willing to accept her as a patient. Any physician asked about his qualifications and experience, or those of a colleague, should therefore answer honestly. The patient is also entitled to decide what to do about errors, both medically and legally. But to do so, she must know that an error was actually committed.[16] This does not mean that physicians must broadcast their colleagues' flaws at every opportunity. I will discuss specifics below, but in general, physicians are morally obligated and legally advised to be frank about errors that harm patents, even where litigation might result.[17]

Legal reasons for exposing incompetent or unethical practices go well beyond the patient's right to seek fair compensation for negligent injuries. Most states have statutes requiring physicians to report impaired or otherwise questionable colleagues. Though these statutes are rarely enforced, reports to state medical boards have increased markedly in the last few years.[18] Reporting statutes are supplemented by three other doctrines: the duty to warn, the doctrine of fraudulent concealment, and *qui tam.*

The duty to warn is admittedly imprecise and variable. First appearing as psychiatrists' duty to warn third parties of dangers posed by their patients,[19] the duty has expanded over the years. Some scholars see a common-law duty to warn those persons, including patients, who may be endangered by an impaired physician.[20] Where this approach is enforced by courts, a physician who fails to warn could find herself liable for the injuries that the miscreant physician causes.[21] Other cases post a duty to warn the colleague directly so as to avoid negligent care in the first place, as where an assisting surgeon sees that the lead surgeon is doing a procedure incorrectly.[22]

The doctrine of fraudulent concealment requires that when a physician knows he or another physician has caused a patient injury, whether or not through negligence, he should disclose it. A failure to disclose—whether actively by deliberate deception, or passively by merely being silent—can constitute fraud. The duty has been applied only to physicians actually caring for that patient, not to uninvolved physicians who just happen to hear about the situation through casual conversation.

In *Lopez v. Sawyer*, for instance, a woman receiving radiation treatments after her mastectomy developed severe burns, pain, nausea, pulmonary fibrosis, and spontaneous rib fractures requiring multiple hospitalizations. She was not aware that her care had been negligent until, during one hospitalization for reconstructive surgery, she overheard a physician tell his colleagues, "And there you see, gentlemen, what happens when the radiologist puts a patient on the table and goes out and has a cup of coffee."[23] In cases like *Lopez*, where the failure to disclose does not lead to further injury, the fraud may only mean that the statute of limitations restricting the patient's time for bringing a lawsuit does not begin to run until the patient has or should have discovered the fraud.[24]

Fraudulent concealment can also be separate tort, particularly if the concealment leads to further injury for the patient. Even a physician who did not cause the original injury, but only helped to conceal it from the patient, can be found liable for the fraud and also, in certain cases, for conspiracy and other torts leading to punitive as well as compensatory damages. In *Sperandio v. Clymer*, surgeons did not inform the patient that the orthopedic procedure they planned to do on his hip was a pediatric procedure that had never been tried on an adult. The surgery went badly, and the patient required further reconstructive surgery. Just prior to one such procedure a third physician warned the hospital that the patient was considering litigation, whereupon the hospital canceled the surgery. All three physicians were found liable for conspiracy and fraudulent concealment.[25]

Because the physician-patient relationship is fiduciary, this legal duty to disclose colleagues' errors does not permit the physician to wait until the patient asks questions. Rather, one must be affirmatively forthcoming with the information.[26]

Qui tam is a Latin expression meaning "one who sues on behalf of the king as well as himself." In a 1986 revision of the False Claims Act, Congress encouraged citizens to help prosecute those who defraud the government by promising them a share of any money recovered. In the case of medicine, such fraud could include billing for noncovered services, double billing, poor quality care, or unnecessary services.[27] While the prospect of profit may not be a noble motive for physicians to help ferret out corrupt uses of federal health-care dollars, it nevertheless promises to be a significant mechanism for rooting out some unethical conduct.[28]

Physicians also have economic reasons to be vigilant about their profession. Cost-containment mechanisms require that physicians and patients consider carefully the economic as well as the medical wisdom of their plans. Less care need not mean worse care, but physicians must now be vigilant to spot cost cutting at the expense of quality.

One form of cost containment is particularly hazardous: economic incentives.

Through bonuses, perks, and penalties, physicians may be induced to discharge patients early, minimize the use of tests and consultants, or maximize profitable procedures. In other cases a physician may create conflicts of interest by investing in facilities, in-office or freestanding, to which she refers her own patients. Such conflicts of interest provide myriad opportunities for exploiting and poorly serving patients.

These points of ethics, law, and economics require that physicians act against incompetent and unethical colleagues, awkward and difficult though that may be. However, it is far less evident just what actions may be appropriate under what circumstances.

ASSESSING THE ERRANT COLLEAGUE

In assessing an errant colleague it is useful to consider competence before proceeding to ethics. It is sorely tempting to ignore the incompetent colleague. "Anyone can make a mistake." "There but for the grace of God go I." "We've all been careless at one time or another." Although sometimes such reflections are quite right, it would be wrong to overlook all errors just because some do not warrant alarm. We need to identify five levels of adverse outcome, distinguishing ordinary mishaps and sad stories from real mistakes indicating incompetence.

The first level of adverse outcome is the complete accident, independent of any human decision or action. A sudden power failure or unusual equipment malfunction can thwart a delicate operative procedure.

At the second level, a physician's well-justified decision unexpectedly turns out badly. Penicillin may be entirely appropriate for a patient with a bacterial infection sensitive to penicillin and no known history of drug allergy. If that patient subsequently suffers an anaphylactic reaction, the outcome is adverse but the physician's decision was not faulty in any way. In this category we also find the expected iatrogenicity of necessary treatments. Chemotherapy for cancer can cause devastating side effects. But if the chance for benefit is acceptable and the patient is willing, these adverse outcomes do not indicate poor practice.

On level three are those instances, so common throughout medicine, where good physicians disagree. They can differ about whether to recommend coronary artery bypass surgery on a patient with a serious three-vessel disease whose emphysema adds a serious surgical risk. Or they can differ about whether the superior antimicrobial coverage of a broad-spectrum antibiotic is worth risking its increased nephrotoxicity in a patient with compromised renal function. The examples are legion, because medicine is inherently uncertain and fallible. Where it happens that a physician's well-founded decision later turns out to be incorrect, we have no basis for criticism. A physician's care is best judged not by an outcome that cannot be certainly predicted, but by the reasoning that he brought to a difficult question.

At level four the physician exercises poor, though not outrageously bad, judgment or skill. Every physician makes such errors, even if only rarely. One misses seeing a lesion on an X-ray that, retrospectively, is painfully obvious. Or one might do too cursory a history and physical examination, missing signs that were both visible and important. Or one forgets to ask the patient about allergies or to note them in the chart. These cases especially prompt the physician observing some error by a colleague to shudder, "There but for the grace of God go I." Here incompetence is marked not by the commission of a lone error, but by a pattern of them.

At the fifth level are egregious violations of the expected quality of care. The surgeon reads the X-ray backward, or doesn't consult it at all, and operates on the wrong leg.[29] A pediatrician injects twenty times the lethal dose of lidocaine into an eleven-month-old infant in order to lance a boil—and then fails to help the dying child because he does not know how to perform basic cardiopulmonary resuscitation.[30] Dr. Revici claims that he can cure breast cancer without surgery by prescribing vinegar, baking soda, soft-boiled eggs, and coffee.[31]

These five classifications must be applied with care. A bad outcome does not imply error. Nor does the bare fact that a physician has done something differently from oneself or one's closest colleagues entail that he is either wrong or generally incompetent. The important question is not how prevalent his practices are, but whether there are respected physicians who agree with him. The law's concept is "reputable minority." Or we could borrow a term from Benjamin Freedman's discussion of research ethics: we are looking for "clinical equipoise," a situation in which there is "no consensus within the expert clinical community about the comparative merits of the alternatives."[32]

A physician uncertain how to evaluate a colleague's competence should share her concern with one or more trusted colleagues, taking care not to violate the anonymity of the person about whom she is speaking. She can thereby gather something of a "reality check" on the standards of evaluation by which she is appraising that physician's questionable care. Having done so, she should limit her attention to level-five errors, and to level-four errors that appear to be part of a pattern.

In appraising the ethical quality of conduct, it is useful to note that good ethical decision making can be remarkably similar to good medical decision making. In some cases one's best efforts do not go well. One may communicate carefully, thoroughly, and respectfully with a patient about his diagnosis and his treatment options. But if the patient is from a very different culture, he may find such discussions disturbing or even insulting, in ways that the physician could not have anticipated.[33] Such cases would correspond roughly to adverse medical outcomes of levels one and two, above.

At other times one's ethical duties, just like medical standards, are not clear. The essence of an ethical dilemma is the conflict of one or more important values, with no resolution available that honors them all. If a patient refuses an urgently needed medical intervention, such as antibiotics for bacterial meningitis, the physician can only honor his autonomy at the expense of his medical well-being and vice versa. In genuine moral dilemmas, one must bring the best thought and argument one can to a situation in which fundamental uncertainty preempts an obviously correct answer. As noted in the discussion of medically adverse outcomes on level three, the quality of a difficult decision in these situations is a function of the quality of the reasoning one brings to it. And where good people of good will can differ, there is no basis for condemnation or correction.

In some instances, however, it is quite clear that a colleague has violated a fundamental norm. Here, too, we can compare moral error with medical error. Medically incompetent care violates accepted standards. Admittedly those standards can change over the years, as physicians' collective knowledge and skill increases. But medicine cannot be practiced without some shared concept of what constitutes appropriate management. Therefore, those who practice medicine must meet its basic standards of quality and keep abreast of its growth and development. As noted above, deviations below medical standards vary An error of moderately bad judgment (level four) is not the same as outrageous malpractice (level five).

In the like manner, medicine as a profession embraces ethical standards. Physicians are expected to elevate patients' interests above the self-interest that normally guides the marketplace. Self-interest neither can nor must be erased, of course, and the tension between altruism and self-interest is probably the most fundamental ethical challenge of medicine.[34] Because medicine does embrace ethical standards, it is possible at least sometimes to identify instances in which a physician deviates from those standards. Not all deviations are of the same character, however, just as a moderately bad judgment is to be distinguished from outrageous malpractice, so must we distinguish levels among ethical misconduct.

On a fairly mundane level are misdeeds arising not out of evil intent, but from ignorance, thoughtlessness, or insensitivity. These surely are the majority of ethical infractions in the medical profession. The physician may want to do good, but may be misguided in some way, or unable for some reason to do what he knows he should. An internist, for instance, might refuse to tell patients truthfully about diagnoses of life-threatening illness or other disturbing information. Or a surgeon may refuse to honor patients' DNR requests because he doesn't believe in them. An oncologist may steer all his patients toward last-ditch, aggressive experimental treatment, even those who are clearly dying and in desperate need of comfort and solace: "I'm a fighter, and so are all my patients."

The misdeeds of misguidance and insensitivity are fundamentally different from outrageous, deliberate moral wrong—the commission of moral evil, if you will. In medicine that evil would consist in the calculated use of physician's knowledge and power to exploit patients or others for personal gain. A psychiatrist has sex with a desperately dependent female patient A surgeon capitalizes on his patients' ignorance to secure their consent to unnecessary, dangerous, lucrative procedures. An internist exploits her power of prescription and her authority to file insurance claims to profit from fraudulent billings.

Physicians who violate traffic laws or shoplift also commit wrongs, but these are not the stuff of professional self-policing. Rather, peer supervision, lest it degrade into generic vigilantism, should generally be limited to misconduct that arises out of the special status and duties of physicians as professionals.

Accordingly, as one evaluates a colleague for possible ethical misconduct, one must consider several dimensions. First, one must determine how clearly the conduct violates the accepted ethical standards of medicine and the community. As noted above, many ethical dilemmas do not admit of clear resolution, and people of good conscience can differ. Collegial scrutiny must be confined to instances of clear violation.

Second, one must consider the seriousness of the violation. In most cases, this is a function of the seriousness of the actual or potential harm that may occur as a result of the wrongdoing. In other cases an action is intrinsically wrong, regardless of whether it is likely to cause anyone direct physical or psychological harm. Many uses of placebos, or other lies to a patient, are wrong even if they do not cause harm. Intrinsic wrongs and harms alike can vary in their seriousness. The psychiatrist who engages in sexual relations with a patient is likely to precipitate profound, lasting damage.[35] The physician who prescribes an unnecessary lab test to enhance his profits has also done wrong, but the harm to the patient is substantially less.

The seriousness of the harm also depends on the likelihood that harm will occur. Where the psychiatrist has sex with a patient, the harm is virtually certain, not speculative. In contrast, some misdeeds are less likely to injure patients and may be, on that dimension at least, morally less serious. The physician who accepts one costly gift from a pharmaceutical representative has arguably done wrong. Yet this lone episode is not as likely to corrupt his decision making and harm patients as a wide-scale acceptance of such gratuities.

Obviously, these guidelines do not tell the physician precisely which conduct is unethical, or which unethical conduct warrants his or her intervention. No formula can do that. Still, they represent foundations on which concerned physicians can begin their inquiry. And they help one to delimit the kinds of problem that are, and are not, fit subjects for collegial scrutiny.

RESPONDING TO THE ERRANT COLLEAGUE

One cannot decide how to respond to an errant colleague without determining first precisely to what one is responding. Where ignorance or lack of skill is the problem then education, not punishment or discipline, is the answer. Where poor ethics is misguided, not evil, then moral education may be in order In contrast, responsibility and retribution are appropriate for deliberate exploitation. Such unethical conduct is committed by free agents who do or should know better and who could have done other than as they did.

Therefore, one's first step in pursuing a problematic colleague is to "diagnose," beginning with careful factual investigation. One cannot judge whether someone's care is incompetent without knowing the circumstances. The man who obviously has appendicitis by the time he presents to the emergency room may only have had vague symptoms of upset stomach when he saw his local physician a few hours earlier. Analogously, ostensibly unethical conduct may have a deeper source. The oncologist who is a fighter may be emotionally unable to accept death without feeling desperately like a failure. The family physician who never truthfully shares bad news may fear that he cannot cope with a patient's horrified response; he may not know how—with what words—to convey bad news in away that helps the patient address the future with hope alongside realism. The internist may appear to defraud an insurance company, but on closer inspection, she may have judged this to be the only way of securing badly needed resources for her patient. Such an explanation does not entirely excuse her conduct, yet an earnest desire to help the patient is far preferable, morally, to mere greed.

When careful investigation concludes that a colleague has committed a serious error, one is obligated to act. Sometimes one can resolve the problem alone. A careful investigation, for instance, may itself be the resolution. A consultant might phone the primary care physician to learn the detailed information that can help him both to evaluate the patient and to appraise the referring physician. At the same time, the follow-up information he then provides about the patient may be just the extra bit of education the primary physician needs to improve her future management of similar cases. Such discussions need not be accusatory or condescending, because both physicians can learn from each other.

Similarly, if one feels that a colleague is not sufficiently honest with his patients, one may help that physician by sharing stories about the kinds of communication that seem most effectively to help patients participate intelligently in their own care. One can portray the indignity and helplessness felt by patients whose wishes are ignored, and narrate accounts of the ways in which well-meaning physicians may have disserved patients by failing to honor the patients' values.

Arguably, the medical profession as a whole needs to develop a more constructive approach to error than the punitive, litigation-wary atmosphere that currently prevails. Perhaps the most eloquent discussion of this problem comes from Dr. David Hilfiker: "Everyone makes mistakes, of course, but the potential consequences of our medical mistakes are so overwhelming that it is almost impossible for practicing physicians to deal with their errors in a psychologically healthy fashion."[36]

Not only is the possibility of committing serious error a constant threat, but in medicine one is taught to reproach oneself even for minor deviations below optimal care. To compound the problem, medical education usually does not prepare physicians well to deal with their errors. Precision, accuracy, and completeness are emphasized, often with an unrealistic neglect of medicine's enormous fallibilities and uncertainties. And those who have erred are encouraged mainly to determine how they could have been better, not helped to face the emotional guilt of having done less than the best for their patients.[37]

This rather punitive approach need not dominate. In any enterprise, the assumption that error is the product of bad performers' incompetence or carelessness yields a system of inspections and penalties that inspires evasiveness, defensiveness, and conflict. A far better approach, some suggest, is a "continuous improvement" in which people are presumed to be capable and motivated, so that error presents a welcome opportunity for improvement.[38]

Admittedly, continuous improvement is no panacea. Some physicians are seriously incompetent, and some are truly unethical. Their problems are not reducible to organizational imperfection. Still, a more constructive, mutually helpful attitude toward error might improve performance and reduce unproductive defensiveness.

In responding to an errant colleague an individual can be most effective by acting alone in situations permitting informal resolution, and in those requiring immediate corrective action. If one witnesses a colleague disclosing confidential patient information to entertain friends at a cocktail party, one can take that physician aside and remind him of the moral rules. Similarly, ethical problems arising from ignorance or insensitivity must be handled immediately. Only the person who is present and assisting in a surgery can correct an error before it becomes a disaster.[39] In other cases the concerned physician can seek informal help from a colleague. A pediatrician, even one who is hospital chief of staff, may be "eaten for lunch" if he complains directly to a prominent surgeon about his mortality rates. But a word to that surgeon's own department chairman could be highly effective.[40]

Though many situations can thus be managed with one-on-one collegial support, other occasions require more serious or long-term action. The morally misguided physician may refuse to recognize that his poor communication can harm patients; the out-of-date practitioner may shun informal education. And the most egregious wrongs and malpractice usually require explicit correction or sanctions. In such contexts, formal group action has important virtues. A committee can more easily assemble the breadth of information needed to establish, for instance, that a pattern of problems is occurring rather than just an occasional mistake. Further, an established peer review group is in a better position to be fair. Several people, with their differing perspectives and questions, are more likely than any one individual to look at all sides of a question. And an official committee has greater power than any private parry to gain access to necessary records and other information. Finally, careful due process by a formal body may be less likely to prompt antitrust or other legal problems.

Once one has decided that it will be better to take his concerns to a formal body rather than to manage the problem by himself, he must still consider to which body he should turn. Where incompetence is the problem, hospital committees are usually preferable because they have powerful reasons to ensure both that serious peer review is undertaken and that it is careful and fair.

Hospitals' peer review is not just a requirement of the Joint Commission on Accreditation of Healthcare Organizations. In a competitive market, it is also economically imperative to have a highly qualified staff whose excellence can attract patients and their revenues. Legally, the doctrine of corporate negligence places on hospitals a direct duty to patients to select and maintain a competent staff.

Hospitals have long borne vicarious liability for the actions of their employees, such as nurses or laboratory technicians. But until recently they could not be held liable for the actions of staff physicians, who are independent contractors over whom hospitals have no direct control. Many jurisdictions, however, have now determined that hospitals have a corporate responsibility to their patients to use reasonable care in selecting staff physicians, to review the medical care given to their patients, and to suspend or restrict the privileges of physicians found to be incompetent.[41] As noted by the Supreme Court of Florida, "the hospital is in a superior position to supervise and monitor physician performance and is, consequently, the only entity that can realistically provide quality control."[42]

Hospitals also must ensure that such review is carried out fairly, else they will not enjoy immunity against antitrust litigation. Because each physician being evaluated is likely to be known to the members of the peer review committee, it is usually possible to assemble a more complete factual picture, and to be flexible in helping an errant physician to improve the quality of his care. The flexibility is in marked contrast to state medical boards, for example, which are mainly restricted to actions regarding the physician's license, and whose findings typically must meet a strong burden of proof, namely, the "clear and convincing" rather than "preponderance of the evidence" standard. These limits account, in part, for the great difficulty that state medical boards have had in effectively addressing physician incompetence.[43]

Hospital-based peer review is an important but not sole solution to physician incompetence. Not all physicians practice in hospitals, and physicians on hospital peer review committees may be reluctant to weed out their own colleagues. Therefore other approaches are also important, such as the peer supervision undertaken by malpractice insurance companies or health insurers, as noted above.

Where unethical conduct is the problem one can, as with incompetence, consult hospital committees. Hospital committees need to know about unethical physicians to take appropriate credential actions or other measures. They also can address more subtle infractions such as a chronic refusal to honor patients' advance directives. In general, such cases must represent violations of hospital policies or of fairly clear ethics guidelines. Considerations of due process require that the hospital state its expectations in advance, before it can cite breaches of those standards as justifications for disciplinary proceedings. The hospital can cite its DNR policy, for instance, as a basis on which to proceed with their further investigation and potential sanctions. Such sanctions can be very flexible, ranging from mandated education, to formal censure, to suspension of certain privileges, to removal from the hospital staff. Other avenues include medical societies, which can revoke an errant physician's membership—an action that must now be entered into the National Practitioner Data Bank.

Serious or systematic ethical misconduct requires serious, formal accord. Such cases should be presented to bodies that have social and legal authority to protect all potential patients from that physician. State medical boards can revoke or limit the physician's license and should be consulted if the unethical conduct threatens patient welfare or otherwise challenges the physician's right to practice. Crimes, such as rape or fraud, should be reported to appropriate legal authorities.

INTEGRITY OF ONE, INTEGRITY OF ALL

Whether one addresses a colleague's incompetence informally by oneself or takes those concerns to higher authorities, two principles surely must apply. First, problems of collegial competence and ethics should not be ignored. Admittedly, investigating colleagues is difficult. One often remains unsure whether he has all pertinent facts, partly because of medicine's inherent complexity, and partly because of the need to be discreet in any such inquiry. And one may fear the whistleblower's common fate of bringing more trouble on oneself than on the bad colleague. It is sorely tempting to ignore such problems. And yet "due process" does not mean "do nothing." If medicine as a profession is to retain its authority to supervise its own, it must use that power or lose it.

Second, one must address the problem directly and not pass it on to someone else, as by sending the incompetent colleague elsewhere with one's warmest recommendations.[44] The point seems obvious, yet deserves emphasis. Donal Billig, a naval surgeon whose incompetence eventually resulted in criminal convictions for involuntary manslaughter and negligent homicide, was hired at Bethesda Naval Hospital in part because he had favorable letters of reference from three professors of surgery—one at Harvard and two at Tufts—who even at that date had good reason to doubt his skills.[45]

The moral management of errant colleagues poses one of the most difficult, yet important issues a physician can face. Traditional professional virtues such as compassion, conscientiousness, honesty, and fidelity are familiar mandates for the care of patients. Here, however, physicians must call on the more difficult virtues of courage, integrity, and wisdom. The incentives to ignore such problems are nearly overwhelming, as one fears the dual dangers of being either the agent or the recipient of unfair accusations and reprisals. Yet there is no choice. One's own professional integrity is compromised when one permits the integrity of one's profession to be compromised. And the care of all patients is jeopardized if physicians do not care about their own profession.

The author acknowledges with gratitude the very helpful comments provided on earlier drafts by Robert J. Levine and the editors and reviewers of the Hastings Center Report.

REFERENCES

1. American Medical Association. *Current Opinions of the Judicial Council.* Chicago, IL: American Medical Association; 1984.

2. Gray J, "Why bad doctors aren't kicked out of medicine," *Medical Economics,* 1992;69(2):126–149; Page L, "MD scalp hunting? Discipline puts heat on state boards," *American Medical News,* May 11, 1992:3,37–38; Fisher JE, "The chemically dependent physician: liability for colleagues and hospitals in California," *San Diego Law Review,* 1984;2:431–453; Walzer RS, "Impaired physicians: an overview and update of the legal issues," *Journal of Legal Medicine,* 1990;11:131–198.

3. Gray, "Why bad doctors aren't kicked out of medicine"; Walzer, "Impaired physicians."

4. Tarlov AR, Ware JE, Greenfield S, et al., "The medical outcomes study," *JAMA,* 1989;262:925–30; Banta HD, Thacker SB, "The case for reassessment of technology: once is not enough," *JAMA,* 1990;264:235–240; Leape LL, Brennan TA, Laird N, et al., "The nature of adverse events in hospitalized patients: results of the Harvard Medical Practice Study II," *New England Journal of Medicine,* 1991;324:377–384.

5. *Viloria v. Sobol,* 547 N.Y.S. 2d 688 (A.D. 3 Dept. 1989).

6. Hamilton J, "Board disciplines 2 local physicians," *Memphis Commercial Appeal,* October 21, 1990.

7. "Suspension of VA MD delayed pending investigation," *American Medical News,* March 13, 1987:18; McCormick B, "MD says her whistle-blowing led to a court-martial," *American Medical News,* October 14, 1991:8; Page L, "Two physicians claim whistle-blowing led to retaliation," *American Medical News,* March 23–30, 1992:14; Page L, "Stakes are high when you blow the whistle," *American Medical News,* April 27, 1992:3,80–81.

8. Curran WJ, "Medical peer review of physician competence and performance: legal immunity and the antitrust laws," *New England Journal of Medicine,* 1987;316:597–598.

9. *Patrick v. Burget,* 108 S.Ct. 1658 (1988); Curran WJ, "Legal immunity for peer review programs: new policies explored," *New England Journal of Medicine,* 1989;320:233–235; Havighurst CC, "Professional peer review and the antitrust laws," *Case Western Reserve Law Review,* 1986;36:1117–1179.

10. Curran, "Legal immunity"; Iglehart JK, "Congress moves to bolster peer review: the Health Care Quality Improvement Act of 1986," *New England Journal of Medicine,* 1989;320:233–235.

11. Curran, "Medical peer review"; Iglehart, "Congress moves to bolster peer review"; Bierig JR, Portman RM, "The Health Care Quality Improvement Act of 1986," *St. Louis Law Journal,* 1988;32:977–1014; Horner SL, "The Health Care Quality Improvement Act of 1986: its history, provisions, applications and implications," *American Journal of Law and Medicine,* 1990;16:453–498; Mullan F, Politzer RM, Lewis CT, et al., "The National Practitioner Data Bank: report from the first year," *JAMA,* 1992;268:73–79.

12. Schwartz WB, Mendelson DN, "The role of physician-owned insurance companies in the detection and deterrence of negligence," *JAMA,* 1989;262:1342–1346; "High-risk physicians aided in Oregon," *American Medical News,* March 6, 1987:15.

13. Jost TS, "Regulatory approaches to problems in the quality of medical care: diagnosis and prescription," *University of California Davis Law Review,* 1989;22:593–608.

14. Kusserow RP, Handley EA, Yessian M, "An overview of state medical discipline," *JAMA,* 1987;257:820–824.

15. King JH. *The Law of Medical Malpractice.* 2d ed. St. Paul, MN: West Publishing; 1986.

16. *Sutlive v. Hackney,* 297 S.E.2d 515 (Ga. App. 1983).

17. Peterson LM, Brennan T, "Medical ethics and medical injuries: taking our duties seriously," *Journal of Medical Ethics,* 1990;1:207–211; American College of Physicians, "American College of Physicians ethics manual," *Annals of Internal Medicine,* 1992;117:956.

18. Gray, "Why bad doctors aren't kicked out of medicine"; Fisher, "The chemically dependent physician"; Walzer, "Impaired physicians."

19. *Tarasoff v. Regents of the University of California,* 551 P.2d 334 (1976).

20. Gostin LO, "The AIDS Litigation Project: a national review of court and human rights commission decisions, part 1: the social impact of AIDS," *JAMA,* 1990;263:1961–1970; Walzer, "Impaired physicians."

21. Fisher, "The chemically dependent physician"; King, *Law of Medical Malpractice.*

22. *McMillin v. L.D.L.R.,* 645 S.W.2d 836 (Tex. App. 1982). The physician may also be obliged to warn about his own inadequacies. One court recently held that a surgeon's failure to disclose his chronic alcohol abuse was a violation of the patient's right to make an informed consent to the proposed surgery. The condition does, after all, create a "material risk associated with the surgeon's ability to perform" the procedure. *Hidding v. Williams,* 578 So.2d 1192 (La. App. 5 Cir 1991), at 1196.

23. *Lopez v. Sawyer,* 100 A.2d 563 (N.J. 1973), at 565.

24. *Sutlive v. Hackney, Pashley v. Pacific Electric Co.,* 153 P.2d 325 (Ca. 1944); *Muller v. Thaut,* 430 N.W.2d 884 (Neb. 1988); *Keithley v. St. Joseph's Hospital,* 696 P.2d 435 (N.M.App. 1984).

25. *State Ex Rel. Spe... ... v. Ch...* ... 99 ... p. 19...

26. Furrow BR, Johnson SH, Jost TS, Schwartz RL. *Health Law ...; Materials, and Problems.* St. Paul, MN: West Publishing, 1987. King, *Law of Medical Malpractice.*

27. Hsia DC, "Qui tam: suing physicians who make false claims," *Annals of Internal Medicine,* 1991;114:1050–1053.

28. McCormick B, "Doctors to see more 'whistle-blower' suits," *American Medical News,* July 1, 1991:1,10,11.

29. *Spero v. Board of Regents of the State University of New York,* 551 N.Y.S. 2d 532 (A.D. 3 Dept. 1990).

30. Feinberg B, "Doctor's license suspended: action involves infant's death," *Memphis Commercial Appeal,* October 6, 1989.

31. *Revici v. Commissioner of Education,* 546 N.Y.S. 2d 240 (A.D. 3 Dept. 1989).

32. Freedman B, "Equipoise and the ethics of clinical research," *New England Journal of Medicine,* 1987;317:144.

33. Pellegrino ED, "Is truth-telling to the patient a cultural artifact?" *JAMA,* 1992;268:1734–1735.

34. Jonsen AR, "Watching the doctor," *New England Journal of Medicine,* 1983;308:1531–1535.

35. Carr M, Robinson GE, "Fatal attraction: the ethical and clinical dilemma of patient-therapist sex," *Canadian Journal of Psychiatry,* 1990;35:122–127; Council on Ethical and Judicial Affairs, AMA, "Sexual misconduct in the practice of medicine," *JAMA,* 1991;266:2741–2745.

36. Chren MM, Landefield CS, Murray TH, "Doctors, drug companies, and gifts," *JAMA,* 1989;262:3448–3451.

37. Hilfiker D, "Facing our mistakes," *New England Journal of Medicine,* 1984;262:3448–3451.

38. Ibid.

39. Berwick DM, "Continuous improvement as an ideal in health care," *New England Journal of Medicine,* 1989;320:53–56; Lorh KM, Schroeder SA, "A strategy for quality assurance in health care," *New England Journal of Medicine,* 1990;322:707–712; Kritchevsky SB, Simmons BP, "Continuous quality improvement: concepts and applications for physician care," *JAMA,* 1991;266:1817–1823.

40. "Navy cardiac surgeon gets 4-year prison sentence," *American Medical News,* March 14, 1986:13; *McMillin v. L.D.L.R.,* 645 S.W.2d 836 (Tex. App. 1982).

41. Holoweiko M, "Hospital peer review: not just for bad apples anymore," *Medical Economics,* 1991;68(16):150–163.

42. Fisher, "The chemically dependent physician."

43. *Insinga v. LaBella,* 543 So.2d 209 (Fla. 1989), at 214; *Corleto v. Shore Memorial Hospital,* 350 A.2d 534 (N.J. Super. 1975).

44. Kusserow, Handley, Yessian, "An overview of state medical discipline"; Gray, "Why bad doctors aren't kicked out of medicine."

45. Broad W, Wade N. *Betrayers of the Truth.* New York: Simon and Schuster; 1982; Stitham S, "Educational malpractice," *JAMA,* 1991;266:905–906; *Walton v. Jennings Community Hospital, Inc.,* 875 F.2d 1317 (7th Cir. 1989).

46. "Navy cardiac surgeon gets 4-year prison sentence"; "Manslaughter and negligent homicide by a Navy surgeon: a banquet of consequences," *Law, Medicine, & Health Care,* 1985;13:258.

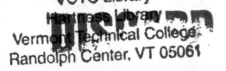